Distal Radial Access

Gregory A. Sgueglia
Editor

Distal Radial Access

Scientific Foundations and Applied Techniques

Springer

Editor
Gregory A. Sgueglia
Division of Cardiology
Sant'Eugenio Hospital
Rome, Italy

ISBN 978-3-031-89924-9 ISBN 978-3-031-89925-6 (eBook)
https://doi.org/10.1007/978-3-031-89925-6

This Springer imprint is published by the registered company Springer Nature Switzerland AG
The registered company address is: Gewerbestrasse 11, 6330 Cham, Switzerland

To my Princesses,
who illuminate the essence of life daily

Preface

Distal Radial Access (DRA) stands as one of the most intriguing and influential innovations in interventional medicine in recent years. It is this exciting advancement that inspired the creation of the *Distal Radial Access* book, a comprehensive exploration of this transformative technique.

The importance of DRA cannot be overstated. Transradial access (TRA) has already demonstrated its life-saving potential across the spectrum of coronary artery disease and offers numerous additional benefits to both patients and healthcare systems. As such, its use has expanded across all interventional specialties. However, as its adoption grows, conventional TRA may become a victim of its own success due to the cumulative risk of radial artery occlusion, a complication that increases with each repeat attempt, ultimately jeopardizing future radial access and its associated benefits.

In this context, DRA emerges as a logical evolution, providing a means to maintain radial artery patency while offering further important benefits. Most notably, DRA does not require specialized equipment, only a thorough understanding of when, why, and how to implement it.

The *Distal Radial Access* book is divided into five distinct sections, each carefully designed to provide a thorough understanding of DRA from multiple perspectives. The first section lays the core knowledge, revealing the rationale behind DRA and its unique characteristics. This foundational section is critical as it addresses key anatomical and physiological principles that are often overlooked by novices, potentially leading to premature dropouts and missed opportunities for patient care.

The second section focuses on the practical and technical aspects of DRA, covering a spectrum from the simplest to the most complex situations. Readers will find invaluable tips and techniques for facilitating access, avoiding complications, improving success rates, and overcoming common challenges. The third section presents current evidence on the unique efficacy and safety profile of DRA, while the fourth section explores advanced applications. The final section provides guidance on how to seamlessly integrate DRA into clinical practice and highlights upcoming developments.

All chapters are specifically relevant to DRA, with a seamless flow of knowledge and experience between them, creating a cohesive and comprehensive resource. I am particularly pleased the *Distal Radial Access* book has contributions from other interventional disciplines, fostering a dynamic exchange of ideas and practices.

Each chapter has been carefully co-authored by two independent experts, ensuring a comprehensive and multifaceted exploration of the topic. This systematic editorial approach not only broadens the range of perspectives but also provides a form of consensus on aspects of DRA that are still evolving.

The creation of the *Distal Radial Access* has been a substantial undertaking, requiring countless hours of research, writing, and collaboration. I extend my deepest gratitude to all of the contributing authors, whose dedication and expertise have been invaluable in shaping a resource that I sincerely hope will play a pivotal role in advancing the understanding and widespread adoption of DRA within the medical community.

Mastering DRA represents a rare opportunity to improve patient care and outcomes at no additional cost. It embodies our commitment to continuing professional development and honing our skills as physicians and interventionalists. By embracing DRA, we are not just adopting a new technique, we are refining our approach to patient care and enhancing the potential for improved clinical outcomes.

Rome, Italy Gregory A. Sgueglia

Contents

Contributors

Pierfrancesco Agostoni Hartcentrum, Ziekenhuis Netwerk Antwerpen, Middelheim, Antwerp, Belgium

Adel Aminian Department of Cardiology, Centre Hospitalier Universitaire de Charleroi, Charleroi, Belgium

Giovanni Amoroso Department of Cardiology, OLVG Hospital, Amsterdam, The Netherlands

Anastasios Apostolos Faculty of Medicine, Department of Cardiology, University of Patras, University Hospital of Patras, Patras, Greece

First Department of Cardiology, Medical School, National and Kapodistrian University of Athens, Hippocration General Hospital of Athens, Athens, Greece

Avtandil Babunashvili Interventional Cardiology and Angiology Faculty of the first Moscow Medical Academy, Moscow, Russian Federation

Ivo Bernat Department of Cardiology, University Hospital and Faculty of Medicine Pilsen, Charles University, Pilsen, Czech Republic

Francesco Bianchini Department of Cardiovascular Sciences, Fondazione Policlinico Universitario Agostino Gemelli IRCCS, Rome, Italy

Francesco Burzotta Department of Cardiovascular Sciences, Fondazione Policlinico Universitario Agostino Gemelli IRCCS, Rome, Italy

Mauricio G. Cohen Interventional Cardiology, Cleveland Clinic Florida, Weston, FL, USA

Giuseppe Colletti Cardiovascular Department, Clinique Saint Joseph, Arlon, Belgium

Thierry Corcos Department of Cardiology, American Hospital of Paris, Neuilly-sur-Seine, France

Angela Di Giorgio Department of Cardiovascular Sciences, Fondazione Policlinico Universitario Agostino Gemelli IRCCS, Rome, Italy

Kareem El Naamani Department of Neurosurgery, Thomas Jefferson University Hospital, Philadelphia, PA, USA

Christopher M. Fernandez Heart and Vascular Center, University of Chicago Medicine, Chicago, IL, USA

Enrique A. Flores Georgia Heart Specialists, Conyers, GA, USA

Tom J. Ford Gosford Hospital, Gosford, NSW, Australia

Gabriele L. Gasparini IRCCS Humanitas Research Hospital, Rozzano, Italy

Ian C. Gilchrist Dartmouth Hitchcock Medical Center, Geisel School of Medicine at Dartmouth, Lebanon, NH, USA

Harkanwar S. Gill Department of Radiology and Radiological Science, Medical University of South Carolina, Charleston, SC, USA

Juan F. Granada Cardiovascular Research Foundation, New York, NY, USA

Marcelo Guimaraes Department of Radiology and Radiological Science, Medical University of South Carolina, Charleston, SC, USA

Stefan Harb University Heart Center, Medical University of Graz, Graz, Austria

Haydn Hoffman Department of Neurosurgery, State University of New York Upstate Medical University, Syracuse, NY, USA

Juan F. Iglesias Department of Cardiology, Geneva University Hospitals, Geneva, Switzerland

Pascal Jabbour Department of Neurosurgery, Thomas Jefferson University Hospital, Philadelphia, PA, USA

Aleksandr Kaledin Endovascular Surgery Department, Northwestern State Medical University named after I.I. Mechnikov, Saint-Petersburg, Russian Federation

Sasko Kedev Department of Cardiology, Faculty of Medicine, University of Ss. Cyril and Methodius, Skopje, Republic of North Macedonia

Ferdinand Kiemeneij Bussum, The Netherlands

Yongcheol Kim Division of Cardiology, Yonsei University College of Medicine and Cardiovascular Center, Yongin Severance Hospital, Yongin, Republic of Korea

Darren Klass Cleveland Clinic Lerner College of Medicine of Case Western Reserve University, Cleveland Clinic London, London, UK

Anna Luisa Kuhn Department of Radiology, Division of Neurointerventional Radiology, University of Massachusetts Medical Center, Worcester, MA, USA

Azeem Latib Division of Cardiology, Montefiore Medical Center, Albert Einstein College of Medicine, New York, NY, USA

Bong-Ki Lee Division of Cardiology, Kangwon National University Hospital, Chuncheon, Republic of Korea

Jin Bae Lee Department of Cardiology, Daegu Catholic University Medical Center, Daegu, Republic of Korea

Jun-Won Lee Division of Cardiology, Department of Internal Medicine, Yonsei University Wonju College of Medicine, Wonju, Republic of Korea

Sang Yeub Lee Heart & Brain Hospital, Chung-Ang University Gwangmyeong Medical Center, Gwangmyeong, Republic of Korea

Takashi Matsukage Department of Cardiology, Shonan Oiso Hospital, Oiso, Japan

Sandeep Nathan Heart and Vascular Center, University of Chicago Medicine, Chicago, IL, USA

James Nolan Cardiovascular Research Group, Keele University, Keele, Staffordshire, UK

Andrea Pacchioni Division of Cardiology, Azienda Ospedaliera Universitaria Integrata Verona, Verona, Italy

Samir B. Pancholy The Wright Center for Graduate Medical Education, Scranton, PA, USA

Tejas Patel Apex Heart Institute, Ahmedabad, Gujarat, India

Ajit S. Puri Department of Radiology, Division of Neurointerventional Radiology, University of Massachusetts Medical Center, Worcester, MA, USA

Sunil V. Rao New York University Langone Health System, New York, NY, USA

Sudhir Rathore Frimley Health NHS Foundation Trust, Camberley, Surrey, UK

Karim Ratib University Hospitals of North Midlands, NHS Trust, Stoke-on-Trent, UK

Stefano Rigattieri Division of Cardiology, Sant'Andrea University Hospital, Rome, Italy

Zoltan Ruzsa Department of Internal Medicine, Division of Invasive Cardiology, University of Szeged, Szeged, Hungary

Christian F. Said Gosford Hospital, Gosford, NSW, Australia

Shigeru Saito Department of Cardiology, Shonan Kamakura General Hospital, Kanagawa, Japan

Karsten Schenke Agaplesion Bethesda Krankenhaus Bergedorf, Hamburg, Germany

Alessandro Sciahbasi Interventional Cardiology, Sandro Pertini Hospital, Rome, Italy

Ignacio M. Seropian Hospital Italiano de Buenos Aires, Buenos Aires, Argentina

Gregory A. Sgueglia Division of Cardiology, Sant'Eugenio Hospital, Rome, Italy

Jasmeet Singh Department of Radiology, Division of Neurointerventional Radiology, University of Massachusetts Medical Center, Worcester, MA, USA

Grigorios Tsigkas Faculty of Medicine, Department of Cardiology, University of Patras, University Hospital of Patras, Patras, Greece

Carlo Tumscitz Azienda Ospedaliero Universitaria di Ferrara, Arcispedale Sant'Anna, Cona, Italy

Claudiu Ungureanu Cardiovascular Department, Jolimont Hospital, La Louvière, Belgium

Marco Valgimigli Cardiocentro Ticino Institute and Università della Svizzera Italiana (USI), Lugano, Switzerland

Mladen I. Vidovich Jesse Brown Veterans Affairs Medical Center, University of Illinois at Chicago, Chicago, IL, USA

Fuminobu Yoshimachi Department of Cardiology, Tokai University Hachioji Hospital, Hachioji City, Tokyo, Japan

Part I

Foundation of Distal Radial Access

Introduction

1

Ferdinand Kiemeneij

In 2016, I had the opportunity to learn about the origins, methods, and outcomes of the pioneering distal radial access (DRA) technique presented by Dr. Farshad Roghani-Dhekordi, an interventional cardiologist at Isfahan University of Medical Sciences, during the Third Isfahan Transradial Course in Isfahan, Iran. His work was based on the pioneering work of Dr. Babunashvili [1] and Dr. Kaledin [2]. Although I had not previously considered using the radial artery in the radial fossa as a primary method, I felt strongly motivated to explore and incorporate left DRA as the default technique for several potential benefits in my practice [3]. The subsequent discussions I had with many colleagues, all experts in conventional transradial techniques, were reminiscent of something I had seen before.

Transradial access (TRA) for coronary interventions (TRI) was introduced in 1992 as an alternative to the traditional transfemoral arterial access (TFA) technique. The main advantages of TRA over TFA were its potential to reduce major local bleeding complications and mortality, improve hemostasis, shorten immobilization and hospital stay, decrease inconvenience and suffering for patients, and improve cost-benefit.

However, the radial artery being smaller, more distal, and more tortuous made the technique more challenging for interventionalists who were trained and experienced in TFA. This often resulted in the need to switch to the femoral artery in case of failure to reach the coronary arteries, subjecting the patient to increased risk for major bleeding and mortality. The adoption of TRA required a significant learning curve for operators and raised questions about its clinical effectiveness and potential risks. Early studies in the first 5 years after the introduction of TRA showed promising results but were limited by small sample sizes, low statistical power, single-center design, and comparisons with a well-established technique performed by low-volume operators. These limitations hindered the acceptance of TRA by the medical community and the industry.

Despite these challenges, the adoption of TRA has continued to grow to a level where it has been established as the standard of care in the field of interventional cardiology. The input of many excellent clinicians and researchers and of the medical industry developing and manufacturing superb dedicated products has played a pivotal role.

Despite all this, the Achilles heel of TRA appears to be radial artery occlusion (RAO). Although mostly without clinical sequelae, this complication limits its future use for other inter-

F. Kiemeneij (✉)
Bussum, The Netherlands

G. A. Sgueglia (ed.), *Distal Radial Access*, https://doi.org/10.1007/978-3-031-89925-6_1

ventions. The recommended 5% RAO threshold, proposed in the "Best practices for the prevention of radial artery occlusion after transradial diagnostic angiography and intervention: an international consensus paper" [4], is outdated and too high in my opinion. This threshold is not recommendable since we are at a point where we can come close to 0%. This 5% RAO incidence should only function as the basis from which we are expected to do better. DRA is one of those strategies, which has been confirmed in the DISCO RADIAL trial which reported a 0.3% RAO rate after DRA [5].

Interestingly, a similar scenario of hindered acceptance by the medical community and the industry is happening right now with the rapidly growing popularity of DRA among enthusiasts, referred to as "believers" just as in the early days of TRA. DRA as compared to TRA will not improve mortality like TRA does when compared to TFA. But it provides better service to the patient by offering extremely low risk for RAO, patient convenience during and after the procedure, improved operator convenience during left radial access, short and simple hemostasis, improved patient independence from postoperative care, shorter hospital stay, cost-effectiveness, and last but not least reduction of nurse intensity times. It can be considered a significant refinement of the conventional approach via the forearm part of the radial artery. Today, I personally see a start in the forearm as a missed chance to serve the patient better.

Indeed, it is worth noting that DRA again is more challenging than forearm TRA, just like conventional TRA is more demanding than TFA. This is due to the smaller diameter in the area of the anatomical snuffbox and the presence of one more curve in the artery at the transition of the dorsum of the hand to the forearm. The success rate is usually over 90%. A crossover from DRA to a point of about 3–5 cm more proximal is not a clinically and technically very relevant issue for patient and operator, and it brings the patient the major advantages of radial access. I wonder why so many patients in the DISCO RADIAL trial [5] crossed over to TFA (25% [12 of 48] of failures in DRA).

The consequence of crossover from DRA to PRA has substantially less impact on patient and operator, and I recommend crossover to the homo- or contralateral radial artery in case of DRA access failure. Once DRA has been mastered, operators have acquired improved technical skills and will notice that conventional TRA seems much easier than before.

Without randomized controlled trials, the use of DRA may become somewhat controversial, as is often the case with innovative techniques that are not yet supported by scientific evidence but only by early pioneers exploring the feasibility of the new approach and its limitations.

However, the call for evidence-based practice should not discourage clinicians from exploring new approaches. While it is important to consider the available evidence, it should not be used as an excuse to stick to routines. Instead, clinicians should be open to new ideas and consider the potential benefits for their patients, using their own logical thinking and experiences to guide their decision-making.

One key difference with the early TRA era is that, in the first 5 years, DRA became rapidly popularized thanks to social media platforms and that there is now a wealth of information available, potentially positioning DRA as the future default procedure.

Interestingly, interventional radiologists and neurointerventional specialists, not being exposed to previous experience in TRA, frequently make the transition from femoral to radial directly in the anatomical snuffbox.

This wealth of information available on DRA has led to a continuous cycle of improvement and empowerment, creating more experts, innovators, and researchers. This, in turn, results in better techniques and ultimately leads to improved patient care. It is a truly beautiful cycle of growth, maturation, and advancement in interventional cardiology.

For this reason, it was decided to publish this book written by experts in the field of DRA. It is intended for medical professionals such as invasive and interventional cardiologists, interventional radiologists, neurointerventional specialists, and vascular surgeons who are interested in learning about this approach. A collection of updated information on all relevant issues is provided in a logical structure ranging between history and future, practical and technical aspects, basic and advanced use, efficacy and safety, and how to start a program and how to overcome the learning curve.

With the information presented in this book, readers will be equipped to become experts in their field and provide the highest level of technique and service to their patients. We encourage you to delve into each chapter and discover the knowledge contained within, empowering you to excel in your profession.

References

1. Babunashvili A, Dundua D. Recanalization and reuse of early occluded radial artery within 6 days after previous transradial diagnostic procedure. Catheter Cardiovasc Interv. 2011;77:530–6.
2. Kaledin AL, Kochanov IN, Seletskiy SS, Arharov IV, Burak TY, Kozlov KL. Peculiarities of arterial access in endovascular surgery in elderly patients. Adv Gerontol. 2014;27:115–9.
3. Kiemeneij F. Left distal transradial access in the anatomical snuffbox for coronary angiography (ldTRA) and interventions (ldTRI). EuroIntervention. 2017;13:851–7.
4. Bernat I, Aminian A, Pancholy S, Mamas M, Gaudino M, Nolan J, et al. Best practices for the prevention of radial artery occlusion after transradial diagnostic angiography and intervention: an international consensus paper. JACC Cardiovasc Interv. 2019;12:2235–46.
5. Aminian A, Sgueglia GA, Wiemer M, Kefer J, Gasparini GL, Ruzsa Z, et al. Distal versus conventional radial access for coronary angiography and intervention: the DISCO RADIAL trial. JACC Cardiovasc Interv. 2022;15:1191–201.

Current Status

2

Sunil V. Rao and Claudiu Ungureanu

2.1 Introduction

Following Avtandil Babunashvili's pioneering work in 2011 to introduce distal radial artery access (DRA) for reopening forearm radial arteries occluded following previous catheterization procedures [1], this innovative approach has gained increasing acceptance in the medical community [2] and has been extensively tested in a variety of clinical scenarios. Numerous observational studies and registries have evaluated the clinical outcomes associated with DRA [3–13], and recent randomized controlled trials have compared this unique approach to conventional transradial access (TRA) [14–16].

Early investigation of this novel approach was driven primarily by the need to provide a safe and valid alternative for vascular access, particularly in cases where transfemoral access or TRA is challenging. Initial results and data on DRA have been encouraging, confirming the feasibility of this innovative technique and demonstrating a consistently high success rate with no significant safety concerns [17].

S. V. Rao (✉)
New York University Langone Health System, New York, NY, USA
e-mail: sunil.rao@nyulangone.org

C. Ungureanu
Cardiovascular Department, Jolimont Hospital, La Louvière, Belgium

Adoption of DRA was further fueled by the proliferation of social media posts [18] promoting the perceived benefits of this approach:

- Improved operator comfort due to better ergonomic positioning of the left hand and wrist.
- Very low incidence of radial artery spasm, which could be explained by several mechanisms, one of the most important being the avoidance of puncturing the forearm radial artery, which is more likely to cause local injury and vasoconstriction that increases with the number of attempts.
- Shorter time to hemostasis with easier and more reliable compression owing to the favorable anatomy (superficial arterial course and bone floor of the anatomical snuffbox area).
- The absence of compression of large venous vessels also reduces the risk of venous stasis during compression, making compression safer.
- Significant reduction in forearm radial artery occlusion (RAO), with almost complete prevention in almost all patients, regardless of the radial hemostasis method used.
- Very low risk of access site bleeding and vascular complications. In addition, the distal radial artery is located in the dorsal subcutaneous space, superficial to the fascial compartments of the hand and the muscle surrounding the first intermetacarpal space, which limits the functional consequences in case of bleeding.

G. A. Sgueglia (ed.), *Distal Radial Access*, https://doi.org/10.1007/978-3-031-89925-6_2

- Greater stability of the guiding catheter with the use of the sheathless technique, where the system is naturally secured first by the position of the hand, which has a curvilinear trajectory, and also by the mechanical force and friction between the distal radial artery and the guiding catheter.

2.2 Rationale for Distal Radial Access

The major advantage of DRA is the protection of the forearm radial artery by avoiding mechanical injury related to the puncture and ultimately preventing its occlusion [19]. Another factor contributing to the exceptionally low rates of RAO is the well-developed anastomotic network connecting deep and superficial arterial branches within the wrist and hand region, which ensures continuous circulation of arterial blood flow along the forearm radial artery [19, 20]. Notably, an optical coherence tomography imaging study confirmed the very low probability of acute vascular injury of the proximal radial artery during DRA interventions using 6-Fr guiding catheters. Intimal tears of the radial artery were observed in only 2.2% of cases, and nonobstructive intraluminal thrombus was detected in 8.7% of patients (see also Chap. 4) [21].

2.3 Current Adoption of Transradial Access

The use of TRA for coronary angiography and intervention is associated with fewer vascular complications, bleeding, and mortality compared to femoral access [22]. These benefits have contributed to the adoption of TRA by the majority of the interventional community as the default strategy across the spectrum of coronary interventions, whether elective or emergent, conventional or complex, and for all patients regardless of age, gender, or other differences [23, 24].

Even in the current era, where the dedicated equipment for TRA has improved significantly with dedicated hydrophilic sheaths and catheters, as well as the increased use of different techniques to allow the use of large-bore guiding catheters and crossing of tortuous vascular anomalies, access site crossover to femoral access still ranges from 4.6% to 10% [25, 26].

Failure of TRA is most commonly related to the small size of the radial artery, spasm, and the presence of tortuosity, but also to occlusion of the artery or reduction in arterial caliber related to previous catheterization procedures. Notably, the rate of radial artery occlusion increases by about 5% with each subsequent access to the same radial artery [27].

Recently, DRA has been proposed to overcome these issues by puncturing the radial artery more distally in the anatomical snuffbox or in the first intermetacarpal space. Indeed, DRA was quickly considered an alternative to conventional TRA, and this approach has become increasingly popular since 2017, when Ferdinand Kiemeneij published his first experience with left DRA in the anatomical snuffbox [28].

Actually, anesthesiologists were the first to use DRA as an alternative site for perioperative blood pressure monitoring in pediatric and adult cardiac patients in case of failure to puncture conventional vascular sites, as reported by Amato et al. in 1977 [29] and Pyles et al. in 1982 [30].

In recent years, the DRA has gained increasing popularity worldwide as a primary access and not exclusively as an alternative approach for interventional cardiology and radiology procedures, performing efficiently in the entire spectrum of percutaneous vascular procedures without major safety issues reported in published registries or trials to date.

2.4 Current Medical Evidence for Using Distal Radial Access

Several registries have published clinical data on the use of DRA in routine daily practice.

Al-Azizi et al. reported no complications and a 98.3% success rate in performing DRA for diagnostic and coronary angioplasty in all five operators involved in this study, highlighting the reproducibility of the technique [3]. Hemostasis was achieved with a conventional radial band, and no bleeding was reported.

Kim et al. reported a good feasibility of 88.0% for coronary angiography and percutaneous coronary intervention (PCI) compared to the conventional radial approach [4]. The failed cases were related to difficult puncture of the distal radial artery and difficult wiring. The DRA approach was used in 2 (1.5%) patients undergoing emergency coronary angiography for ST-elevation myocardial infarction and 56 (42.4%) patients with non-ST-elevation acute coronary syndrome (including unstable angina).

The success and safety of DRA are reproducible at the operator and center level with reports published worldwide from different countries.

Gajurel et al. included 190 patients for coronary procedures by TRA and DRA in Nepal with similar rates of successful cannulation in both groups and no complication in the DRA group [5].

The Turkish experience was reported by Soydan et al. in 54 patients treated with coronary interventions, showing similar results to previous studies regarding the safety and feasibility of DRA [31].

In the Polish prospective registry, Wretowski et al. included 195 patients after screening 320 patients for a suitable, well-palpable distal radial pulse [6]. The rate of successful cannulation was 89.4% after puncture failure in nine patients or wire not crossing in 14 patients.

In the Chinese registry, Yu et al. studied 92 patients and showed an excellent cannulation success rate of 95.7% [7]. The access time of 2.3 ± 1.78 minutes was similar to previous studies. Exclusion criteria were the absence of pulse, distal arterial occlusion as demonstrated by ultrasound, or other proximal vascular disease such as arterial malformation.

The first Greek experience with DRA published by Ziakas et al. included 49 patients [8]. The authors had a failure rate of 10.2% and a puncture time of 3.9 ± 4.1 min. In their experience, manual hemostasis was significantly shorter compared to device hemostasis (11 ± 7 versus 198 ± 42 min, $p < 0.001$).

2.4.1 Expanded Use of Distal Radial Access and Competency Enhancement

DRA appears to be feasible and safe, as it has been demonstrated in all these registries around the world in a broad population of patients with coronary or noncoronary pathologies treated by catheterization in acute or elective settings. Another important question to be answered is whether DRA could be used as a standard strategy in routine clinical practice (see also Chap. 15).

In the Brazilian prospective observational registry, Oliveira et al. enrolled 435 consecutive patients for coronary diagnostic angiography and/or angioplasty over 6 months and showed that DRA was a reliable and safe approach with only 3.0% access site crossovers and no major complications [9].

In terms of technical details, the distal radial artery was punctured mainly in the anatomical snuffbox using a 20-G micropuncture cannula over the needle without ultrasound guidance.

Achim et al. recently published their experience with DRA in conventional coronary and peripheral interventions involving more than 1200 patients [32]. Ultrasound guidance was used in all patients, resulting in a very high success rate of 97%. After performing 150 cases, operators reached a plateau DRA success rate of over 96%. The authors highlighted the limited puncture time of 1.26 ± 1.1 minutes with a low number of attempts of 2.28 ± 0.67 using a conventional puncture kit, considering that the use of ultrasound contributed to this performance.

Hadjivassiliou et al. also strongly recommended the use of ultrasound guidance for several reasons, to safely perform the puncture with a single anterior wall crossing, avoiding the risk of tendon and radial nerve damage, after recognizing all surrounding structures [33]. The ultrasound exploration allows easy recognition of the scaphoid floor, the extensor pollicis longus, and the extensor pollicis brevis, which helps to easily identify the distal radial artery and the puncture site, ideally in a non-angulated segment to avoid multiple punctures.

The Japanese experience published by Mizuguchi et al. showed a very low incidence of RAO of 0.4% at 1 month after ultrasound evaluation, without bleeding or vascular complications [34]. Another important finding was the post-procedural dilatation of the distal radial artery 1 day after DRA compared to baseline (2.7 ± 0.5 mm vs. 2.4 ± 0.5 mm, $p < 0.001$). The authors also highlighted the benefits of using ultrasound, not systematically as in previous studies, but more selectively in patients with a low distal radial pulse or after an initial failed attempt. The rate of vascular access conversion was extremely low at 0.4%, conversion to contralateral DRA, which could be explained by the technical versatility of the operators to puncture within the anatomical snuff box in 58.8% (134 patients) and the dorsum of the hand in 41.2% (94 patients).

Lee et al. evaluated 200 consecutive patients with DRA for coronary procedures and showed that the puncture and fluoroscopy times were relatively short (3.0 ± 2.8 min and 11.3 ± 18.4 min, respectively) [10]. There were very few complications (7.9%), mostly minor hematomas. This study also addressed the question of the learning curve and optimal training for cannulation of the distal radial artery. After 150 cases, operators reached a plateau DRA success rate of over 95%, similar to previous studies, but only using conventional techniques without ultrasound guidance. The pitfalls of DRA were the small diameter of the artery, weak pulse, and advanced age, which contribute to cannulation failure or delayed punctures.

2.4.2 Complex Settings and Procedures

The DRA has been used in a variety of clinical settings and for almost all types of coronary interventions (Fig. 2.1), as highlighted by the following reports.

In the American Progress-CTO registry, Nikolakopoulos et al. compared 120 chronic total occlusion (CTO) PCIs performed via DRA with 2625 CTO PCIs performed via the proximal radial artery (TRA) and indicated that the use of DRA in CTO PCI has steadily increased over time and is associated with favorable outcomes (see also Chap. 20) [11].

The pitfalls of DRA related to the small size of this artery compared to the wrist radial artery could make access difficult or impossible for some patients, but no specific data were reported in this registry. Large 7-Fr guiding catheters were used in only 2% of patients, and there was no report on the need for specific techniques to overcome these anatomical limitations.

One of the solutions has been proposed in a prospective observational registry where a new technique named RailTracking uses a long dilator Railway system (Cordis) to reduce the entry profile of the guiding catheter by tapering the entire system and improving the transition zone, trackability, and crossing in normal but especially in difficult anatomies [35]. This technique has been tested in 20 consecutive complex coronary interventions such as CTO PCI, left main coronary artery PCI, rotational atherectomy, coronary lithotripsy, and multivessel PCI without any cross-

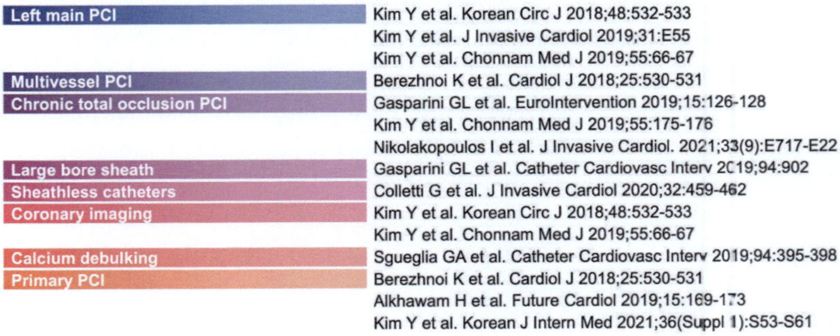

Fig. 2.1 Snapshot of reports and registries focused on distal radial access in complex percutaneous coronary intervention settings. *PCI* percutaneous coronary intervention

over to another vascular access (see also Chap. 19) [12].

Another solution proposed by Gasparini et al. for CTO PCI, where large-bore guiding catheters are often required, is the use of an introducer sheath with a reduced outer diameter related to a thin-walled specific technology such as the Glidesheath Slender (Terumo) [13].

Similar to the previous report by Babunashvili, a Korean experience was published by Bae et al. regarding the use of the distal right radial artery as a bailout technique in a case of proximal radial artery occlusion after previous catheterization [36]. Distal radial access allowed the radial artery to be wired, and after percutaneous transluminal angioplasty using a 2.0-mm balloon catheter, proximal vessel patency was restored (see also Chap. 23).

Several reports on this topic have been published by different authors. Kontopodis et al. [37] described the use of the left DRA in a patient with end-stage renal disease and a functioning arteriovenous fistula in the right arm, with no femoral access due to severe peripheral disease and with an occluded proximal radial artery [37]. Catheterization was performed safely through the left DRA, which was considered by the authors to be the only viable vascular access in this specific situation.

Sheikh et al. were faced with a difficult vascular access to the left arm vessels for PCI of the left anterior descending artery through the left mammary artery [38]. The patient had no palpable left radial pulse at the wrist and weak femoral pulses. The left DRA was successfully used, and the authors were able to perform PCI of the distal left anterior descending artery.

Sgueglia et al. reported a first experience with coronary shockwave lithotripsy through a 5-Fr guiding catheter inserted through the distal radial artery, which may allow a safer procedure in patients with a small radial artery [39]. This article brings new possibilities and arguments in the direction of slender procedures and techniques through the distal radial artery. Considering the slightly smaller size of the distal radial artery and the other anatomical features, more tortuous with higher variability of its course and topography, there is an interest in developing miniaturized materials suitable for this new vascular access (see also Chap. 18).

2.4.3 Noncoronary Interventions

Di Cesare et al. described for the first time the use of DRA for balloon aortic valvuloplasty in ten patients [40]. The procedure was performed in selected patients where the distal radial artery could accommodate an 8-Fr sheath. No complications were reported, and a 30-day color Doppler ultrasound demonstrated patency of the distal radial artery in 89% of cases.

This approach may be an interesting option for patients with femoral artery calcifications or lesions considered at high risk for vascular complications (see also Chap. 22).

The RADCAR-DISTAL study published by Nardai et al. evaluated the feasibility of DRA for carotid artery stenting in an all-comer population using a sheathless coronary guiding system [41]. All patients in the DRA group achieved procedural success from the primary access using ultrasound-guided cannulation, and only one patient had a major access site complication: an arteriovenous fistula requiring surgical treatment (see also Chap. 24).

Finally, DRA is increasingly being used for neurointerventional procedures and has been used successfully for diagnostic cerebral angiography and interventions for hemorrhagic pathology and ischemic stroke, as shown in a meta-analysis of seven studies including 348 (75.8%) diagnostic cerebral angiograms and 111 (24.2%) interventions published by Hoffman et al. (see also Chap. 25) [42].

2.5 Distal Radial Access vs. Conventional Transradial Access Randomized Controlled Trials

While RAO has little or no clinical impact on digital perfusion or functional outcomes, it is a major predictor of unsuccessful radial artery cannulation and increased rates of crossover to the femoral approach.

Preservation of proximal radial artery patency remains an important goal in the cath lab because of the importance of maintaining the radial artery as a potential conduit for future access or use as a bypass graft. In addition, in some patients with severe peripheral disease and previous unilateral radial artery harvesting or arteriovenous fistulas for hemodialysis, the radial artery may be the only or safest vascular access for coronary interventions. In these exceptional cases, it is critical to prioritize RAO prevention with the widest range of solutions at our disposal [43].

In fact, DRA stands out for its minimal impact on the proximal radial artery, both in terms of flow disruption and mechanical injury, resulting in a lower rate of RAO.

One of the pivotal trials, the Distal vs. Conventional Radial Access (DISCO RADIAL) trial, marked a significant milestone as it was the first large-scale, prospective, multicenter, international, randomized, controlled trial comparing DRA with conventional TRA in patients undergoing percutaneous coronary intervention using a 6-Fr thin-walled introducer sheath [16]. Surprisingly, the study failed to demonstrate the superiority of DRA over conventional TRA in reducing RAO due to the extremely low occurrence of the primary endpoint in both study groups, possibly due to the rigorous and consuming protocol that requires state-of-the-art methods to ensure radial artery patency in the conventional TRA group.

Conversely, the similar Distal Radial Approach to Prevent Radial Artery Occlusion (DAPRAO) trial on 282 patients randomized between TRA and DRA showed a notable difference in RAO incidence [14]. The rates of RAO at both 24 h and 30 days were significantly different, being 8.4% and 5.6% in the TRA group and only 0.7% in both time points in the DRA group.

In the large single-center Anatomical sNuffbox for Coronary anGiography and IntervEntions (ANGIE) trial, 1042 patients were randomized to either DRA or TRA [15]. The results showed a significantly lower RAO rate in the DRA group compared to the TRA group, 3.7% vs. 7.9% ($p < 0.014$). It is important to note that not all patients underwent vascular ultrasound follow-up, with evaluation rates of 78.0% for the DRA group and 74.8% for the TRA group.

Recently, Ferrante et al. reported the results of a study-level meta-analysis of 14 randomized clinical trials and 6208 participants comparing DRA vs. TRA using rigorous methods [17]. The primary outcome of interest was RAO at the longest available follow-up. In the pooled data, DRA conferred an average 64% lower risk of RAO (1.6% vs. 5.2%) with a number needed to treat of 30. Patients with DRA also had fewer major hematomas, with a 49% lower risk compared to TRA (see also Chap. 16).

A subsequent network meta-analysis confirmed the superiority of DRA in significantly reducing RAO compared with conventional TRA and also demonstrated an advantage over ulnar access. In addition, point estimates indicated a trend in favor of DRA over conventional TRA with respect to a lower incidence of radial artery spasm. These results further strengthen the evidence supporting the use of DRA to minimize access site complications and improve overall procedural outcomes [44].

2.6 Additional Advantages of Distal Radial Access

In addition, DRA may facilitate early discharge after coronary interventions, with a shorter hemostasis time than TRA and very low rates of access-related bleeding. In the DISCO RADIAL trial, the post-procedural hemostasis time was 180 min (134–292) for the TRA group and 153 min (105–242) for the DRA group ($p < 0.001$), although a dedicated hemostasis device was used in only 88% of the DRA patients [16]. Similar conclusions had also been found in previous publications.

Aoi et al. reported an even shorter hemostasis time after DRA of 104.7 min (120.8 min for PCI and 91.7 min for diagnostic) in their series of 408 patients but used a dedicated compression device in all patients [45].

Koutouzis et al., who preferred manual compression, showed a faster time to hemostasis in the DRA group compared to TRA-treated patients (568 ± 462 s vs 841 ± 574 s, $p = 0.002$) [46].

In the ANGIE trial, the time to hemostasis was twice as short in the DRA group compared to the TRA group (60 vs. 120 min; $p < 0.001$), suggesting that the smaller diameter of the distal radial artery and its more superficial course compared to the proximal radial artery make compression much easier [15].

2.7 Current Limitations of Distal Radial Access

The pitfalls and drawbacks of DRA are well described in the published studies and are related to the difficulty of puncturing the distal radial artery with higher failure rates and longer times to successful radial puncture and sheath insertion as well as more puncture attempts. The crossover rate with DRA is approximately two to three times higher than with conventional TRA, with mostly similar results reported in the DISCO RADIAL, DAPRAO, or ANGIE trials.

Notably, the KOrean Distal Radial Access (KODRA) registry, the largest DRA study to date, reported an overall success rate of 94.4%, with most crossovers to ipsilateral conventional TRA, preserving the initial upper extremity access strategy [47]. This success rate is consistent with results from the DRA arm of the DISCO RADIAL and the RadIal Vs femorAL access for coronary intervention (RIVAL) trial [48]. A comprehensive analysis identified a weak distal radial pulse and limited operator experience as the only independent predictors of puncture failure, highlighting the importance of experience and encouraging operators to complete the DRA learning curve [49].

The use of special equipment including alternative wires and sheaths has the potential to increase the success rate of cannulation, wiring, and crossing of the distal radial artery.

Ultrasound-guided puncture could accelerate the learning curve and reduce the number of cases needed to achieve a high success rate in distal radial artery cannulation. In addition, even experienced operators can see the benefits of ultrasound in improving the likelihood of successful cannulation while reducing the number of attempts when faced with challenging scenarios such as cases with smaller artery diameters, weaker pulses, or tortuous courses.

Interestingly, a recent network meta-analysis comparing four different vascular access approaches for percutaneous coronary procedures found that the crossover rate for DRA compared to conventional TRA was lower than the crossover rate for conventional TRA compared to femoral access [44].

References

1. Babunashvili A, Dundua D. Recanalization and reuse of early occluded radial artery within 6 days after previous transradial diagnostic procedure. Catheter Cardiovasc Interv. 2011;77:530–6.
2. Sgueglia GA, Lee BK, Cho BR, Babunashvili A, Lee JB, Lee JW, et al. Distal radial access: consensus report of the first Korea-Europe transradial intervention meeting. JACC Cardiovasc Interv. 2021;14:892–906.
3. Al-Azizi KM, Grewal V, Gobeil K, Maqsood K, Haider A, Mohani A, et al. The left distal transradial artery access for coronary angiography and intervention: a US experience. Cardiovasc Revasc Med. 2019;20:786–9.
4. Kim Y, Ahn Y, Kim I, Lee DH, Kim MC, Sim DS, et al. Feasibility of coronary angiography and percutaneous coronary intervention via left snuffbox approach. Korean Circ J. 2018;48:1120–30.
5. Gajurel RM, Sahi R, Shrestha H, Thapa S, Khanal R. Initial experience on anatomical snuff box approach for coronary angiogram & percutaneous coronary intervention in a tertiary care center Nepal. World J Cardiovasc Dis. 2018;8:578–87.
6. Wretowski D, Krakowian M, Labyk A, Pruszczyk P, Roik M. Very distal transradial approach (VITRO) for coronary interventions. Postepy Kardiol Interwencyjnej. 2019;15:42–5.
7. Yu W, Hu P, Wang S, Yao L, Wang H, Dou L, et al. Distal radial artery access in the anatomical snuffbox for coronary angiography and intervention: a single center experience. Medicine. 2020;99:e18330.
8. Ziakas A, Koutouzis M, Didagelos M, Tsiafoutis I, Kouparanis A, Gossios T, et al. Right arm distal transradial (snuffbox) access for coronary catheterization: initial experience. Hell J Cardiol. 2020;61:106–9.
9. Oliveira MDP, Navarro EC, Kiemeneij F. Distal transradial access as default approach for coronary angiography and interventions. Cardiovasc Diagn Ther. 2019;9:513–9.

10. Lee JW, Park SW, Son JW, Ahn SG, Lee SH. Real-world experience of the left distal transradial approach for coronary angiography and percutaneous coronary intervention: a prospective observational study (LeDRA). EuroIntervention. 2018;14:e995–1003.
11. Nikolakopoulos I, Patel T, Jefferson BK, Sheikh AM, Jaber W, Samady H, et al. Distal radial access in chronic Total occlusion percutaneous coronary intervention: insights from the PROGRESS-CTO registry. J Invasive Cardiol. 2021;33:E717–22.
12. Colletti G, Auslender J, De Meester A, Aminian A, Kayaert P, Ungureanu C. Feasibility and safety of performing complex coronary interventions by distal radial artery using the railway sheathless vascular system. J Invasive Cardiol. 2020;32:459–62.
13. Gasparini GL, Garbo R, Gagnor A, Oreglia J, Mazzarotto P. First prospective multicentre experience with left distal transradial approach for coronary chronic total occlusion interventions using a 7 Fr Glidesheath Slender. EuroIntervention. 2019;15:126–8.
14. Eid-Lidt G, Rivera Rodriguez A, Jimenez Castellanos J, Farjat Pasos JI, Estrada Lopez KE, Gaspar J. Distal radial artery approach to prevent radial artery occlusion trial. JACC Cardiovasc Interv. 2021;14:378–85.
15. Tsigkas G, Papageorgiou A, Moulias A, Kalogeropoulos AP, Papageorgopoulou C, Apostolos A, et al. Distal or traditional transradial access site for coronary procedures: a single-center, Randomized study. JACC Cardiovasc Interv. 2022;15:22–32.
16. Aminian A, Sgueglia GA, Wiemer M, Kefer J, Gasparini GL, Ruzsa Z, et al. Distal versus conventional radial access for coronary angiography and intervention: the DISCO RADIAL trial. JACC Cardiovasc Interv. 2022;15:1191–201.
17. Ferrante G, Condello F, Rao SV, Maurina M, Jolly S, Stefanini GG, et al. Distal vs conventional radial access for coronary angiography and/or intervention: a meta-analysis of randomized trials. JACC Cardiovasc Interv. 2022;15:2297–311.
18. Serruys PW, Onuma Y. Twitterature: will social media have an impact on scientific journals? EuroIntervention. 2018;14:e962–4.
19. Sgueglia GA, Di Giorgio A, Gaspardone A, Babunashvili A. Anatomic basis and physiological rationale of distal radial artery access for percutaneous coronary and endovascular procedures. JACC Cardiovasc Interv. 2018;11:2113–9.
20. Sgueglia GA, Santoliquido A, Gaspardone A, Di Giorgio A. First results of the distal radial access Doppler study. JACC Cardiovasc Imaging. 2021;14:1281–3.
21. Kim Y, Lee SY, Lee DI, Lee JH, Kim SM, Bae JW, et al. Assessment of the conventional radial artery with optical coherent tomography after the snuffbox approach. Cardiol J. 2021;28:849–54.
22. Ferrante G, Rao SV, Juni P, Da Costa BR, Reimers B, Condorelli G, et al. Radial versus femoral access for coronary interventions across the entire Spectrum of patients with coronary artery disease: a meta-analysis of randomized trials. JACC Cardiovasc Interv. 2016;9:1419–34.
23. Neumann FJ, Sousa-Uva M, Ahlsson A, Alfonso F, Banning AP, Benedetto U, et al. 2018 ESC/EACTS Guidelines on myocardial revascularization. Eur Heart J. 2019;40:87–165.
24. Lawton JS, Tamis-Holland JE, Bangalore S, Bates ER, Beckie TM, Bischoff JM, et al. 2021 ACC/AHA/SCAI guideline for coronary artery revascularization. Circulation. 2022;145:e18–114.
25. Rao SV, Bernat I, Bertrand OF. Clinical update: remaining challenges and opportunities for improvement in percutaneous transradial coronary procedures. Eur Heart J. 2012;33:2521–6.
26. Rao SV, Cohen MG, Kandzari DE, Bertrand OF, Gilchrist IC. The transradial approach to percutaneous coronary intervention: historical perspective, current concepts, and future directions. J Am Coll Cardiol. 2010;55:2187–95.
27. Sakai H, Ikeda S, Harada T, Yonashiro S, Ozumi K, Ohe H, et al. Limitations of successive transradial approach in the same arm: the Japanese experience. Catheter Cardiovasc Interv. 2001;54:204–8.
28. Kiemeneij F. Left distal transradial access in the anatomical snuffbox for coronary angiography (ldTRA) and interventions (ldTRI). EuroIntervention. 2017;13:851–7.
29. Amato JJ, Solod E, Cleveland RJ. A "second" radial artery for monitoring the perioperative pediatric cardiac patient. J Pediatr Surg. 1977;12:715–7.
30. Pyles ST, Scher KS, Vega ET, Harrah JD, Rubis LJ. Cannulation of the dorsal radial artery: a new technique. Anesth Analg. 1982;61:876–8.
31. Soydan E, Akin M. Coronary angiography using the left distal radial approach – an alternative site to conventional radial coronary angiography. Anatol J Cardiol. 2018;19:243–8.
32. Achim A, Kakonyi K, Jambrik Z, Nagy F, Toth J, Sasi V, et al. Distal radial artery access for coronary and peripheral procedures: a multicenter experience. J Clin Med. 2021;10:5974.
33. Hadjivassiliou A, Kiemeneij F, Nathan S, Klass D. Ultrasound-guided access to the distal radial artery at the anatomical snuffbox for catheter-based vascular interventions: a technical guide. EuroIntervention. 2021;16:1342–8.
34. Mizuguchi Y, Izumikawa T, Hashimoto S, Yamada T, Taniguchi N, Nakajima S, et al. Efficacy and safety of the distal transradial approach in coronary angiography and percutaneous coronary intervention: a Japanese multicenter experience. Cardiovasc Interv Ther. 2020;35:162–7.
35. Ungureanu C, Gasparini GL, Aminian A, Blaimont M, Dumitrascu S, Lepiece C, et al. RailTracking: a novel technique to overcome difficult anatomy during transradial approach. J Invasive Cardiol. 2022;34:E757–62.

36. Bae DH, Lee SY, Lee DI, Kim SM, Bae JW, Hwang KK. Percutaneous angioplasty at previous radial puncture site via distal radial access of anatomical snuffbox. Cardiol J. 2019;26:610–1.
37. Kontopodis E, Rigatou A, Tsiafoutis I, Lazaris E, Koutouzis M. Snuffbox to the rescue: distal transradial approach for cardiac catheterisation after failed ipsilateral radial puncture. Kardiol Pol. 2018;76:1491.
38. Sheikh AR, Abdelaal E, Sastry S, Karim S, Zeb M. Novel distal left radial artery access in anatomical snuffbox for recanalization of proximal radial artery total occlusion and percutaneous coronary intervention through left internal mammary artery. Circ Cardiovasc Interv. 2018;11:e006579.
39. Sgueglia GA, Gioffre G, Piccioni F, Gaspardone A. Slender distal radial five French coronary shockwave lithotripsy. Catheter Cardiovasc Interv. 2019;94:395–8.
40. Di Cesare A, Tonet E, Campo G, Tumscitz C. Snuffbox approach for balloon aortic valvuloplasty: a case series. Catheter Cardiovasc Interv. 2021;97:E743–7.
41. Narcai S, Vegh E, Orias V, Nemes B, Toth J, Huttl A, et al. Feasibility of distal radial access for carotid interventions: the RADCAR-DISTAL pilot study. EuroIntervention. 2020;15:1288–90.
42. Hoffman H, Jalal MS, Masoud HE, Pons RB, Rodriguez Caamano I, Khandelwal P, et al. Distal transradial access for diagnostic cerebral angiography and neurointervention: systematic review and meta-analysis. AJNR Am J Neuroradiol. 2021;42:888–95.
43. Bernat I, Aminian A, Pancholy S, Mamas M, Gaudino M, Nolan J, et al. Best practices for the prevention of radial artery occlusion after transradial diagnostic angiography and intervention: an international consensus paper. JACC Cardiovasc Interv. 2019;12:2235–46.
44. Maqsood MH, Yong CM, Rao SV, Cohen MG, Pancholy S, Bangalore S. Procedural outcomes with femoral, radial, distal radial, and ulnar access for coronary angiography: a network meta-analysis. Circ Cardiovasc Interv. 2004;17:e014186.
45. Aoi S, Htun WW, Freeo S, Lee S, Kyaw H, Alfaro V, et al. Distal transradial artery access in the anatomical snuffbox for coronary angiography as an alternative access site for faster hemostasis. Catheter Cardiovasc Interv. 2019;94:651–7.
46. Koutouzis M, Kontopodis E, Tassopoulos A, Tsiafoutis I, Katsanou K, Rigatou A, et al. Distal versus traditional radial approach for coronary angiography. Cardiovasc Revasc Med. 2019;20:678–80.
47. Lee JW, Kim Y, Lee BK, Yoo SY, Lee SY, Kim CJ, et al. Distal radial access for coronary procedures in a large prospective multicenter registry: The KODRA Trial. JACC Cardiovasc Interv. 2024;17:329–40.
48. Jolly SS, Yusuf S, Cairns J, Niemelä K, Xavier D, Widimsky P, et al. Radial versus femoral access for coronary angiography and intervention in patients with acute coronary syndromes (RIVAL): a randomised, parallel group, multicentre trial. Lancet. 2011;377:1409–20.
49. Sgueglia GA. Distal radial access evolution: from randomized controlled trials to the real world and beyond. JACC Cardiovasc Interv. 2024;17:341–4.

Anatomic Basis

3

Thierry Corcos, Francesco Bianchini, and Francesco Burzotta

3.1 Introduction

A thorough understanding of upper extremity arterial anatomy is essential for successful radial access and navigation. This chapter provides a comprehensive overview of the relevant anatomy, beginning with the axillary artery and progressing distally through the brachial and radial arteries. It examines the course, relationships, and key anatomical landmarks of these arteries and discusses common anatomical variants and their potential impact on radial access procedures. By mastering this anatomical knowledge, interventional cardiologists can optimize their technique, minimize complications, and improve overall procedural success rates for radial access procedures.

3.2 Axillary Artery

The axillary artery begins at the distal edge of the first rib and ends at the distal edge of the teres major tendon, continuing the subclavian artery [1–3]. It traverses the axilla distally and inferiorly, describing a superior convexity with the arm at the side (Fig. 3.1). The artery initially lies deep in the axilla, inferior to the anterior border of the deltoid, partially covered by the pectoralis minor and more distally by the pectoralis major. As it passes anterior to the teres major, it becomes superficial and palpable in the axilla, being covered only by skin and fascia in its most distal portion.

The axillary artery is conventionally divided into three parts based on its relationship to the pectoralis minor muscle. The axillary vein lies parallel to the axillary artery and is located anteriorly or inferiorly to the artery along the course of the artery through the axilla.

The first (proximal) part extends from the lateral border of the first rib to the medial border of the pectoralis minor and is approximately 2.5 cm long. It is bordered superiorly by the anterior deltoid muscle and covered anteriorly by skin, fascia, pectoralis major muscle, and clavipectoral fascia. Posteriorly, it is bordered by the first intercostal space, the serratus anterior, and the medial cord of the brachial plexus. The axillary vein lies medially. This part gives rise to the superior thoracic artery.

The second (posterior) portion, approximately 3 cm long, lies deep into the pectoralis minor. It passes anterior to the subscapularis muscle and is surrounded by the cords of the brachial plexus. The axillary vein lies medially. This portion gives rise to the thoracoacromial and lateral thoracic arteries.

T. Corcos
Department of Cardiology, American Hospital of Paris, Neuilly-sur-Seine, France

F. Bianchini · F. Burzotta (✉)
Department of Cardiovascular Sciences, Fondazione Policlinico Universitario Agostino Gemelli IRCCS, Rome, Italy
e-mail: francesco.burzotta@unicatt.it

G. A. Sgueglia (ed.), *Distal Radial Access*, https://doi.org/10.1007/978-3-031-89925-6_3

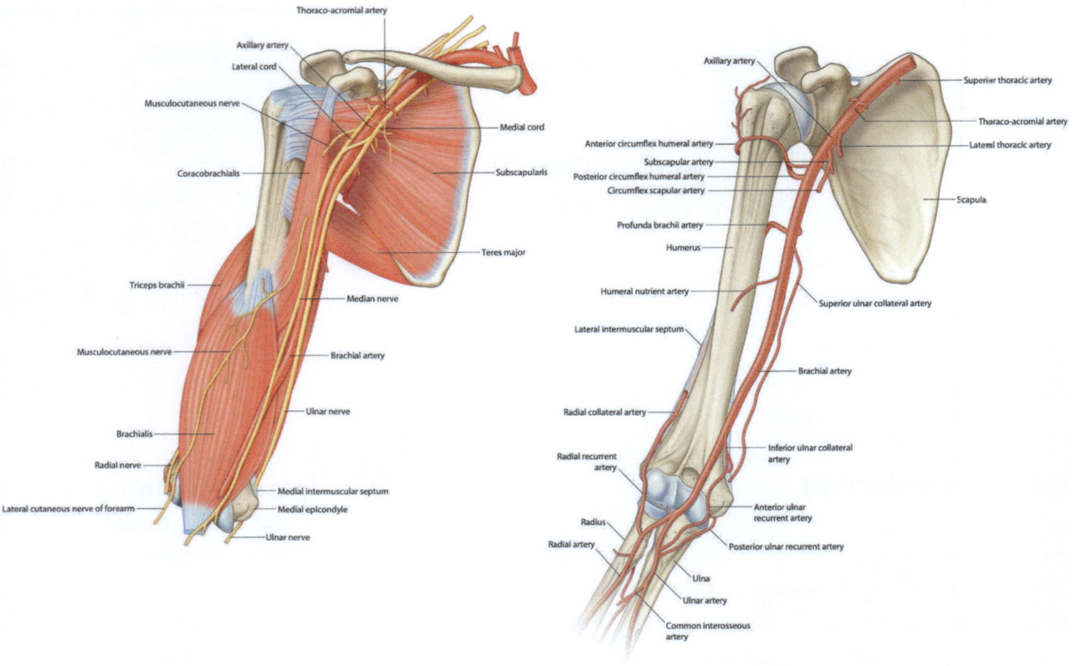

Fig. 3.1 Anterior view of the axillary and brachial arteries with relevant surrounding anatomical structures. (Reproduced from Drake et al. [2])

The third (distal) part, approximately 7.5 cm long, extends from the lateral border of the pectoralis minor to the distal border of the teres major tendon. Anteriorly, it is covered proximally by the pectoralis major and becomes subcutaneous distally. Posteriorly, it is covered by the subscapularis, latissimus dorsi, and teres major. The axillary vein lies medially. Branches of the brachial plexus surround this portion: the median nerve laterally, the ulnar and medial brachial cutaneous nerves medially, and the radial and axillary nerves posteriorly. This portion gives rise to the subscapular artery and the anterior and posterior humeral circumflex arteries.

3.3 Brachial Artery

The brachial artery, a continuation of the axillary artery, begins at the distal margin of the teres major and ends approximately 1 cm distal to the elbow, where it divides into the radial and ulnar arteries (Fig. 3.1). It runs along the medial aspect of the arm, becoming more anterior distally [1–3].

The artery is superficial and palpable along its course, covered only by skin and fascia. It passes deep to the bicipital aponeurosis. In the proximal arm, the median nerve lies anterior to the brachial artery, crossing it mid-arm to lie medial to the elbow. The ulnar nerve is initially medial to the artery but separates from it distally.

In the proximal arm, the brachial artery passes along the medial head of the triceps and the insertion of the coracobrachialis and then continues along the brachialis muscle. More distally, the biceps brachii lies lateral to the artery. Two venae comitantes closely follow the artery. At the elbow, the brachial artery courses anteriorly to cross the mid-portion of the cubital fossa anteromedially to the brachialis muscle.

3.4 Radial Artery

As the brachial artery bifurcates into the ulnar and radial arteries approximately 1 cm distal to the elbow joint, just below the cubital fossa, it provides dual vascular supply to the hand (Fig. 3.2). This bifurcation marks the origin of two critical arterial pathways that supply the forearm and hand [1, 2].

The ulnar artery (Fig. 3.1) follows an oblique downward course, reaching the ulnar aspect of the forearm at a point approximately midway between the elbow and the wrist. It then courses along the ulnar border to the wrist, traverses the transverse carpal ligament on the radial side of the pisiform bone, and immediately distal to this bone gives rise to a deep palmar branch. The ulnar artery then continues across the palm to form the superficial palmar arch, which is variably completed by an anastomotic branch from the radial artery.

Although the radial artery appears to be a continuation of the brachial artery due to its slightly lateral course, it is typically smaller in caliber than the ulnar artery [1]. For descriptive purposes, the course of the radial artery is traditionally divided into three anatomical segments: the forearm, wrist, and hand. Originating at the bifurcation, the radial artery extends from the neck of the radius to the anterior aspect of the styloid process (Fig. 3.3).

In the proximal forearm, the radial artery runs along the medial aspect of the radius, deep to the brachioradialis muscle. As it progresses through the middle and distal portions of the forearm, it transitions to an anterior position relative to the radius, becoming progressively more superficial. Throughout its forearm course, the artery passes superficial to several important anatomical structures, including the biceps tendon, the supinator muscle, the pronator teres muscle, the radial origin of the flexor digitorum superficialis, the flexor

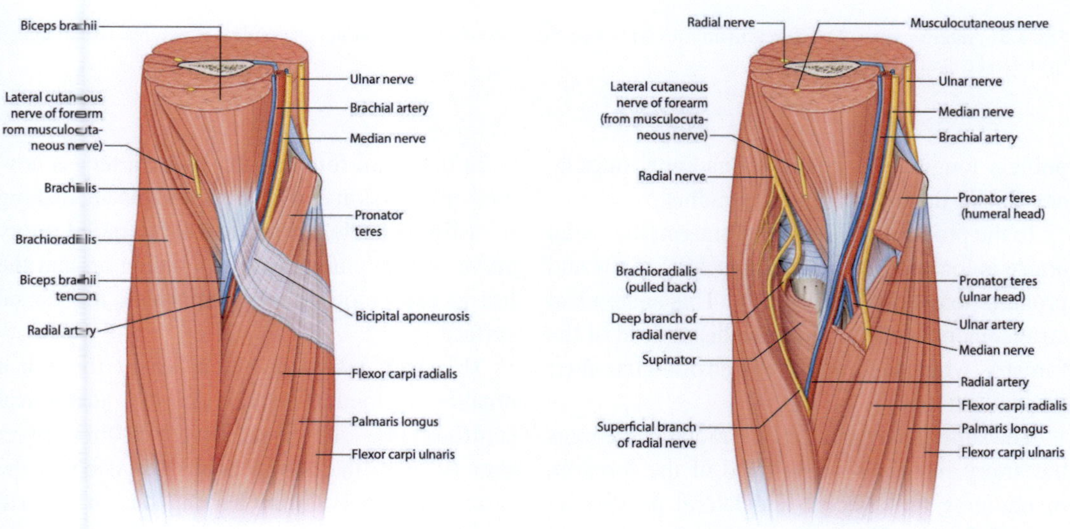

Fig. 3.2 Contents of the cubital fossa. (Reproduced from Drake et al. [2])

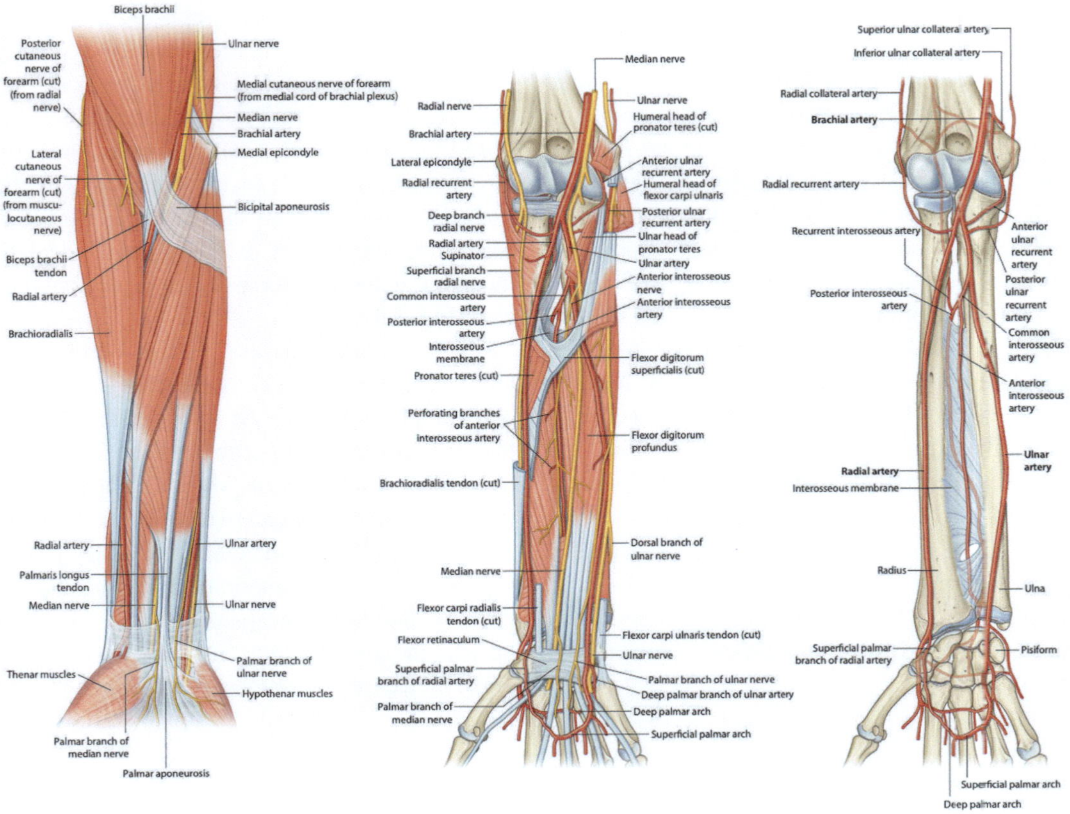

Fig. 3.3 Anterior view of the forearm arteries with superficial and deep surrounding anatomical structures. (Reproduced from Drake et al. [2])

pollicis longus, the pronator quadratus muscle, and finally the distal end of the radius.

In the proximal third of the forearm, the radial artery is located between the brachioradialis and pronator teres muscle (Fig. 3.3). This anatomical arrangement continues into the distal third of the forearm, where these muscles transition into their respective tendons.

The superficial branch of the radial nerve joins the artery in the proximal third of the forearm, maintaining an adjacent and lateral position in the middle third. Throughout its course, the radial artery is accompanied by a pair of venae comitantes, which closely follow its path.

In the distal forearm, the radial artery is covered only by skin and antebrachial fascia, making it easily palpable. At the wrist, the radial artery curves dorsally and distally, winding around the lateral aspect of the wrist to reach the dorsal surface.

This path takes the radial artery through a notable anatomical landmark: the anatomical snuffbox [4]. The artery traverses this space, superficial to the carpal bones but deep to the extensor tendons. After leaving the anatomical snuffbox, the radial artery continues its course superficially in the first intermetacarpal space on the back of the hand before entering the palmar

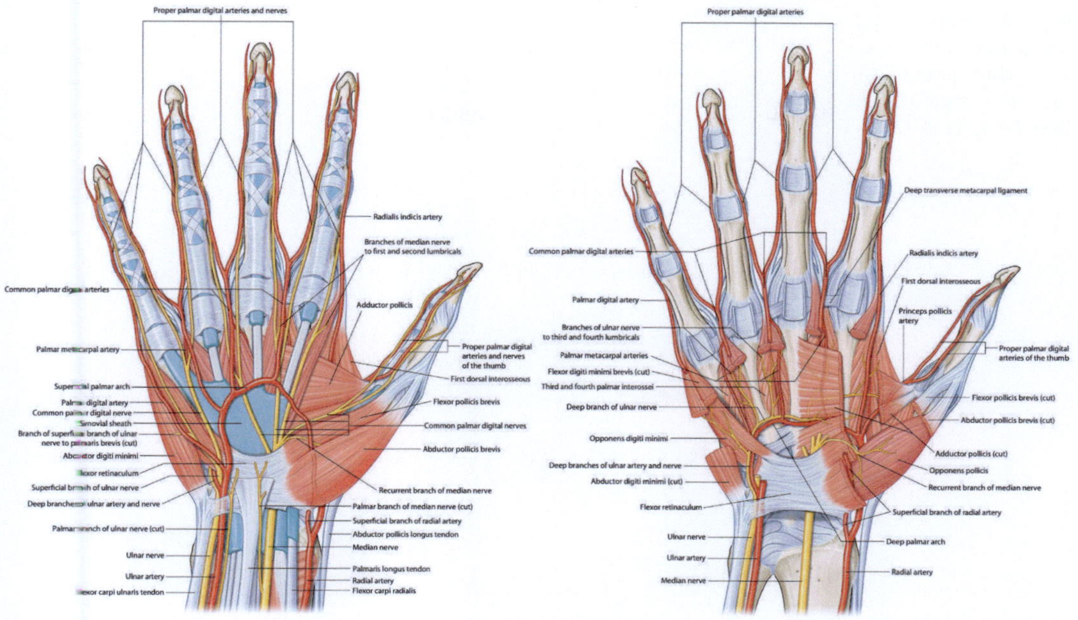

Fig. 3.4 Superficial and deep arteries of the palmar hand with surrounding anatomical structures. (Reproduced from Drake et al. [2])

aspect [5]. It then crosses the deep palm transversely, passing between the oblique and transverse heads of the adductor pollicis muscle [2]. The artery then passes through the transverse head of this muscle and reaches the base of the small finger metacarpal [1, 3]. At this point, it forms a variable anastomosis with the deep palmar branch of the ulnar artery, completing the deep palmar arch (Fig. 3.4).

Throughout its extensive course, the radial artery gives rise to several important branches and participates in important anastomoses. In the proximal forearm, it gives rise to the recurrent radial artery. Further along, it provides several small muscular branches to surrounding tissues. In the distal forearm and wrist, it gives rise to several carpal branches that form dorsal and palmar transverse anastomoses with homologous branches of the ulnar artery (Fig. 3.5) [3].

The radial artery also forms important anastomoses with the anterior and posterior interosseous arteries in the distal forearm, which in turn anastomose with the ulnar artery and contribute to the vascular network of the distal radius.

A relatively small but significant branch, the superficial palmar branch, arises just distal to the carpus. This branch continues into the palmar aspect of the wrist and usually contributes to the formation of the radial aspect of the superficial palmar arch (Fig. 3.4).

The palmar arches are critical to the digital blood supply. The interconnected palmar metacarpal and common palmar digital arteries, which arise from the deep and superficial palmar arches, respectively, serve as the primary source of blood supply to the digits [1–4].

This extensive anastomotic network between the radial and ulnar arterial systems is of great clinical importance, as it ensures the preservation of blood supply to the digits even in cases of transient or persistent radial artery occlusion [2].

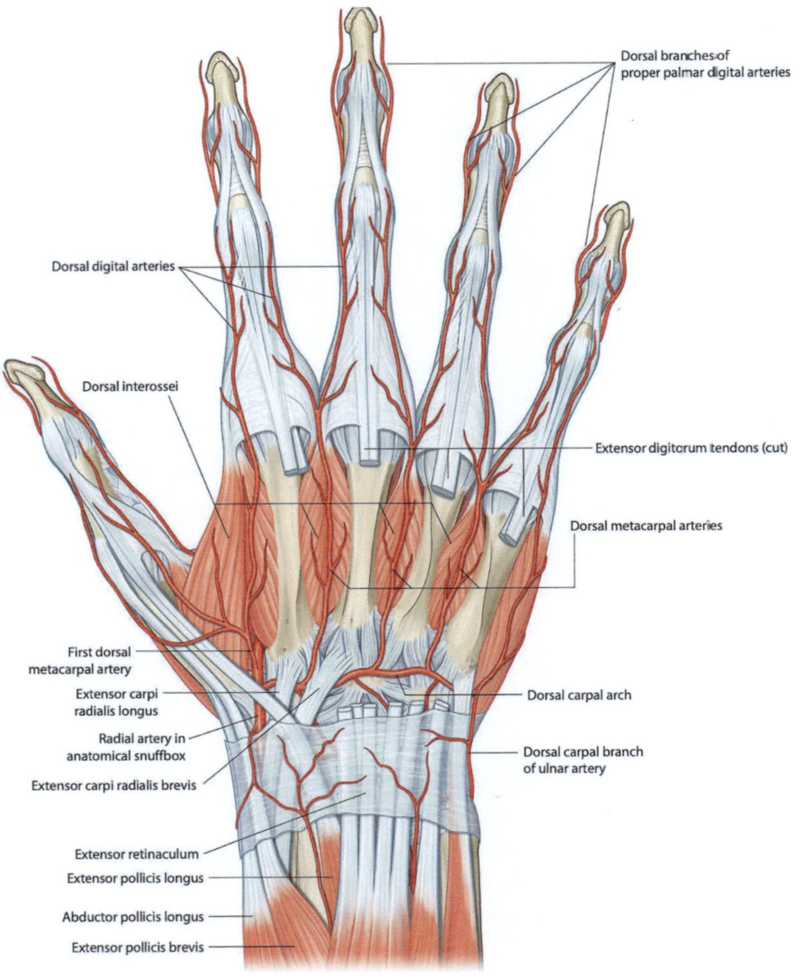

Fig. 3.5 Arteries of the dorsal hand with surrounding anatomical structures. (Reproduced from Drake et al. [2])

3.5 Anatomical Snuffbox

The anatomical snuffbox, also known as the radial fossa, is a well-defined triangular depression located on the dorsolateral aspect of the wrist. This region is bounded by three prominent tendons: the extensor pollicis longus tendon medially (ulnar side) and the extensor pollicis brevis and abductor pollicis longus tendons laterally (radial side). The floor of this compartment consists of the scaphoid and trapezium carpal bones, which provide a bony substrate for the overlying soft tissues (Fig. 3.6).

This anatomical region is traversed by the distal radial artery, accompanied by the superficial branch of the radial nerve. The cephalic vein, if present, may also be visible beneath the skin, although its course may be variable.

The radial artery, after emerging from under the brachioradialis tendon, traverses the floor of the snuffbox in a superficial plane. This superficial course makes the artery easily palpable and accessible for cannulation. The extensor pollicis longus tendon serves as an important anatomical landmark, separating the anatomical snuffbox from the first intermetacarpal space where the distal radial artery can be accessed on the dorsal hand [6]. As the radial artery progresses distally, it passes between the two heads of the first dorsal interosseous muscle to reach the palmar aspect of the hand. Here, it contributes to the formation of the deep palmar arch.

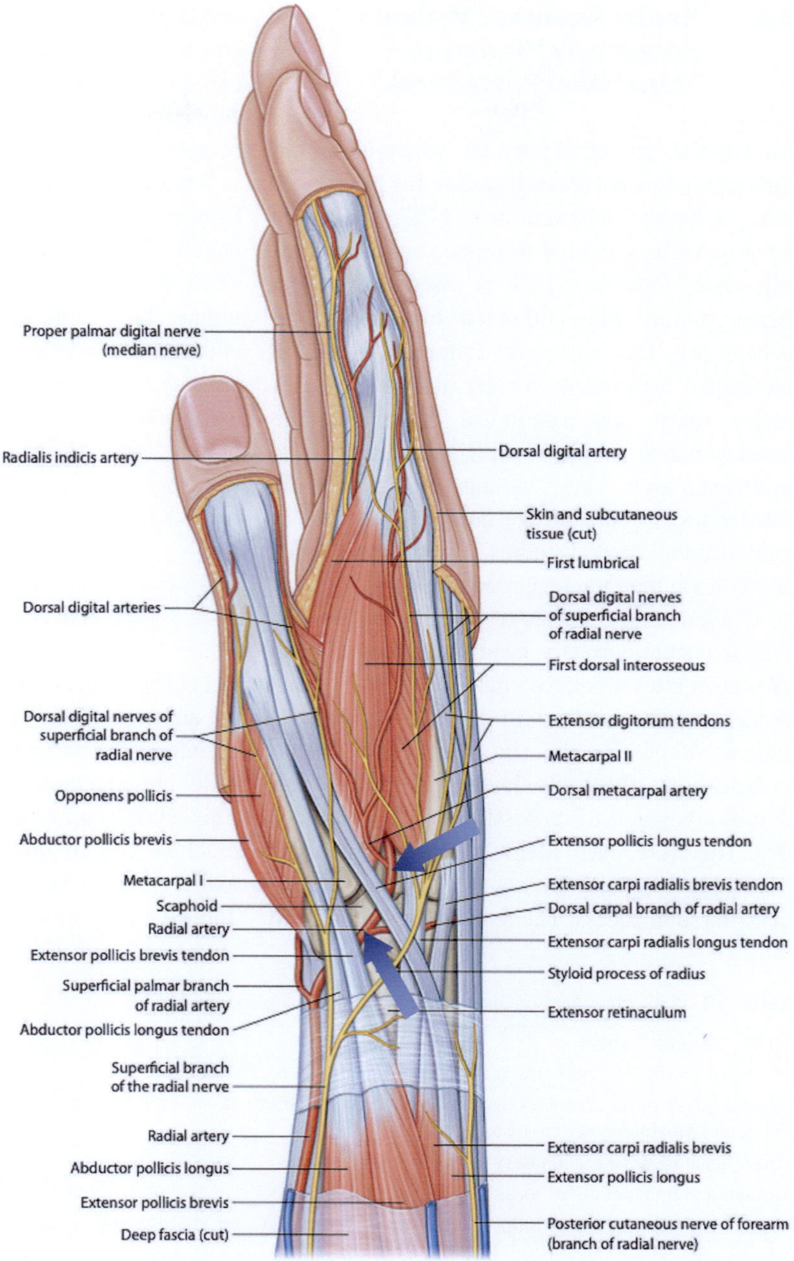

Fig. 3.6 Distal radial artery puncture sites (blue arrows) and relevant surrounding anatomical structures. (Adapted from Drake et al. [2])

Two specific sites have been identified where the radial pulse can be reliably palpated: within the anatomical snuffbox and on the dorsum of the hand. These sites represent alternative puncture points for distal radial access (Fig. 3.6) that offer comparable advantages to conventional transradial access [6] because the distal radial artery accessed in either the anatomic snuffbox or on the dorsum of the hand is the continuation of the same radial artery accessed in the forearm [7].

3.6 Radial Anatomic Variants Potentially Hindering Transradial Procedures

Transradial access (TRA) has emerged as an alternative to transfemoral access for percutaneous coronary intervention (PCI), primarily because of its potential to reduce vascular complications. However, TRA is associated with a higher failure rate compared to transfemoral access [8]. This increased failure rate can be attributed to several factors, including radial artery spasm and anatomical variants of the brachio-radial, axillo-subclavian arterial axis, and aortic arch. These variants pose navigation challenges in reaching the coronary arteries, as evidenced by several studies of patients undergoing PCI via the radial approach [9–11].

Contemporary studies of patients undergoing PCI for acute coronary syndromes report radial crossover rates of approximately 8%. This occurrence is associated with patient discomfort, increased radiation exposure, and delayed revascularization, ultimately leading to worse outcomes compared to successful radial access [12, 13]. Therefore, early identification of patients at high risk for radial crossover is critical to successful radial access. The recently developed and validated MATRIX score aims to predict radial crossover in patients undergoing PCI for acute coronary syndromes [14] and may help operators anticipate and manage radial access-related complications.

Traditional anatomic classifications derived from postmortem studies have limitations in the context of TRA procedures. These classifications often describe variants that do not significantly impact TRA (e.g., anomalous courses of radial and brachial arteries in relation to muscles and nerves). Furthermore, they fail to report on tortuosity and atherosclerotic disease of radial and brachial arteries, which are frequently identified by angiography and can affect transradial procedures.

3.7 Operative ABC Classification

Recognizing the importance of identifying different anatomical variants for successful transradial coronary interventions, a simplified "operative" ABC classification has been proposed [15, 16]. This classification extends beyond the radial-brachial axis to include the assessment of the axillary-subclavian axis and the aortic arch. Table 3.1 lists ten potential angiographic variants

Table 3.1 ABC classification and anatomic variant prevalence

ABC anatomic variant	Prevalence
Group A: radio-brachial arterial axis	
Radial artery pulse absent (congenital absence of the artery or acquired occlusion due to previous injury or occlusive atherosclerotic disease)	0.3%
Significant (>50%) radial artery atherosclerotic stenosis	0.4%
Radial and brachial artery tortuosity (bending >45°)	4.9%
Radial and brachial artery loops (360° loop in the arterial course not located at anastomotic sites)	0.4%
Radio-ulnar loops (360° loop at the anastomosis with brachial-ulnar artery)	0.7%
High origin of the radial artery from brachial or axillary artery	2.9%
Group B: axillary-subclavian-anonymous arterial axis	
Severe tortuosity (bending >90°)	1.5%
Significant (>50%) atherosclerotic stenosis of the axillary-subclavian anonymous arterial axis	0.4%
Group C: aortic arch	
Retro-esophageal right subclavian artery (arteria lusoria) (right subclavian artery arising from the distal and posterior margin of the horizontal part of the aortic arch at its junction with the descending aorta, less frequently from the proximal descending aorta)	0.2%
Aortic arch elongation (aortic arch elongation creating distal dislodgement of the anonymous trunk and changes in the ascending aorta anatomy)	0.1%

Burzotta et al. [16]

Table 3.2 Transradial access failure according to each ABC variant

ABC anatomic variant	TRA failure rate	OR (95% CI)	*p*
(A) Radial artery occlusion	100%	–	<0.0001
(A) Significant radial artery atherosclerotic stenosis	15.4%	27.3 (5.7–130.6)	0.0037
(A) Radial and brachial artery tortuosities	7.6%	12.3 (6.0–24.9)	0.0001
(A) Radial or brachial artery loop	14.3%	25.0 (5.3–118.6)	0.0043
(A) Radio-ulnar loops	30.4%	65.6 (24.5–175.9)	<0.0001
(A) High origin of the radial artery	11.7%	19.8 (9.4–41.4)	0.0001
(B) Severe tortuosities of epi-aortic vessels	15.4%	27.3 (11.5–64.9)	<0.0001
(B) Significant atherosclerotic stenosis of epi-aortic vessels	12.5%	21.4 (4.6–100.1)	0.0056
(C) Arteria lusoria	12.5%	21.4 (2.5–181.8)	0.0013
(C) Aortic arch elongation	66.6%	449.7 (44.9–4501.4)	<0.0001

Burzotta et al. [16]
CI confidence interval, *OR* odds ratio, *TRA* transradial access

Table 3.3 Anatomic variants distribution in the right vs left arm

Variant	Right ($n = 610$)	Left ($n = 610$)	*p*	OR (95% CI)
Any anatomic variant	65 (10.7%)	40 (6.6%)	0.02	6.7 (3.8–11.4)
Arm arterial axis level variants				
Type A variant only	57 (9.3%)	38 (6.2%)	<0.001	7.2 (4.1–12.7)
Type B variant only	24 (3.9%)	14 (2.3%)	0.01	8.0 (2.1–30.9)
Combined type A + B variants	10 (1.6%)	6 (1.0%)	0.42	13.2 (1.4–124.9)
Specific anatomic variants				
Radial occlusion	4 (0.7%)	3 (0.5%)	1	0.99 (0.98–1.01)
Severe atherosclerotic radial/brachial disease	5 (0.8%)	6 (1.0%)	0.09	19.9 (2.0–197.4)
Severe radial/brachial tortuosity	33 (5.4%)	16 (2.6%)	0.02	17.5 (8.1–37.7)
Radial/brachial loop	7 (1.1%)	8 (1.3%)	0.11	10 (1.2–96.5)
Radioulnar loop	13 (2.1%)	8 (1.3%)	0.02	11.3 (2.1–58.4)
High origin of radial artery	27 (4.4%)	20 (3.3%)	<0.001	9.2 (3.8–22.2)
Severe axillary/subclavian/anonymous tortuosity	20 (3.3%)	12 (1.96%)	0.22	7.2 (1.9–27.5)
Atherosclerotic axillary/subclavian/anonymous stenosis	6 (0.98%)	7 (1.1%)	0.005	28.3 (4.9–165.5)

Burzotta et al. [17]
CI confidence interval, *OR* odds ratio

encountered during TRA, divided into three subgroups, along with their respective incidences. As reported by Burzotta et al. [15], each of the ten ABC variants has a significantly increased risk of transradial access failure compared to its absence (Table 3.2). A large retrospective study of 610 patients who underwent bilateral angiographic evaluation of upper extremity anatomy showed that the incidence of anatomical variants is higher in the right compared to the left upper extremity vasculature (Table 3.3). Furthermore, bilateral variants occur in less than 8% of patients and are often of similar type and symmetric distribution [17].

3.7.1 Group A: Radial-Brachial Axis Variants

Brachial and radial arteries have a wide range of anatomic variants, but not all are equally important in determining access success. According to the angiographic ABC classification [11, 15], the main variants of this group are summarized below.

Absence of the radial artery pulse (Fig. 3.7a). This condition results from the complete absence of the radial artery, with blood flow supplied by the anterior interosseous or

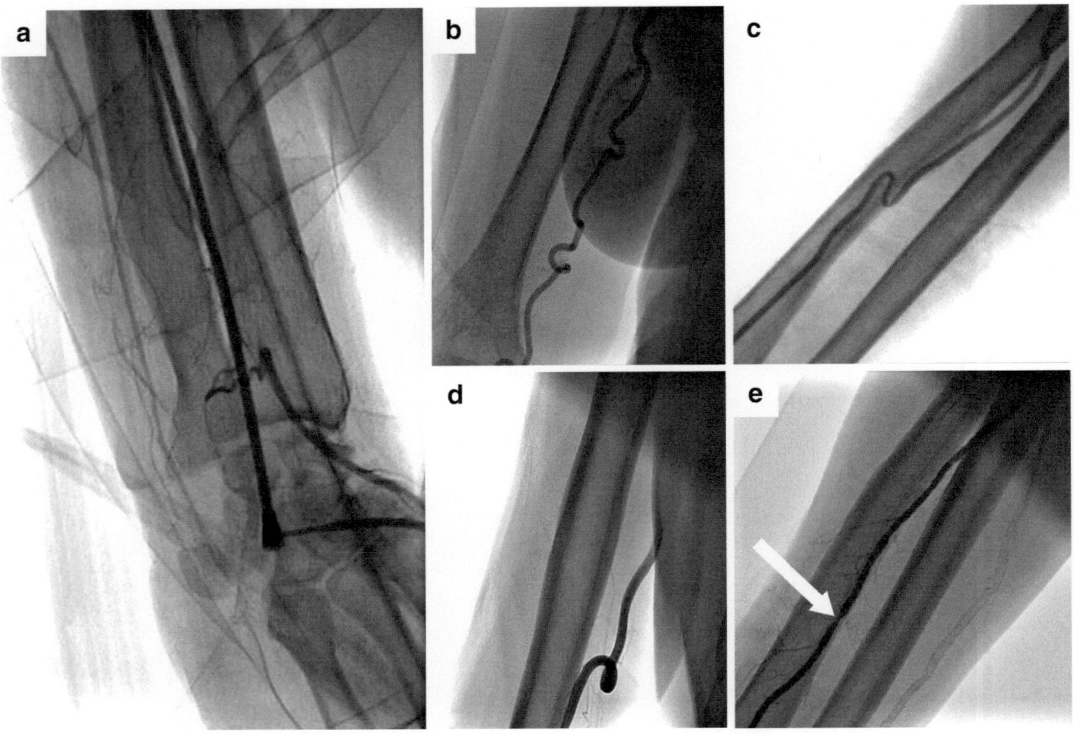

Fig. 3.7 Anatomic variants of the radio-brachial arterial axis. (**a**) Retrograde radial angiography from the sheath showing an occluded distal radial artery. (**b**) High origin of the radial artery from the axillary artery with an extremely tortuous course. (**c**) Radial artery severe tortuosity with "Z-shape." (**d**) Radial artery loop. (**e**) Diffuse radial artery atherosclerosis with a stenosis (white arrow) in the mid portion of the vessel. (Reproduced from Burzotta et al. [11])

median arteries. The etiology may be congenital or acquired, the latter possibly due to previous injury or atherosclerotic occlusive disease [11, 18].

High origin of the radial artery (Fig. 3.7b). This variant is characterized by the radial artery originating proximal to the intercondylar contour of the humerus, which serves as a fixed anatomic landmark representing the proximal edge of the antecubital fossa [11]. These vessels are often smaller in caliber and are associated with increased tortuosity and propensity for vasospasm [18].

Severe tortuosity of the radial and brachial arteries (Fig. 3.7c). Defined as a curvature of more than 45° in the course of the vessel, this variant affects the radial artery more frequently than the brachial artery [18]. The presence of severe tortuosity can significantly complicate catheter navigation and increase the risk of vessel trauma.

Arterial loops (Fig. 3.7d). Loops are defined as a full 360° turn in the course of the artery and can occur in both the brachial and radial arteries. Of all anatomical variations, arterial loops are associated with the highest rate of access failure [18]. These loops present significant challenges to catheter advancement and may require specialized techniques or alternative access sites.

Radial artery atherosclerosis (Fig. 3.7e). Radial artery atherosclerosis can manifest as focal stenosis or diffuse calcification. The presence of atherosclerotic disease can complicate catheter insertion, increase the risk of arterial spasm, and potentially lead to distal embolization during instrumentation.

3.7.2 Group B: Axillary-Subclavian-Anonymous Axis Variants

The axillary-subclavian-anonymous arterial axis has a number of anatomical variations that can significantly impact transradial procedures. These variations can be broadly categorized into two main types.

Tortuosity and loops (Fig. 3.8a). Tortuosity in this arterial segment is defined as a bend greater than 90° in the course of the vessel. Loops represent an extreme form of tortuosity in which the vessel makes a complete 360° turn. These deviations from the normal, relatively straight path can be either congenital or acquired.

Atherosclerotic disease (Fig. 3.8b). The axillary-subclavian-anonymous axis may also be the site of atherosclerotic plaques [11].

3.7.3 Group C: Aortic Arch Variants

The aortic arch exhibits a variety of anatomical variations, which may be further modified by aging and pathological processes such as arterial hypertension, atherosclerosis, and connective tissue disease [11, 16]. Although there are numerous variants, only certain conformations of the aortic arch have a significant impact on the success of percutaneous coronary procedures through a transradial approach.

Retroesophageal right subclavian artery (RORSA) or arteria lusoria (Fig. 3.9a, b). This variation is characterized by an anomalous origin of the right subclavian artery from the distal and posterior border of the horizontal portion of the aortic arch at its junction with the descending aorta or, less commonly, from the proximal descending aorta [11].

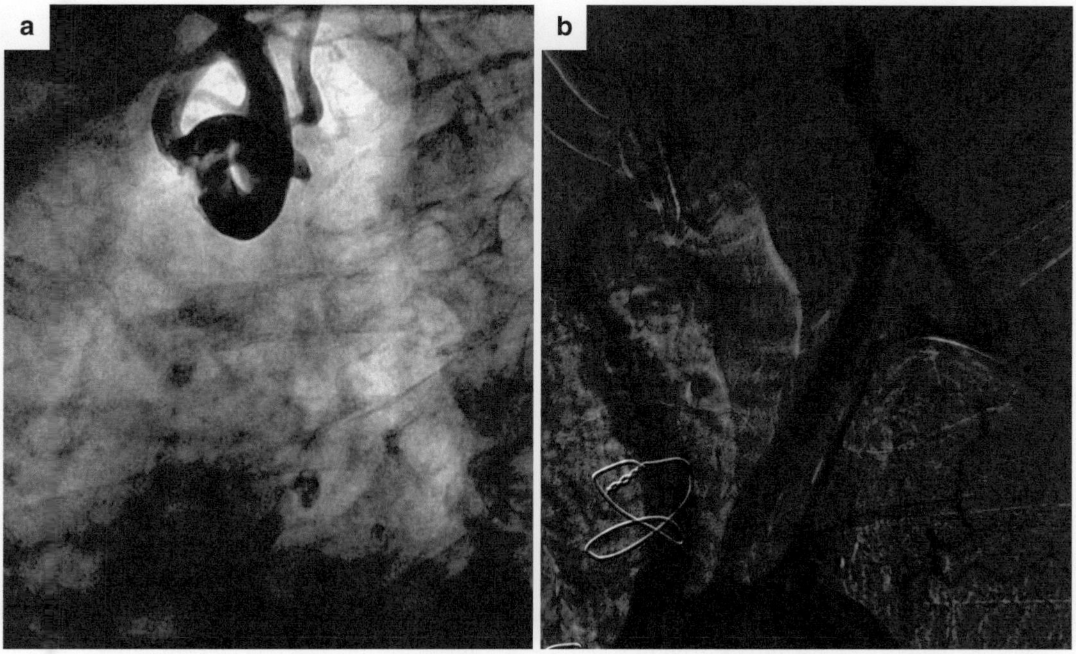

Fig. 3.8 Anatomic variants of the axillary-subclavian-anonymous arterial axis. (**a**) Retrograde angiography from the diagnostic catheter showing severe tortuosity of the subclavian-anonymous arterial axis. (**b**) Severe stenosis of the left subclavian artery. (Reproduced from Burzotta et al. [11])

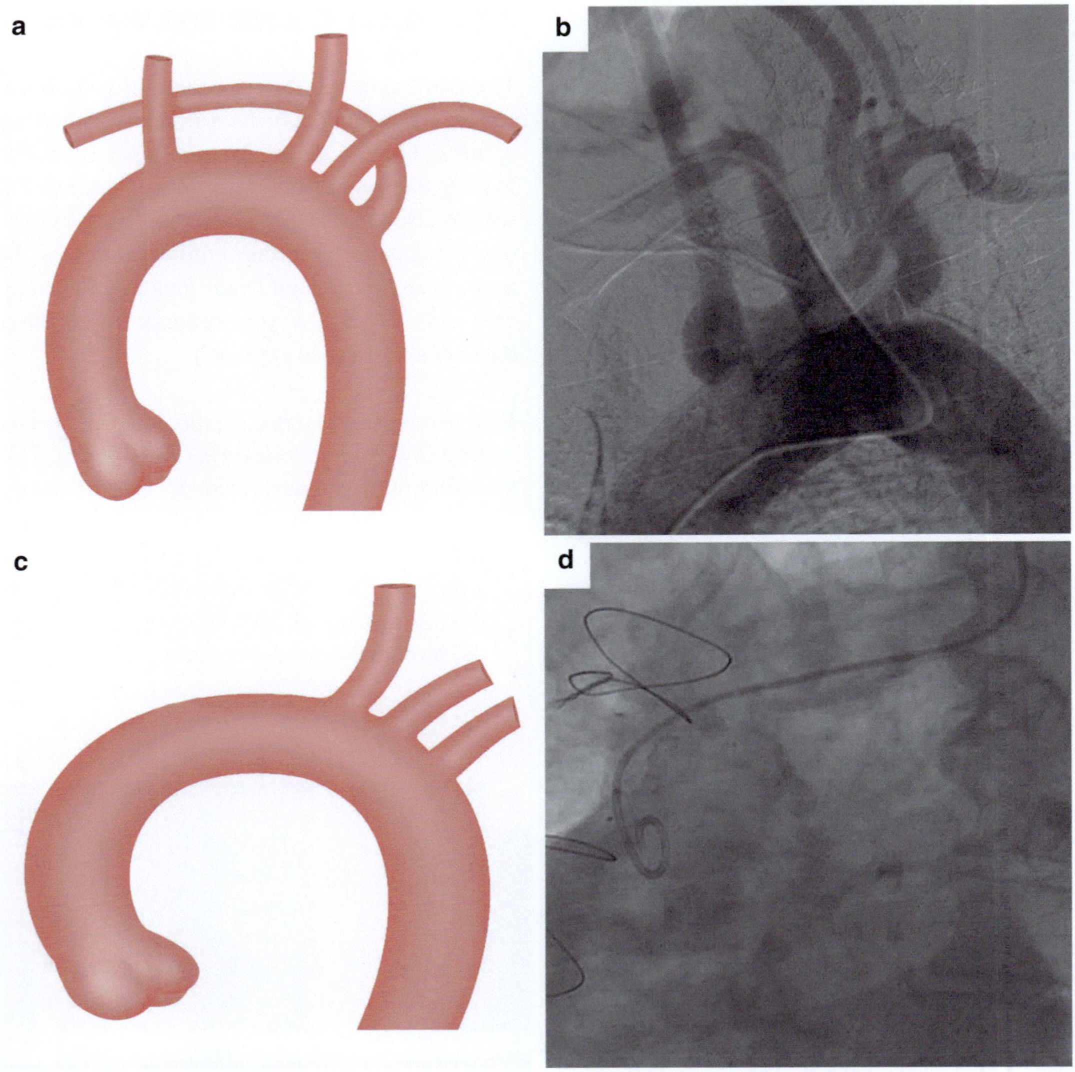

Fig. 3.9 Anatomic variants of the aortic arch. (**a**, **b**) Arteria lusoria. (**c**, **d**) Aortic arch elongation. (Adapted from Burzotta et al. [11])

Aortic arch elongation (Fig. 3.9c, d). This variant is characterized by distal displacement of the brachiocephalic trunk (anonymous trunk) and alteration of the anatomy of the ascending aorta and is generally associated with aging and arterial hypertension [11].

3.8 Tips and Tricks for Managing and Overcoming Upper Arm Variants

As a basic principle, any resistance encountered during wire or catheter advancement should prompt immediate retrograde arterial angiography, as rapid identification of upper extremity arterial anomalies is necessary for rapid, safe, and effective management of the transradial approach [17].

This can typically be performed over the existing cannula, sheath, or catheter, with an anteroposterior view usually providing sufficient information.

The anatomical variants encountered can be broadly classified into three groups: radial-brachial axis (group A), axillary-subclavian-anonymous axis (group B), and aortic arch (group C). Each group presents unique challenges that require tailored approaches [11].

For Group A variants [11, 16, 17], the strategy is largely dictated by vessel caliber. In vessels larger than 2.5 mm in diameter, a 0.035″ hydrophilic wire supported by a 5–6-Fr JR4 diagnostic catheter is typically used. This setup allows for what we call "catheter-oriented wire advancement," a technique that has proven particularly effective in navigating tortuous segments (Fig. 3.10). Conversely, vessels smaller than 2.5 mm or those with sharp angulations

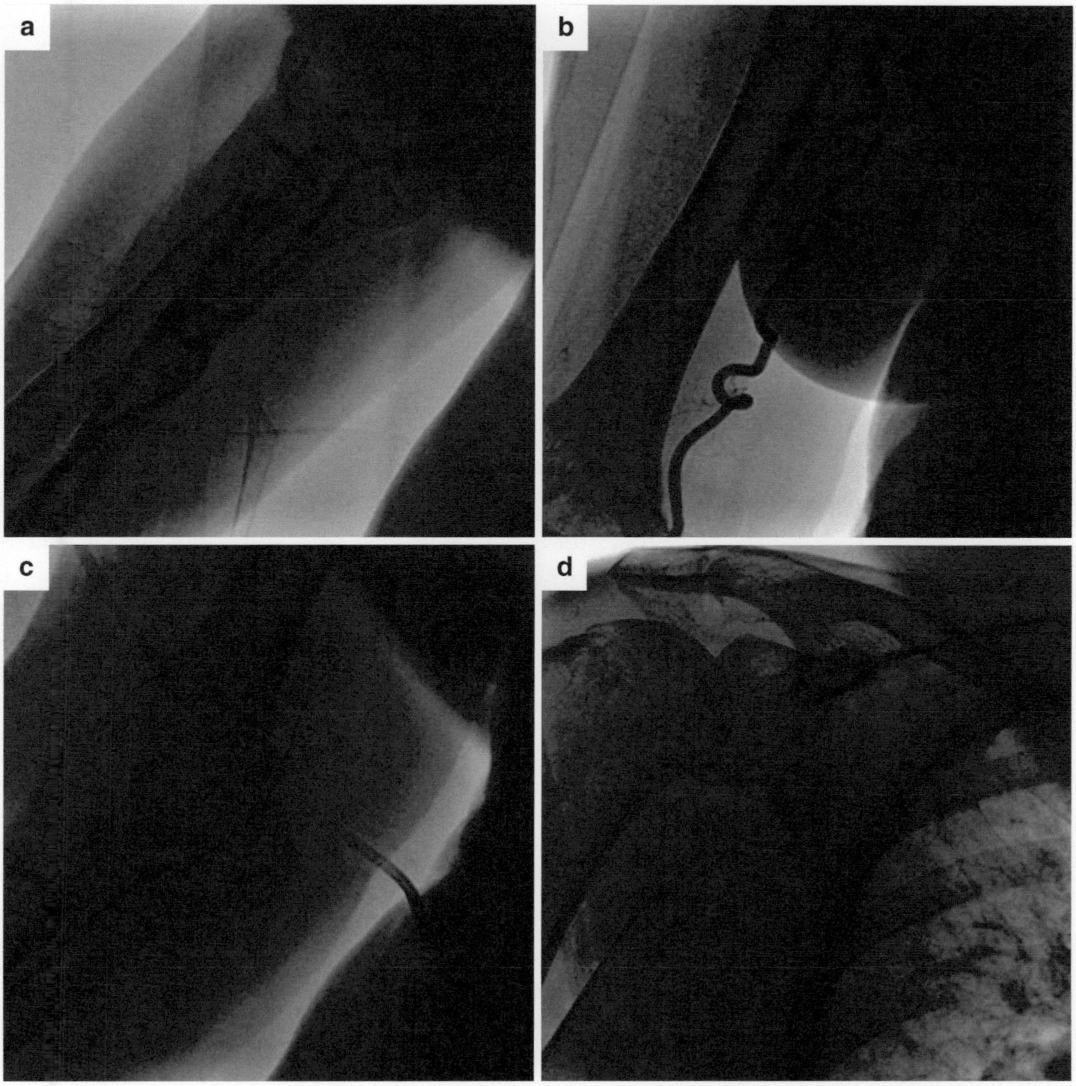

Fig. 3.10 Management of high origin of the radial artery. (**a**, **b**) Baseline angiography. (**c**, **d**) Implementation of the "catheter-oriented wire-advancement" technique with hydrophilic wire supported and directed using a 4-Fr JR4 diagnostic catheter. (Reproduced from Burzotta et al. [11])

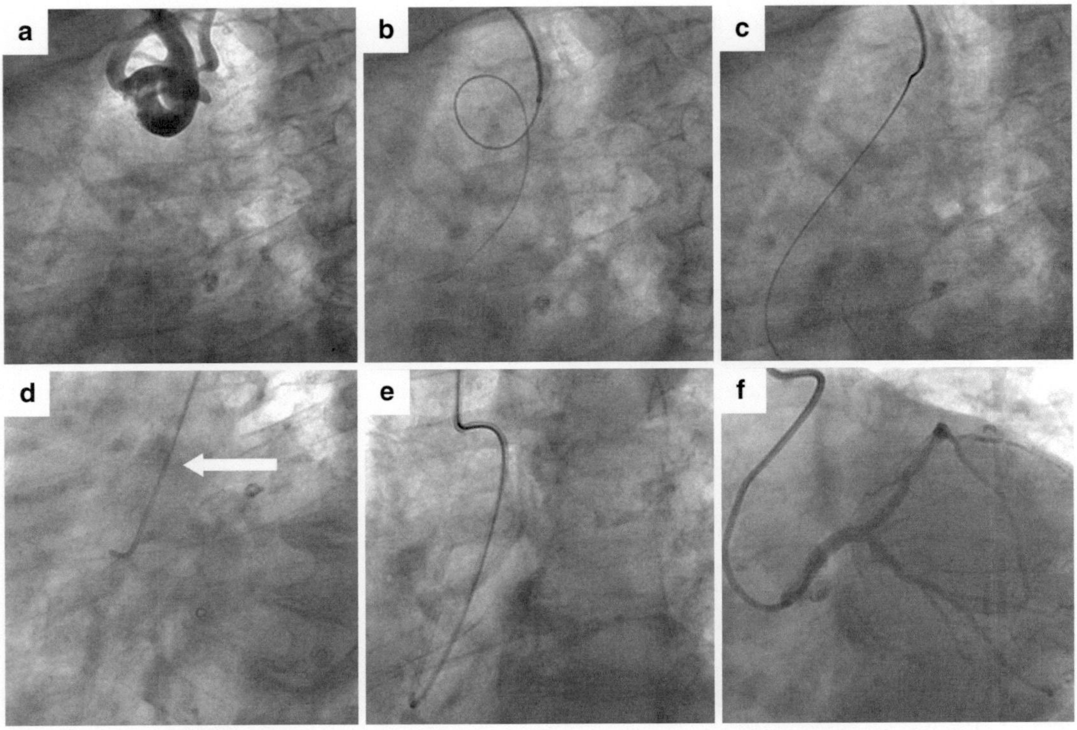

Fig. 3.11 Management of severe tortuosity of subclavian-anonymous arterial axis. (**a**) Baseline angiography. (**b**) Navigation of the tortuosity with a 0.035″ wire supported and directed using a 4-Fr JR4 diagnostic catheter. (**c**) Straightening of the vessel to reach the aortic valve. (**d**) Right coronary artery cannulation with the wire inside the catheter (arrow). (**e**, **f**) Cannulation of the left coronary artery with an XB guiding catheter to increase support and facilitate contrast injections. (Reproduced from Burzotta et al. [11])

require a more delicate approach. Here, a 0.014″ guidewire (such as the Choice PT Extra-support, Boston Scientific, USA) supported by a 4-Fr JR4 diagnostic catheter often proves invaluable. This latter setup is also our go-to strategy when faced with severe arterial spasm. Wire advancement should always be gentle and performed under careful fluoroscopic guidance. The propensity of hydrophilic guidewires to inadvertently enter small branches requires constant vigilance to avoid vessel dissection or perforation.

Perhaps the most challenging of the Group A variants is the presence of arterial loops, which should first be crossed with a 0.035″ or 0.014″ guidewire, followed by a carefully executed straightening maneuver using either the rigid shaft of the wire or the catheter itself.

For Group B variants [11, 16, 17], a 0.035″ wire supported by a JR4 diagnostic catheter is used to navigate to the ascending aorta (Fig. 3.11). This combination provides a balance of support and maneuverability that is often sufficient to overcome the tortuosity often encountered in this segment.

For Group C variants [11, 16, 17], a different diagnostic catheter is often required, either a JL 3.5 or a pigtail catheter, depending on the specific anatomic presentation. An important consideration, especially in cases of extreme tortuosity, is the potential limitation of catheter manipulation. In such scenarios, it is advisable to perform coronary cannulation with the 0.035″ wire still in the diagnostic catheter or exchange it for a guiding catheter to facilitate contrast injection [11, 16, 17].

3.9 Conclusion

A thorough understanding of the arterial anatomy of the upper extremity, from the axillary artery to the intricate network of the hand, is paramount to successful distal radial access procedures. Specific knowledge of the anatomy of the radial artery and its course through the anatomical snuffbox is critical. Recognition of common and clinically significant anatomical variations is also essential, as these can significantly impact the ease and success of radial procedures, often requiring specific strategies and tools to overcome potential obstacles.

By mastering this anatomical knowledge, interventional cardiologists can optimize their techniques, anticipate challenges, and develop effective management strategies. This comprehensive understanding allows procedures to be tailored to individual patients, ultimately increasing procedural success rates and improving outcomes.

As the field continues to evolve, this anatomical foundation will remain paramount to the advancement of techniques and technologies in radial access.

References

1. Gabella G. Blood vessels. In: Williams PL, editor. Gray's anatomy: the anatomical basis of medicine and surgery. 38th ed. New York: Churchill Livingstone; 1995.
2. Drake R, Vogl AW, Mitchell A, Tibbitts RM, Richardson PE. Gray's Atlas of anatomy. 2nd ed. Philadelphia: Churchill Livingstone; 2015.
3. Doyle JR, Botte MJ. Surgical anatomy of the hand and upper extremity. Philadelphia: Lippincott Williams & Wilkins; 2003.
4. Sgueglia GA, Di Giorgio A, Gaspardone A, Babunashvili A. Anatomic basis and physiological rationale of distal radial artery access for percutaneous coronary and endovascular procedures. JACC Cardiovasc Interv. 2018;11:2113–9.
5. Hoppenfeld S, de Boer P, Buckley R. Surgical exposures in orthopaedics: the anatomic approach. 5th ed. Philadelphia: Wolters Kluwer; 2016.
6. Sgueglia GA, Lee BK, Cho BR, Babunashvili A, Lee JB, Lee JW, et al. Distal radial access: consensus report of the first Korea-Europe transradial intervention meeting. JACC Cardiovasc Interv. 2021;14:892–906.
7. Corcos T. Distal radial access for coronary angiography and percutaneous coronary intervention: a state-of-the-art review. Catheter Cardiovasc Interv. 2019;93:639–44.
8. Jolly SS, Amlani S, Hamon M, Yusuf S, Mehta SR. Radial versus femoral access for coronary angiography or intervention and the impact on major bleeding and ischemic events: a systematic review and meta-analysis of randomized trials. Am Heart J. 2009;157:132–40.
9. Yokoyama N, Takeshita S, Ochiai M, Koyama Y, Hoshino S, Isshiki T, et al. Anatomic variations of the radial artery in patients undergoing transradial coronary intervention. Catheter Cardiovasc Interv. 2000;49:357–62.
10. Valsecchi O, Vassileva A, Musumeci G, Rossini R, Tespili M, Guagliumi G, et al. Failure of transradial approach during coronary interventions: anatomic considerations. Catheter Cardiovasc Interv. 2006;67:870–8.
11. Burzotta F, de Vita M, Trani C. How to manage difficult anatomic conditions affecting transradial approach coronary procedures? Indian Heart J. 2010;62:238–44.
12. Le May M, Wells G, So D, Chong AY, Dick A, Froeschl M, et al. Safety and efficacy of femoral access vs radial access in ST-segment elevation myocardial infarction: the SAFARI-STEMI Randomized Clinical Trial. JAMA Cardiol. 2020;5:126–34.
13. Gragnano F, Branca M, Frigoli E, Leonardi S, Vranckx P, Di Maio D, et al. Access-site crossover in patients with acute coronary syndrome undergoing invasive management. JACC Cardiovasc Interv. 2021;14:361–73.
14. Gragnano F, Jolly SS, Mehta S, Branca M, van Klaveren D, Frigoli E, et al. Prediction of radial crossover in acute coronary syndromes: derivation and validation of the MATRIX score. EuroIntervention. 2021;17:E971–80.
15. Burzotta F, Trani C, de Vita M, Crea F. A new operative classification of both anatomic vascular variants and physiopathologic conditions affecting transradial cardiovascular procedures. Int J Cardiol. 2010;145:120–2.
16. Burzotta F, Brancati MF, Trani C, Tommasino A, Porto I, Niccoli G, et al. Impact of radial-to-aorta vascular anatomical variants on risk of failure in transradial coronary procedures. Catheter Cardiovasc Interv. 2012;80:298–303.
17. Burzotta F, Brancati MF, Porto I, Saffioti S, Aurigemma C, Niccoli G, et al. Comparison of right and left upper limb arterial variants in patients undergoing bilateral transradial procedures. Circ Cardiovasc Interv. 2015;8:e002863.
18. Lo TS, Nolan J, Fountzopoulos E, Behan M, Butler R, Hetherington SL, et al. Radial artery anomaly and its influence on transradial coronary procedural outcome. Heart. 2009;95:410–5.

Physiological Rationale

4

Angela Di Giorgio and Avtandil Babunashvili

4.1 Current Appraisal of Transradial Access

Transradial access (TRA) is associated with a reduced risk of procedure-related complications, comprising bleeding, vascular complications, and major adverse cardiovascular events, including mortality, compared with transfemoral access [1–3]. Notably, this remarkable improvement in outcomes occurs across the full spectrum of patients with coronary artery disease and is of particular importance when percutaneous procedures are not expected to provide a prognostic benefit [4]. Other advantages of TRA, such as increased post-procedural comfort and faster ambulation, are primarily relevant to the patient, while cost-effectiveness is more relevant to the healthcare system [5, 6]. Because of its broad benefits, TRA is recommended as the standard approach for interventional procedures with a class IA recommendation in both European and American guidelines for coronary revascularization [7, 8].

A. Di Giorgio (✉)
Department of Cardiovascular Sciences, Fondazione Policlinico Universitario Agostino Gemelli IRCCS, Rome, Italy
e-mail: angela.digiorgio@policlinicogemelli.it

A. Babunashvili
Interventional Cardiology and Angiology Faculty of the first Moscow Medical Academy, Moscow, Russian Federation

In fact, few complications occur after TRA, with radial artery occlusion (RAO) being the most commonly reported, with an incidence of 7.7% in the first 24 h after the transradial procedure [9]. However, because of the dual blood supply to the hand and the extensive carpal and metacarpal anastomoses between the forearm arteries, RAO is not associated with ischemic complications and may be overlooked [10]. Although RAO is sometimes associated with paresthesia, pain, or hand dysfunction, small dedicated studies have failed to support any adverse effect of RAO on hand function [11–13]. The inability to use the same radial artery for future needs is arguably the most significant consequence of RAO [9, 14]. Indeed, an occluded radial artery precludes intra-arterial pressure monitoring, arteriovenous fistula creation for hemodialysis, and the availability of a valuable arterial conduit for surgical vascular reconstruction or coronary artery bypass grafting. More importantly, an occluded radial artery prevents its use for a new percutaneous procedure. In a retrospective study of patients undergoing repeat TRA over 1 year at a Canadian referral catheterization center, 42% of patients had undergone ≥3 repeat percutaneous coronary interventions, with an estimated failure rate of 5% for each attempt (Fig. 4.1a) [15]. These findings are in line with a previous Japanese study, which showed a gradual increase in failure rates from 3.5% to 15.9% in men and from 7.9% to 28.6% in women at the

G. A. Sgueglia (ed.), *Distal Radial Access*, https://doi.org/10.1007/978-3-031-89925-6_4

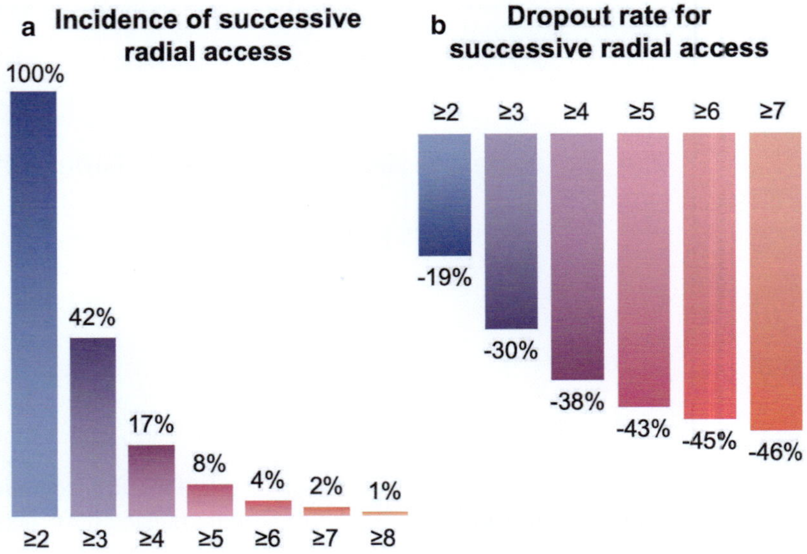

Fig. 4.1 (**a**) Incidence of successive transradial access among consecutive patients who underwent ≥2 repeat transradial coronary procedures between May 2010 and May 2011 at the Quebec Heart-Lung Institute, a high-volume tertiary-level radial center. (**b**) Dropout rate for successive radial access among 812 Japanese population between April 1997 and April 2000

second and fifth TRA procedures, respectively (Fig. 4.1b) [16].

As the likelihood of RAO increases with successive catheterizations, the latter issue is of growing concern given the increasing use of TRA for an increasing number of different indications, potentially leading to multiple percutaneous procedures in the same patient.

Against this background, physiological principles support the distal radial artery (DRA) as a superior access for percutaneous coronary interventions.

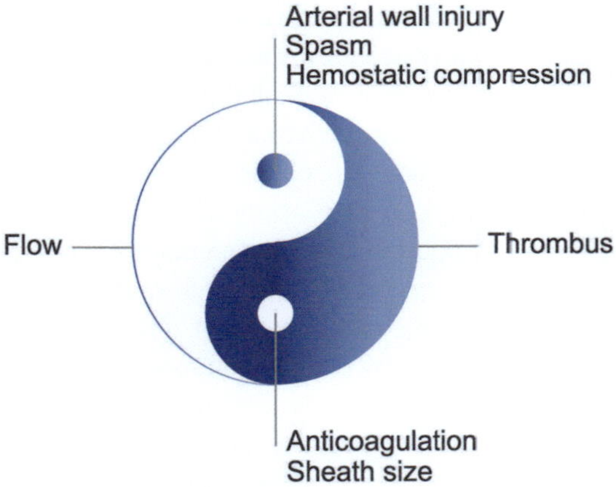

Fig. 4.2 Interacting factors contributing to radial artery occlusion. Persistence of blood flow is of paramount importance in avoiding thrombosis. However, radial artery flow may be compromised by access-related factors such as arterial wall injury, spasm, and hemostatic compression. On the other hand, thrombosis can be thwarted by anticoagulants and, to some extent, by smaller-diameter sheaths. The interplay between these elements is actually more complex because, for example, the use of anticoagulants limits shorter hemostatic compression

4.2 Radial Artery Occlusion

Several interacting mechanisms have been implicated in the occurrence of RAO, a complex process that ultimately leads to thrombosis, as demonstrated by histopathological analysis of the occlusion plug removed from occluded radial arteries [17, 18]. Not surprisingly, flow disruption plays a key role in this interplay of factors (Fig. 4.2). Indeed, in a prospective series of 275 patients undergoing transradial catheterization, absence of flow during hemostasis was the only independent predictor of RAO at follow-up [19]. In another analysis comparing shorter and longer hemostatic compressions in 400 consecutive patients undergoing transradial coronary intervention, occlusive hemostatic was again the only independent predictor of RAO at follow-up [20]. Notably, interventions aimed at maintaining blood flow in the radial artery during hemostasis, including patent hemostasis [21], nitroglycerin administration through the sheath prior to its removal [22], and ipsilateral ulnar artery compression during radial artery hemostasis [23], have all been shown to reduce the rate of RAO.

4.3 Physiological Rationale of Distal Radial Access

Because the DRA is obtained distal to the anastomotic branches that originate in the wrist and proximal hand, it allows for the preservation of flow in the forearm radial artery during hemostatic compression, thereby preventing blood stasis and significantly reducing the risk of proximally extending thrombosis and widespread forearm RAO (Fig. 4.3a, b) [14]. In contrast, if thrombosis occurs at the conventional TRA site, it may extend back to the origin of the radial artery because of the absence of important branching between the forearm arteries that would otherwise allow flow preservation and consequently prevent thrombus growth (Fig. 4.3a, c) [24].

In addition, branches from the radial artery before reaching the anatomic snuffbox create important anastomoses in the wrist and hand that allow optimal distal blood flow even in patients with poor radio-ulnar interaction (Fig. 4.4).

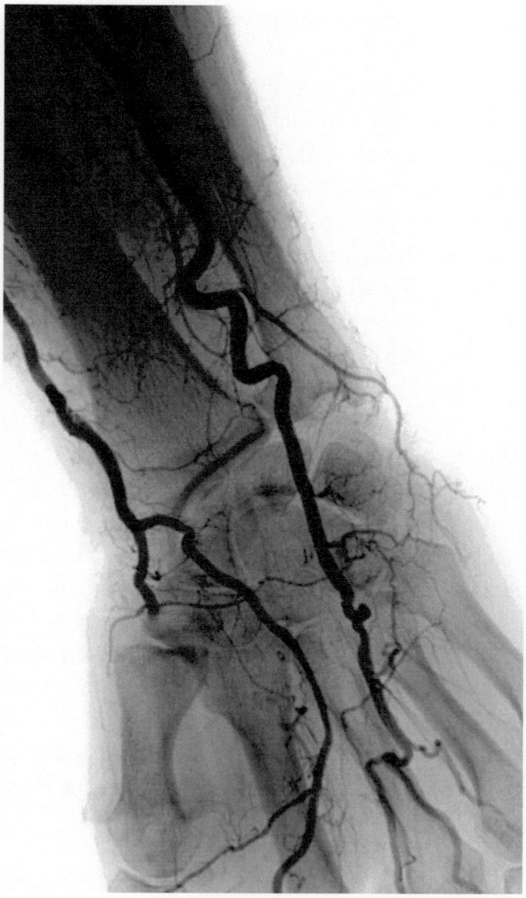

Fig. 4.4 Digital subtraction angiography of the hand during simulated distal radial artery occlusion within the first intermetacarpal space showing persistent blood flow in the metacarpal branches in a case of poor radio-ulnar connection. (Reproduced from Sgueglia et al. [14])

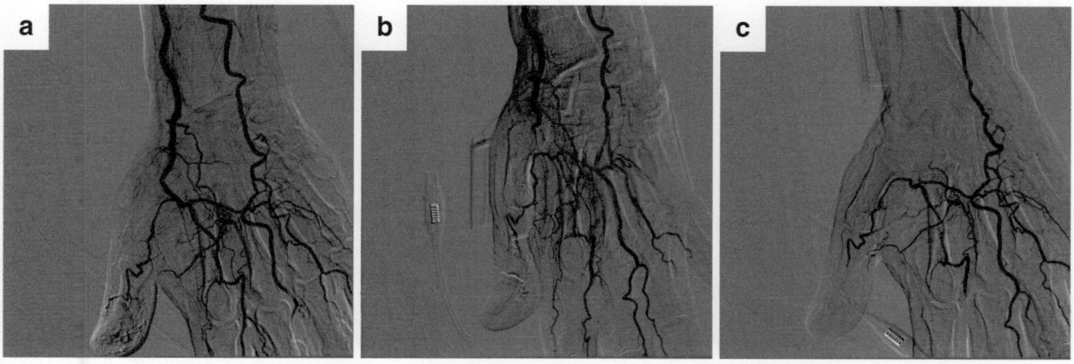

Fig. 4.3 Digital subtraction angiography of the hand. (**a**) At baseline. (**b**) During simulated occlusion of the radial artery within the anatomical snuffbox with a maximally inflated hemostasis device, forearm radial artery flow is maintained. (**c**) During simulated occlusion of the radial artery at the wrist level with a maximally inflated hemostasis device, forearm radial artery flow is interrupted

4.4 Experimental Physiology

The concepts outlined above are supported by the results of the Distal Radial Access Doppler Imaging Study [25], which was a double-crossover, repeated-measures study designed to assess the upstream and downstream physiological effects of simulated RAO as the worst-case scenario of radial artery catheterization at both the wrist and anatomical snuffbox levels bilaterally (Fig. 4.5).

A total of 100 unselected subjects older than 45 years of age in apparently good health with no history of disease were included in the study. Baseline blood flow was measured by pulsed-wave Doppler sampling in the radial artery at an intermediate distance from the elbow and wrist and in the radiodorsal digital artery of the thumb, a direct branch of the radial artery, above the first interphalangeal joint. Assessments were repeated after simulated RAO was effectively achieved with a typical radial hemostasis device maximally inflated for 5 min at the same positions used to achieve hemostasis after transradial catheterization at wrist level or anatomical snuffbox level. After a 15-min interval, measurements were repeated a third time at the same sites after switching to the alternative simulated RAO configuration. The two simulated RAOs for each upper extremity were implemented randomly with a 15-min interval to allow for a return to baseline flow conditions.

The Distal Radial Access Doppler Imaging Study demonstrated virtually unchanged flow in the forearm radial artery during simulated RAO (primary efficacy endpoint) at the anatomic snuffbox level, in contrast to the severe reduction in flow observed during simulated RAO at the wrist level (Fig. 4.6). Indeed, in the forearm radial artery, peak systolic velocity (PSV) showed a significant reduction during simulated RAO at wrist level (24 ± 13% of baseline, $p = 0.001$).

However, PSV remained essentially unchanged during simulated RAO at the anatomical snuffbox level (93 ± 2% of baseline, $p = 0.65$). Overall, the change in PSV in the forearm radial artery was −7.5% during simulated RAO at the anatomical snuffbox level and

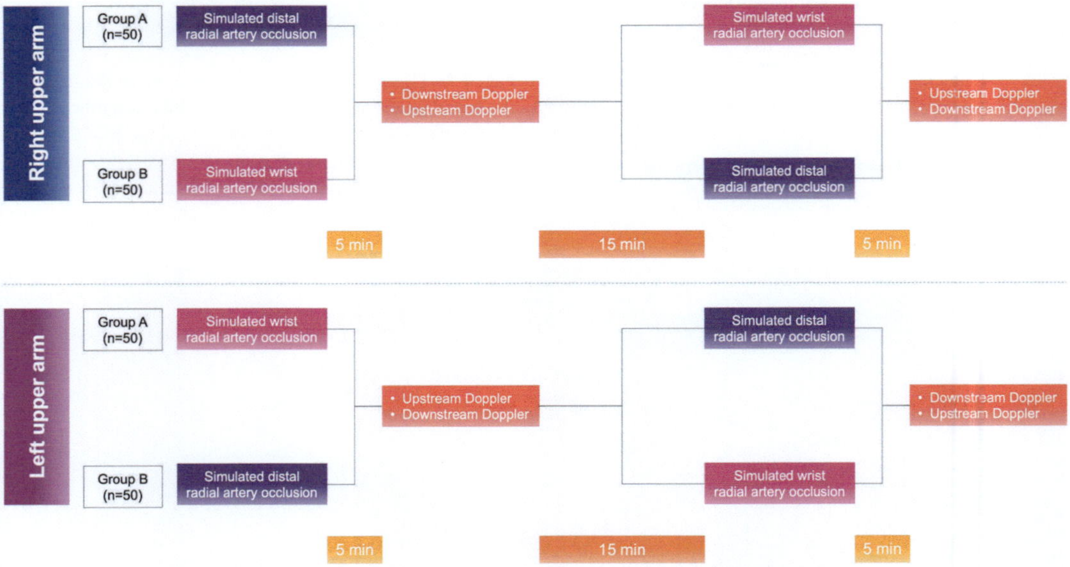

Fig. 4.5 Flowchart of the Distal Radial Access Doppler Imaging Study. Subjects were divided into two groups according to the order in which assessments were performed in both the right and left upper extremities. Blood flow was measured by pulsed-wave Doppler sampling in the forearm radial artery (upstream Doppler sampling) and in the radiodorsal digital artery of the thumb (downstream Doppler sampling) at baseline and after 5 min of simulated radial artery occlusion at the wrist and anatomical snuffbox levels. A 15-min interval was allowed between simulated radial artery occlusions to allow a return to baseline flow conditions

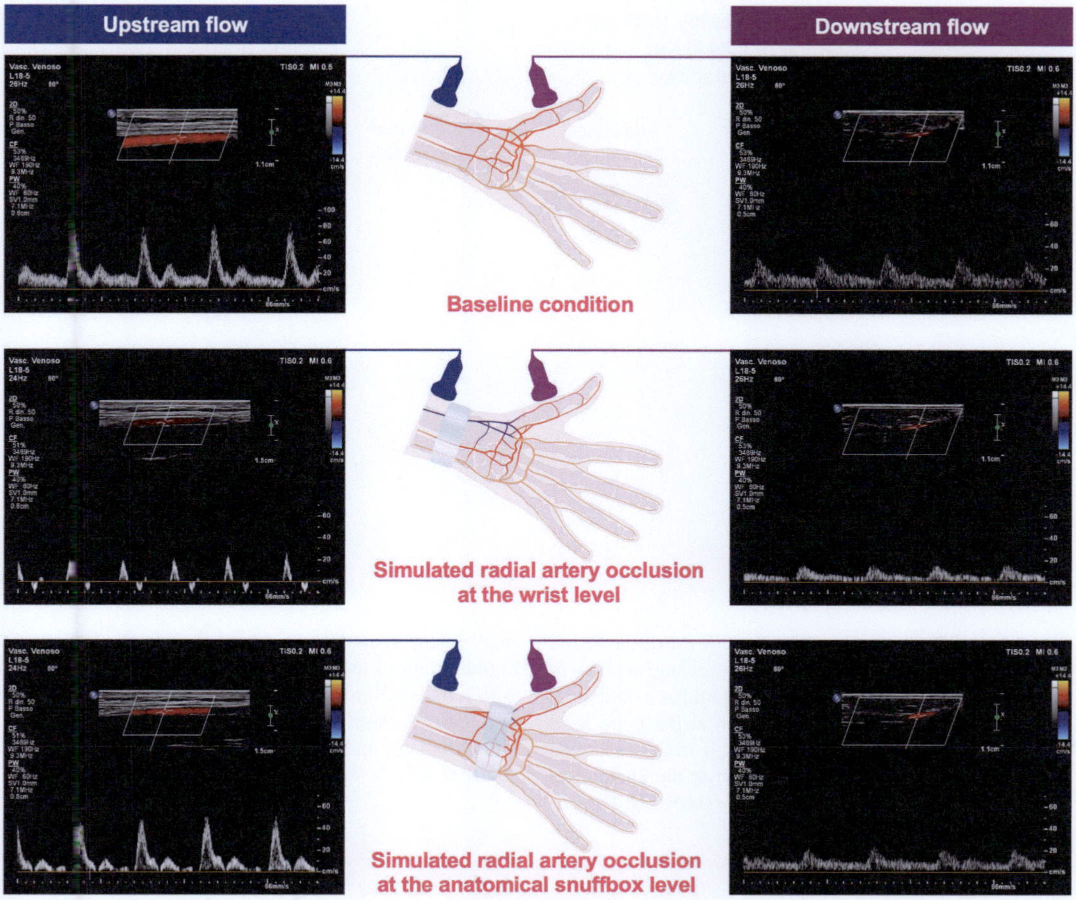

Fig. 4.6 Upstream and downstream flow changes during forearm and distal radial artery occlusion in the Distal Radial Access Doppler Imaging Study. Top row shows the baseline condition. Simulated occlusion with a radial hemostasis device at wrist level (middle row) induces marked flow reduction in both the forearm radial artery and the radiodorsal digital artery of the thumb. In contrast, simulated occlusion with a radial hemostasis device at the anatomical snuffbox level (bottom row) is associated with almost unchanged flow in both upstream and downstream sampling sites. (Modified from Sgueglia et al. [25])

−74.4% during simulated RAO at the wrist level (Fig. 4.7a).

This worst-case scenario suggests that distal TRA can be considered the minimum effective intervention to maintain forearm radial artery patency.

Similarly, the study results demonstrated virtually unchanged flow in the radiodorsal digital artery of the thumb during simulated RAO (primary safety endpoint) at the anatomic snuffbox level, in contrast to the marked reduction in flow observed during simulated RAO at the wrist level (Fig. 4.6). Indeed, PSV in the radiodorsal digital artery of the thumb showed a significant reduction during simulated RAO at the wrist level (68 ± 8% of baseline, $p = 0.001$) and remained essentially unchanged during simulated RAO at the anatomical snuffbox level (95 ± 2% of baseline, $p = 0.71$).

Overall, the PSV change in the radiodorsal digital artery of the thumb was −4.8% during simulated RAO at the anatomical snuffbox level

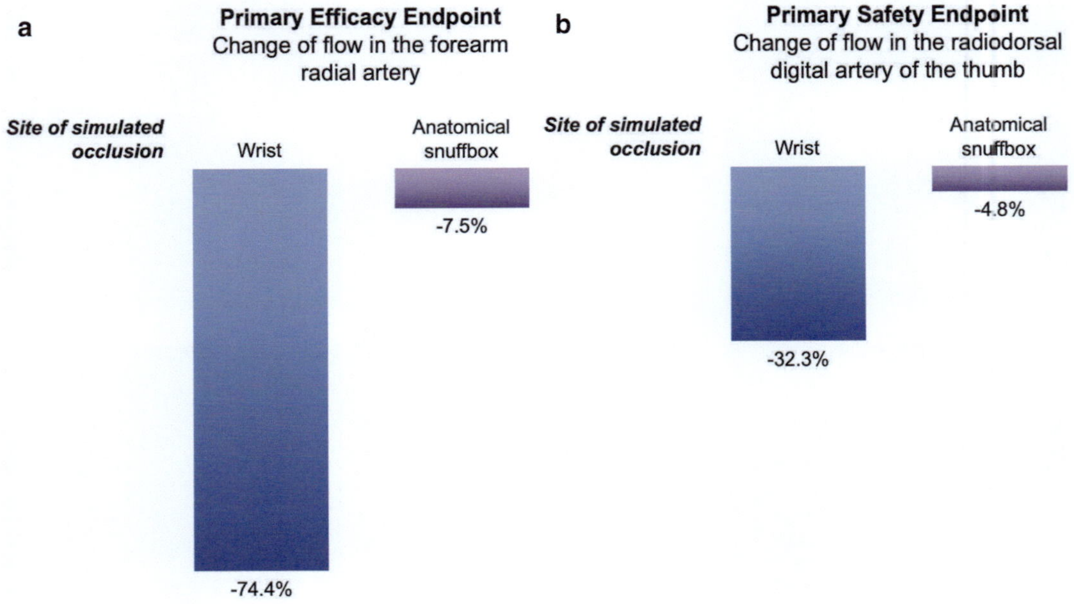

Fig. 4.7 (**a**) The primary efficacy endpoint of the Distal Radial Access Doppler Imaging Study, change in flow in the forearm radial artery, shows a significant reduction with simulated radial artery occlusion at the wrist level (−74.4% vs. baseline, $p = 0.001$) but a trivial reduction with simulated radial artery occlusion at the anatomical snuffbox level (−7.5% vs. baseline, $p = 0.65$), (**b**) The primary safety endpoint, change in flow in the radiodorsal digital artery of the thumb, shows a significant reduction with simulated radial artery occlusion at the wrist level (−32.3% vs. baseline, $p = 0.001$) but a trivial reduction with simulated radial artery occlusion at the anatomical snuffbox level (−4.8% vs. baseline, $p = 0.71$)

and −32.3% during simulated RAO at the wrist level (Fig. 4.7b). These findings also alleviate potential concerns about anastomotic carpal network compromise due to hand compression during actual hemostasis.

Prespecified subgroup comparisons for the primary efficacy endpoint show a consistent change in flow in response to simulated RAO across all subgroups (Fig. 4.8). Interaction testing suggested incidental heterogeneity in the effect of simulated RAO at the anatomical snuffbox level on the primary safety endpoint according to the patient's family history of cardiovascular disease (Fig. 4.9).

Notably, these experimental pathophysiological findings were ultimately translated into a notable reduction in RAO, as demonstrated in randomized controlled trials [26–28] and confirmed by meta-analytic research (see also Chap. 16) [29].

4.5 Other Physiological Characteristics of Distal Radial Access

The distal radial artery has been reported to be between 5.5% and 21.4% smaller than the forearm radial artery by angiography and vascular ultrasound, respectively [30, 31]. Overall, these observations are consistent with the asymmetric geometric reduction of branching arteries according to Murray's law [32]. Consequently, blood flow in the distal radial artery has a lower kinetic energy thus offering the prospect of systematically shorter and nonocclusive hemostasis in order to pursue the lowest probability of RAO [9].

Also, DRA may avert nerve damage related to excessive hemostatic compression [33]. Furthermore, in the anatomical snuffbox, the radial artery runs quite superficially yet in a groove that is lined by the scaphoid and trapezium

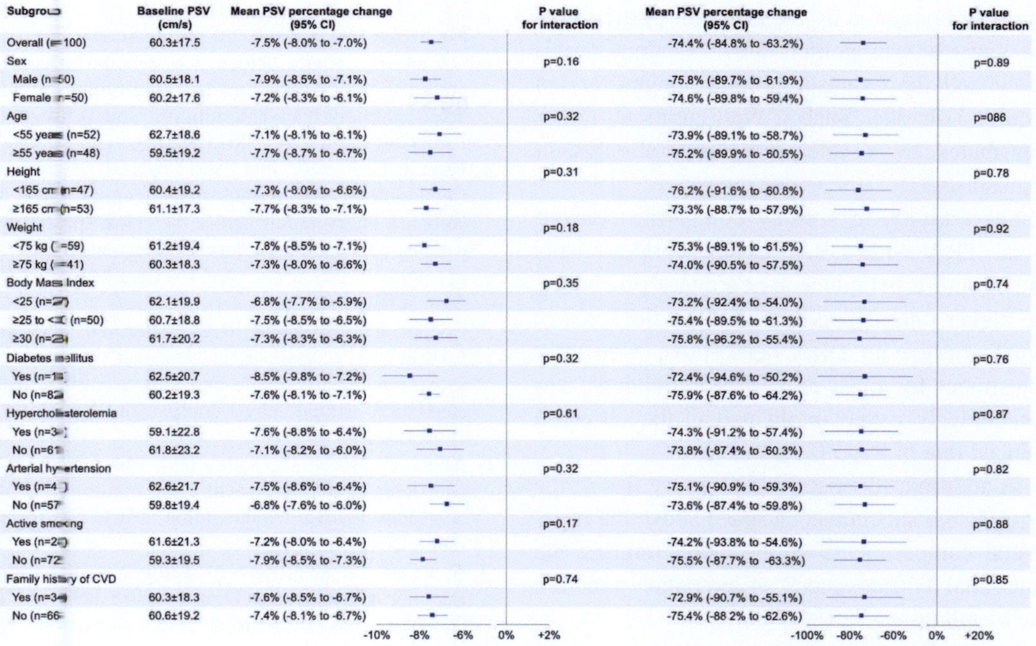

Fig. 4.8 Subgroup analysis for the primary efficacy endpoint of the Distal Radial Access Doppler Imaging Study. Percentage change in various subgroups of peak systolic velocity (PSV) in the forearm radial artery in response to simulated radial artery occlusion at the anatomical snuffbox level (left side of the graph) and at the wrist level (right side of the graph) showing a consistent change in PSV

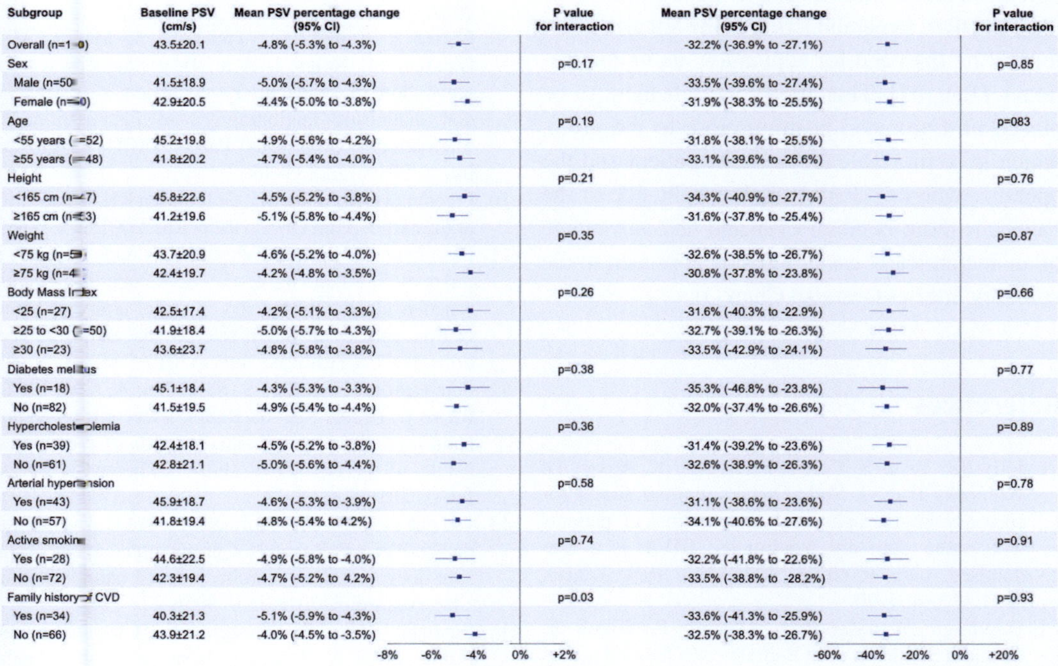

Fig. 4.9 Subgroup analysis for the primary safety endpoint of the Distal Radial Access Doppler Imaging Study. Percentage change in various subgroups of peak systolic velocity (PSV) in the radiodorsal digital artery of the thumb in response to simulated radial artery occlusion at the anatomical snuffbox level (left side of the graph) and at the wrist level (right side of the graph) showing a consistent change in PSV and statistical interaction with the risk factor family history of cardiovascular disease

bones and bounded by the abductor pollicis longus and extensor pollicis brevis tendons proximally and the extensor pollicis longus tendon distally [14, 34]. Such a configuration further contributes to a safe and essentially patent hemostasis.

Interestingly, in a study comparing conventional TRA with DRA in real-world patients undergoing a percutaneous coronary procedure, the higher rate of preserved flow in the forearm radial artery with DRA hemostasis, even after adjustment for most relevant confounders, was speculatively called implicated in the observed reduced rate of RAO [35].

In addition, the distal radial artery lies in the loose dorsal subcutaneous space above the myofascial compartments of the hand, limiting the functional consequences of potential puncture site bleeding.

Finally, DRA allows the patient's right hand to be held between the resting and functional positions, with the wrist slightly deviated medially, the digits moderately flexed, and the thumb partially abducted which favorably allows the least amount of tension on the muscles and tendons of the hands [36]. In DRA, hyperabduction of the left arm is not limited by the need for supination, as in conventional TRA [37]. This allows the left hand to be placed in a pronated position close to the groin, which is comfortable for both the patient and the operator, who can work from the right side of the patient without bending over and take advantage of an anatomically easier left side approach to the coronary arteries (see also Chap. 3).

References

1. Jolly SS, Yusuf S, Cairns J, Niemelä K, Xavier D, Widimsky P, et al. Radial versus femoral access for coronary angiography and intervention in patients with acute coronary syndromes (RIVAL): a randomised, parallel group, multicentre trial. Lancet. 2011;377:1409–20.
2. Valgimigli M, Gagnor A, Calabro P, Frigoli E, Leonardi S, Zaro T, et al. Radial versus femoral access in patients with acute coronary syndromes undergoing invasive management: a randomised multicentre trial. Lancet. 2015;385:2465–76.
3. Ratib K, Mamas MA, Anderson SG, Bhatia G, Routledge H, De Belder M, et al. Access site practice and procedural outcomes in relation to clinical presentation in 439,947 patients undergoing percutaneous coronary intervention in the United Kingdom. J Am Coll Cardiol Intv. 2015;8:20–9.
4. Ferrante G, Rao SV, Juni P, Da Costa BR, Reimers B, Condorelli G, et al. Radial versus femoral access for coronary interventions across the entire spectrum of patients with coronary artery disease: a meta-analysis of randomized trials. JACC Cardiovasc Interv. 2016;9:1419–34.
5. Cooper CJ, El-Shiekh RA, Cohen DJ, Blaesing L, Burket MW, Basu A, et al. Effect of transradial access on quality of life and cost of cardiac catheterization: a randomized comparison. Am Heart J. 1999;138:430–6.
6. Amin AP, House JA, Safley DM, Chhatriwalla AK, Giersiefen H, Bremer A, et al. Costs of transradial percutaneous coronary intervention. JACC Cardiovasc Interv. 2013;68:827–34.
7. Neumann FJ, Sousa-Uva M, Ahlsson A, Alfonso F, Banning AP, Benedetto U, et al. 2018 ESC/EACTS Guidelines on myocardial revascularization. Eur Heart J. 2019;40:87–165.
8. Lawton JS, Tamis-Holland JE, Bangalore S, Bates ER, Beckie TM, Bischoff TM, et al. 2021 ACC/AHA/SCAI guideline for coronary artery revascularization: a report of the American College of Cardiology/American Heart Association Joint Committee on Clinical Practice Guidelines. J Am Coll Cardiol. 2022;79:e21–9.
9. Bernat I, Aminian A, Pancholy S, Mamas MA, Gaudino M, Nolan J, et al. Best practices for the prevention of radial artery occlusion after transradial diagnostic angiography and intervention: an International Consensus Paper. JACC Cardiovasc Interv. 2019;12:2235–46.
10. Freedman DM, Botte MJ, Gelberman RH. Vascularity of the carpus. Clin Orthop Relat Res. 2001;383:47–59.
11. Uhlemann M, Mobius-Winkler S, Mende M, Eitel I, Fuernau G, Sandri M, et al. The Leipzig prospective vascular ultrasound registry in radial artery catheterization: impact of sheath size on vascular complications. JACC Cardiovasc Interv. 2012;5:36–43.
12. Sciahbasi A, Rigattieri S, Sarandrea A, Cera M, Di Russo C, Fedele S, et al. Radial artery occlusion and hand strength after percutaneous coronary procedures: results of the HANGAR study. Catheter Cardiovasc Interv. 2016;87:868–74.
13. van der Heijden DJ, van Leeuwen MAH, Ritt M, van de Ven PM, van Royen N. Chronic radial artery occlusion does not cause exercise induced hand ischemia. J Interv Cardiol. 2018;31:949–56.
14. Sgueglia GA, Di Giorgio A, Gaspardone A, Babunashvili A. Anatomic basis and physiological rationale of distal radial artery access for percutaneous coronary and endovascular procedures. JACC Cardiovasc Interv. 2018;11:2113–9.

15. Abdelaal E, Molin P, Plourde G, Machaalany J, Bataille Y, Brousseau-Provencher C, et al. Successive transradial access for coronary procedures: experience of Quebec Heart-Lung Institute. Am Heart J. 2013;165:325–31.
16. Sakai H, Ikeda S, Harada T, Yonashiro S, Ozumi K, Ohe H, et al. Limitations of successive transradial approach in the same arm: the Japanese experience. Catheter Cardiovasc Interv. 2001;54:204–8.
17. Mamas MA, Fraser DG, Ratib K, Fath-Ordoubadi F, El-Omar M, Nolan J, et al. Minimising radial injury: prevention is better than cure. EuroIntervention. 2014;10:824–32.
18. Pancholy SB. Transradial access in an occluded radial artery: new technique. J Invasive Cardiol. 2007;19:541–4.
19. Sanmartin M, Gomez M, Rumoroso JR, Sadaba M, Martinez M, Baz JA, et al. Interruption of blood flow during compression and radial artery occlusion after transradial catheterization. Catheter Cardiovasc Interv. 2007;70:185–9.
20. Pancholy SB, Patel TM. Effect of duration of hemostatic compression on radial artery occlusion after transradial access. Catheter Cardiovasc Interv. 2012;79:78–81.
21. Pancholy S, Coppola J, Patel T, Roke-Thomas M. Prevention of radial artery occlusion-patent hemostasis evaluation trial (PROPHET study): a randomized comparison of traditional versus patency documented hemostasis after transradial catheterization. Catheter Cardiovasc Interv. 2008;72:335–40.
22. Dharma S, Kedev S, Patel T, Kiemeneij F, Gilchrist IC. A novel approach to reduce radial artery occlusion after transradial catheterization: postprocedural/prehemostasis intra-arterial nitroglycerin. Catheter Cardiovasc Interv. 2015;85:818–25.
23. Pancholy SB, Bernat I, Bertrand OF, Patel TM. Prevention of radial artery occlusion after transradial catheterization: the PROPHET-II randomized trial. JACC Cardiovasc Interv. 2016;9:1992–9.
24. Richter Y, Edelman ER. Cardiology is flow. Circulation. 2006;113:2679–82.
25. Sgueglia GA, Santoliquido A, Gaspardone A, Di Giorgio A. First results of the Distal Radial Access Doppler study. JACC Cardiovasc Imaging. 2021;14:1281–3.
26. Eid-Lidt G, Rivera Rodriguez A, Jimenez Castellanos J, Farjat Pasos JI, Estrada Lopez KE, Gaspar J. Distal radial artery approach to prevent radial artery occlusion trial. JACC Cardiovasc Interv. 2021;14:378–85.
27. Tsigkas G, Papageorgiou A, Moulias A, Kalogeropoulos AP, Papageorgopoulou C, Apostolos A, et al. Distal or traditional transradial access site for coronary procedures: a single-center, randomized study. JACC Cardiovasc Interv. 2022;15:22–32.
28. Aminian A, Sgueglia GA, Wiemer M, Kefer J, Gasparini GL, Ruzsa Z, et al. Distal versus conventional radial access for coronary angiography and intervention: the DISCO RADIAL trial. JACC Cardiovasc Interv. 2022;15:1191–201.
29. Ferrante G, Condello F, Rao SV, Maurina M, Jolly S, Stefanini GG, et al. Distal vs conventional radial access for coronary angiography and/or intervention: a meta-analysis of randomized trials. JACC Cardiovasc Interv. 2022;15:2297–311.
30. Kim Y, Ahn Y, Kim MC, Sim DS, Hong YJ, Kim JH, et al. Gender differences in the distal radial artery diameter for the snuffbox approach. Cardiol J. 2018;25:639–41.
31. Naito T, Sawaoka T, Sasaki K, Iida K, Sakuraba S, Yokohama K, et al. Evaluation of the diameter of the distal radial artery at the anatomical snuff box using ultrasound in Japanese patients. Cardiovasc Interv Ther. 2019;34:312–6.
32. Murray CD. The physiological principle of minimum work. The vascular system and the cost of blood volume. Proc Natl Acad Sci USA. 1926;12:207–14.
33. Ayyaz Ul Haq M, Rashid M, Gilchrist IC, Bertrand O, Kwok CS, Wong CW, et al. Incidence and clinical course of limb dysfunction post cardiac catheterization. Circ J. 2018;82:2736–44.
34. Norimatsu K, Kusumoto T, Yoshimoto K, Tsukamoto M, Kuwano T, Nishikawa H, et al. Importance of measurement of the diameter of the distal radial artery in a distal radial approach from the anatomical snuffbox before coronary catheterization. Heart Vessel. 2019;34:1615–20.
35. Pacchioni A, Mugnolo A, Sanz Sanchez J, Sgueglia GA, Pesarini G, Bellamoli M, et al. Radial artery occlusion after conventional and distal radial access: impact of preserved flow and time-to-hemostasis in a propensity-score matching analysis of 1163 patients. Catheter Cardiovasc Interv. 2022;99:827–35.
36. DeMott L, Flinn SR. Functional anatomy. In: Wietlisbach CM, editor. Cooper's fundamentals of hand therapy: Clinical reasoning and treatment guidelines for common diagnoses of the upper extremity. St. Louis: Elsevier; 2020. p. 21–45.
37. Rao SV, Cohen MG, Kandzari DE, Bertrand OF, Gilchrist IC. The transradial approach to percutaneous coronary intervention: historical perspective, current concepts, and future directions. J Am Coll Cardiol. 2010;55:2187–95.

Hand Circulation Variants for Distal Radial Access

5

Gregory A. Sgueglia and Jun-Won Lee

5.1 Introduction

Historically, a detailed appreciation of the anatomy of the carpus and hand circulation has been largely limited to reconstructive and orthopedic hand surgery. However, with the strong recommendation of guidelines supporting transradial access (TRA) as the standard vascular access for percutaneous coronary procedures to reduce bleeding complications and mortality [1, 2] and the increased benefit of distal radial access (DRA) to further reduce adverse events [3, 4], interventional specialists are called upon to gain a better understanding of the vascular anatomy of the hand.

The purpose of this chapter is to provide a clear and accessible overview of the anatomical variations in hand circulation and to provide the practitioner with the knowledge to effectively apply these findings in the clinical setting.

G. A. Sgueglia (✉)
Division of Cardiology, Sant'Eugenio Hospital, Rome, Italy

J.-W. Lee
Division of Cardiology, Department of Internal Medicine, Yonsei University Wonju College of Medicine, Wonju, Republic of Korea

5.2 Vascular Anatomy of the Wrist and Hand

The vascular supply to the distal radius, ulna, carpus, and hand is primarily provided by four major arteries: the radial, ulnar, anterior interosseous, and posterior interosseous arteries. These vessels form an intricate network of anastomoses, comprising three dorsal and three palmar arches within the carpus (Fig. 5.1). From proximal to distal, these are identified as the radiocarpal, intercarpal, and basal metacarpal arches. Numerous anastomotic connections exist not only between these arches but also between the radial and ulnar arteries and the interosseous arterial network [5–8].

With the exception of the pisiform, each carpal bone typically receives its blood supply from both dorsal and palmar vascular entry points. The majority of carpal bones are supplied by multiple nutrient arteries. In addition to these primary nutrient vessels, numerous smaller penetrating vessels contribute to the rich vascular network of the carpus.

5.2.1 Radial Artery

In the distal forearm, the radial artery gives rise to the first/second intercompartmental supraretinacular artery approximately 5 cm proximal to the radiocarpal joint (Fig. 5.1). This branch passes under the brachioradialis muscle and lies

G. A. Sgueglia (ed.), *Distal Radial Access*, https://doi.org/10.1007/978-3-031-89925-6_5

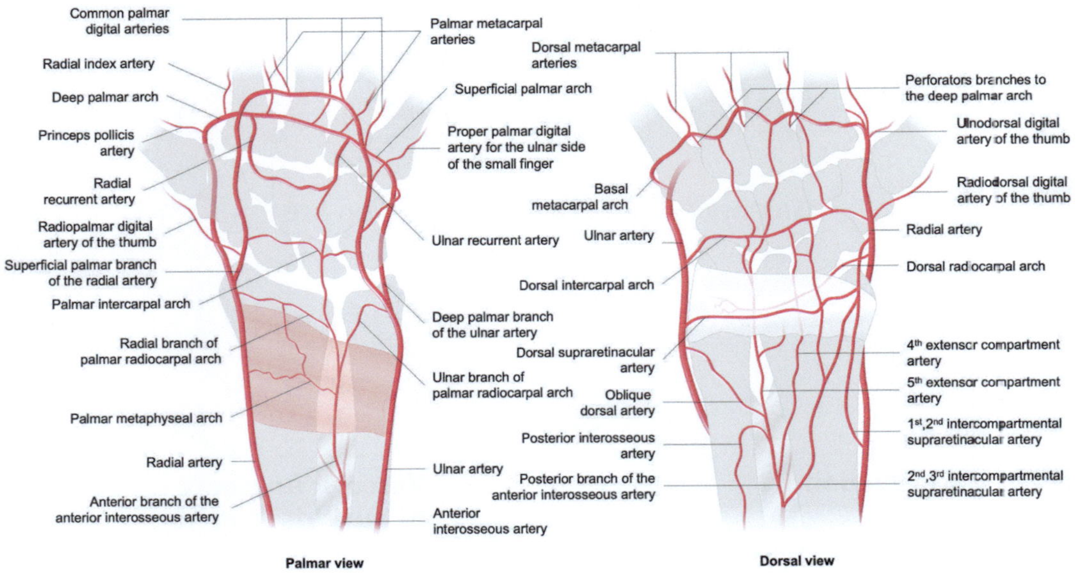

Fig. 5.1 Schematic representation of the arterial supply of the distal radius, distal ulna, and carpus in dorsal and palmar views. (Adapted from Sheetz et al. [5])

over the first/second intercompartmental septum on the dorsal surface of the extensor retinaculum. Distally, it passes under the tendons of the first extensor compartment and rejoins the radial artery (52%), radiocarpal arch (52%), both (13%), or intercarpal arch (19%). The first/second intercompartmental supraretinacular artery also gives off the dorsal supraretinacular arch, which variably connects to the first/second intercompartmental supraretinacular artery, the fourth extensor compartment artery, the fifth extensor compartment artery, or the ulnar artery (Fig. 5.1). In 56% of cases, the first/second intercompartmental supraretinacular artery has a branch that originates proximal to the extensor retinaculum and continues to the floor of the second extensor compartment [5].

The radial artery serves as the most consistent vascular supplier to the carpus giving rise to seven major branches: three dorsal, three palmar, and one terminal (Fig. 5.2) [8].

The most proximal branch, the superficial palmar branch, originates from the radial artery 5–8 mm proximal to the tip of the radial styloid. Due to its trajectory, it may occasionally appear as a small continuation of the radial artery, while the main trunk continues distally, curving dorsally and laterally. The superficial palmar branch courses between the flexor carpi radialis and brachioradialis muscles before contributing to the superficial palmar arch. Just distal to the superficial palmar branch, small palmar scaphoid branches arise, supplying the distal palmar aspect of the scaphoid in the tubercle region [7].

The second branch originates approximately 5 mm distal to the superficial palmar branch and courses toward the ulna. It contributes to the palmar radiocarpal arch, which is the most proximal of three transverse vascular arches supplying the carpus.

A third branch originates at the level of the radiocarpal joint. It courses dorsally and ulnarly, penetrating the radiocarpal ligament deep to the extensor tendons, and supplies the dorsal radiocarpal arch.

The fourth branch arises on the palmar aspect at the level of the scapho-trapezial joint. It supplies the tubercle of the scaphoid and the trapezium before anastomosing with the superficial palmar artery.

This fifth branch, supplying the dorsal ridge of the scaphoid, arises directly from the radial artery in 75% of cases and from the radiocarpal or intercarpal arch in the remaining 25% [6]. It provides

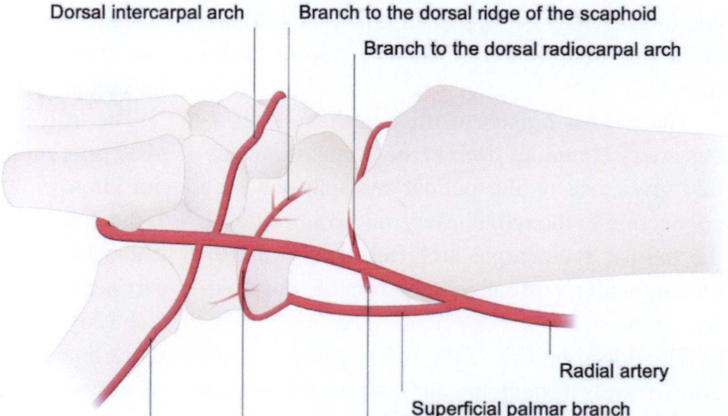

Fig. 5.2 Schematic representation of the arterial supply of the radial aspect of the wrist. (Adapted from Gelberman et al. [6])

blood supply to 70–80% of the scaphoid's proximal and central portions.

The sixth branch emerges 5 mm distal to the scaphoid branch and contributes to the dorsal intercarpal arch.

The final branch originates at the level of the trapezium. It courses distally, supplying the trapezium and the lateral aspect of the thumb metacarpal as the radiodorsal digital artery of the thumb.

In the first intermetacarpal space, the radial artery abruptly dives through the two heads of the first dorsal interosseous muscle to reach the deep palmar hand. At the base of the thumb and index metacarpal, just before forming the deep palmar arch, it gives rise to the first dorsal metacarpal artery. This artery bifurcates, with one branch supplying the medial aspect of the thumb and the other extending along the index metacarpal to supply the dorsoradial aspect of the index finger.

5.2.2 Ulnar Artery

The ulnar artery contributes significantly to the vascular supply of the medial carpus through a network of fine vessels spanning both the dorsal and palmar aspects. Three primary branches emerge proximal to the distal end of the ulna: one contributing to the dorsal radiocarpal arch, one contributing to the palmar radiocarpal arch, and one contributing to the proximal pole of the pisiform and the palmar aspect of the triquetrum (Fig. 5.1).

Additional branches include several smaller vessels supplying the lateral aspect of the pisiform, a branch joining the palmar intercarpal arch; a more distal branch supplying the distal pisiform and medial hamate, which continues dorsally to contribute to the dorsal intercarpal arch; and a branch arising proximal to the origin of the superficial palmar arch, continuing dorsally to supply the basal metacarpal arch.

The deep palmar branch of the ulnar artery arises from the ulnar aspect of the distal ulnar artery near the carpal canal. It travels briefly on the anterior surface of the flexor retinaculum, passing anterior to the ulnar nerve to reach the hypothenar muscles. It then travels between the abductor digiti minimi and flexor digiti minimi brevis, passes through the opponens digiti minimi, and curves laterally into the palm alongside the deep branch of the radial nerve, anastomosing with the radial artery to complete the deep palmar arch (Fig. 5.1).

5.2.3 Anterior Interosseous Artery

The anterior interosseous artery travels along the anterior surface of the interosseous membrane and then divides into a palmar and dorsal branch at the proximal border of the pronator quadratus muscle (Fig. 5.1).

The palmar branch of the anterior interosseous artery continues deep to the pronator quadratus, gives rise to the palmar metaphyseal arch connecting to the radial artery, and contributes to the palmar radiocarpal arch, ultimately anastomosing with recurrent vessels from the deep palmar arch.

The dorsal branch of the anterior interosseous artery travels through the interosseous membrane to supply the dorsal distal radius and contributes to the dorsal carpal network. It continues distally on the interosseous membrane to the carpus, where it supplies the dorsal radiocarpal arch in 89% of cases [6]. It extends small branches radially to supply the lunate and anastomose with radial artery branches, supplying the dorsal ridge of the scaphoid. The dorsal branch of the anterior interosseous artery bifurcates at the intercarpal level, with each branch contributing to the intercarpal arch in 83% of cases [6].

The anterior interosseous artery also gives rise to three arteries that contribute to the vascularity of the distal radius and ulna and anastomose with the carpal vessels [5].

The second/third intercompartmental supraretinacular artery originates proximally from the anterior interosseous artery (48%), the dorsal branch of the anterior interosseous artery (48%), or the palmar branch of the anterior interosseous artery (4%) and runs superficial to the extensor retinaculum directly on the Lister tubercle to anastomose with the dorsal intercarpal arch (94%), the dorsal radiocarpal arch (52%), or the fourth extensor compartment artery (38%). It also has superficial and deep transverse anastomoses with the first/second intercompartmental supraretinacular artery and may branch to the second compartment floor.

The fourth extensor compartment artery originates from the dorsal branch of the anterior interosseous artery (55%) or from the fifth extensor compartment artery (45%) and runs in the fourth compartment just lateral to the posterior interosseous nerve. It anastomoses to the dorsal intercarpal arch (94%), the dorsal radiocarpal arch (59%), the second/third intercompartmental supraretinacular artery (38%), or the fifth extensor compartment artery (34%).

The fifth extensor compartment artery is supplied proximally by the dorsal branch of the anterior interosseous artery and anastomoses distally to the dorsal intercarpal arch in all cases. Distally, it also anastomoses with the fourth extensor compartment artery (34%), the dorsal radiocarpal arch (23%), the second/third intercompartmental supraretinacular artery (9%), or the oblique dorsal artery of the distal ulna (9%).

5.2.4 Posterior Interosseous Artery

In the distal forearm, the posterior interosseous artery forms an anastomotic arch with the dorsal branch of the anterior interosseous artery, contributing to the vascular supply of the distal ulna and dorsal capsule of the distal radioulnar joint.

5.2.5 Dorsal Carpal Network

The dorsal aspect of the carpal region is supplied by three dorsal transverse arches: the radiocarpal, intercarpal, and basal metacarpal transverse arches (Fig. 5.1). The presence of each arch varies from individual to individual [6, 7]. These arches typically have a diameter of approximately 1 mm, with branches measuring less than 1 mm [8]. The central connection between the dorsal arches is provided by the dorsal branch of the interosseous artery, while the radial and ulnar arteries provide radial and ulnar connections.

The *dorsal radiocarpal arch*, the most proximal, is found in 80% of cases and is located at the level of the radiocarpal joint, deep to the extensor tendons. It is primarily formed by the radiocarpal branch of the radial artery, but also by branches of the ulnar artery and the dorsal branch of the anterior interosseous artery [6].

The *dorsal intercarpal arch*, the largest of the dorsal transverse arches and always present, spans the carpal region between the proximal and distal carpal rows and primarily supplies the distal carpal row. This arch is supplied by the radial, ulnar, and anterior interosseous arteries in 53% of cases, the radial and ulnar arteries alone in 20%, and the ulnar and anterior interosseous arteries in 7% [6].

The *basal metacarpal arch* is the most distal of the dorsal transverse arches and is located at the base of the metacarpals, just distal to the carpometacarpal joints. It is the smallest of the dorsal arches and has the greatest variability. It is complete in 27% of cases, absent in 27%, and present only in its radial aspect in 46% [6].

5.2.5.1 Dorsal Metacarpal Arteries

The dorsal metacarpal arteries arise from the dorsal carpal network, except for the first dorsal metacarpal artery, which arises directly from the radial artery. These arteries course distally in the second, third, and fourth intermetacarpal spaces and eventually divide into dorsal digital branches. These branches supply the adjacent dorsal aspects of the index, middle, ring, and small fingers.

The dorsal metacarpal arteries form anastomoses with the deep palmar arch via perforating branches at the metacarpal bases and more distally with the common palmar digital arteries near their bifurcations.

5.2.6 Palmar Carpal Network

The palmar carpal vasculature mirrors its dorsal counterpart featuring three transverse arches: the palmar radiocarpal, palmar intercarpal, and deep palmar arches (Fig. 5.1). These arches are connected longitudinally by the radial, ulnar, anterior interosseous, and deep palmar recurrent arteries [6].

The *palmar radiocarpal arch*, the most proximal of the palmar arches, is consistently present and typically forms a double arch. In 87% of cases, it receives contributions from the radial, anterior interosseous, and ulnar arteries. In the remaining 13%, it is formed solely by the radial and ulnar arteries [6]. This arch is essentially composed of a radial branch and an ulnar branch, which is generally smaller in diameter.

The *palmar intercarpal arch*, situated between the proximal and distal carpal rows, exhibits the most variability. Present in 53% of cases, it receives contributions from the ulnar, radial, and anterior interosseous arteries in 75% of instances and from the ulnar and radial arteries alone in the remaining 25%. This small arch plays a minor role in the nutrient supply to the carpus [6].

The *deep palmar arch* is consistently present and located at the level of the metacarpal bases, approximately 5–10 mm distal to the palmar carpometacarpal joints.

The deep and superficial palmar arches form critical anastomotic networks in the hand vascular system. These arches are of paramount importance in the arterial supply of the hand, as they provide the primary blood supply to all fingers, providing redundancy that is critical to maintaining adequate perfusion in different hand positions and in the event of vascular compromise.

5.2.7 Deep Palmar Arch

The deep palmar arch is primarily formed by the terminal portion of the radial artery (Fig. 5.1). After passing under the abductor pollicis longus and extensor pollicis brevis tendons on the dorsal aspect of the hand, the radial artery penetrates the first (or occasionally the second) interosseous space. It then joins the deep palmar branch of the ulnar artery at the base of the small finger's metacarpal bone [9]. The deep palmar arch lies deep in the palm, superficial to the interosseous muscles, but deep to the extrinsic flexor tendons, lumbricals, and the oblique head of the adductor pollicis. In 83% of cases, it is located proximal to the superficial palmar arch, while in 15% of cases, it is positioned distally [9].

The deep palmar arch provides the primary arterial supply to the distal carpal row through two branches, the radial and ulnar recurrent arteries, which are always present [6]. The radial recurrent artery, slightly smaller, arises just lateral to the index metacarpal base and courses proximally, bifurcating on the palmar aspect of the trapezium. It anastomoses with the ulnar recurrent artery in 45% of cases. The ulnar recurrent artery originates between the bases of the third and fourth metacarpals, coursing proximally in the ligamentous groove between the capitate and hamate, supplying both bones. It anastomoses with the terminal portion of the anterior interosseous artery in 80% of cases [6].

The deep palmar arch also gives off several perforating branches that pass dorsally through the second, third, and fourth interosseous spaces to connect with the dorsal metacarpal arteries.

Three palmar metacarpal arteries arise from the distal edge of the deep palmar arch and extend toward the second, third, and fourth intermetacarpal spaces, anastomosing with the common palmar digital arteries from the superficial palmar arch. These arteries lie superficial to the interosseous muscles but deep to the extrinsic flexor tendons and lumbrical muscles. The princeps pollicis artery arises from the most radial part of the deep palmar arch, continues distally toward the thumb, and divides into the ulnopalmar and radiopalmar digital arteries of the thumb. The radial index artery arises in close proximity to the princeps pollicis artery and continues distally along the radial aspect of the index finger. It may also arise from a common trunk shared with the proximal portion of the princeps pollicis artery. This trunk is then referred to as the first palmar metacarpal artery [10].

5.2.8 Superficial Palmar Arch

The superficial palmar arch originates primarily from the terminal portion of the ulnar artery and is often completed by the superficial branch of the radial artery (Fig. 5.1). Less frequently, it may receive contributions from the princeps pollicis artery, the radialis indicis artery, or, rarely, the median artery. In fact, the formation of the superficial palmar arterial arch has several variations that have been variably classified.

As the ulnar artery enters the palm along the ulnar nerve through Guyon's canal, typically on the lateral aspect of the pisiform and superficial to the flexor retinaculum, it is usually located radially and deep to the ulnar nerve. It continues medially to the hook of the hamate and then curves laterally, forming a distal convexity as it traverses the palm beneath the palmaris brevis muscle and the palmar fascia. The superficial palmar arch typically crosses the palm at the level of the metacarpal diaphysis, slightly proximal to the distal transverse palmar crease [11].

As it extends radially across the palm, the superficial palmar arch remains superficial to the flexor digitorum superficialis and profundus tendons, the lumbrical muscles, and the branches of the median and ulnar nerves. It gives rise to three common palmar digital arteries and the proper digital artery to the ulnar aspect of the small finger. Each common palmar digital artery then divides into two proper palmar digital arteries. A terminal branch of the superficial palmar arch contributes to the vascular supply of the thumb [12, 13].

5.3 Anatomical Variations of Palmar Arches

Standard anatomy textbooks often lack information on important variations in the arterial supply of the hand, despite their significant clinical implications. Our understanding of these variations derives primarily from cadaveric studies, which have been fundamental in revealing the structural diversity of the hand vasculature.

Through meticulous dissection, postmortem studies allow direct visualization of arterial patterns, precise measurements, and identification of even rare variations. In addition, these studies allow the examination of relationships between vascular structures and surrounding tissues. However, the dissection of small vessels, particularly those deeply embedded in the palm muscle, is technically challenging. Furthermore, such studies cannot capture the dynamic aspects of the circulation, may be influenced by postmortem changes, and may not fully represent the diversity observed in living populations.

The vascular patterns of the palmar arches and their interconnecting branches are quite complex and exhibit considerable variability among individuals. Numerous attempts have been made to classify these variations, one of the earliest and most influential being that of Coleman and Anson [14]. Over the years, a variety of techniques and different classification systems have been used in anatomical studies, each with its own advantages and limitations [15]. The lack of a universal classification system has led to variations in the reported frequency of different types of palmar arches [16]. Consequently, the most reliable and consistent information across studies revolves around the prevalence of complete and incomplete arches, a distinction first introduced by Jaschtschinski in 1897 [17].

To accurately represent the prevalence of anatomical variations of the deep and superficial palmar arches, a comprehensive meta-analysis of 36 studies was performed, including a total of 4841 palmar arches [18]. These studies were published between 1961 and 2017, and the majority were cadaveric studies. A complete palmar arch was defined by the presence of a clear anastomosis between the contributing arteries (Fig. 5.3a). In addition, an arch was considered complete if the ulnar artery supplied the thumb. Conversely, an arch was classified as incomplete if there was no anastomosis between the arteries or if the ulnar artery did not adequately supply the ulnar side of the thumb (Fig. 5.3b).

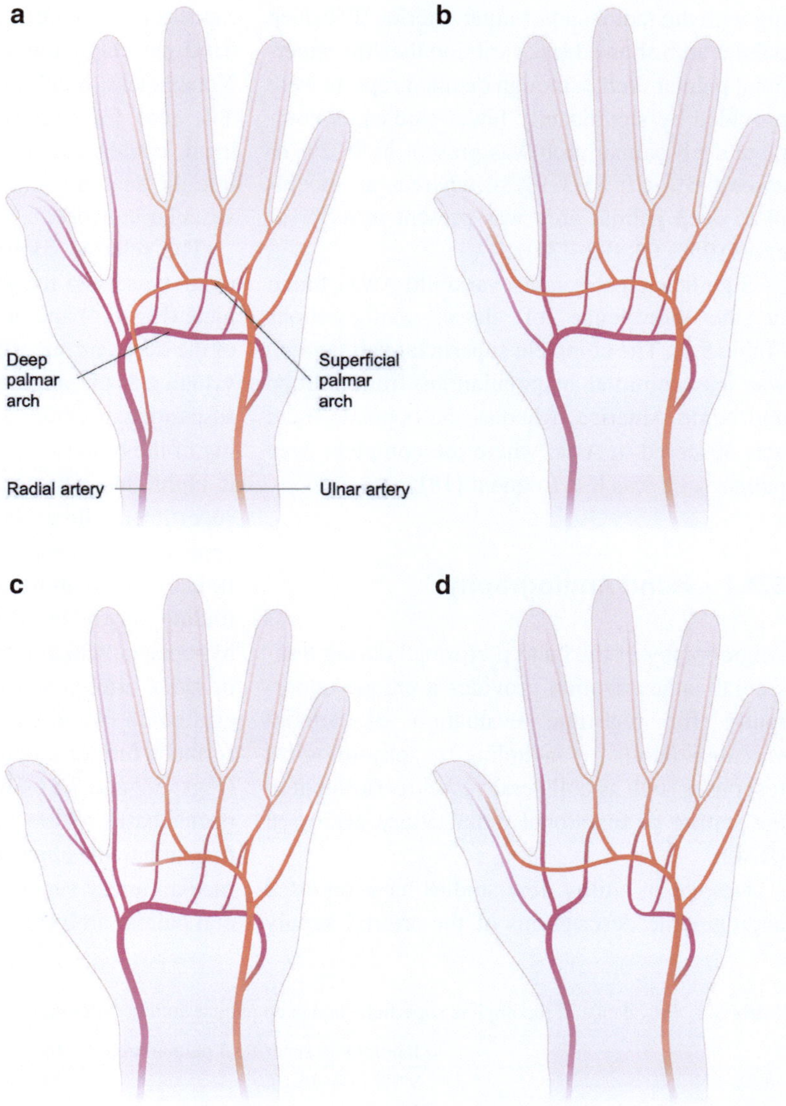

Fig. 5.3 Schematic representations of the major variations in palmar arch anatomy. (**a**) Complete deep and superficial arches, both with radial-ulnar anastomosis. (**b**) Both palmar arches are complete, with the ulnar artery supplying the thumb without radial anastomosis. (**c**) Complete deep palmar arch and incomplete superficial palmar arch without radial-ulnar anastomosis. (**d**) Incomplete deep palmar arch without radial-ulnar anastomosis and a complete superficial palmar arch in which the ulnar artery supplies the thumb without radial anastomosis

The results showed that a complete superficial palmar arch was present in 81.3% of cases (95% CI: 74.7–87.3), while an incomplete superficial palmar arch had a prevalence of 18.7% (95% CI: 12.8–25.5). The most common configuration of a complete superficial palmar arch was an anastomosis between the radial and ulnar arteries, observed in 72.0% of cases (95% CI: 58.0–80.5). Another common configuration was the ulnar artery reaching the ulnar side of the thumb, which accounted for 20.7% of cases (95% CI: 11.2–30.8). In a small proportion of individuals, the median artery persists after birth and contributes to the superficial palmar arch by anastomosing with the radial and/or ulnar arteries. The deep palmar arch showed less variation than the superficial palmar arch, although detailed reports were provided by significantly fewer studies. A complete deep palmar arch was present in 95.2% of cases (95% CI: 85.3–99.3), whereas an incomplete deep palmar arch was present in 4.8% of cases (95% CI: 0.2–13.0).

Significant geographic variability was found in the prevalence of these configurations (Table 5.1). The complete superficial palmar arch was less common in populations from Europe and North America, whereas the opposite trend was observed in Asia, where the complete deep palmar arch was less frequent [18].

5.3.1 Hand Angiography

Angiography of the hand performed during transradial catheterization provides a unique opportunity for real-time evaluation of arterial vascularization, including physiological responses such as collateral vessel recruitment in the setting of functional radial artery occlusion (RAO).

Despite its utility, few studies have reported angiographic descriptions of the arterial supply to the hand [15, 19]. In fact, the procedure has inherent limitations due to its two-dimensional nature. This modality provides a planar projection of the complex three-dimensional vascular architecture, which can lead to interpretive challenges. The superimposition of multiple vessel planes on a single image can conceal subtle anatomical variations and potentially confound the accurate assessment of vessel trajectories. Also, it may be affected by significant vasoreactivity induced by the contrast agent, and arterial spasm may result from the stress induced by both the arterial puncture and the catheterization procedure itself. In addition, the need to temporarily reposition the C-arm for optimal imaging of the hand presents an additional technical challenge. Nonetheless, hand angiography remains a valuable tool for improving our understanding of hand circulation, providing invaluable insight into the anatomy and physiology of this intricate vascular network.

The relative contributions of the radial and ulnar vessels to the formation of both the complete (Fig. 5.4) and incomplete (Fig. 5.5) variants of the deep and superficial palmar arches are well visualized on angiography. However, in vivo assessment provides a more nuanced understanding of the blood supply to the hand. In particular, it highlights how the presence of a noticeable superficial palmar branch of the radial artery appears important for maintaining flow in the forearm radial artery with DRA (Fig. 5.6). Such a finding may be critical in the case of ulnar artery hypoplasia, which may not be known at the time of radial artery catheterization unless a thorough evaluation of the forearm arteries has been performed, further emphasizing the value of DRA (Figs. 5.7 and 5.8). The same is true for the unexpected cases of direct connection of the deep palmar arch to the ulnar artery (Fig. 5.9) or persistent median artery supporting an incomplete superficial palmar arch (Fig. 5.10).

Table 5.1 Prevalence of incomplete superficial and deep palmar arch in different geographical regions

	Incomplete superficial palmar arch	Incomplete deep palmar arch
Asia	9.4% (4.4–16.1%)	18.3% (0.0–45.7%)
North America	18.5% (13.0–24.9%)	1.2% (0.0–3.9%)
Europe	34.5% (17.5–53.7%)	4.7% (0.0–27.7%)

Values are pooled estimates (95% confidence interval)

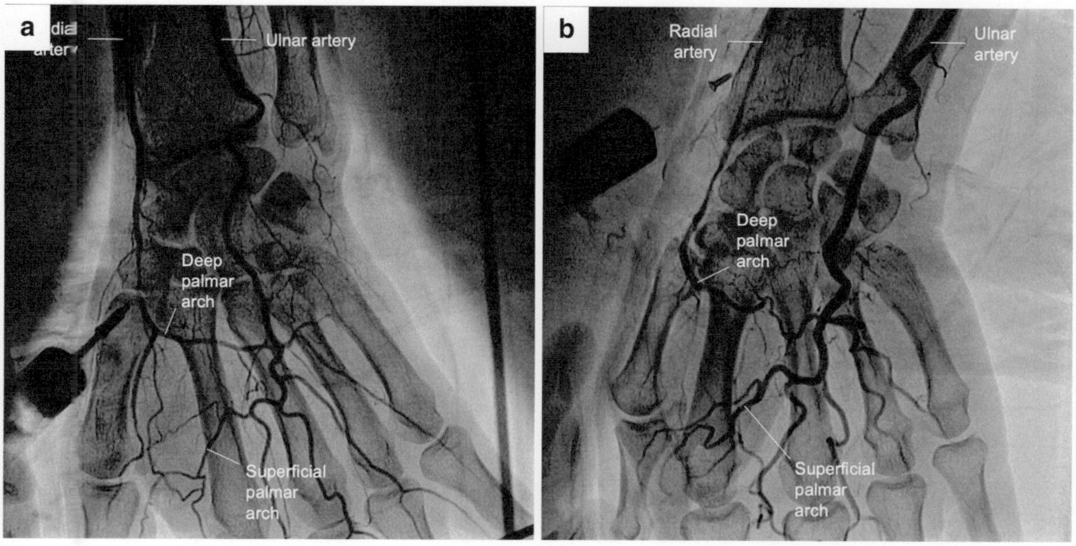

Fig. 5.4 Hand angiography showing (**a**) complete deep and superficial arches, both with radial-ulnar anastomosis. (**b**) Both palmar arches are complete, with the ulnar artery supplying the thumb without radial anastomosis

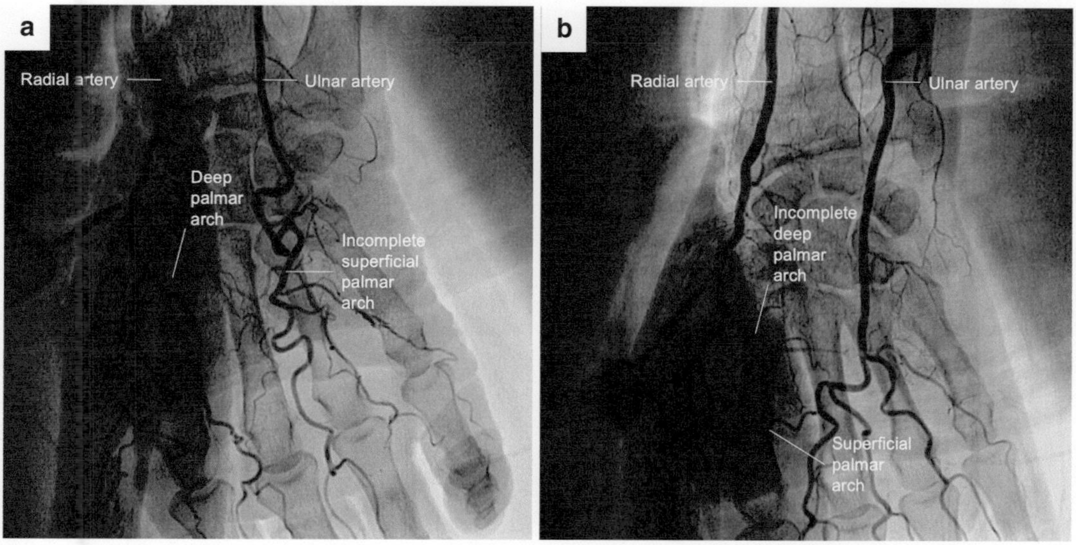

Fig. 5.5 Hand angiography showing (**a**) complete deep palmar arch and incomplete superficial palmar arch without radial-ulnar anastomosis. (**b**) Incomplete deep palmar arch without radial-ulnar anastomosis and a complete superficial palmar arch with radial-ulnar anastomosis

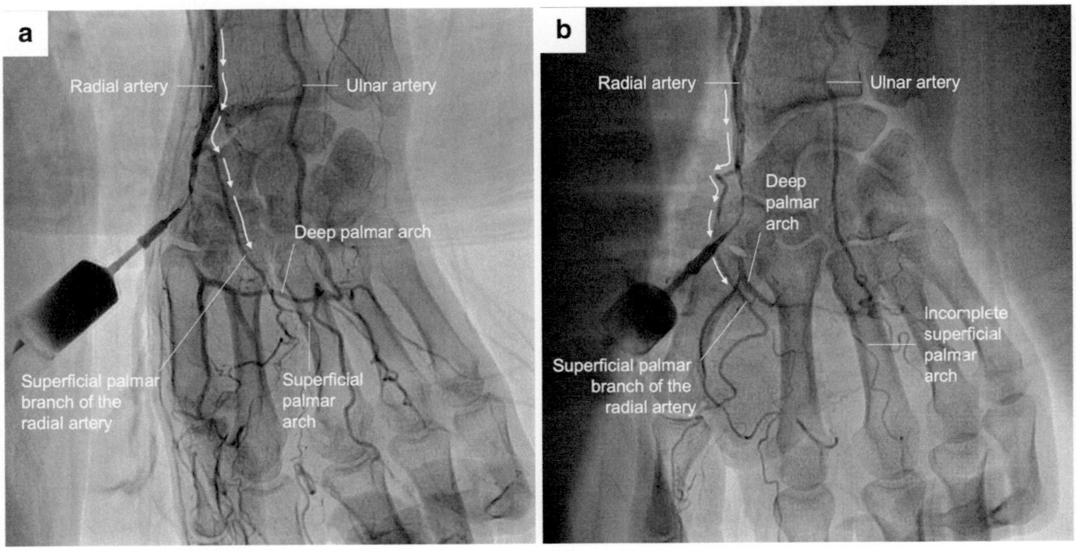

Fig. 5.6 Hand angiography showing the importance of the superficial palmar branch of the radial artery with distal radial access in (**a**) complete superficial arch with radial-ulnar anastomosis and (**b**) incomplete superficial palmar arch without radial-ulnar anastomosis. Arrows indicate the path of persistent flow from the forearm radial artery through the superficial palmar branch of the radial artery despite transient occlusion at the puncture site (spasm)

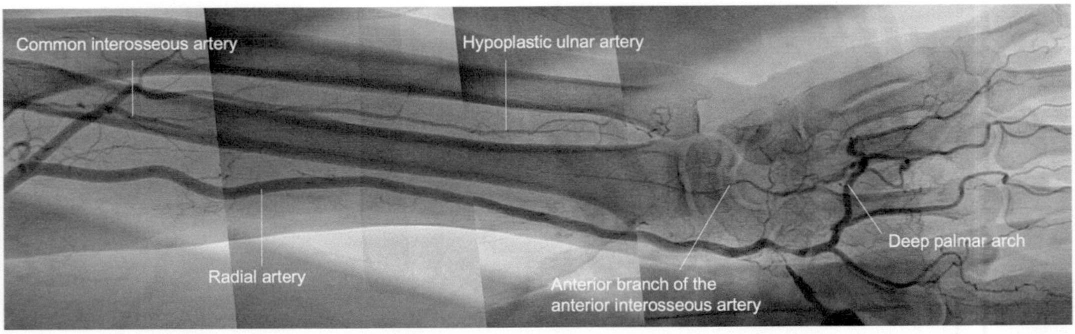

Fig. 5.7 Angiography of the upper extremity showing essential absence of the superficial palmar arch due to hypoplasia of the ulnar artery and concomitant absence of a noticeable superficial palmar branch of the radial artery

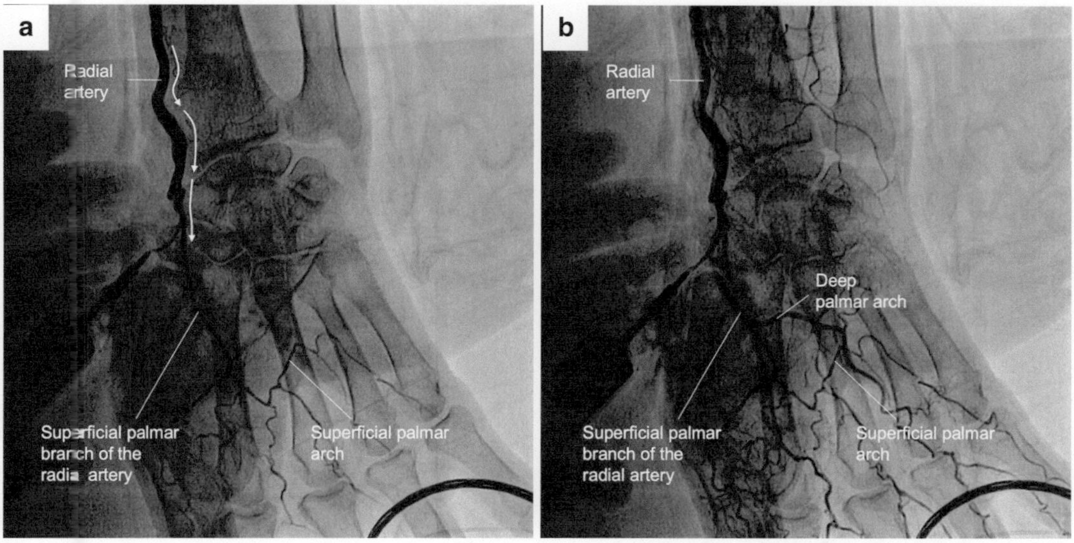

Fig. 5.8 Hand angiography showing hypoplasia of the ulnar artery and highlighting the importance of the superficial palmar branch of the radial artery with distal radial access to both support the superficial palmar arch and ensure flow persistence in the forearm radial artery with distal radial access. Arrows indicate the path of persistent flow from the forearm radial artery through the superficial palmar branch of the radial artery despite transient occlusion at the puncture site (spasm)

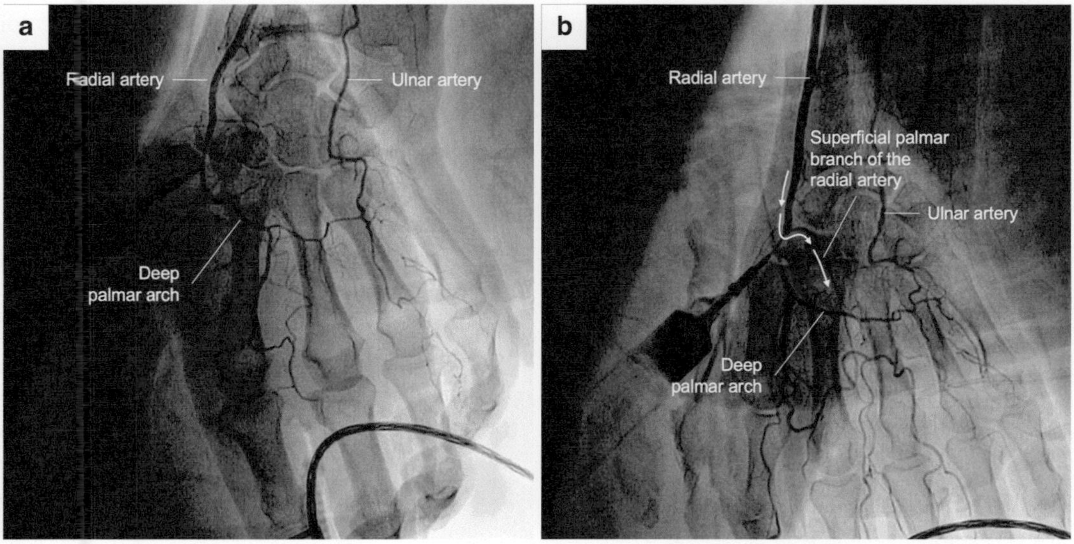

Fig. 5.9 Hand angiography showing essential absence of the superficial palmar arch with direct connection of the deep palmar arch to the ulnar artery and (**a**) concomitant absence of a noticeable superficial palmar branch of the radial artery. (**b**) Noticeable superficial palmar branch of the radial artery, which appears to be important to ensure flow persistence in the forearm radial artery with distal radial access. Arrows indicate the path of persistent flow from the forearm radial artery through the superficial palmar branch of the radial artery despite transient occlusion at the puncture site (spasm)

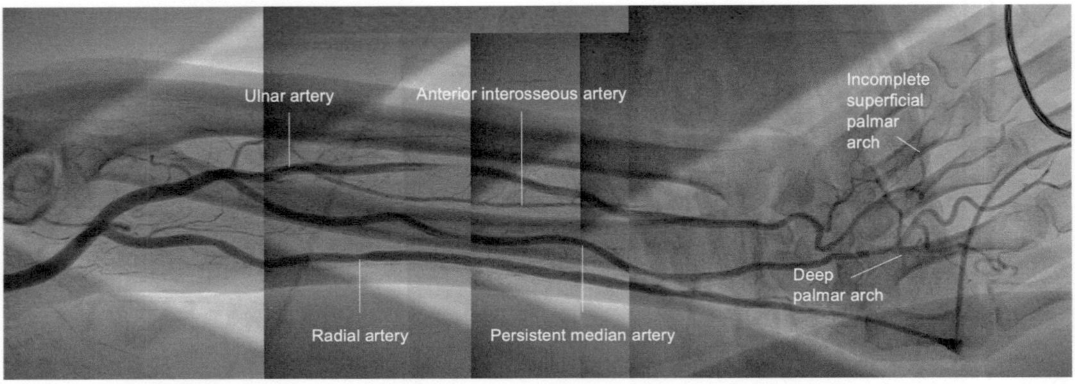

Fig. 5.10 Angiography of the upper extremity showing persistent median artery supporting an incomplete superficial palmar arch and concomitant absence of a noticeable superficial palmar branch of the radial artery

5.4 Assessing Collateral Circulation of the Hand

The evaluation of hand vascularization has been a crucial aspect of vascular medicine for decades. Initially developed for patients with arterial disease, these assessment techniques have found applications in various clinical scenarios, including preoperative evaluation for radial artery harvesting in coronary artery bypass grafting, reconstructive surgery, and, more recently, for patient selection in transradial catheterization procedures. The utility of different assessment methods varies depending on the specific purpose of evaluating hand vascularization.

5.4.1 Allen's Test

In 1929, Edgar Van Nuys Allen introduced a noninvasive method to assess the patency of hand arterial supply in patients with thromboangiitis obliterans [20]. The original technique involved bilateral compression of the radial arteries while the patient's hands were elevated and fisted for 1 min, facilitating the reduction of blood content within the hands. Upon opening the hands, the return of color indicated patency of the uncompressed ulnar arteries.

In the early 1950s, Wright adapted the Allen test for the assessment of collateral circulation prior to arterial cannulation [21]. This modified version involves the examiner compressing both ulnar and radial arteries while the patient clenches their fist, causing the hand to pale. After 30 s, the patient opens their hand, and the examiner releases pressure on the ulnar artery while maintaining compression on the radial artery. The return of normal color to the hand indicates adequate collateral circulation, while a lack of color change is considered a positive or abnormal result.

It is crucial that the patient avoids hyperextension of the fingers while opening the hand. Excessive digital abduction can potentially reduce perfusion to the palmar arch, possibly leading to a false-negative result [22].

Patient-related issues such as pallor, uncooperativeness, or unconsciousness may affect the test's accuracy. Individual anatomical variations, particularly in forearm arterial anatomy, can also influence the results. Procedural aspects present additional challenges, with observer bias in assessing the return of normal hand coloration being a significant concern. Furthermore, incomplete occlusion of the radial artery during testing may lead to false-negative results.

A comparative study with vascular ultrasound in 93 coronary artery bypass graft patients demonstrated varying sensitivity and specificity at different cut-off times. A 6-s cut-off yielded 54.5% sensitivity and 91.7% specificity, while a 3-s cut-off increased sensitivity to 100% but reduced specificity to 27% [23].

Despite its limitations, the Allen test has been used for years to select patients for TRA, excluding many patients from its benefits. However, a comprehensive study demonstrated the feasibility and safety of transradial catheterization across all the Allen test results, challenging its utility and essentially leading to its discontinuation in patient selection for TRA [24]. In addition, the study demonstrated the dynamic nature of the hand collateral circulation that can be recruited during and after transradial procedures, particularly in patients with poor baseline collateral circulation.

In contemporary practice, the reverse modified Allen test, which involves releasing compression over the radial artery rather than the ulnar artery, has emerged as a valuable tool for assessing radial artery patency in patients with a history of transradial catheterization (Fig. 5.11) [25].

5.4.2 Barbeau's Test

To address the limitations of the modified Allen test, Gérald Barbeau developed an enhanced method in 2004 to improve the sensitivity of the assessment of hand collateral circulation [26]. This technique involves attaching a pulse oximeter to the thumb or forefinger and recording the oxygen saturation and pulsatile blood flow waveform at baseline and after compression of the radial artery for 2 min. The results are classified into four types:

- Type A: no damping of the pulse waveform immediately after radial artery compression with a constant oximetric reading.
- Type B: damping of the pulse waveform with a constant oximetric reading.
- Type C: loss of pulse waveform and oximetric reading followed by recovery within 2 min.
- Type D: loss of pulse waveform and oximetric reading without recovery within 2 min.

Types A, B, and C are considered indicative of patency of the ulnopalmar arch, while type D is considered abnormal.

The reverse Barbeau test, performed by releasing compression from the radial artery, is indicated to assess the patency of the radial artery during hemostasis compression. It aids in identifying and reducing excessive compression of the hemostasis device to achieve patent hemostasis in conventional transradial procedures [27].

5.4.3 Diagnostic Techniques

While the Allen and Barbeau tests provide valuable qualitative assessments of hand circulation, several quantitative methods have emerged to improve diagnostic accuracy, particularly in the context of coronary artery bypass grafting, where the radial artery may be considered a conduit [28, 29].

5.4.3.1 Digital Plethysmography

It quantifies changes in blood volume in the finger caused by arterial pulsations, typically using infrared light and photoelectric sensors. Advanced photoplethysmographic techniques incorporate a pressure cuff placed at the base of the finger. When inflated to subdiastolic pressures, this cuff occludes venous outflow while permitting arterial inflow, allowing pressure-volume curve analysis.

5.4.3.2 Laser Perfusion Imaging

This technique utilizes the Doppler effect applied to laser light scattered by erythrocytes in the tissue microcirculation (laser Doppler perfusion imaging, LDPI) or the speckle pattern created by the interference of laser light scattered by moving erythrocytes in the tissue microcirculation (laser speckle contrast imaging, LSCI). The methods use a noncontact scanning laser beam to create a two-dimensional map of tissue perfusion over an extended area. The laser perfusion imaging technique can effectively visualize superficial perfusion patterns over the palm or dorsum of the hand (Fig. 5.12).

5.4.3.3 Vascular Ultrasound

Vascular ultrasound has become an important tool in the assessment of collateral circulation in

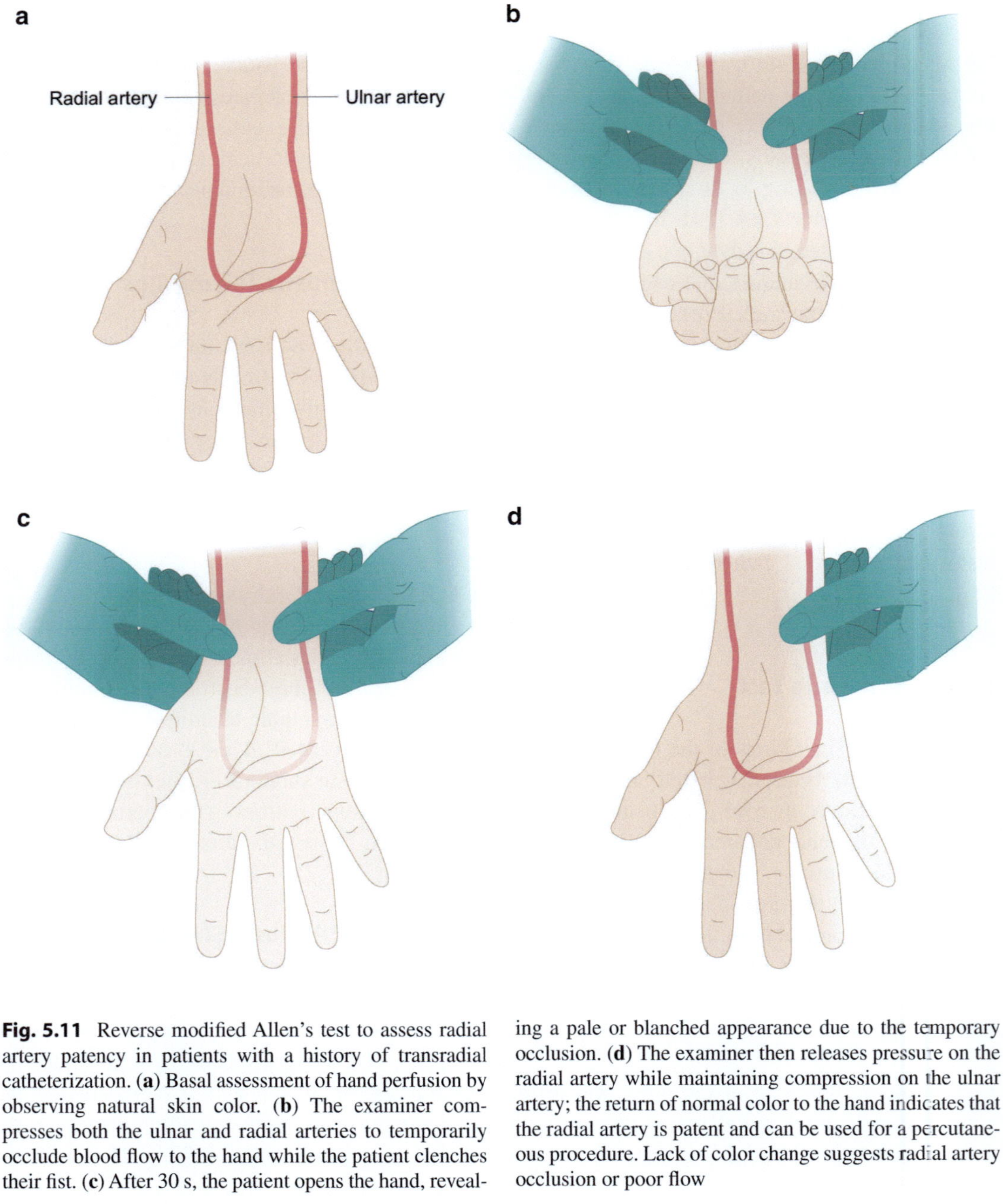

Fig. 5.11 Reverse modified Allen's test to assess radial artery patency in patients with a history of transradial catheterization. (**a**) Basal assessment of hand perfusion by observing natural skin color. (**b**) The examiner compresses both the ulnar and radial arteries to temporarily occlude blood flow to the hand while the patient clenches their fist. (**c**) After 30 s, the patient opens the hand, revealing a pale or blanched appearance due to the temporary occlusion. (**d**) The examiner then releases pressure on the radial artery while maintaining compression on the ulnar artery; the return of normal color to the hand indicates that the radial artery is patent and can be used for a percutaneous procedure. Lack of color change suggests radial artery occlusion or poor flow

the hand, providing both anatomical and functional insight. High-frequency ultrasound allows direct visualization of the radial and ulnar arteries, palmar arches, and digital vessels while providing quantitative data on blood flow velocities and directionality.

These techniques allow the evaluation of flow changes during provocative maneuvers, potentially increasing their diagnostic sensitivity. However, factors such as ambient temperature and patient motion can affect the results. In addition, the accuracy of these methods depends on the expertise of the operator and the proper interpretation of the results. Finally, they require specialized equipment and additional time for setup and interpretation.

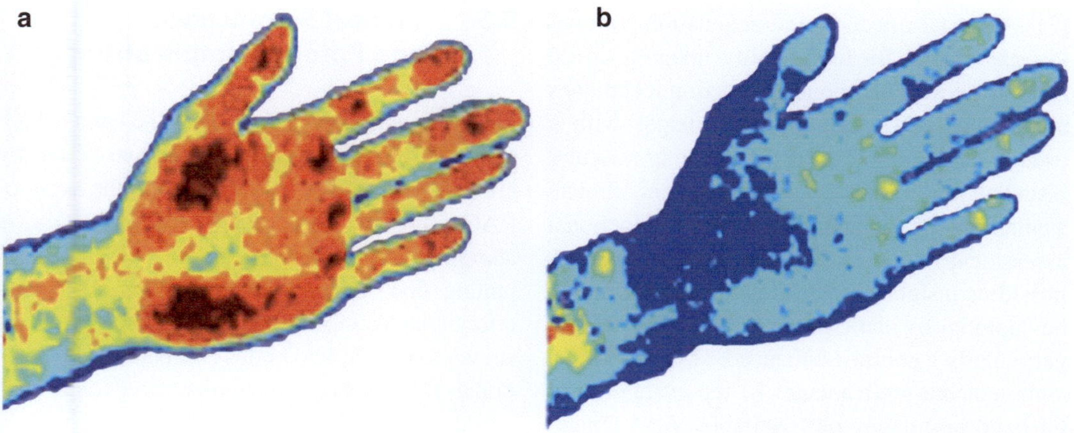

Fig. 5.12 Laser perfusion imaging (**a**) at baseline and (**b**) after simulated occlusion of both radial and ulnar arteries

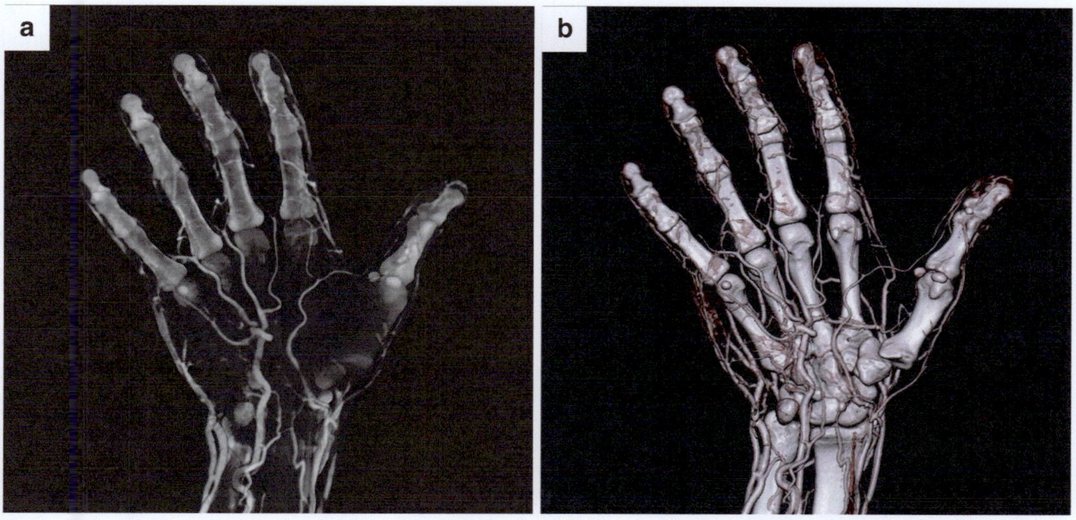

Fig. 5.13 Computed tomography (CT) angiography of the hand showing the complex arterial network of the hand with an incomplete superficial palmar arch. (**a**) 3D maximum intensity projection angio CT and (**b**) 3D volume-rendered angio CT

5.4.4 Advanced Imaging Techniques

Computed tomography angiography (CTA) and magnetic resonance angiography (MRA) have proven to be efficient methods for evaluating hand vasculature, providing high-resolution vascular images. Recent advances in CT techniques, such as dynamic CTA and super high-resolution CTA (SHR-CTA), have increased the utility of CTA in hand vascular imaging [30]. To ensure optimal image quality, hand imaging should be performed as a distinct procedure rather than as part of a comprehensive upper extremity imaging protocol (Fig. 5.13). Indeed, while single-scan upper limb CTA can adequately visualize arteries up to the distal portions of the radial and ulnar arteries, it is insufficient for further evaluation due to temporal and spatial resolution limitations. Of note, a method for simultaneous CTA of the coronary and radial arteries without increasing the use of contrast has recently been reported

[31]. Optimal injection and acquisition parameters are crucial for high-quality imaging of the hand arteries. When bone subtraction techniques are applied, CTA can produce images with a pseudo-angiographic effect, enhancing vascular visualization. In particular, the recent clinical availability of dynamic CTA allows functional assessment of the arterial network of the hand, providing insights into flow dynamics that cannot be captured by static imaging. Similarly, MRA, particularly contrast-enhanced MRA, offers complementary advantages in the evaluation of the hand vasculature [30]. Suitably, MRA images can be analyzed with or without subtraction techniques, allowing for improved contrast resolution and visualization of background structures, respectively. Of note, recent technological advances, coupled with emerging safety concerns regarding gadolinium-based contrast agents, have led to a growing interest in contrast-free imaging modalities (Fig. 5.14) [32]. Despite their advantages, these modalities are limited by cost, availability, and, in the case of CTA, radiation exposure and potential contrast-related complications.

5.5 Clinical Significance and Potential Implications

The redundant vascularization of the hand, which supports the safety of conventional TRA by allowing alternative blood supply in the event of RAO and preventing ischemic complications, is also the basis for the efficacy of DRA in maintaining flow and patency in the forearm radial artery (see also Chap. 4). In fact, DRA has been shown to reduce RAO rates compared to conventional TRA in both randomized trials and real-world settings [2, 33].

A complete superficial palmar arch has been proposed as a critical anatomic feature providing a path of lower resistance to blood flow in the event of transient or persistent distal RAO at the puncture site, thereby preserving forearm radial artery flow [34]. However, regional data on the prevalence of complete and incomplete deep and superficial palmar arches reveal ethnic differences that challenge the universal importance of a complete superficial palmar arch [18]. This is further supported by the observed rates of RAO following distal radial access (DRA), which are

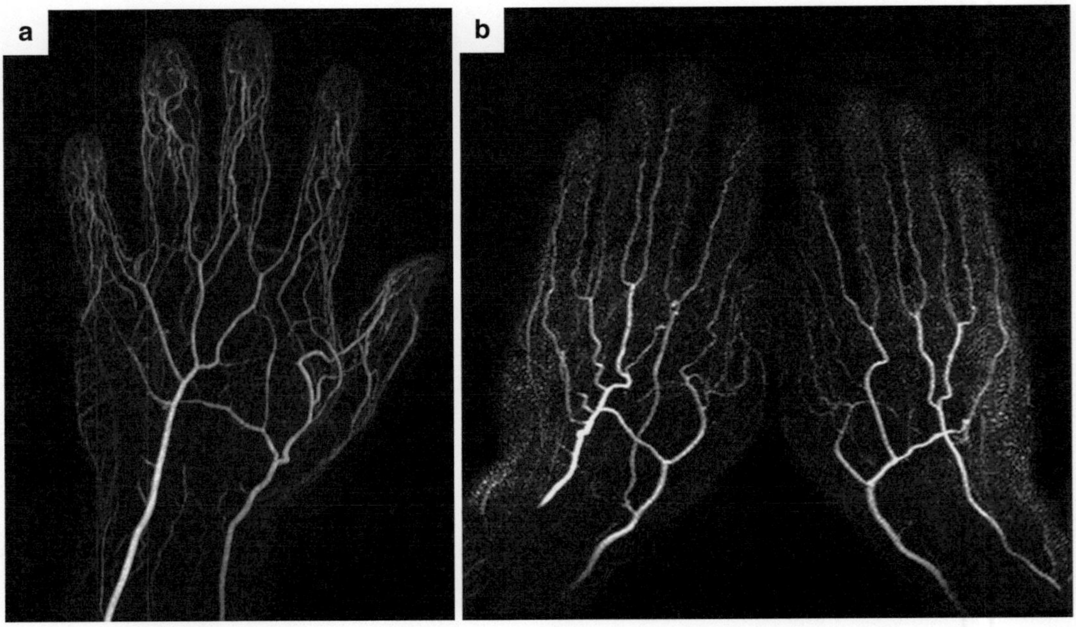

Fig. 5.14 Magnetic resonance angiography of the hand implementing (**a**) contrast-enhanced and (**b**) nonenhanced maximum intensity projection

remarkably low and consistent across European and Asian populations [33, 35].

Such uniformity of outcomes suggests that other factors are at play. A closer examination of the anatomy reveals the rich and intricate anastomotic network of the wrist and hand, further supporting the value of DRA. Real-time in vivo angiographic observation of blood flow highlights the critical importance of prominent anastomotic branches arising from the radial artery proximal to the distal puncture site, which can provide alternative pathways for blood flow to maintain upstream flow and downstream perfusion in the event of puncture site RAO [36].

However, several knowledge gaps persist. It is unknown whether the overall anatomy of DRA inherently protects against occlusive hemostasis and thus ensures flow persistence. Also, while the primary advantage of DRA may be that its puncture site is distal to one or more noticeable branches arising from the radial artery more proximally, the role of these branches in preserving flow, their dynamic recruitment in the event of RAO, and their potential contribution to the few observed cases of RAO with DRA have yet to be fully elucidated.

In addition, the feasibility and utility of using vascular ultrasound to assess these branches and select the optimal site for DRA have not been explored, and it is unclear whether the poor visualization of such branches observed on angiography could be beneficial in identifying patients who may require a modified hemostasis protocol. Current evidence suggests that DRA reduces RAO independent of the hemostasis protocol, but due to the low incidence of RAO, no significant signal has emerged to confirm this hypothesis.

References

1. Neumann FJ, Sousa-Uva M, Ahlsson A, Alfonso F, Banning AP, Benedetto U, et al. 2018 ESC/EACTS guidelines on myocardial revascularization. Eur Heart J. 2019;40:87–165.
2. Lawton JS, Tamis-Holland JE, Bangalore S, Bates ER, Beckie TM, Bischoff TM, et al. 2021 ACC/AHA/SCAI guideline for coronary artery revascularization: a report of the American College of Cardiology/American Heart Association Joint Committee on Clinical Practice Guidelines. J Am Coll Cardiol. 2022;79:e21–9.
3. Sgueglia GA, Lee BK, Cho BR, Babunashvili A, Lee JB, Lee JW, et al. Distal radial access: consensus report of the first Korea-Europe transradial intervention meeting. JACC Cardiovasc Interv. 2021;14:892–906.
4. Ferrante G, Condello F, Rao SV, Maurina M, Jolly S, Stefanini GG, et al. Distal vs conventional radial access for coronary angiography and/or intervention: a meta-analysis of randomized trials. JACC Cardiovasc Interv. 2022;15:2297–311.
5. Sheetz KK, Bishop AT, Berger RA. The arterial blood supply of the distal radius and ulna and its potential use in vascularized pedicled bone grafts. J Hand Surg. 1995;20A:902–14.
6. Gelberman RH, Panagis JS, Taleisnik J, Baumgaertner M. The arterial anatomy of the human carpus. Part I: the extraosseous vascularity. J Hand Surg Am. 1983;8:367–75.
7. Grettve S. Arterial anatomy of the carpal bones. Acta Anat. 1955;25:331–45.
8. Freedman DM, Botte MJ, Gelberman RH. Vascularity of the carpus. Clin Orthop Relat Res. 2001;383:47–59.
9. Olave E, Gabrielli C, Del Sol N, Rodriques CF, Prates JC. A biometric study on the relationships between the deep palmar arch and the superficial palmar arch, the distal wrist and palmar creases. Folia Morphol (Warsz). 1998;57:383–8.
10. Bianchi H. Anatomy of the radial branches of the palmar arch: variations and surgical importance. Hand Clin. 2001;17:139–46.
11. Olave E, Prates JC, Gabrielli C, Mandiola E. Perforating branches: important contribution to the formation of the dorsal metacarpal arteries. Scand J Plast Reconstr Surg Hand Surg. 1998;32:221–7.
12. Bianchi HF, Leiro R. The arterial trunk of the thumb-index digital collaterals. Surg Radiol Anat. 1987;9:63–7.
13. Erbil M, Aktekin M, Denk CC, Onderoglu S, Sürücü HS. Arteries of the thumb originating from the superficial palmar arch: five cases. Surg Radiol Anat. 1999;21:217–20.
14. Coleman SS, Anson BJ. Arterial patterns in the hand based upon a study of 650 specimens. Surg Gynecol Obstet. 1961;113:409–24.
15. Gokhroo R, Bisht D, Gupta S, Kishor K, Ranwa B. Palmar arch anatomy: Ajmer Working Group classification. Vascular. 2016;24:31–6.
16. Feigl GC, Petrac M, Pixner T, Ulz H, Mörth C, Dreu M. The superficial palmar arch and median artery as an example of misleading results due to a small number of investigated specimens or the use of different classifications. Ann Anat. 2012;194:389–95.
17. Jaschtschinski SN. Morphologie und Topographie des Arcus volaris sublimis und profundus des Menschen. Anat Hefte. 1897;7:161–88.
18. Zarzecki MP, Popieluszko P, Zayachkowski A, Pękala PA, Henry BM, Tomaszewski KA. The surgical

anatomy of the superficial and deep palmar arches: a meta-analysis. J Plast Reconstr Aesthet Surg. 2018;71:1577–92.
19. van Leeuwen MAH, Hollander MR, van der Heijden DJ, van de Ven PM, Opmeer KHM, Taverne YJHJ, et al. The ACRA Anatomy Study (Assessment of Disability After Coronary Procedures Using Radial Access): a comprehensive anatomic and functional assessment of the vasculature of the hand and relation to outcome after transradial catheterization. Circ Cardiovasc Interv. 2017;10:e005753.
20. Allen EV. Thromboangiitis obliterans: methods of diagnosis of chronic occlusive arterial lesions distal to the wrist with illustrative cases. Am J Med Sci. 1929;178:237–44.
21. Wright I. Vascular diseases in clinical practice. Chicago: Year Book Medical Publishers; 1952.
22. Greenhow DE. Incorrect performance of Allen's test—ulnar-artery follow erroneously presumed inadequate. Anesthesiology. 1972;37:356–7.
23. Jarvis MA, Jarvis CL, Jones PR, Spyt TJ. Reliability of Allen's test in selection of patients for radial artery harvest. Ann Thorac Surg. 2000;70:1362–5.
24. Valgimigli M, Campo G, Penzo C, Tebaldi M, Biscaglia S, Ferrari R. Transradial coronary catheterization and intervention across the whole spectrum of Allen test results. J Am Coll Cardiol. 2014;63:1833–41.
25. Foreman A, de Almeida JR, Gilbert R, Goldstein DP. The Allen's test: revisiting the importance of bidirectional testing to determine candidacy and design of radial forearm free flap harvest in the era of trans radial endovascular access procedures. J Otolaryngol Head Neck Surg. 2015;44:47.
26. Barbeau GR, Arsenault F, Dugas L, Simard S, Larivière MM. Evaluation of the ulnopalmar arterial arches with pulse oximetry and plethysmography: comparison with the Allen's test in 1010 patients. Am Heart J. 2004;147:489–93.
27. Pancholy S, Coppola J, Patel T, Roke-Thomas M. Prevention of radial artery occlusion-patent hemostasis evaluation trial (PROPHET study): a randomized comparison of traditional versus patency documented hemostasis after transradial catheterization. Catheter Cardiovasc Interv. 2008;72:335–40.
28. Chloros GD, Smerlis NN, Li Z, Smith TL, Smith BP, Koman LA. Noninvasive evaluation of upper-extremity vascular perfusion. J Hand Surg Am. 2008;33:591–600.
29. Habib J, Baetz L, Satiani B. Assessment of collateral circulation to the hand prior to radial artery harvest. Vasc Med. 2012;17:352–61.
30. Blum AG, Gillet R, Athlani L, Prestat A, Zuily S, Wahl D, et al. CT angiography and MRI of hand vascular lesions: technical considerations and spectrum of imaging findings. Insights Imaging. 2021;12:16.
31. Tamaoki H, Yoshimachi F, Sakurai T, Shin T, Ikari Y. Simultaneous computed tomographic angiography of the coronary and radial arteries. Cardiovasc Interv Ther. 2020;35:185–93.
32. Miyazaki M, Lee VS. Nonenhanced MR angiography. Radiology. 2008;248:20–43.
33. Lee JW, Kim Y, Lee BK, Yoo SY, Lee SY, Kim CJ, et al. Distal radial access for coronary procedures in a large prospective multicenter registry: The KODRA trial. JACC Cardiovasc Interv. 2024;17:329–40.
34. Sgueglia GA, Di Giorgio A, Gaspardone A, Babunashvili A. Anatomic basis and physiological rationale of distal radial artery access for percutaneous coronary and endovascular procedures. JACC Cardiovasc Interv. 2018;11:2113–9.
35. Aminian A, Sgueglia GA, Wiemer M, Kefer J, Gasparini GL, Ruzsa Z, et al. Distal versus conventional radial access for coronary angiography and intervention: the DISCO RADIAL trial. JACC Cardiovasc Interv. 2022;15:1191–201.
36. Sgueglia GA, Santoliquido A, Gaspardone A, Di Giorgio A. First results of the Distal Radial Access Doppler Study. JACC Cardiovasc Imaging. 2021;14:1281–3.

Part II

Practical and Technical Aspects

6 Patient Selection and Preparation

Christopher M. Fernandez, Karim Ratib, and Sandeep Nathan

6.1 Introduction

Transradial access (TRA) for catheter-based interventions offers a number of advantages over transfemoral access (TFA) including a reduction in major bleeding and vascular access site complications and earlier time to ambulation [1–3].

Distal radial access (DRA), particularly left DRA, offers favorable ergonomics for the operator working from the right side of the patient, facilitating cannulation of bypass grafts (especially the left internal mammary artery), avoiding the tortuosity and angulation more typically associated with the right subclavian and brachiocephalic arteries, and allowing catheter selection/manipulation that more closely approximates TFA than right TRA.

Compared to the conventional TRA, DRA is also associated with the additional benefit of maintaining blood flow through the superficial palmar arch which appears to reduce the risk of more proximal radial artery occlusion (RAO) (see also Chap. 4) [4].

While there are other putative benefits of DRA covered elsewhere in this text, specific patient and procedural factors may contribute to technical challenges from the outset, impacting timely case completion and, in turn, discouraging the novice DRA operator. A focused but thorough preprocedural evaluation and patient preparation are both critical to ensuring the highest probability of successful DRA case performance. We will briefly review factors that influence a patient's candidacy for DRA and discuss the salient points of patient preparation.

C. M. Fernandez · S. Nathan (✉)
Heart and Vascular Center, University of Chicago Medicine, Chicago, IL, USA
e-mail: snathan@medicine.bsd.uchicago.edu

K. Ratib
University Hospitals of North Midlands, NHS Trust, Stoke-on-Trent, UK

6.2 Patient Selection

Evaluating a patient's candidacy for DRA is an important prerequisite in order to avoid frustration and access site crossover once the patient has already been prepped. The evaluation is straightforward and can be broken down into patient characteristics and procedural factors.

6.2.1 Patient Characteristics

Given the proximity of the DRA site to the conventional TRA site, many of the same patient factors that make a good conventional TRA candidate also make a good DRA patient. Some of these factors include the presence of a prominent, palpable, radial pulse in or distal to the anatomical snuffbox, the absence of prior injury or surgical instrumentation at the site, and type A–C patterns on a Barbeau test, although many con-

G. A. Sgueglia (ed.), *Distal Radial Access*, https://doi.org/10.1007/978-3-031-89925-6_6

sider this latter test unnecessary for any type of radial access given its lack of discriminatory ability to predict adverse vascular events after catheterization [5].

In addition to the aforementioned advantages of TRA over TFA, certain patient characteristics should further convince the operator to specifically choose DRA. The optimal distal puncture site within the anatomical snuffbox, bounded by the extensor pollicis brevis and extensor longus tendons, offers both a very shallow entry into the radial artery and easy compressibility over the scaphoid or trapezium carpal bones. The shallow entry may be advantageous in morbidly obese patients, where DRA puncture into a deeper vessel and placement of a hemostasis band may be complicated by excessive soft tissue and forearm girth. Therefore, patients considered at high risk for bleeding due to thrombocytopenia, uninterrupted anticoagulation, or other bleeding diathesis may be better candidates for DRA.

In addition, patients who have previously had a RAO as a result of radial cannulation should be considered at risk for further occlusion, and therefore, the use of the ipsilateral DRA for subsequent access may mitigate the loss of another radial access. Also, DRA may be preferable in other important scenarios where preservation of the proximal radial artery is paramount, such as patients who may require a fistula for hemodialysis and patients who are likely to require arterial grafts for coronary bypass.

Patients with unfavorable anatomic features at the conventional TRA site, such as scar tissue, prior carpal tunnel release surgery, or inability to supinate the forearm due to orthopedic issues, contractures, etc., may also be considered better candidates for DRA than the conventional TRA.

Ideally, the evaluation of the patient's candidacy for DRA should also include a brief ultrasound evaluation of the site to examine the size, course, and anomalies of the radial artery and to ensure that the vessel is overlying a compressive bony surface within the optimal puncture zone [4]. Several studies have demonstrated a slightly smaller radial artery size at the distal site compared to the conventional site and a smaller distal radial size in females compared to males, which may affect sheath size or overall candidacy [6–8]. As a general rule, it is helpful to know the outer diameter of the radial sheaths most commonly used in your cath lab, as the outer diameter of the sheath should not exceed the inner diameter of the radial artery to avoid overstretch injury to the vessel and resultant RAO [9].

While proximal radial loops and tortuosity are not absolute contraindications to the transradial approach, ultrasound assessment in skilled hands can help navigate around these issues.

Finally, it should be noted that occasionally the point of maximal radial pulsation is actually distal to the anatomical snuffbox, and thus, ultrasound will help in this regard as well (see also Chap. 8) [7].

Despite the advantages of DRA, there are certain patient-related factors that should prompt consideration of an alternative access point. These include patients with known distal vaso-occlusive disease, symptomatic Raynaud's syndrome, thromboangiitis obliterans, very small radial artery size on ultrasound, radiobrachial anatomy known to be noncrossable from previous catheterization attempts, active arteriovenous fistulae, and patients being considered for coronary artery bypass grafting with planned radial artery harvesting (the latter two being relative contraindications).

Other factors that make the specific choice of DRA less desirable include significant radial artery calcification, tortuosity, or disease at the puncture site and prior trauma or orthopedic procedures that have either altered radial anatomy, created significant scar tissue, or made hand positioning impossible [10].

Anecdotally, it has been noted that unfavorable anatomic characteristics of the radiobrachial vasculature are rarely mirrored in the contralateral arm, and therefore, difficult anatomy in one arm should not automatically preclude TRA in the other arm [11].

6.2.2 Procedural Factors

Before attempting DRA, several procedural factors should also be considered. First, the operator should consider the urgency of obtaining vascular access and his or her personal experience and skill, recognizing that obtaining DRA may be somewhat more time-consuming than conventional TRA, especially in the early stages of DRA adoption (see also Chap. 26). For primary percutaneous coronary interventions (PCI) where time is of the essence, only experienced DRA operators should consider using this approach.

A study by Roh JW et al. found that at least 200 DRA cases were required to achieve proficiency commensurate with more experienced DRA operators [12]. While no randomized controlled trial has compared DRA to conventional TRA in primary PCI, a recent registry has published data on DRA access during coronary procedures, including ST-elevation myocardial infarction (STEMI), and suggests that DRA is safe and feasible in STEMI [13]. In non-emergent PCI and diagnostic cases, operators have greater luxury of time to obtain access. A recent single-center randomized study demonstrated lower rates of RAO and a shorter time to hemostasis but a higher crossover rate and longer procedure time with DRA (14 min vs. 11 min) compared to conventional TRA [14]. As such, new DRA operators can expect a longer time to access and a higher crossover rate, especially in the early learning stages.

Due to the slightly smaller size of the radial artery in the distal segment, the equipment requirements for a DRA case should generally not exceed what is feasible with a 6-Fr guiding catheter. While this allows for virtually all sizes of coronary balloons and stents, all intravascular imaging and physiology platforms, and devices for a variety of complex and two-stent PCI techniques, it may preclude some large-bore atherectomy devices and devices for various advanced techniques for complex or chronic total occlusion PCI. To allow for larger bore devices, other techniques such as sheathless access and thin-walled 7-Fr sheaths have been used over DRA (see also Chaps. 18 and 19). A final consideration is the fact that DRA adds several centimeters to the required catheter length compared to conventional TRA. While this is not a concern in routine cases, it can be a factor in very tall individuals and when performing radial-to-peripheral interventions of the superficial femoral artery and below. In such cases, an ultrasound-guided high puncture of the more proximal radial artery may be preferable, taking care to avoid the body of the brachioradialis muscle or cannulation in a location that precludes successful hemostasis after the procedure.

6.3 Patient and Procedure Preparation

Once the patient has been assessed for DRA candidacy, the patient and supplies can be prepared. A list of supplies (including some optional items) for a typical DRA case is provided in Table 6.1.

After the patient is placed supine on the cath lab table, the left wrist is pronated, and the arm is elevated and adducted on towels or a foam wedge. The left forearm is typically positioned across the abdomen so that the left DRA site is easily accessible to the operator. An optional flexing arm board may be used to maintain wrist positioning,

Table 6.1 Recommended supplies for distal radial access

Chlorohexidine or similar topical antimicrobial prep
Bendable arm board or wrist support (optional)
Sterile drape with appropriate fenestration
Sterile towels
Sterile scissors
Ultrasound system with linear vascular probe
Sterile ultrasound probe cover
Sterile ultrasound gel
4- or 5-Fr micropuncture kit (optional, typically packaged with a 21-G × 4-cm needle and 0.018″ guidewire)
Low profile (preferably thin-walled) hydrophilic radial sheath (typically 5 or 6 Fr with a 0.021″ guidewire)
Sterile gauze
Transparent adhesive dressing to secure sheath
Syringe (5 cc) with 25-G skin needle
Lidocaine hydrochloride (or similar local anesthetic) for infiltration
Nitroglycerin (200 mcg/mL concentration) for local infiltration and intra-arterial vasodilation after sheath insertion

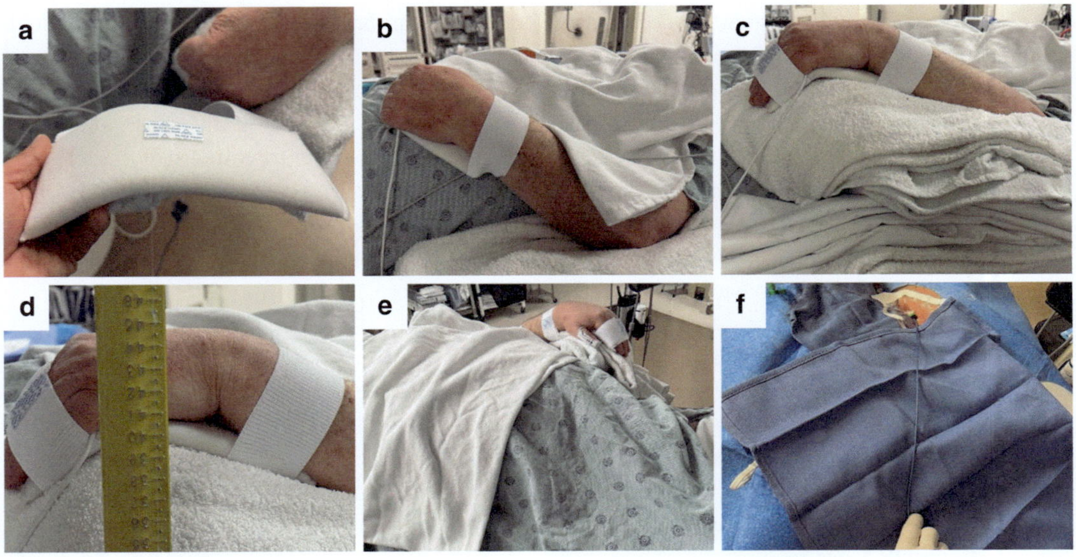

Fig. 6.1 Positioning of the patient's arm for left distal radial access should strike a balance between patient comfort and favorable ergonomics for the interventional operator, typically working from the right side of the patient. (**a**) An optional disposable, bendable arm board (Dale Medical Products, Franklin, MA) with elastic band fasteners may be bent and secured on the palmar surface. (**b**) The arm is then positioned with the left shoulder flat against the mattress, the elbow slightly bent, and the forearm pronated and adducted. (**c**) The forearm rests comfortably on either a foam wedge or an elevation comprised of towels or blankets, (**d**) at approximately 35–45 cm above the surface of the mattress depending on operator preference. (**e**) The puncture site should thus be elevated above the patient's abdomen and easily accessible from the operating position, (**f**) allowing catheters and interventional equipment to be laid across the patient's legs and comfortably manipulated

but it is not mandatory. A detailed illustration of these steps is shown in Fig. 6.1.

The dorsum of the hand and volar aspect of the forearm (ipsilateral proximal radial site for rapid conversion in case of DRA access failure) are then cleansed with chlorohexidine or topical antimicrobial scrub according to local standard of care and draped in a sterile fashion with the fenestration of the drape positioned over the planned puncture site. Because determining the optimal puncture site can sometimes be difficult once the patient is draped, it may be helpful to mark the skin at the ultrasound-guided puncture site with either an indelible marker or by indenting the skin with a needle cap prior to draping the arm.

In addition to preparing the distal radial artery, we also prepare at least one backup access site (in addition to the ipsilateral proximal radial site as noted).

After the patient is draped, the table, flat panel detector, and supplies are positioned to minimize interference with efficient DRA access.

Ultrasound guidance for access, while not mandatory, can help minimize the number of puncture attempts and reduce the time to successful access. Therefore, its use is recommended, and the ultrasound screen should be positioned so that it is clearly visible to the operator. A linear vascular ultrasound probe capable of high-resolution images at low penetration depths is typically used with a sterile probe cover placed over the probe.

The flat panel detector is then positioned over the distal forearm with a slight cranial angulation and contralateral tilt (i.e., left DRA = shallow RAO/cranial angulation) to provide the operator with an unobstructed view of the access site and the ability to use fluoroscopic guidance for guidewire manipulation and advancement as needed (Fig. 6.2).

Unlike left DRA, right-side DRA does not require adduction of the forearm over the abdomen, as most operators work from the right side of the patient. Elevating the right forearm to

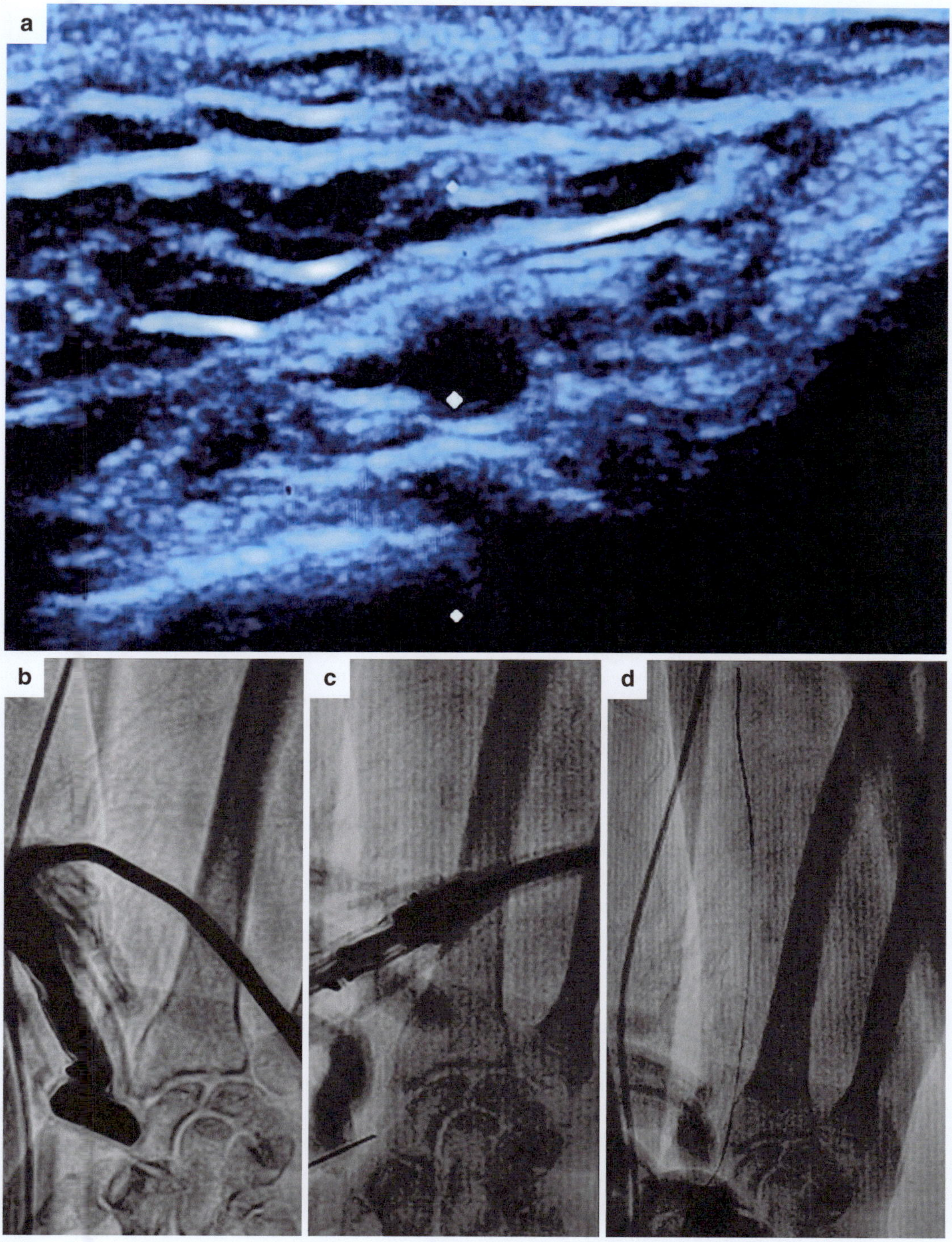

Fig. 6.2 (**a**) Vascular ultrasound guidance (Fujifilm SonoSite SII ultrasound system with a L25x linear 13–6 MHz probe) of distal radial access with the patient arm positioned to allow predictable entry into a centered vessel without excessive needle angulation. (**b**) Fluoroscopic position of the ultrasound probe over the anatomical snuffbox. (**c**) Fluoroscopic view of a beveled micropuncture needle used to gain anterior wall access to the distal radial artery. (**d**) Fluoroscopic view of a 0.018″ × 40 cm nitinol micropuncture wire advanced into the radial artery

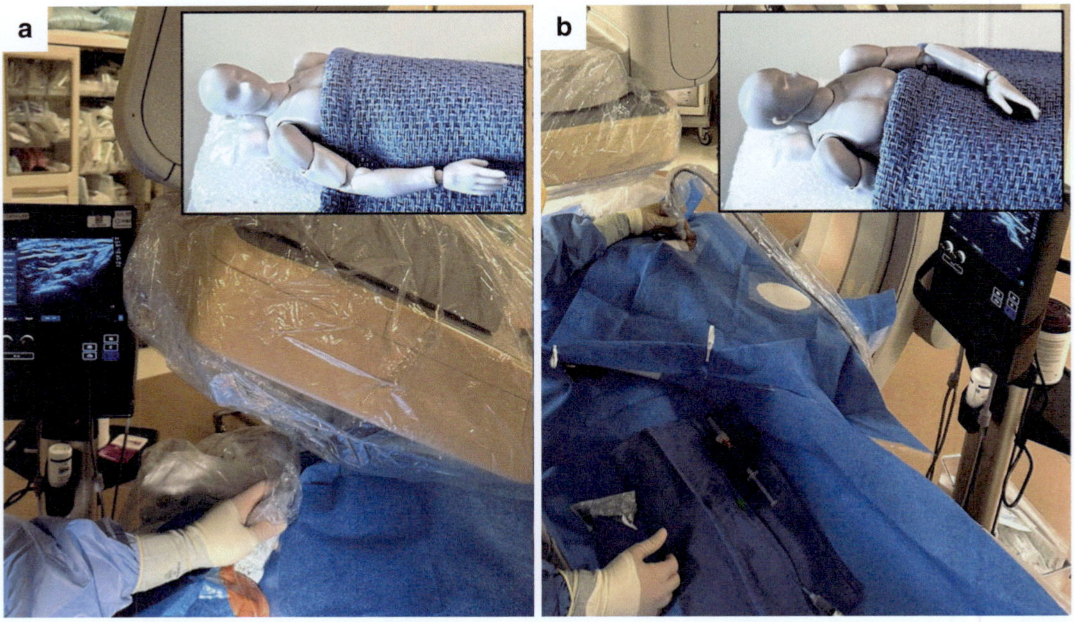

Fig. 6.3 Positioning of the arm for distal radial access will vary slightly based on the left vs. right side approach. (**a**) For right distal radial access, the straightened right arm is fully pronated and elevated slightly on a foam wedge or towels, to approximate the elevation of the patient's adjacent right thigh, and secured in place using surgical tape across the dorsum of the extended digits. (**b**) With left distal radial access, greater elevation of the pronated hand, along with flexion at the elbow and adduction of the forearm, may be necessary to facilitate ergonomics for the operator; in the case of significantly obese patients, exaggerating the aforementioned positioning to allow the pronated hand to rest on the lower abdomen helps ensure that the case may be performed without having to lean over the patient (inset images show suggested arm positions as demonstrated on an articulating anatomical model)

approximate the height of the patient's right hip/thigh provides comfort for both the patient and the operator and creates a work surface on which to place interventional equipment. Figure 6.3 illustrates optimal arm positioning for both left DRA and right DRA.

Once the arm is prepped and draped and the patient is sedated, the distal radial site can be infiltrated with local anesthetic with or without nitroglycerin prior to access attempts. In the case of small radial caliber and/or radial spasm as a result of repeated puncture attempts, subcutaneous infiltration with 200–400 mcg of nitroglycerin (200 mcg/mL concentration) may serve as a valuable adjunct with no systemic effect on blood pressure. A more detailed discussion of ultrasound-guided and conventional puncture is provided in Chaps. 7 and 8.

6.4 Conclusions

Over the past three decades, the transradial approach for catheter-based vascular interventions has demonstrated significant clinical advantages over the transfemoral approach.

More recently, DRA has emerged as an important iterative adaptation of the root technique, gaining acceptance due to its potential safety advantages over the conventional radial approach as well as favorable ergonomics for operators working from the right side of the patient.

While there are technical challenges and a learning curve as with any new technique, following a routine for pre-procedural assessment and patient setup will help improve the chances of a successful approach and reduce frustration and otherwise avoidable challenges.

References

1. Nathan S, Rao SV. Radial versus femoral access for percutaneous coronary intervention: implications for vascular complications and bleeding. Curr Cardiol Rep. 2012;14:502–9.
2. Hirai T, Conway BD, Paul J, Klass D, Blair J, Nathan S. Frontiers in transradial catheterization and intervention: challenges and advances in the “new gold standard” for vascular access. Curr Cardiovasc Risk Rep. 2017;11:37.
3. Jhand A, Atti V, Gwon Y, Dhawan R, Turagam MK, Mamas MA, et al. Meta-analysis of transradial vs transfemoral access for percutaneous coronary intervention in patients with ST elevation myocardial infarction. Am J Cardiol. 2021;141:23–30.
4. Hadjivassiliou A, Kiemeneij F, Nathan S, Klass D. Ultrasound-guided access to the distal radial artery at the anatomical snuffbox for catheter-based vascular interventions: a technical guide. EuroIntervention. 2021;16:1342–8.
5. Mason PJ, Shah B, Tamis-Holland JE, Bittl JA, Cohen MG, Safirstein J, et al. An update on radial artery access and best practices for transradial coronary angiography and intervention in acute coronary syndrome: a scientific statement from the American Heart Association. Circ Cardiovasc Interv. 2018;11:e000035.
6. Lee JW, Son JW, Go TH, Kang DR, Lee SJ, Kim SE, et al. Reference diameter and characteristics of the distal radial artery based on ultrasonographic assessment. Korean J Intern Med. 2022;37:109–18.
7. Hadjivassiliou A, Cardarelli-Leite L, Jalal S, Chung J, Liu D, Ho S, et al. Left distal transradial access (ldTRA): a comparative assessment of conventional and distal radial artery size. Cardiovasc Intervent Radiol. 2020;43:850–7.
8. Lee L, Kern J, Bair J, Rosenberg J, Lee M, Nathan S. Clinical determinants of radial artery caliber assessed at the time of transradial cardiac catheterization using routine prospective radiobrachial angiography. Cardiovasc Revasc Med. 2018;19:939–43.
9. Gupta S, Nathan S. Radial artery use and reuse. Preserving radial latency after transracial catheterization procedures. Card Interv Today 2015;May/June:49–56.
10. Sgueglia GA, Di Giorgio A, Gaspardone A, Babunashvili A. Anatomic basis and physiological rationale of distal radial artery access for percutaneous coronary and endovascular procedures. JACC Cardiovasc Interv. 2018;11:2113–9.
11. Lee L, Kern J, Blair J, Rosenberg J, Lee M, Nathan S. Routine prospective use of forearm angiography in transradial cardiac catheterization: incidence of radial artery anatomic variants and predictors of procedural success. J Am Coll Cardiol. 2018;71:A1267.
12. Roh JW, Kim Y, Lee OH, Im E, Cho DK, Choi D, et al. The learning curve of the distal radial access for coronary intervention. Sci Rep. 2021;11:13217.
13. Oliveira MD, Navarro EC, Caixeta A. Distal transradial access for coronary procedures: a prospective cohort of 3,683 all-comers patients from the DISTRACTION registry. Cardiovasc Diagn Ther. 2022;12:208–19.
14. Tsigkas G, Papageorgiou A, Moulias A, Kalogeropoulos AP, Papageorgopoulou C, Apostolos A, et al. Distal or traditional transradial access site for coronary procedures: a single-center, randomized study. JACC Cardiovasc Interv. 2022;15:22–32.

7 Conventional Puncture

Sang Yeub Lee and Ian C. Gilchrist

7.1 Introduction

Distal radial access (DRA) has been shown to offer numerous benefits over conventional transradial access (TRA) for patients undergoing catheterization procedures.

Experienced transradial operators may find that there are no significant differences between DRA and conventional TRA, except for the location of the puncture site. This means that operators who are already skilled in TRA should have no trouble adapting to DRA. Meanwhile, femoral operators may appreciate the fact that left DRA offers a similar catheterization approach as femoral access, with the added benefit of being ergonomically favorable.

Given these advantages, it is increasingly clear that DRA should be encouraged as the first-choice access for all patients undergoing catheterization procedures. By adopting DRA as a standard approach, clinicians can help reduce complications, improve patient comfort, and enhance the overall quality of care.

S. Y. Lee
Heart & Brain Hospital, Chung-Ang University Gwangmyeong Medical Center, Gwangmyeong, Republic of Korea

I. C. Gilchrist (✉)
Dartmouth Hitchcock Medical Center, Geisel School of Medicine at Dartmouth, Lebanon, NH, USA

7.2 Patient Assessment

When preparing to perform a DRA procedure, it is important for the operator to conduct a thorough assessment of the radial artery. This assessment should include palpation of the vessel to evaluate the pulse, tortuosity, and size of both the distal and forearm radial arteries [1].

Due to the location of the distal radial artery within the hand anastomotic network, testing for vessel collateralization is not applicable in this case. However, ultrasound imaging can be a useful tool for assessing the diameter of the distal radial artery and its precise location within the adjacent tissues [2–4]. This can help the operator to select an appropriate puncture site and minimize the risk of complications such as arterial spasm or occlusion. In addition to aiding with the assessment of the radial artery, ultrasound can also be helpful in identifying potential alternative access sites in the event of failure (see also Chap. 8).

Overall, a careful and comprehensive assessment of the radial artery is crucial for ensuring the success and safety of a distal radial access procedure. Vessel assessment using palpation and ultrasound can minimize the risk of complications and improve the overall outcome of vascular access.

G. A. Sgueglia (ed.), *Distal Radial Access*, https://doi.org/10.1007/978-3-031-89925-6_7

7.3 Arm and Hand Position

For left-side access, the left hand is typically placed either on the left groin or next to the left hip [1, 5, 6], while for right-side access, the arm is placed along the patient's body in a neutral position with the lateral (radius) side facing upward (see also Chap. 6) [7, 8].

Some operators may choose to place the patient's left upper arm over a pillow and bend the elbow slightly so that the left hand naturally rests on the left groin, which can be a more comfortable position for a number of patients. Additionally, while most operators stand on the patient's right side to perform both right and left DRA, left-handed operators may prefer to stand on the left side when performing left-side access (Fig. 7.1) [9].

In certain emergency situations, such as hemodynamic instability, femoral access may need to be considered as an alternative. However, with DRA procedures, both femoral access sites can easily be made available.

Ultimately, the positioning of the arm and hand should be tailored to the specific access side and the operator's preference (Fig. 7.2) [1, 5, 6].

As adduction favors the upshift of the distal radial artery in the anatomical snuffbox (Fig. 7.3), some operators ask the patient to grasp the thumb under the other four fingers to bring the distal radial artery to the surface of the fossa radialis [1]. An alternative approach is to use a pre-shaped arm board with a plastic mandrel (DRAWS device, Davies Precision Machining) that the patient can grasp to optimize the positioning of the thumb and fingers, as shown in Fig. 7.4.

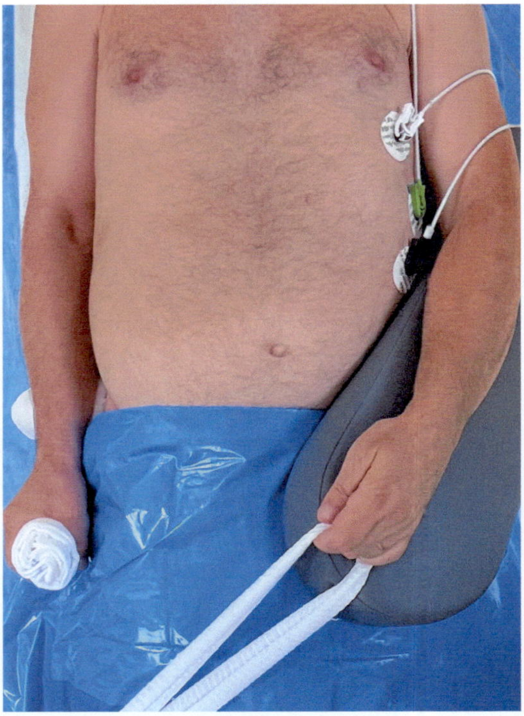

Fig. 7.2 Patient's right- and left-hand position for distal radial access

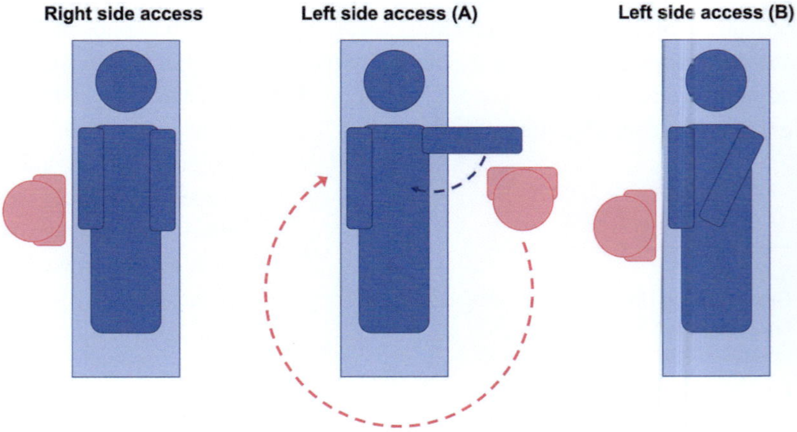

Fig. 7.1 Cath lab and operator setups for right and left distal radial access

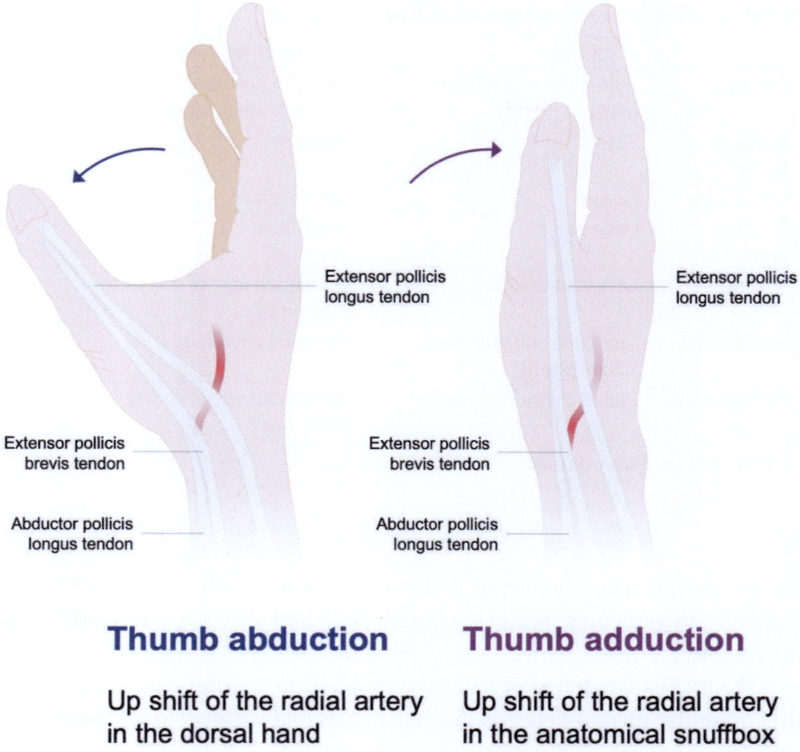

Fig. 7.3 Distal radial artery upshift

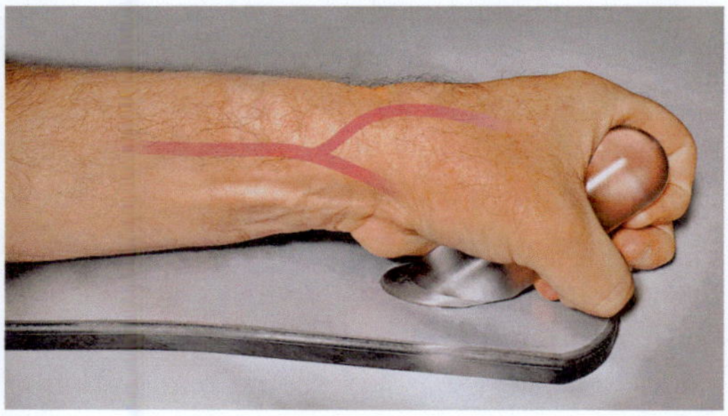

Fig. 7.4 Setup of a dorsal radial positioning board (DRAWS device, Davies Precision Machining, Lebanon, PA). The overlapping red indicates the course of the distal and forearm radial arteries. Note the plastic mandrel for hand grip and the slight medial flexion/lateral extension provided by the angulation of the board to optimize exposure of the region of interest

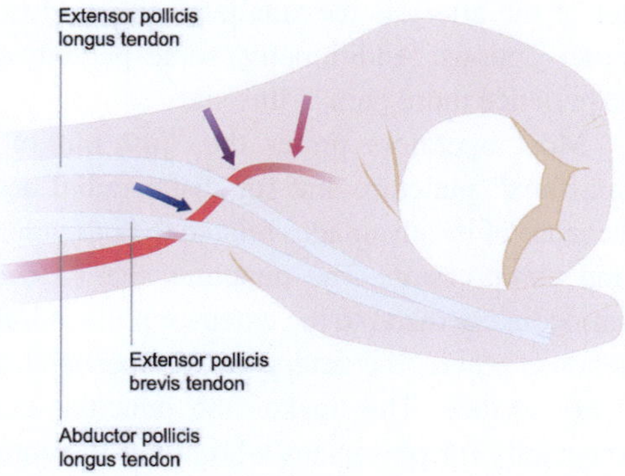

Fig. 7.5 The puncture sites for distal radial access: blue arrow, within the anatomical snuffbox; purple arrow, just outside the anatomical snuffbox; and magenta arrow, far distal radial artery

7.4 Puncture Sites

When performing DRA procedures, operators have three options for puncture: within the anatomical snuffbox, just outside the anatomical snuffbox, and far distal radial artery (Fig. 7.5) [10]. Each option has its own advantages and disadvantages that the operator should consider before making a decision (Table 7.1).

The in-snuffbox puncture site offers the largest vessel size, reducing the risk of arterial spasm during the procedure. Additionally, the potential risk of tendon injury is lower at this site.

Table 7.1 Strength and weakness of each puncture point

	In snuffbox	Just out of the snuffbox	Far distal radial
Location	Within the anatomical snuffbox	Distal to the extensor pollicis longus tendon	Between first and second metacarpal bone
Puncture angle	Sharp	Shallow	Shallow
Vessel size	Larger	Intermediate	Smaller
Puncture depth	Deepest	Superficial	Superficial
Advantage	Less tendon injury	Greater chance of anterior puncture	Less tendon injury
Disadvantage	More difficult guidewire advancement	Potential tendon injury	Potentially more painful
Compression	Radial artery in a groove	Superficial vessel course Bony floor	Lack of bony structure beneath

Courtesy of Dr. Jun-Won Lee

However, the artery is deeper and may be more difficult to puncture, requiring more skill and experience.

The far distal radial artery, located over a leaning muscular surface between the first and second metacarpal bones, is a superficial site that is easily accessible for puncture. However, the diameter of the artery is the smallest compared to the other options. Additionally, some patients may experience more pain at this site.

Most operators prefer the "just out of the snuffbox" puncture site for distal radial access because of its advantages related to both puncture and compression. The puncture site is located immediately distal to the extensor pollicis longus tendon, where the artery runs superficial to a bony surface. This makes the puncture easier, especially for physicians who prefer the anterior wall puncture technique. Compression can also be performed more easily at this site due to the close bone floor underneath.

The choice of puncture site in DRA should be carefully considered based on the individual patient's anatomy and the operator's skill level, by weighing the advantages and disadvantages of each option, to maximize the likelihood of a successful and safe approach.

7.5 Skin Preparation and Local Anesthesia

After disinfection and local anesthesia with lidocaine to prevent pain to surrounding anatomic structures, subcutaneous injection of nitroglycerin at the puncture site may promote radial artery vasodilation and facilitate vessel access. The depth of the infiltration of the numbing agent varies according to the puncture technique and puncture site (shallow in the case of the anterior wall technique of a very superficial artery, deeper in the case of a more profound vessel and of through-and-through technique).

In addition, the superficial course of the dorsal radial artery has led to the exploration of alternative methods for pain relief. One such method is the use of topical anesthetic creams, which can be applied to the skin over the wrist and distal puncture sites at least 30 minutes before the procedure (Fig. 7.6). These creams contain a combination of lidocaine and prilocaine, which work together to numb the skin and reduce pain during the puncture [5]. This can greatly improve patient comfort and satisfaction during the procedure.

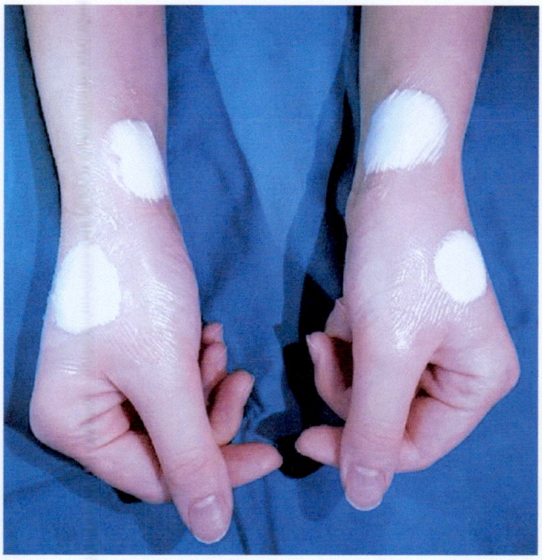

Fig. 7.6 Skin preparation for distal radial access with white topical anesthetic cream applied

7.6 Puncture Technique

At the operator's discretion, a small skin incision may be made to avoid damaging superficial structures before puncture and insertion of the introducer sheath [5].

After pinching the distal radial artery with the fingers of the other hand to minimize its movement, the distal radial artery around the bony surface is punctured with a 20-G venipuncture catheter needle or a 21-G open steel needle at an angle of approximately 30 or 45° according to the puncture site (Fig. 7.7). This technique minimizes periosteal pain from the needle tip and facilitates puncture of the anterior arterial wall [1, 5, 6, 9]. The operator's preference or experience dictates whether a bare access needle or a catheter-covered needle (venipuncture catheter) is used.

In a two-piece needle-and-catheter system, the metal needle is removed, and a straight, flexible 0.025″ plastic guidewire is inserted through the venipuncture catheter. The mini guidewire is advanced carefully into the vessel lumen without force to avoid arterial dissection and perforation. If resistance is felt, the guidewire is retracted and rotated to avoid damaging small arterial branches rising between the puncture site and the forearm radial artery. Adduction of the thumb straightens the radial artery and may reduce the risk of guidewire misdirection. Shaping the tip of the mini guidewire may help overcome the tortuosity of the distal radial artery [3]. If the guidewire does not pass, a 0.018 or 0.014″ guidewire is a suitable alternative.

When using a one-piece bare steel needle system, a through-and-through puncture is usually not recommended to avoid periosteal pain due to the proximity of the bone to the posterior arterial wall. After a successful puncture, a flexible, soft, J-shaped 0.21″ metal wire is inserted. Then, a 4–5-Fr introducer sheath is placed along the wire for diagnostic catheterization; however, 6–7-Fr sheaths are suggested for coronary intervention. If the size of the distal radial artery is less than 2.5 mm [11], a sheathless 6.5-Fr guide catheter (Asahi) or a thin-walled introducer sheath (Glidesheath Slender, Terumo; Prelude IDeal, Merit Medical; RAIN, Cordis) is a good alternative [12].

Administering a spasmolytic agent immediately after placement of the sheath introducer is beneficial to prevent spasm and radial artery occlusion [3].

Once the vascular sheath is in place, the procedure should proceed as for conventional TRA.

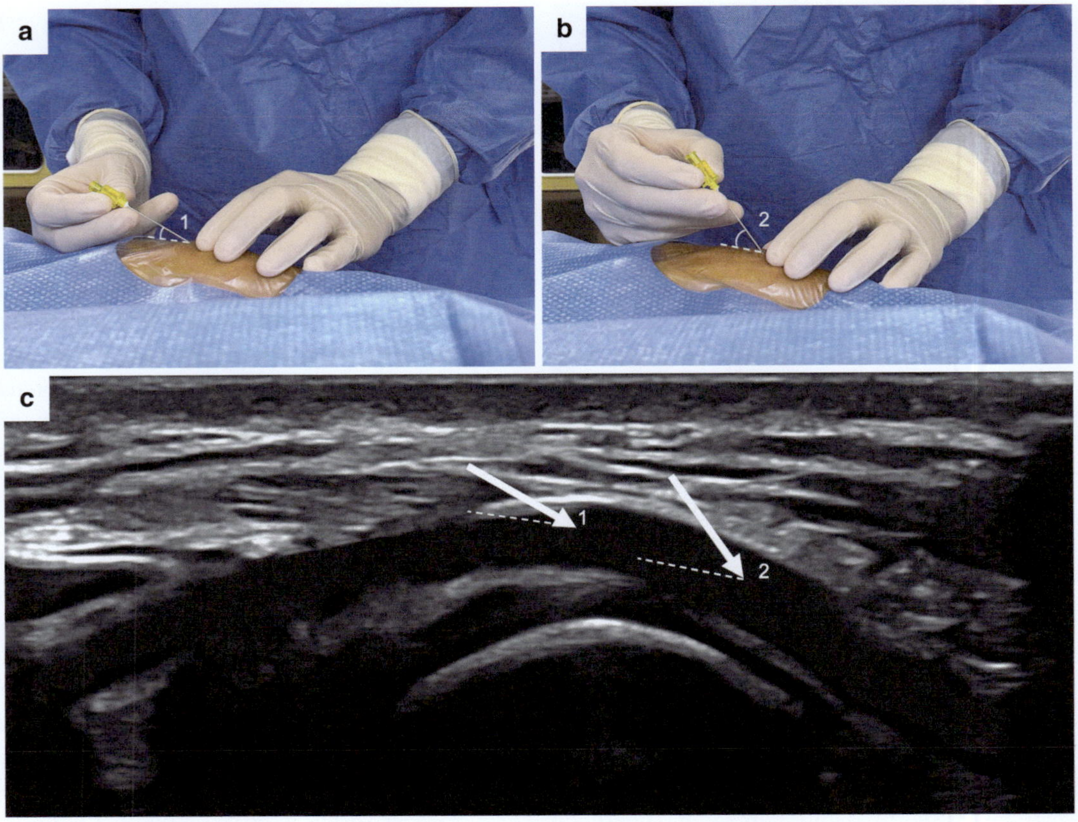

Fig. 7.7 (**a**) Operator position and needle angle (approximately 30°) for distal radial access in the first intermetacarpal space (distal to the extensor pollicis longus tendon). (**b**) Operator position and needle angle (approximately 45°) for distal radial access in the anatomical snuffbox. (**c**) Projection of the needle trajectories on a transverse ultrasound image showing how a different entry angles to the skin (white dashed lines) promotes a better entry angle to the curvilinear artery

7.7 Conclusions

With its many advantages and increasing evidence base, DRA is a safe and effective alternative to conventional TRA. Proper patient selection, adequate training and expertise, and meticulous technique are critical to ensure success and minimize complications. Indeed, familiarity with the anatomical landmarks, careful patient positioning, appropriate use of needles and wires, and administration of spasmolytic agents can all contribute to the success of the puncture for DRA.

References

1. Kiemeneij F. Left distal transradial access in the anatomical snuffbox for coronary angiography (ldTRA) and interventions (ldTRI). EuroIntervention. 2017;13:851–7.
2. Mori S, Hirano K, Yamawaki M, Kobayashi N, Sakamoto Y, Tsutsumi M, et al. A comparative analysis between ultrasound-guided and conventional distal Transradial access for coronary angiography and intervention. J Interv Cardiol. 2020;2020:7342732.
3. Sgueglia GA, Santoliquido A, Gaspardone A, Di Giorgio A. First results of the Distal Radial Access Doppler study. JACC Cardiovasc Imaging. 2021;14:1281–3.

4. Hadjivassiliou A, Kiemeneij F, Nathan S, Klass D. Ultrasound-guided access to the distal radial artery at the anatomical snuffbox for catheter-based vascular interventions: a technical guide. EuroIntervention. 2021;16:1342–8.
5. Lee JW, Park SW, Son JW, Ahn SG, Lee SH. Real-world experience of the left distal transradial approach for coronary angiography and percutaneous coronary intervention: a prospective observational study (LeDRA). EuroIntervention. 2018;14:e995–1003.
6. Kim Y, Ahn Y, Kim I, Lee DH, Kim MC, Sim DS, et al. Feasibility of coronary angiography and percutaneous coronary intervention via left snuffbox approach. Korean Circ J. 2018;48:1120–30.
7. Valsecchi O, Vassileva A, Cereda AF, Canova P, Satogami K, Fiocca L, et al. Early clinical experience with right and left distal transradial access in the anatomical snuffbox in 52 consecutive patients. J Invasive Cardiol. 2018;30:218–23.
8. Ziakas A, Koutouzis M, Didagelos M, Tsiafoutis I, Kouparanis A, Gossios T, et al. Right arm distal transradial (snuffbox) access for coronary catheterization: initial experience. Hell J Cardiol. 2020;61:106–9.
9. Sgueglia GA, Lee BK, Cho BR, Babunashvili A, Lee JB, Lee JW, et al. Distal radial access: consensus report of the first Korea-Europe transradial intervention meeting. JACC Cardiovasc Interv. 2021;14:892–906.
10. Roh JH, Lee JH. Distal radial approach through the anatomical snuff box for coronary angiography and percutaneous coronary intervention. Korean Circ J. 2018;48:1131–4.
11. Lee JW, Son JW, Go TH, Kang DR, Lee SJ, Kim SE, et al. Reference diameter and characteristics of the distal radial artery based on ultrasonographic assessment. Korean J Intern Med. 2022;37:109–18.
12. Gasparini GL, Garbo R, Gagnor A, Oreglia J, Mazzarotto P. First prospective multicentre experience with left distal transradial approach for coronary chronic total occlusion interventions using a 7 Fr Glidesheath Slender. EuroIntervention. 2019;15:126–8.

Ultrasound-Guided Puncture

8

Enrique A. Flores and Darren Klass

8.1 Introduction

The use of ultrasound for vascular access is sporadic outside of radiology, where it is considered the standard of care for vascular access. In fact, in other disciplines, the use of ultrasound for vascular access is often considered cumbersome, expensive, and time-consuming.

However, once an operator is comfortable using ultrasound, the time it takes to gain access is no longer than it takes with palpation, even in emergency situations where time is crucial. A misconception about ultrasound is that it slows the operator down. The benefit to the patient is immeasurable in terms of the number of access attempts, time to access, and failed access [1, 2], and there is no risk to the patient as the operator becomes comfortable with the procedure [3].

E. A. Flores
Georgia Heart Specialists, Conyers, GA, USA

D. Klass (✉)
Cleveland Clinic Lerner College of Medicine of Case Western Reserve University, Cleveland Clinic London, London, UK

8.2 Ultrasound Visualization of the Advantageous Distal Radial Artery Anatomy

The distal segment of the radial artery, which runs between the styloid process of the radius and the soft tissue depression between the thumb and the first index finger, lies superficially just above a row of carpal bones with minimal intervening muscle. Ultrasound imaging of the stylo-scaphoid-trapezium corridor below the distal radial artery trajectory reveals a "bumpy" bony surface floor that curves downward and upward along the trajectory. The distal radial artery above this bony floor also moves up, down, and sideways along the valleys and hills created by the connection between the radius, carpal, and metacarpal bones. This anatomy allows for precise and effective hemostasis by applying a light compressive force to the distal radial artery resting on a firm floor created by the scaphoid and trapezium bones.

In contrast, with conventional transradial access (TRA), there are no superficial horizontal bones at the wrist to apply light pressure against. This is because the anterior surface of the radial bone lies deeper and at an angle relative to the superficial course of the radial artery, with layers of muscle and tendon separating the radial artery from the surface of the radial bone (Fig. 8.1). The greater separation of the radial artery from the anterior surface of the radius bone explains the greater compression force necessary to achieve

G. A. Sgueglia (ed.), *Distal Radial Access*, https://doi.org/10.1007/978-3-031-89925-6_8

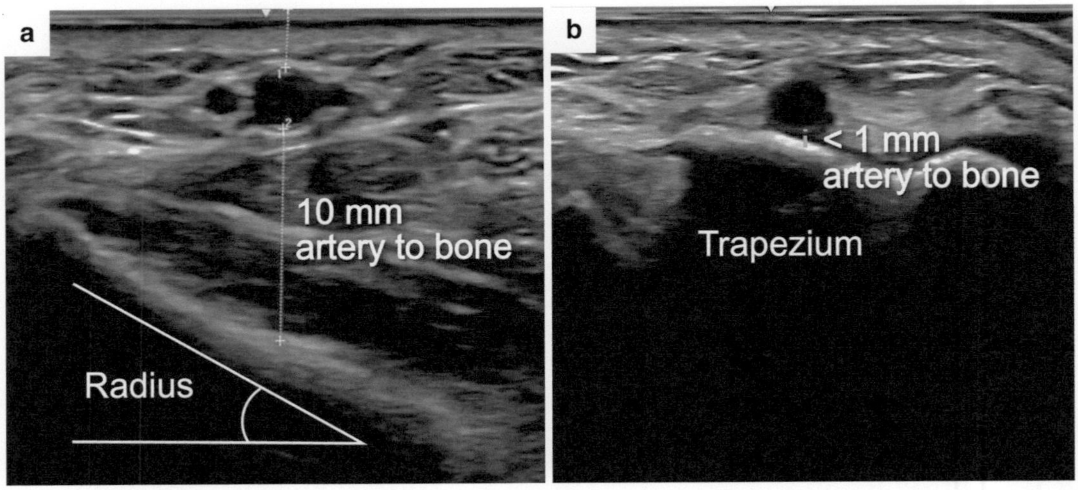

Fig. 8.1 (**a**) Ultrasound images of the radial artery at the wrist in the axial view showing the vessel 10 mm away from the anterior surface of the radius and separated by muscle and soft tissue; in addition, the anterior surface of the radius runs at an angle relative to the radial artery, adding to the challenge of achieving hemostasis. (**b**) The distance of the distal radial artery from the trapezium is ten times less than the distance of the forearm radial artery from the radius

hemostasis of the conventional TRA at the wrist, which is at least twice that required to achieve hemostasis of distal radial access (DRA).

8.3 Challenges of Distal Radial Access

DRA presents more challenges than conventional TRA, which are well addressed with ultrasound guidance.

1. The optimal access site is shorter than for conventional TRA, which means less margin for error. The distal radial artery should be accessed above the carpal bones to ensure good hemostasis, including rapid and light compression, which almost certainly contributes to fewer complications compared to conventional TRA. The vessel, although palpable in the interosseous space of the thumb and the index finger, is not a desirable site for access because there are no bones below to assist in hemostasis, which increases the risk of bleeding.
2. The anatomical snuffbox has three tendons that form its borders; these tendons may be superficial to the distal radial artery, and failure to identify these tendons at the time of puncture may result in pain during the procedure and tendinitis after the procedure. Identification and avoidance of these tendons are essential and can only be reliably done with ultrasound.
3. The distal radial artery is smaller than at the conventional access site in the wrist, and although not clinically significant, this does increase the complexity of access, particularly if palpation is used. Utilizing ultrasound for access improves access rates and decreases the incidence of hematomas [1].
4. The vessel traverses the anatomical snuffbox from medial to lateral, making DRA more challenging than conventional TRA. Needle insertion does not necessarily translate into easy wire passage, as the needle may enter the vessel from lateral to medial, making wire passage suboptimal and leading to loss of access and hematoma formation. Elderly patients, especially women, are prone to osteoarthritis with osteophyte formation, which often leads to displacement of the vessel, further complicating the procedure. Also, older patients are more prone to ectasia and

tortuosity of their vessels. Evaluation with ultrasound shows the path of the radial artery, and the operator can adjust the puncture site or direction of the needle based on the anatomy.

5. The distal radial artery is superficial, and therefore, a small hematoma can compress it enough to make access extremely difficult. Access success decreases with repeated attempts due to hematoma formation, focal dissection, or focal intramural hematoma.
6. The periosteum of the underlying carpal bones is extremely sensitive, and contact with the needle causes discomfort to the patient. Single wall puncture, although not shown to be safer than double wall puncture, eliminates this risk.
7. The overall complexity of access is greater with DRA than with conventional TRA, but the use of ultrasound improves the success rate [4, 5] and mitigates the steep DRA learning curve. This technique is also more likely to be adopted as the risk of conversion to conventional TRA is minimized [6].

8.4 The Physics of Ultrasound

Ultrasound uses high-frequency sound waves to produce images. The sound waves are generated by a transducer (probe), which converts electrical energy into mechanical energy in the form of sound. The sound waves then travel through the body, encountering different types of tissues and reflecting this sound back to the transducer at different speeds depending on the tissue, which converts the returning waves back into an electrical signal. The speed at which the sound returns to the transducer ultimately determines the brightness (echotexture/reflectivity of the tissue on the image).

This is why fat is bright, and flowing blood and fluid are dark, relative to adjacent muscle in the snuffbox. These basic concepts are important to the operator, especially when identifying an acute thrombus or hematoma surrounding the vessel.

The frequency of ultrasound waves used in medical imaging ranges from 2 to 18 MHz. The higher the frequency, the higher the resolution of the image produced. However, high-frequency waves are more easily absorbed by tissue, which can limit their penetration depth. For this reason, vascular access requires a higher-frequency transducer in the range of 9–16 MHz. This provides high-resolution images of the superficial vessel being accessed.

Some important concepts to understand are the properties of sound waves, including reflection, refraction, and attenuation (Fig. 8.2). Reflection occurs when a sound wave encounters a boundary between two tissues with different acoustic impedances, causing some of the energy to be reflected back to the transducer. Refraction occurs when a sound wave passes through a medium with varying density, causing the wave to bend and not necessarily return to the transducer. Attenuation refers to the loss of energy from a sound wave as it passes through a medium. These concepts are responsible for the change in

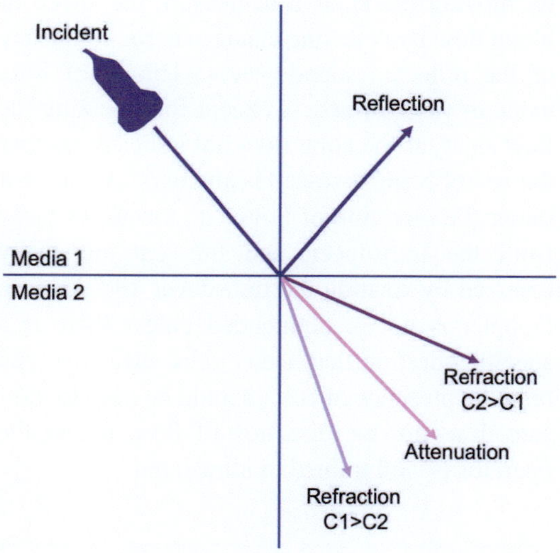

Fig. 8.2 Interaction of ultrasound waves with tissues. When a sound wave encounters a boundary between two tissues with different acoustic impedances, some of the energy is reflected back to the transducer. When an ultrasound wave strikes the interface between two media at an angle other than 90°, the transmitted wave is refracted; when the velocity of an ultrasound wave in media 1 is greater than that in media 2 (C1 > C2), the angle of reflection is decreased, and when the velocity of an ultrasound wave in the media 1 is less than in media 2 (C1 < C2), the angle of reflection is increased. Attenuation refers to the loss of energy from a sound wave as it passes through a medium

image quality due to the position of the transducer on the skin, such as angulation, or poor contact between the skin and transducer, as well as the inherent properties of the tissue itself. For example, air in tissue is a poor conductor of sound and causes severe image degradation. If air is inadvertently introduced into the tissue, image quality can be degraded to the point where a previously identified vessel is no longer visible. This can occur if air is inadvertently injected into the tissue during local anesthetic instillation.

The image produced by an ultrasound machine is created by analyzing the intensity and timing of returning echoes. The echoes are used to create a map of tissue density, which can be displayed as a bidimensional image, which is the most common, also known as B-mode ultrasound. Doppler ultrasound is used to visualize blood flow using the Doppler effect to measure the speed of the flow. The Doppler effect uses the shift in frequency of an ultrasound wave caused by moving blood. It can measure the speed of blood flow by detecting changes in the frequency of the reflected sound waves. This is of little value in vascular access except for assessing the flow itself, as the color does not indicate whether the vessel being assessed is an artery or vein, but rather the direction of flow, i.e., toward or away from the transducer, and this can be easily reversed by rotating the transducer 180 degrees. Doppler is not recommended unless there is a specific question that needs to be answered, and only the presence of color should be used to indicate flow, not the direction of flow, unless the operator is well trained in ultrasound.

8.5 Choosing the Equipment

When deciding on the type of ultrasound system to purchase or rent, there are a number of factors to consider.

1. The type of work the machine will be used for.
2. Ease of mobility of the machine (will the machine remain in one area or will it be moved around).
3. Detail of image required (vascular access only or for diagnostic assessment).
4. Need for documentation of images in the patient's record.

Once these questions have been answered, the decision becomes easier as many of the devices available are designed for vascular access only, with ease of use and portability as the primary considerations.

8.5.1 Procedure Specific Devices

Lumify (Philips) This consists of a transducer, compatible with both Android and iOS platforms, that plugs into a tablet or phone and acts as a screen interface. This system allows any device to be used with the transducer once an app is downloaded. It is then up to the user to decide on the type of transducer to purchase based on the application. This system allows for easy portability and is well suited for point-of-care ultrasound (POCUS).

Butterfly iQ+ (Butterfly Network) This device consists of a wirelessly charged transducer that connects to a tablet or smartphone and includes POCUS features such as needle visualization, which can be helpful for novice users. The system includes multiple presets for specific exams and is portable for use in the procedure room or clinic.

Clarius (Clarius Mobile Health) This portable system is wireless and compatible with both Android and iOS. The transducer houses a rechargeable battery and has a variety of transducer options. The advantage of this device is its wireless design, which can be beneficial in the clinical setting, especially in difficult situations where the placement of the tablet for image assessment is more versatile without a connecting cable. In addition, preparation for procedures is easier as the device can be placed in a bag and left on the table for the duration of a case, which can be helpful in situations where the radial artery requires further assessment.

VScan Air/Extend (GE HealthCare) Vscan Air consists of a wireless dual-headed probe that integrates both curved and linear array transducers and is an app that can be installed on Android or iOS mobile devices. Vscan Extend is a handheld ultrasound imaging system that is wired to a dual-headed probe that integrates both sector and linear transducers. Both of these pocket-sized systems provide real-time blood flow imaging and are particularly useful for interventional guidance.

8.5.2 Versatile Devices

Sonosite (Fujifilm Sonosite) This family of devices includes a range of options for the end user and is more suited to a practice where the device is used for more than vascular access or could potentially be used for other diagnostic testing. The Sonosite SII is specifically designed for a small footprint and can be used in a variety of hospital environments. It has a touch screen but allows the end user to adjust the image and is suitable for users with ultrasound experience.

Acuson Freestyle (Siemens Healthcare) This device was the world's first wireless interventional and point-of-care ultrasound (POCUS) system, allowing scanning up to 3 m from the unit and an easy transition between wireless transducers. This system is purchased with three transducers and is designed to be versatile, not just a single-procedure device. However, if total body vascular access is part of the clinical practice, this option provides the transducers needed for any vascular access site, including a curvilinear transducer for larger femoral access patients.

8.6 Choosing a Transducer

Ultrasound transducers convert electrical energy to acoustic energy and vice versa. Ultrasound transducers vary in construction, frequency range, and applications. The most common types of ultrasound transducers are linear, curvilinear, sector, and phased array.

For vascular access purposes, linear transducers are the most versatile and practical; if ultrasound is used solely for vascular access, a linear transducer is almost sufficient for use. The caveat to this is when femoral access is required as a bailout or for a more complex procedure or when radial access is not possible. In these cases, the patient's body habitus may preclude the use of a linear transducer due to the lack of adequate tissue penetration, and the use of a lower-frequency curved transducer, typically used for abdominal imaging, may be required.

Linear transducers have a straight probe and are primarily used for superficial imaging. They have a high frequency range (9–16 MHz) and provide good resolution but are limited in their ability to image deeper tissues and are therefore limited in femoral access in larger patients.

Curvilinear transducers have a curved probe and are used for obstetrical, gynecological, and abdominal imaging. They have a moderate frequency range (1–6 MHz) and provide a wider field of view than linear transducers. This may be necessary for larger patients for femoral access, but it is important to remember that deeper penetration also means lower resolution and therefore lower image quality.

Sector transducers have a wedge-shaped probe and are used for cardiac applications. They have a low frequency range, providing good depth penetration but lower resolution.

Phased array transducers consist of multiple individual elements that can be activated individually to produce a focused beam in any direction. Used primarily for deep tissue imaging, they provide excellent resolution but have a limited field of view and are not required for vascular access.

8.7 Scanning Technique

Before scanning, ultrasound gel should be applied liberally to the skin; the gel acts as a sound conductor, so the better the contact, the better the image. If there is poor contact on the skin, the image is degraded and often leads to difficulty in interpretation. The gel is water soluble and will not block the needle during puncture.

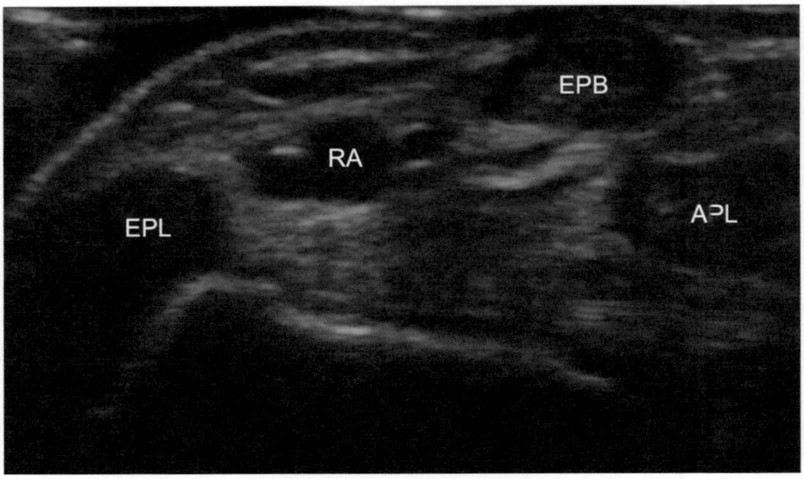

Fig. 8.3 Ultrasound image showing the extensor and abductor pollicis tendons forming the borders of the anatomical snuffbox and the radial artery. *APL* abductor pollicis longus tendon, *EPB* extensor pollicis brevis, *EPL* extensor pollicis longus tendon

The transducer should be held lightly against the skin, making sure to maintain good contact with the gel. If too much downward pressure is applied, the vessel will be compressed, and structures will be distorted, ultimately making the puncture difficult, if not impossible. This is especially important in patients with low cardiac output, where even very light pressure can result in vessel compression (Fig. 8.3).

Probe orientation is critical: if the probe is incorrect, any lateral movement on the screen will be opposite to the direction of movement on the skin, making the puncture extremely difficult. If the operator is familiar with the anatomy and comfortable with ultrasound, this can be done by moving the transducer from medial to lateral and assessing the movement of the structures to determine the correct orientation. If the operator is new or unfamiliar with the anatomy, the simplest technique is to tap the plate and watch the screen to determine which side of the probe corresponds to which side of the screen. If the left side of the probe is tapped, it should correspond to the left side of the screen; if not, the probe must be rotated 180°.

The initial image obtained at the start of the scan must be optimized for good visualization. The distal radial artery is superficial, and therefore, the amount of penetration should be adjusted accordingly to maximize the radial artery in the image and remove the deeper structures 1 cm deeper into the underlying cortical bone. This is done by adjusting the depth (penetration of the sound into the tissue). The depth should be decreased to a point where the artery is in the near field (closest to the transducer). The focus of the image (the point where the ultrasound beam is maximized in the image) can also be changed so that the ultrasound beam is focused on the radial artery. The focus is shown as a small triangle on the side of the screen and can be moved to be in the near field (close to the transducer) or far field (farther from the transducer). For DRA, the focus will always be on the near field. The next parameter to adjust is the gain (brightness of the image); increasing the gain will produce a brighter (whiter) image. This is not always desirable, as if the image is too bright, structures may be obscured. Many ultrasound machines have an auto gain option and can be adjusted at any time during the procedure; depth and focus must be adjusted manually.

8.8 Planning Distal Radial Access with Ultrasound

Performing arterial ultrasound imaging of the six available arterial access sites in the arms (left-right distal radial arteries, forearm radial arteries, and ulnar arteries) in the office, cardiac observation unit, or catheterization laboratory prior to preparation and draping to select the optimal access will improve procedural efficiency and

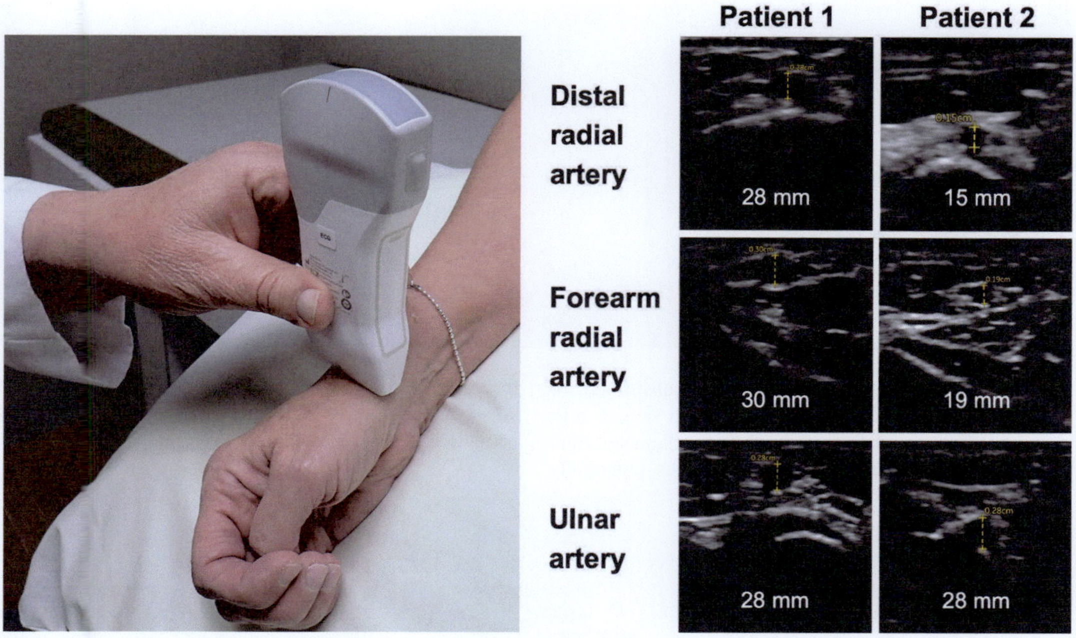

Fig. 8.4 Ultrasound information to help select the optimal arterial access for the planned procedure. In patient 1, the diameter of both the distal and forearm radial artery and the ulnar artery is similar in diameter, making the distal radial artery the most attractive arterial access option. In contrast, patient 2 has a small, diameter distal radial artery, a slightly larger right forearm radial artery, and an even larger ulnar artery

hospital throughput (Fig. 8.4). A detailed assessment of the forearm radial artery can be performed until it is seen to join the brachial artery at the level of the elbow [7]. The vessel can be assessed for size, patency, and the presence of a radial loop. This can help guide device selection, and different wires and catheters can be selected if a known radial loop must be crossed. This may be performed in lieu of a radial angiogram. The additional time and effort required for ultrasound-guided planning will help the operator identify the most appropriate artery for cannulation and avoid sheath-to-artery mismatch, which could result in radial artery occlusion (RAO). Ultrasound imaging of all six options in advance will also help identify the best crossover site in the event of an index access failure.

Current ultrasound devices can provide the percentage of the vessel occupied by the selected sheath by manually measuring the vessel diameter. For example, a 6-Fr sheath occupies 80% of a 2.3-mm-diameter DRA (Fig. 8.5).

There are several options for DRA puncture along the scaphoid and trapezium bone corridors (Fig. 8.6). The best site for needle puncture is generally where the artery is the largest in caliber, superficial, with little soft tissue but a nearly straight bony floor below, and at a location with the least amount of atherosclerotic plaque in the vessel wall.

One author's preferred DRA puncture site is above the trapezium bone. At this site, the DRA is closest to the supporting bone below and closest to the skin above (Fig. 8.7). In this location, the trapezium and the DRA are superficial so that the artery rests on a nearly flat or convex surface of the bone. A line can be drawn across the wrist with a demographic marker to indicate the separation of the carpal and metacarpal bones (Fig. 8.8). This is most easily done along the side of the operator's finger perpendicular to the anatomical snuffbox.

The second DRA puncture site is proximal to the carpal-metacarpal separation line, at the true snuffbox space over the scaphoid. Here, the DRA is deeper from the skin and lies in a more irregular, slightly more difficult space to puncture compared to the trapezium site (Fig. 8.9). At this most

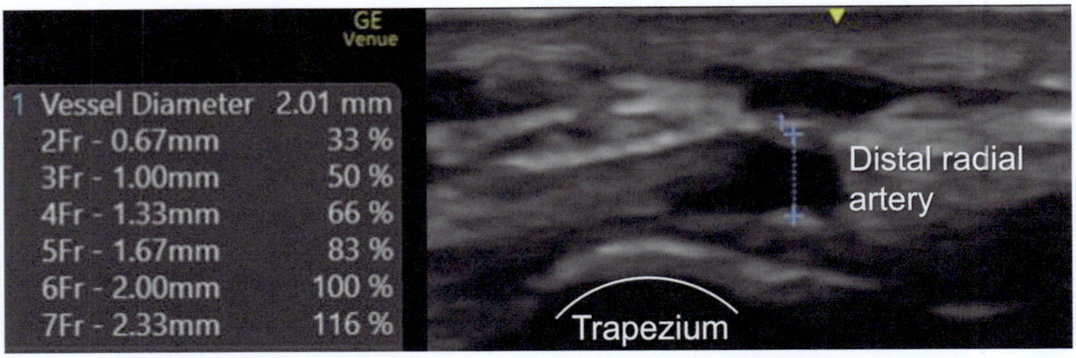

Fig. 8.5 Sheath-to-artery ratio could be substituted for the vessel diameter occupied by the sheath size. A 6-Fr sheath will occupy 100% of the 2.0-mm-diameter right distal radial artery of this patient and thus potentially increase the risk of radial artery occlusion. If diagnostic angiography without intervention is anticipated in this patient, a 5-Fr sheath should be preferred

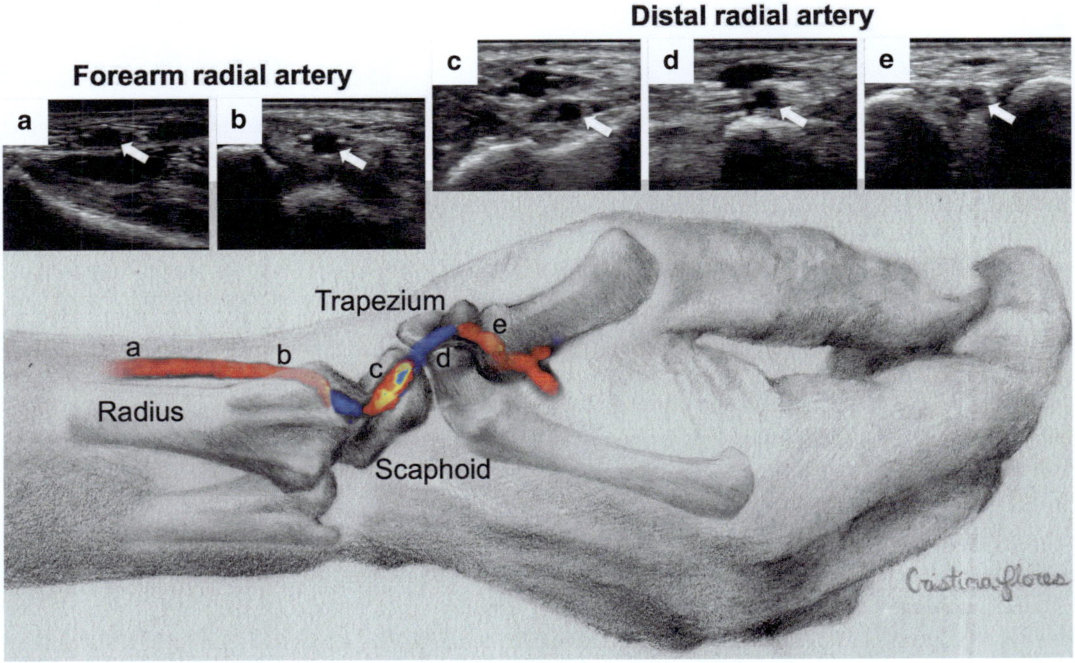

Fig. 8.6 (**a**, **b**) Ultrasound imaging of the forearm radial artery. (**c–e**) Ultrasound imaging of the distal radial artery of the right hand in the axial (cross-sectional) plane (top, grayscale) and in the longitudinal plane (bottom, color Doppler). The radial artery passes over the radius (**a**), and the distal radial artery dips and gets close to the scaphoid (**c**) before turning up again to go over the trapezium bone (**d**) and then turns down between the first and second metacarpal bones (**e**); note the lack of soft tissue underneath the distal radial artery and its proximity to the bone

proximal entry site, the DRA has already branched to the hand, so an undesirable vessel occlusion here avoids causing hand ischemia [8].

The third site is more distal, at the first intermetacarpal space, just before the DRA dives anteriorly into the hand, between the first and second metacarpal bones (Fig. 8.10). This is also the preferred reentry site if occlusive DRA dissection occurs when attempting to access the more proximal trapezium or scaphoid sites.

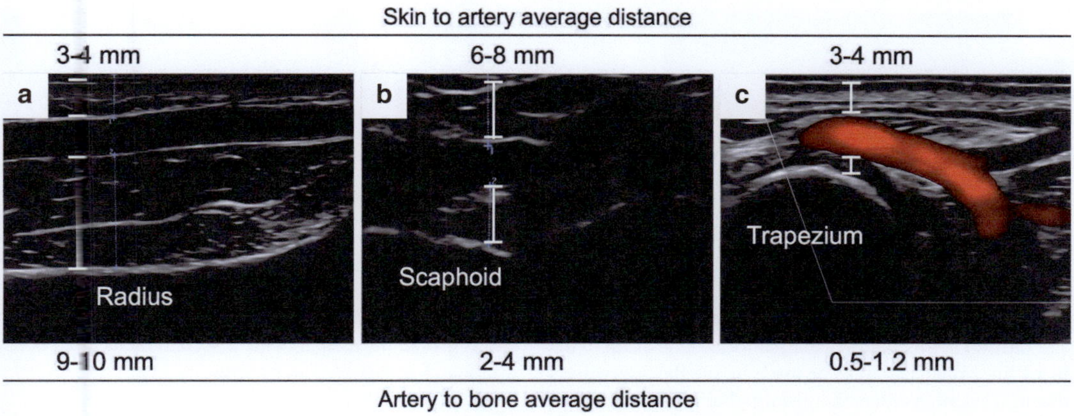

Fig. 8.7 (**a**) The forearm radial artery is ten times farther from the radius than the distal radial artery at the trapezium. (**b**) The distal radial access at the scaphoid is twice as far from both the skin and the bone compared to the distal radial access at the trapezium. (**c**) The distal radial artery (red) at the trapezium is the ideal puncture site because it is closest to the supporting bone (<1.2 mm)

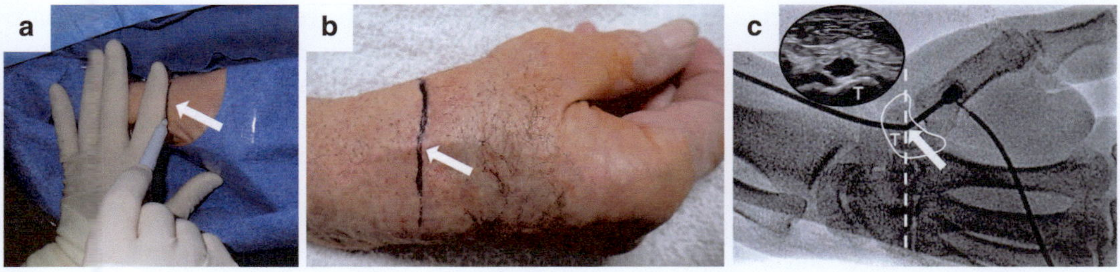

Fig. 8.8 The preferred distal radial artery puncture site (arrow) is above the trapezium. (**a**, **b**) The axial plane of the distal radial artery at the trapezium is marked by a black line drawn across the wrist separating the carpal (left of line) from the metacarpal (right of line) bones. (**c**) Radiographic image shows the sheath entry site (arrow) in the distal radial artery above the trapezium; the dotted white line corresponds to the black line drawn on the skin; in the inset, the axial ultrasound view of the distal radial artery shows the optimal puncture site above the trapezium bone. *T* trapezium

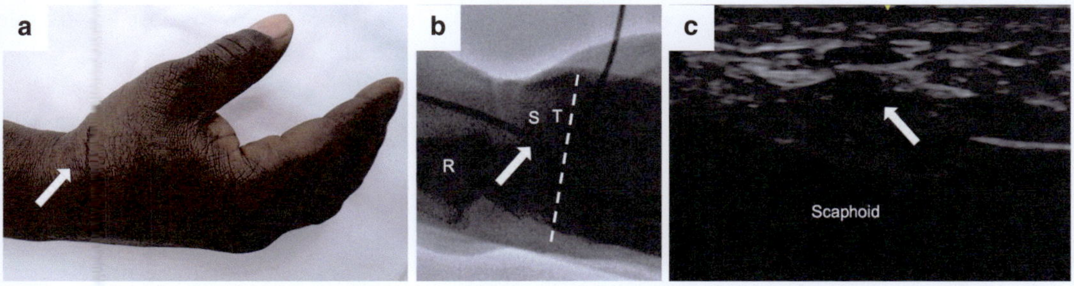

Fig. 8.9 (**a**) Distal radial artery puncture site at the anatomical snuffbox (arrow) is proximal to the black line separating the carpal bones from the metacarpal bones. (**b**) The radioscopic image shows the sheath entering the distal radial artery at the scaphoid, proximal to the separation line. (**c**) The ultrasound image shows the axial view of the distal radial artery (arrow) above the scaphoid. The sheath at the snuffbox site often enters the artery at a steep angle due to the depth and small compartment size and could kink, especially in patients with protuberant metacarpal bones; also note the more abundant soft tissue between the distal radial artery and the scaphoid. *R* radius, *S* scaphoid, *T* trapezium

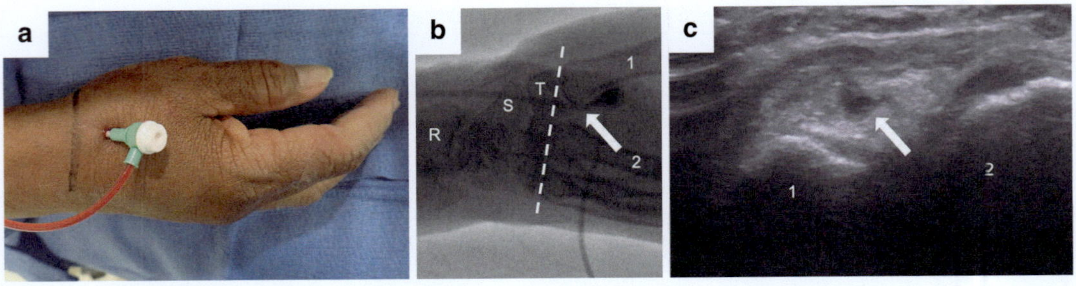

Fig. 8.10 (**a**, **b**) The third distal radial artery puncture site (arrow) at this intermetacarpal location is distal to the black line drawn and must be made before the artery dives down. (**c**) demonstrates the distal radial artery (arrow) in the intercarpal space, just before entering the interosseous space. *1* first metacarpal bone, *2* second metacarpal bone, *R* radius, *S* scaphoid, *T* trapezium

8.9 Ultrasound Assessment

It is important to have a structured, methodical approach to accessing the radial artery in the snuffbox. The scan should begin as distally as necessary to facilitate the identification of key landmarks. The snuffbox contains arteries, veins, and tendons that all need to be identified, and it is often easier to start more distally than proximally (Fig. 8.11). Assessment should begin in the first dorsal intermetacarpal space between the thumb and the index finger, which contains the first dorsal interosseous muscle. If the vessel is very small or the patient has poor cardiac output, a subcutaneous injection of nitroglycerin will aid with vasodilation and facilitate assessment of the vessel. It is recommended that a Doppler assessment be performed to confirm vessel patency, especially in patients with previous radial artery access or poor output. Thrombosed radial arteries may appear patent if the thrombus is of low reflectivity, and although a thrombosed vessel does not preclude puncture, it is important for the operator to be aware of this prior to puncture and to have a very clear image of the needle in the vessel prior to wire advancement to reduce the risk of dissection. A good understanding of the structures in the snuffbox is essential. The boundaries of the anatomical snuffbox should be identified as the three tendons of the thumb. Tendons appear as well-defined structures of intermediate shades on the grayscale image. They may appear round and contain very small bright dots corresponding to the tendon fibers on the axial image. These must be identified and avoided, as accidental puncture is painful for the patient and can lead to postoperative tendinitis. The superficial branches of the radial nerve run in the roof of the snuffbox and can be visualized with ultrahigh-frequency ultrasound. These do not appear to cause any trouble when punctured.

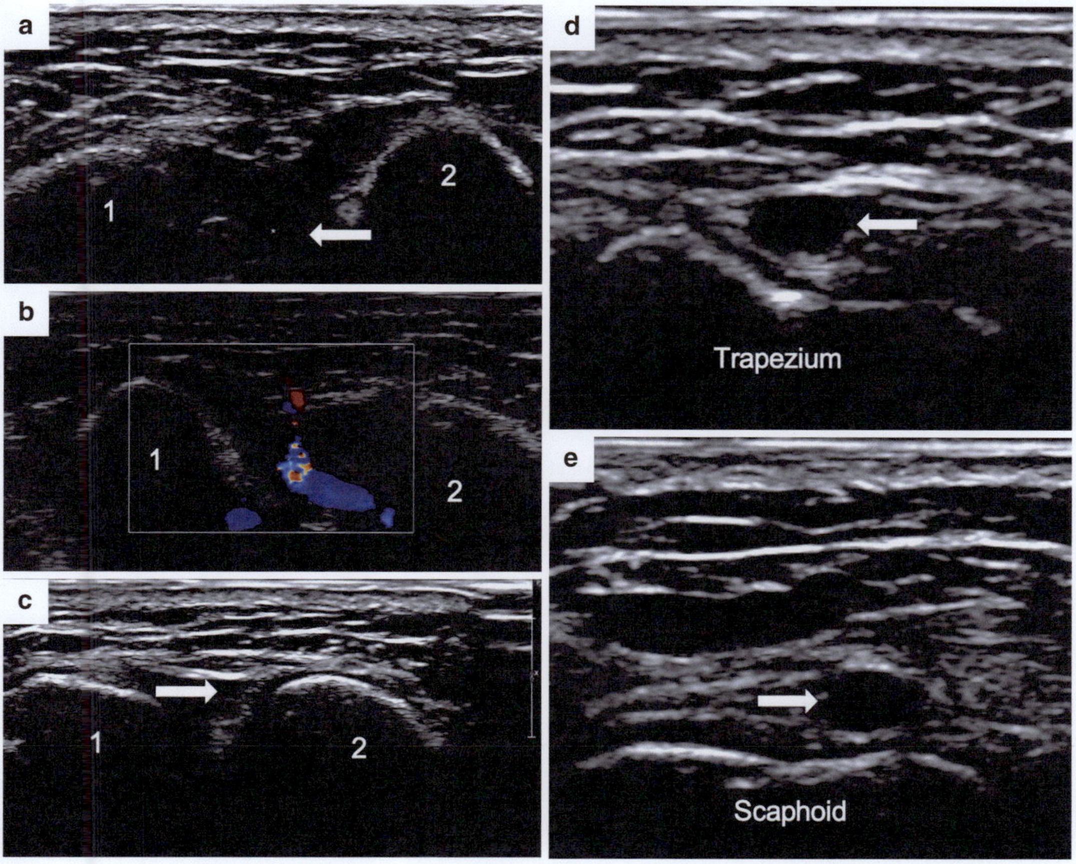

Fig. 8.11 (**a**) In the first intermetacarpal space, the distal radial artery is palpable but is deep (arrow), and hemostasis is difficult in this location. (**b**) Color vascular ultrasound showing flow in the deep distal radial artery and a small princeps pollicis artery above it (the box on the image is generated using Doppler and is the defined region of interest, which can be manually adjusted). (**c**) The distal radial artery (arrow) is superficial over the bases of the thumb and index finger metacarpals, but the bones are prone to osteoarthritis and osteophytes at this site which can distort the vessel path (note that the focus marked X on the right side of the picture is optimized for the depth of the tissue being visualized and centered on the vessel). (**d**) Distal artery over the trapezium. (**e**) Distal artery over the scaphoid is superficial, and both bones are flat and ideal for hemostasis. *1* first metacarpal bone, *2* second metacarpal bone

8.10 Subcutaneous Anesthesia

Once a satisfactory puncture site has been selected, the skin should be infiltrated with local anesthetic solution. Many operators choose different amounts to inject. The amount of lidocaine required is typically 1–2 mL, except when the DRA is very close to the skin. In such cases, more lidocaine is infiltrated into the subcutaneous tissue to increase the separation space between the skin and the DRA, thus facilitating ultrasound visualization of the puncture needle as it moves down and reaches the target entry site. If the operator is less experienced with ultrasound and there is a higher likelihood of a double wall puncture or the needle touching the periosteum during attempts to puncture the vessel, more solution is recommended. Actually, 5–10 mL is recommended to anesthetize the periosteum deep into the vessel as accidental contact can cause significant pain. It is preferable and safer to perform the deeper infiltration under ultrasound guidance to avoid patient discomfort and inadvertent arterial puncture. This allows the operator

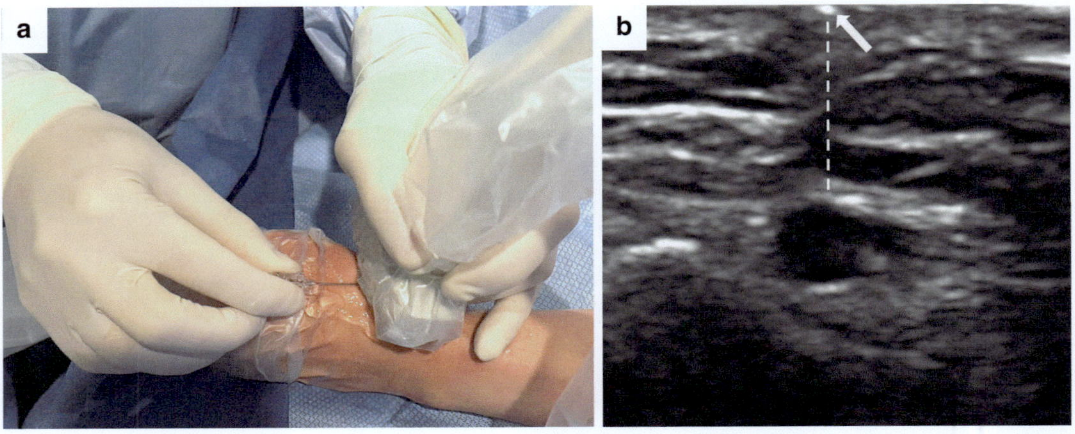

Fig. 8.12 (**a**, **b**) By placing the needle flat on the skin and the ultrasound probe over it, a shadow (dotted line) is created by the needle, which can then be moved manually from side to side until it is over the vessel, and this site is used for puncture; the needle itself can be seen as a bright dot (arrow)

to deliver the solution in a methodical manner and ensure that the vessel is surrounded by local anesthetic. Due to the superficial nature of the artery and the shallow bottom of the snuffbox, it is important to remember that a large infusion of anesthetic solution could be misinterpreted as a hematoma by post-procedural care staff in relatively short procedures where the solution has not had sufficient time to absorb.

8.11 Arterial Puncture

The arm should be in a pronated position. The radial artery is best accessed with a 21-G needle using a single wall puncture technique, which is preferred for DRA as it causes no trauma to the periosteum and can be easily performed using ultrasound [7]. To ensure that the skin entry site is directly over the vessel, a useful technique is to place the needle flat on the skin with the transducer over it and move it from side to side until the needle is directly over the vessel (Fig. 8.12). This can be seen on the ultrasound image as the needle will cast an acoustic shadow directly below it on the image. This shadow should then fall directly over the vessel. At this point on the skin, the needle should then be raised and angled in preparation for the puncture. The needle should be angled from an ulnar to a radial direction, approximately 30° to the radial artery in the horizontal plane and 45–60° in the vertical plane (Fig. 8.13). This steep puncture is used for two reasons: (1) to ensure that the skin entry site is over the arterial puncture site, which makes the ultrasound-guided puncture more reliable and eliminates the need to move the probe as the needle passes through the tissue in the artery, and (2)

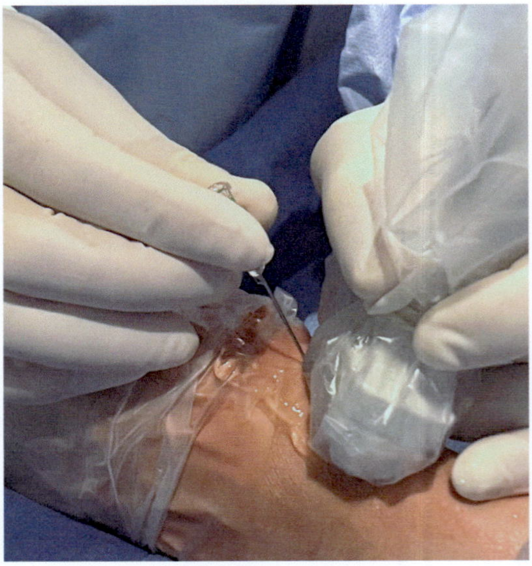

Fig. 8.13 Steep angle used for puncture to ensure that the skin entry site is over the arterial puncture site. Note that the operator's little finger is placed on the patient's arm to support the weight of the probe so as not to exert too much pressure on the vessel and compress it

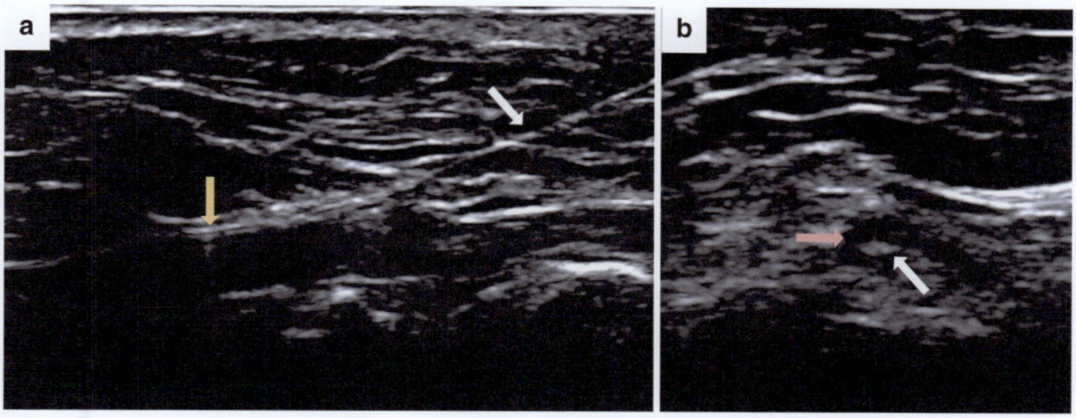

Fig. 8.14 (**a**) Longitudinal puncture in which the needle remains in plane throughout. The hollow needle is well visualized (white arrows), along the wire exiting the needle tip and advancing into the vessel (yellow arrow). (**b**) Transverse puncture with the out-of-plane needle tip as the only visualized part of the needle (white arrow) in the vessel (orange arrow)

to aid in good placement of the hemostasis device after the procedure.

The puncture can be performed in either the longitudinal or axial plane (Fig. 8.14). In the longitudinal plane, the entire length of the needle can be visualized through the subcutaneous tissue into the vessel.

This is called in-plane imaging because the needle is continuously positioned within the ultrasound beam. This is preferred by many operators but requires more skill and experience with ultrasound, as the needle must remain perfectly in the beam at all times to ensure that the tip is always visualized. Once operators have mastered this technique, many prefer it to the transverse or axial technique.

The alternative technique (out-of-plane imaging) images the vessel in the axial (cross-sectional) plane. This allows the operator more latitude in needle positioning as the needle passes through the wide part of the beam, but because the needle is perpendicular to the ultrasound beam, only the part that passes through the beam can be visualized. The operator must understand the limitations of this technique and ensure that the tip of the needle is always visible. To master this technique, the probe must be manipulated on its short axis to allow the needle tip to flow into the vessel without physically changing its position on the skin.

Ultrasound imaging of the DRA at the puncture site should show the needle entering the artery at the optimal 12 o'clock position (Fig. 8.15). The needle tip should make an indentation in the vessel wall before entering the true lumen. The pressure of the ultrasound probe against the artery should be reduced at the time of the needle artery puncture to allow a larger vessel diameter by decompression of the lumen and free passage of the needle wire into the artery. Entering the DRA at 12 o'clock with direct ultrasound visualization almost guarantees that the needle wire will advance freely into the distal radial artery.

A common operator error is to move the needle and the ultrasound probe simultaneously. This can be very confusing to the operator and should be avoided. Once an appropriate arterial access site has been selected, the probe should not be moved from its position on the skin but should be manipulated in the same position by angling the probe in its short or long axis. While stationary, the probe can be tilted on either its long axis (heel-toe movement) or short axis (toggle movement) to locate the needle tip. The most common movement for tip location is the toggle movement for both longitudinal and axial access techniques.

Moving the probe along the length of the vessel to locate the needle tip often results in punc-

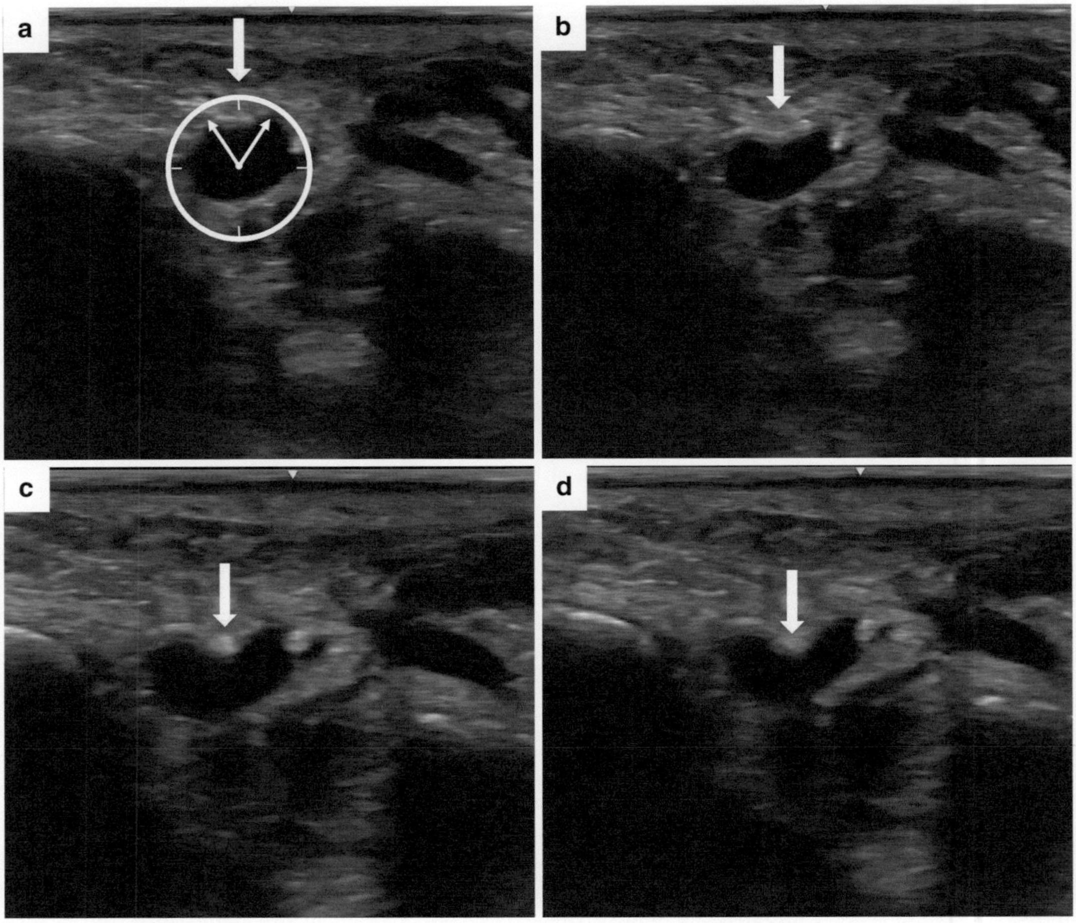

Fig. 8.15 (**a**) Ultrasound images of the distal radial artery in the axial (cross-sectional) plane showing needle entry at the optimal "12 o'clock" mark. (**b–d**) Arrow showing the gradual entry of the 21-G needle in the distal radial artery; needle puncture at any other site could result in puncture failure due to vessel dissection and trauma after entry of the needle wire into the subintimal space

turing the vessel where the needle tip is located, rather than at the desired puncture site above the carpal bones.

Learning to coordinate perfect alignment between the ultrasound transducer beam and the moving needle can be frustrating, but this frustration is overcome with practice. Having a midline mark on the transducer probe that matches a midline on the ultrasound screen can help.

The intravascular position is confirmed when the needle position is satisfactory on the ultrasound image and blood is seen with a steady trickle or steady pulsatile flow through the hub. The amount of blood flow from the needle hub is often related to the position of the needle tip. At a minimum, there should be a steady trickle of blood from the hub; if this is not present, the needle is probably not truly intravascular and may be against the side wall of the vessel. It is important not only to watch the screen for needle tip position but also to watch the hub for blood flow. It is not uncommon in early experience to watch the needle on the vessel wall and lose the tip as it enters the vessel and searches the screen for the tip without looking at the hub with free-flowing blood. Once in a satisfactory position, the needle should be held securely and the ultrasound probe released.

The wire used can affect the ease of advancement through the vessel. Soft spring-coiled wires have a higher incidence of failure because they provide no support for the sheath as it passes over the radial styloid. A stainless steel–reinforced wire provides support for the sheath and is much easier to advance through the vessel.

The backflow of blood in the needle hub does not guarantee the intraluminal placement of the needle tip. Resistance encountered when advancing the wire into the distal radial artery should be interpreted as unsuccessful access, unless overcome by gentle rotation and manipulation of the needle while gently probing with the wire, leading to its subsequent unopposed entry into the distal radial artery, ideally confirmed by ultrasound in the longitudinal plane. If resistance to advancement of the needle wire persists, the needle and wire should be removed and finger compression applied until the site ceases to bleed. Re-puncture should be attempted at a more distal or proximal site in the carpal corridor.

In some cases, the bevel may be against the back or side wall, preventing the wire from advancing. The needle angle can also be adjusted if the rotation of the bevel does not allow the wire to pass easily. This may occur when a lateral to medial puncture is made. If resistance is noted as the wire exits the needle, this may be due to the wire advancing into the superficial palmar branch; ultrasound can then be used to assess the wire position. If the puncture is made distal to the anatomical snuffbox, over the base of the metacarpals, or in the first intermetacarpal space, the wire may track into a lateral branch of the deep palmar arch. If this occurs, adduction of the thumb will straighten the artery and reduce the chance of wire misdirection. Occasionally, extreme tortuosity of the distal radial artery or osteoarthritis can create uncomfortable resistance to wire advancement. When this occurs and intraluminal positioning of the wire cannot be confirmed with ultrasound, crossover to conventional TRA may be considered.

Once the wire is advanced, the volar aspect of the wrist should be assessed with ultrasound to confirm the correct position of the wire in the forearm radial artery prior to sheath insertion. Alternatively, fluoroscopy may be used to confirm wire position, depending on operator preference. Once the needle wire is certainly in the radial artery lumen, the sheath is inserted. The operator can maintain a 30-degree separation angle of the sheath relative to the skin by placing a rolled gauze under the sheath.

8.12 Tips for Successful Ultrasound-Guided Distal Radial Access

1. Novice ultrasound users may benefit from practicing cannulation in a gel phantom block to master vessel puncture under ultrasound visualization (Fig. 8.16). Ultrasound training block models are readily available for purchase online.

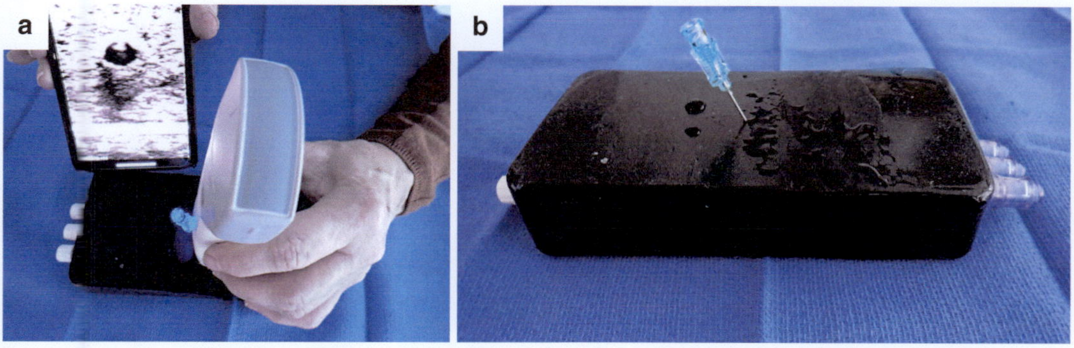

Fig. 8.16 Beginners can practice ultrasound-guided needle puncture using a commercially available gel phantom block model

2. Locate the optimal site for the distal radial artery puncture by asking the patient to place their hand (right or left) in a straight prone position as if holding a drink. Any tilting of the hand that could "spill the drink" could alter the familiar bony landmarks and result in delayed or inadvertent arterial puncture outside the distal radial artery corridor. Drawing a line along the separation between the carpal and metacarpal bones, as described earlier, is beneficial in finding the optimal distal radial artery puncture site with ultrasound (Fig. 8.8). This is especially helpful when access is needed quickly and efficiently, such as in patients with ST-elevation myocardial infarction.
3. The needle tip with the bevel up should enter the distal radial artery between 11 and 1 o'clock on the vessel wall, but ideally at 12 o'clock. The needle tip should create an indentation or notch at the edge of the vessel wall as it approaches the arterial wall as seen by ultrasound (Fig. 8.15c, d).
4. If the needle wire does not advance freely despite good blood return, do not push because the wire is likely subintimal and the distal radial artery is likely dissected. A linear red thrombus often adheres to the needle wire when it is withdrawn. Distal radial artery cannulation in the true lumen is still possible in the same hand by puncturing with ultrasound at the site of dissection if a rounded residual central lumen with color flow is still present (Fig. 8.17e). The arterial dissection is seen as "onion rings" on ultrasound imaging with occasional color Doppler flow in the remaining central lumen (Figs. 8.17f and 8.18). Subsequent access more distal to the initial puncture site, at the first intermetacarpal space, is often effective in cannulating the distal radial artery, and the needle wire will cross the dissection and remain in the true lumen without adverse consequences (Fig. 8.17i).
5. If the puncture needle is seen crossing vertically along the distal radial artery without imprinting the 12 o'clock notch in the vessel wall, the needle tip is extraluminal, and the puncture attempt will be unsuccessful. This "phantom puncture" sign means that the needle is outside the lumen, anterior or posterior to the intended puncture site. Puncture failure occurs due to the tortuosity and natural angulation of the distal radial artery. By tilting the ultrasound transducer downward, the artery will generally appear slightly deeper in the field of view and is likely to allow good alignment between the transducer and the needle tip to facilitate entry into the distal radial artery at the intended site. This phantom effect does not occur when puncturing the radial artery at the wrist because the artery is straight at this site with no angulation (Fig. 8.18).
6. If the distal radial artery is very close to the skin, infiltration of lidocaine at the puncture site will separate the distal radial artery from the skin, allowing more space for the needle tip to be seen on ultrasound imaging as it is directed toward the vessel wall for entry at the 12 o'clock mark.

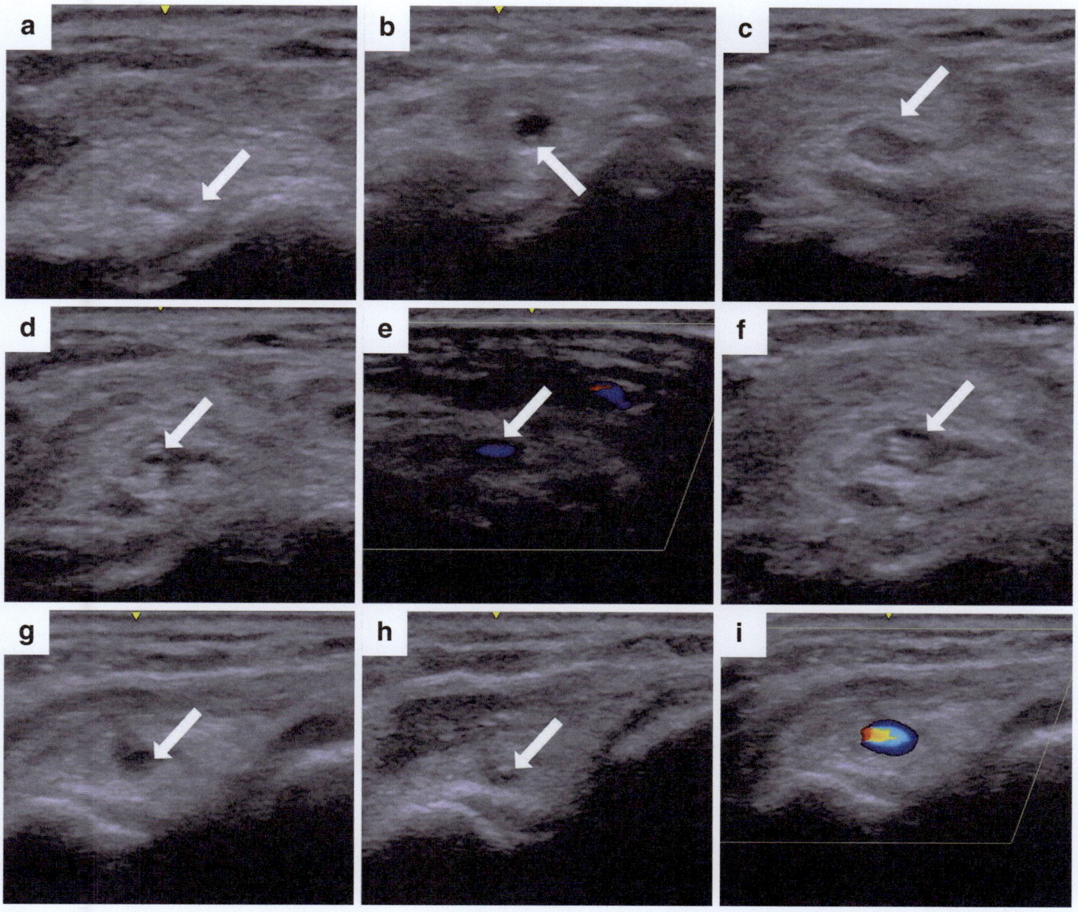

Fig. 8.17 Ultrasound images of distal radial artery dissection at the trapezium puncture site and subsequent successful vessel re-cannulation after reentering the artery more distally at the intermetacarpal space. (**a**) The needle tip (arrow) enters the distal radial artery outside the 11–1 o'clock mark. (**b**) The needle wire (arrow) entering the subintimal space. (**c**) Haziness in the distal radial artery occurs due to thrombus formation. (**d**, **e**) The dissected distal radial artery shows multiple vessel wall layers and a small central lumen. (**f**) The dissected DRA shows the "onion ring sign" with multiple layers of echo lucent confluent lines like an onion split in half. (**g**) Re-puncture of the distal radial artery more distally, at the intermetacarpal space. (**h**) Optimal intraluminal positioning of the wire. (**i**) Normal color Doppler flow in the distal radial artery before discharge

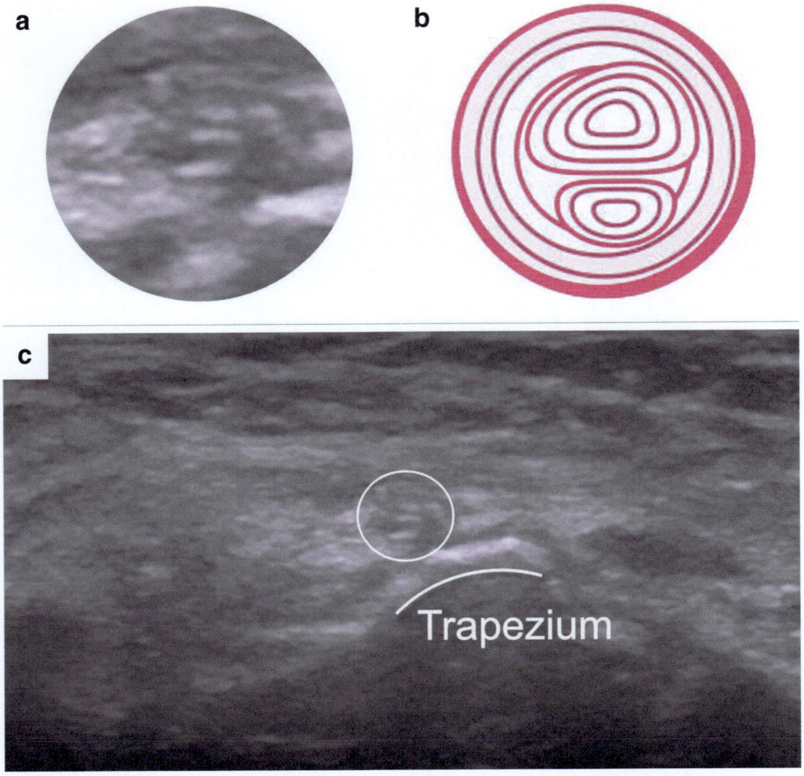

Fig. 8.18 (**a**, **b**) The "onion ring sign" in an axial ultrasound view of the distal radial, with multiple confluent echogenic lines and loss of the true arterial lumen, reflects the appearance of an onion cut cross-sectionally. (**c**) Dissection of the distal radial artery occurred above the trapezium, and successful reentry of the wire into the true lumen was achieved after puncturing the artery at the first intermetacarpal space

8.13 Conclusions

Ultrasound imaging of the distal radial artery above the carpal bones facilitates vascular puncture at the anatomical segment that is ideal for hemostasis. The distal radial artery over the trapezium in the hand as seen by ultrasound is the optimal access site due to its proximity to the bone below and the short distance to the skin above. In comparison, the conventional TRA at the wrist is at the same distance from the skin but has no immediate transverse bone underneath to resist pressure during hemostasis, and there are layers of muscle tissue that can bleed and collect blood. This anatomical difference between the carpal bone and the wrist bone, as observed by ultrasound imaging, is one of the fundamental advantages of DRA in hemostasis and hematoma prevention.

Acknowledgements Enrique A. Flores wishes to thank Robert Todd, RVT, for his superb assistance in obtaining several of the ultrasound images included in this chapter and his continuous support of our 6-year quality improvement project by conducting routine post-procedure ultrasound imaging, Drew Imhulse from Emory Healthcare media services for his advice and assistance in organizing the chapter and the figures, and Michelle Kienholz for her suggestions and editorial assistance. Also, special thanks are given to Cristina A. Flores, MD, for drawing her dad's hands and most sincere thanks to the catheterization laboratory team at Piedmont Rockdale Hospital in Conyers and to our patients for their incredible support in developing and improving these DRA access protocols for diagnostic angiograms and interventions.

Enrique Flores can be contacted at eflores075@gmail.com.

References

1. Nguyen P, Makris A, Hennessy A, Jayanti S, Wang A, Park K, et al. Standard versus ultrasound-guided radial and femoral access in coronary angiography and intervention (SURF): a randomised controlled trial. EuroIntervention. 2019;15:e522–30.
2. Seto AH, Roberts JS, Abu-Fadel MS, Czak SJ, Latif F, Jain SP, et al. Real-time ultrasound guidance facilitates transradial access: RAUST (Radial Artery access with Ultrasound Trial). JACC Cardiovasc Interv. 2015 8:283–91.
3. Roberts J, Manur R. Ultrasound-guided radial artery access by a non-ultrasound trained interventional cardiologist improved first-attempt success rates and shortened time for successful radial artery cannulation. J Invasive Cardiol. 2013;25:676–9.
4. Mori S, Hirano K, Yamawaki M, Kobayashi N, Sakamoto Y, Tsutsumi M, et al. A comparative analysis between ultrasound-guided and conventional distal transradial access for coronary angiography and intervention. J Interv Cardiol. 2020;2020:7342732.
5. Flores E. Making the right move: use of the distal radial artery access in the hand for coronary angiography and percutaneous coronary intervention. Cath Lab Digest. 2018;26:16–25.
6. Maitra S, Baidya DK, Ray BR, Chowhan G, Bhattacharjee S. Comparison of ultrasound guided dorsal radial artery cannulation and conventional radial artery cannulation at the volar aspect of wrist: a pilot randomized controlled trial. J Vasc Access. 2022;24:1463–68.
7. Hadjivassiliou A, Kiemeneij F, Nathan S, Klass D. Ultrasound-guided access to the distal radial artery at the anatomical snuffbox for catheter-based vascular interventions: a technical guide. EuroIntervention. 2021;16:1342–8.
8. Sgueglia GA, Di Giorgio A, Gaspardone A, Babunashvili A. Anatomic basis and physiological rationale of distal radial artery access for percutaneous coronary and endovascular procedures. JACC Cardiovasc Interv. 2018;11:2113–9.

Advanced Distal Radial Access

9

Fuminobu Yoshimachi and Gregory A. Sgueglia

9.1 Introduction

Transradial access (TRA) is currently associated with very low rates of access site bleeding, vascular complications, and mortality [1] and has been endorsed by European and American guidelines for myocardial revascularization [2, 3]. Radial artery occlusion (RAO) and poor ergonomics of left-side access are the main limitations of TRA [4]. The former, although clinically silent, does not allow the same radial artery to be used for another coronary procedure, while the latter is cumbersome for both patient and operator. In both cases, the better outcomes observed with TRA may be offset. Distal radial access (DRA) has been introduced into interventional practice as an alternative access for percutaneous procedures, favoring persistence of flow in the forearm radial artery, shorter hemostasis, and comfortable left side access (see also Chap. 4) [5–7].

Puncture of a different site after recent TRA has also been proposed as another important indication for distal TRA to avoid recurrent injury to the same arterial segment. As discussed in more detail in Chaps. 3 and 7, DRA offers two relevant additional puncture sites where the radial artery pulse can be felt in the anatomical snuffbox, between the abductor pollicis longus and extensor pollicis brevis tendons proximally and the extensor pollicis longus tendon distally, and on the dorsum of the hand just distal to the extensor pollicis longus tendon [5].

9.2 Secondary Distal Radial Access

Previous observational studies have shown that TRA can be performed multiple times [8, 9], but the failure to reuse the same TRA increases with each subsequent procedure. Therefore, in patients undergoing multiple transradial percutaneous procedures, especially in a short period of time, implementing secondary DRA using the different puncture sites in a sequential manner represents a more advanced strategy to minimize the impact of repeated radial artery punctures.

Typically, the need for a second procedure occurs at least 1 day after the hemostatic compression is removed. Yet TRA is a valuable option for urgent secondary ipsilateral TRA when wrist compression cannot be removed because of ongoing hemostasis [10]. This is the case of acute stent thrombosis occurring very soon after coronary stenting by conventional TRA. Such a com-

F. Yoshimachi
Department of Cardiology, Tokai University Hachioji Hospital, Hachioji City, Tokyo, Japan

G. A. Sgueglia (✉)
Division of Cardiology, Sant'Eugenio Hospital, Rome, Italy

G. A. Sgueglia (ed.), *Distal Radial Access*, https://doi.org/10.1007/978-3-031-89925-6_9

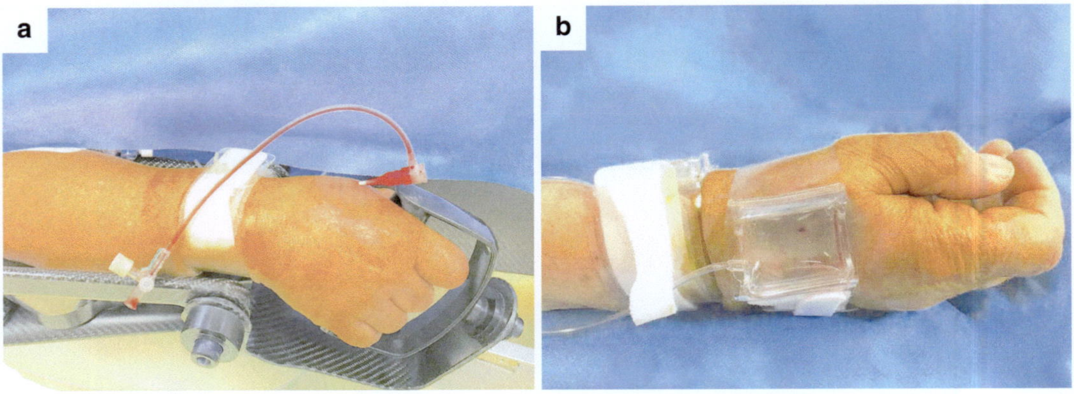

Fig. 9.1 (**a**) Distal radial access in the dorsum of the hand for an urgent coronary procedure in a patient with acute stent thrombosis and ongoing ipsilateral compressive hemostasis after a conventional transradial procedure ended less than half an hour earlier. (**b**) After the procedure, distal radial access hemostasis is easily performed with a second compressive device noninterfering with the one placed over the wrist hence strengthening the safety and efficacy of secondary distal radial access even very early after conventional transradial access

plication can occur after both elective and urgent coronary procedures and requires immediate secondary revascularization and maximal antithrombotic therapy. Conventional TRA, which has shown the most striking reduction in adverse outcomes and mortality in patients with acute coronary syndromes, may be hampered by ongoing hemostasis for ipsilateral radial artery catheterization.

Against this background, DRA in such a complex and highly unfavorable setting warrants the important advantage of conventional TRA despite the inaccessibility of the wrist for another arterial access. Careful implementation of patent hemostasis at the end of the first procedure seems important to allay concerns about potential injury to the forearm radial artery under the hemostatic device and to ensure the safe advancement of the sheath introducer inserted through the DRA. However, our experience supports the lack of interaction between the two hemostatic devices at the wrist and hand level, underscoring the safety and efficacy of secondary DRA even in the earliest period after conventional TRA and even with effective quadruple antithrombotic therapy (Fig. 9.1).

9.3 Adjunctive Distal Radial Access

Because DRA expands the options for puncture sites along the same radial artery, it is sometimes the case that one of these sites is already in use for another application. These may include arterial lines, which are most commonly used in intensive care settings to monitor blood pressure directly and in real time and to easily obtain samples for arterial blood gas analysis. There are several scenarios in which a patient may arrive at the catheterization laboratory with an arterial line inserted into the radial artery at the wrist. In most cases, the patient is expected to be at high risk, and therefore, the greatest potential benefit may be gained from a transradial rather than transfemoral approach. Very usefully, DRA can be used without major drawbacks in patients with an arterial line previously placed in the radial artery at the wrist level (Fig. 9.2). The availability of an adjunctive vascular access option such as DRA helps to adapt to a complex clinical situation while retaining all the safety benefits of transradial access [11].

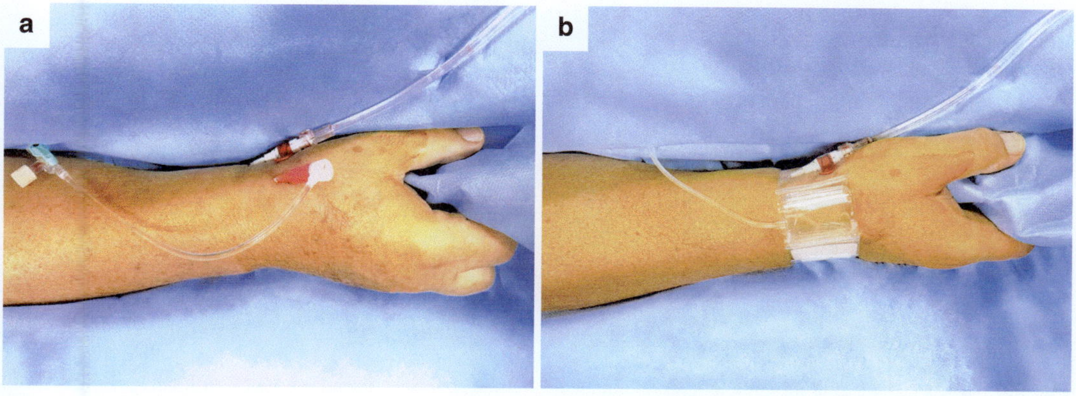

Fig. 9.2 (**a**) Distal radial access in the anatomical snuffbox in a patient with an ipsilateral 20-G arterial line for invasive arterial pressure monitoring previously placed in the right radial artery at the wrist level. (**b**) Remarkably, the smooth plastic band of the hemostatic device does not hinder invasive pressure monitoring

9.4 Dual-Access Techniques

In some other circumstances, it is the percutaneous procedure itself that requires the use of two catheters. This is most often the case in the treatment of chronic total occlusions (CTOs), which requires contralateral imaging or a retrograde approach. The use of two catheters inserted along the same arterial pathway was first proposed about 10 years ago by Fuminobu Yoshimachi in his Retro 555 technique, which consisted of the simultaneous insertion of a 5-Fr introducer sheath in the radial artery to advance a 5-Fr guiding catheter for the antegrade approach and a 7.5-Fr sheathless guiding catheter in the brachial artery for the retrograde approach.

This technique later evolved into the BUSHI DO (Bipoint Uni-lateral SHeathless catheter Insertion via Distal & prOximal radial artery) technique. In the initial report by Yoshimachi et al., a 3-Fr diagnostic catheter and a 5-Fr guiding catheter were inserted sheathless through DRA in the dorsum of the hand and conventional TRA at the level of the wrist, respectively [12], although the two puncture sites may actually be in the anatomical snuffbox and the dorsum of the hand (Fig. 9.3). The steps of the BUSHI DO technique are shown in Table 9.1.

A further iteration was proposed by Sgueglia et al., who introduced the OTRANTO (One-point TRANstradial TwO-sheathless catheter insertion) technique, which consists of the simultaneous insertion of two sheathless guiding catheters through the same radial access. In the first report, two 5-Fr guiding catheters were inserted through

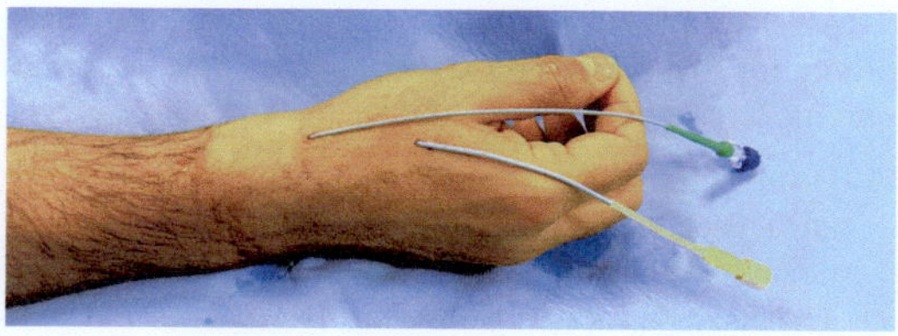

Fig. 9.3 Two 5-Fr guiding catheters simultaneously inserted through distal radial access in the dorsum of the hand and in the anatomical snuffbox, respectively, using the BUSHI DO (Bipoint Unilateral SHeathless catheter Insertion via Distal and prOximal radial artery) technique

Table 9.1 Steps of the BUSHI DO (Bipoint Unilateral SHeathless catheter Insertion via Distal and prOximal radial artery) technique for percutaneous coronary intervention of chronic total occlusions

1. Proximal puncture secured with a peripheral intravenous catheter
2. Distal puncture
3. Sheathless advancement of the antegrade guiding catheter from the distal puncture site[a]
4. Sheathless advancement of the retrograde coronary catheter from the proximal puncture site[a]

[a]If the catheter is advanced using the BAT (balloon-assisted tracking) technique, it is recommended to use first the dilator of a corresponding size radial introducer sheath

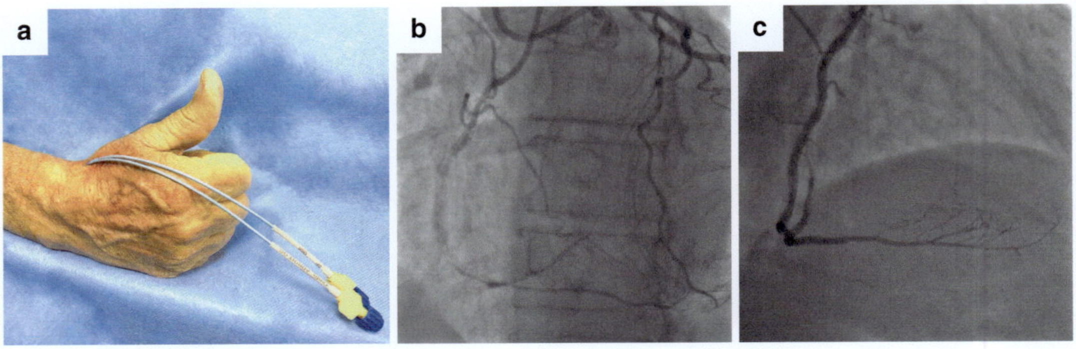

Fig. 9.4 (**a**) Two 5-Fr guiding catheters simultaneously inserted through a single distal radial access in the anatomical snuffbox using the OTRANTO (One-point TRANsradial TwO sheathless catheters insertion) technique. (**b**) Baseline angiography with dual injection showing the target right coronary total chronic occlusion. (**c**) Final result after the successful implementation of an antegrade strategy

Table 9.2 Steps of the distal OTRANTO (One-point TRANsradial TwO sheathless catheters insertion) technique for the percutaneous coronary intervention of chronic total occlusions

1. Distal radial artery puncture secured with a radial introducer sheath of a size corresponding to the largest coronary catheter intended to be used
2. Advancement of two guidewires (guidewire diameter to be selected according to the intended sheathless catheter advancement technique)
3. Removal of the radial introducer sheath
4. Sheathless advancement of the first coronary catheter
5. Sheathless advancement of the second coronary catheter[a]

[a]If necessary, a guidewire can be exchanged for a larger or smaller one using a peripheral intravenous catheter

conventional TRA to perform a unique intravascular lithotripsy kissing balloon for the treatment of a highly calcified left main coronary artery bifurcation in a very complex patient [13]. The distal OTRANTO technique was then implemented via DRA for percutaneous CTO treatment (Fig. 9.4). The detailed procedural steps of the OTRANTO technique are shown in Table 9.2.

With the OTRANTO technique, insertion of the second sheathless catheter may be more cumbersome than with the BUSHI DO technique, especially when balloon-assisted tracking is used instead of a dedicated long dilator (see also Chap. 19). In contrast, the OTRANTO requires only one vascular access and hemostasis.

The BUSHI DO and OTRANTO techniques were initially described in situations where other vascular access was unavailable or considered too risky. Although they are certainly limited to pragmatic procedures in selected cases, their knowledge is important if one needs to overcome vascular access limitations or is willing to strive for transradial access even in the most complex situations. Both have been carefully designed to maintain safety as their greatest advantage, with only one artery potentially compromised by the catheterization procedure. Importantly, the sheathless delivery of the two guiding catheters allows the thickness of the sheath introducer to be saved. Even when using two sheathless 5-Fr guiding catheters, their combined cross-sectional area is less than that of a single thin-walled 6-Fr sheath introducer (Fig. 9.5), resulting in minimal trauma to the vessel and preserving radial artery patency.

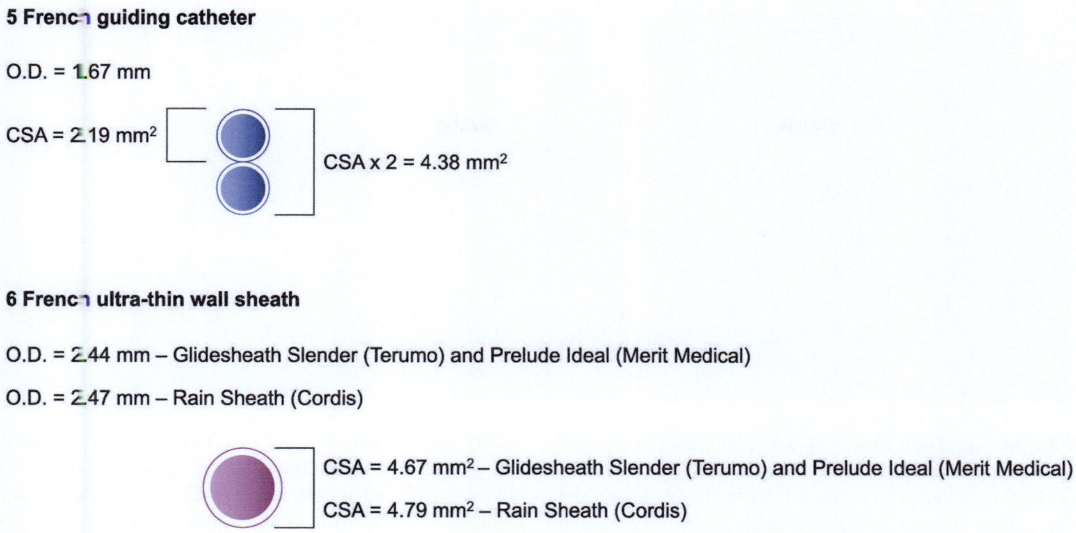

Fig. 9.5 Two 5-Fr guiding catheters simultaneously inserted in the same artery yield a total cross-sectional area (CSA) of 4.38 mm², which is 7–9% less than the 4.67–4.71 mm² CSA of a single 6-Fr thin-walled sheath introducer which has the smallest outer diameter of any of the 6-Fr introducer sheaths currently available

9.5 Radial Artery Flow Enhancement

In an experimental physiology study in unselected subjects, simulated occlusion of the distal radial artery was associated with effective persistence of flow in the forearm radial artery, in contrast to the marked impairment of flow observed with simulated occlusion at the wrist level [14]. Similar behavior was observed when the flow was assessed in the radiodorsal digital artery of the thumb, a dependent branch of the distal radial artery. These findings support distal radial access as a safer and more effective intervention to maintain forearm radial artery patency (see also Chap. 4).

Despite such significant observations, incidental procedural findings such as refractory spasm, retrograde dissection, or radial artery anomaly can raise significant concerns about loss of radial artery patency, which paradoxically is the primary reason for performing DRA. In such situations where radial artery blood flow is potentially compromised, it may be beneficial to perform ipsilateral ulnar artery occlusive compression, which is intended to increase radial flow through the release of vasodilator mediators according to flow-mediated dilation (Fig. 9.6). The clinical value of ipsilateral ulnar artery compression in addition to a patent hemostasis protocol was previously demonstrated by the PROPhylactic Hyperperfusion Evaluation Trial (PROPHET) II, which showed a significant reduction in RAO compared to conventional hemostasis with the implementation of the patent hemostasis protocol alone [15]. However, despite such an effective performance in a large randomized controlled trial, the adoption of ipsilateral ulnar artery compression as a technique to prevent RAO is limited by the lack of a dedicated device that allows for radial artery patent hemostasis at the wrist level and simultaneous ulnar artery occlusive compression. In contrast, if ipsilateral ulnar artery compression is indicated after DRA, a second hemostatic device can be easily placed on the medial side of the wrist to induce ulnar artery occlusive compression when maximally inflated (Fig. 9.6c) [16].

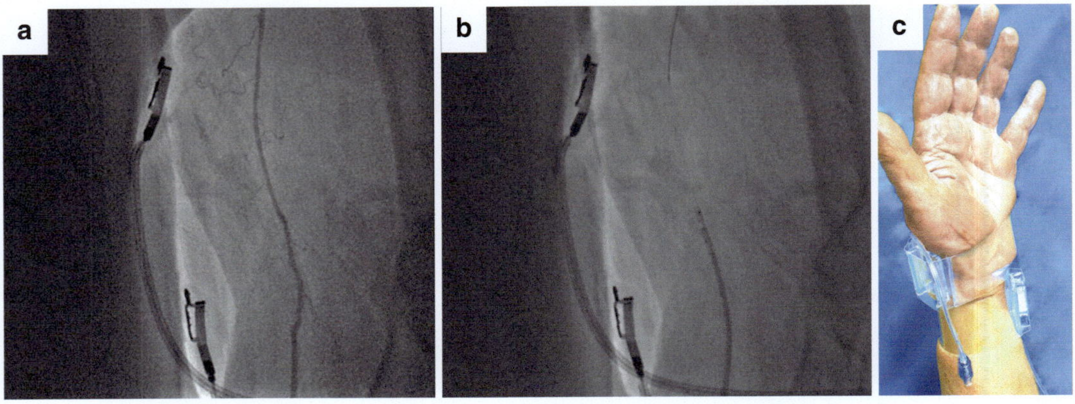

Fig. 9.6 (**a**) High origin of a hypoplastic radial artery hampering the advancement of a 5-Fr guiding catheter for ad hoc percutaneous coronary intervention of a focal left circumflex stenosis in a patient with acute coronary syndrome. (**b**) After nitroglycerin administration, the guiding catheter was finally advanced using the BAT (balloon-assisted tracking) technique, and the left circumflex artery was successfully treated. (**c**) To minimize the risk of radial artery occlusion, a hemostatic device with minimal inflation was applied to the anatomical snuffbox to ensure hemostasis of the distal radial access, and a second hemostatic device was used for ulnar artery compression to favor flow in the radial artery

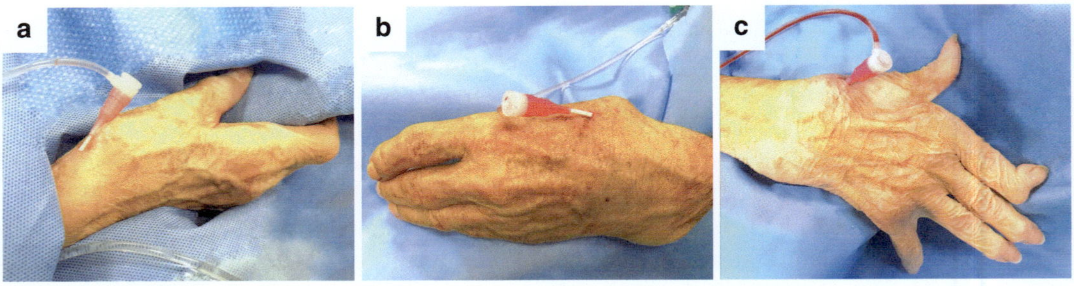

Fig. 9.7 (**a–c**) In patients with varying degrees of hand deformity, distal radial access is possible after careful preprocedural evaluation

9.6 Distal Radial Access in Unfavorable Hand Anatomies

The improved patient ergonomics afforded by left DRA also supports right DRA, especially for subjects with orthopedic problems who are more comfortable with their hand in a neutral position rather than in the difficult or inaccessible supination position that would otherwise be required for conventional TRA. However, congenital or hereditary conditions, injuries resulting in joint dislocations or fractures, or acquired diseases such as osteoarthritis or rheumatoid arthritis can cause various hand deformities that can severely interfere with proper hand position and anatomical relationships even when DRA is performed. In fact, such conditions may be amenable to effective and safe DRA, provided that a careful preprocedural assessment of the likely possible hand position and altered course of the distal radial artery is performed (Fig. 9.7). It is also prudent to test the fit of the available hemostatic device on the deformed hand prior to DRA puncture. With some care, the experienced operator will be able to warrant DRA even in these unfortunate cases. The procedural steps for DRA in hand deformities are summarized in Table 9.3.

Ultrasound guidance has been shown to significantly increase the success rate of DRA compared to a conventional palpation-based approach

Table 9.3 Steps of the distal radial access in unfavorable hand anatomy

1. Assessment for distal radial artery course and anatomical relationships
2. Test for a working hand position for distal radial access
3. Appraisal of the hemostatic device placement
4. Distal radial artery puncture at the most accessible site

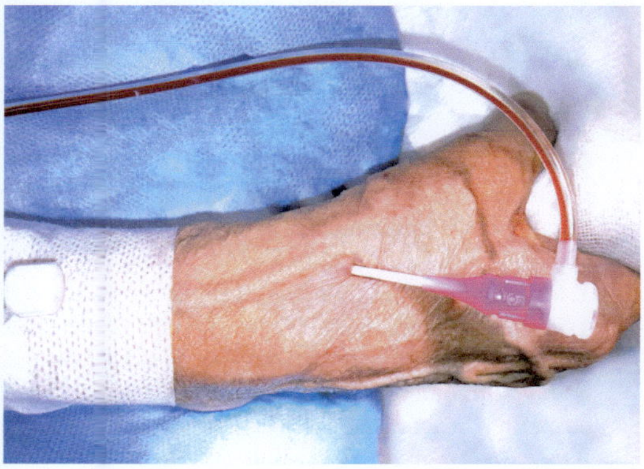

Fig. 9.8 Distal radial access in a patient with a dilated cephalic vein overhanging the distal radial artery in the anatomic snuffbox. Ultrasound-guided puncture appears essential to ensure safe access in such a peculiar condition

[17] and may be a useful tool to improve DRA in patients with hand deformities (see also Chap. 8). In addition, vascular ultrasound appears to be essential in the presence of abnormal anatomical structures that prevent a straightforward DRA puncture (Fig. 9.8).

Finally, in conditions such as poststroke paralysis or spasticity that challenge smooth catheter delivery through the upper extremity vasculature, fluoroscopy-guided tracking is critical to overcoming difficulties and ensuring safety (Fig. 9.9).

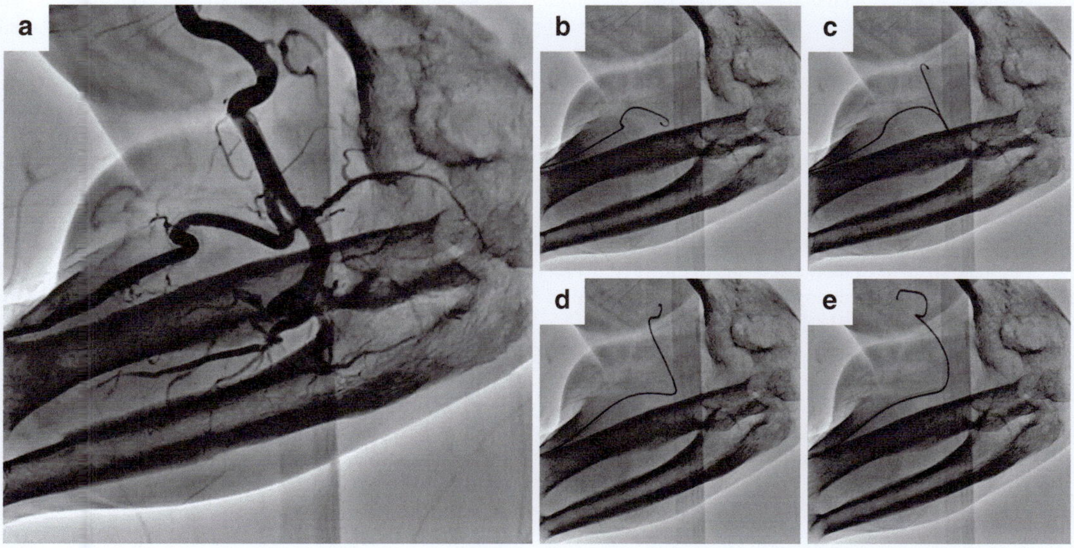

Fig. 9.9 (**a**–**e**) Fluoroscopy-guided tracking is critical to overcoming difficulties and ensuring safety when faced with significant challenges to smooth catheter delivery through the upper extremity vasculature, such as in poststroke upper limb spasticity

9.7 Conclusions

Although it has only recently been introduced in interventional practice, DRA has already established itself as the safest arterial access ever and a worthy alternative to traditional TRA. Moreover, proper knowledge and experience allow for overcoming potential limitations and developing innovative applications to unveil the full range of opportunities offered by DRA.

References

1. Ferrante G, Rao SV, Juni P, Da Costa BR, Reimers B, Condorelli G, et al. Radial versus femoral access for coronary interventions across the entire spectrum of patients with coronary artery disease: a meta-analysis of randomized trials. JACC Cardiovasc Interv. 2016;9:1419–34.
2. Neumann FJ, Sousa-Uva M, Ahlsson A, Alfonso F, Banning AP, Benedetto U, et al. 2018 ESC/EACTS guidelines on myocardial revascularization. Eur Heart J. 2019;40:87–165.
3. Lawton JS, Tamis-Holland JE, Bangalore S, Bates ER, Beckie TM, Bischoff TM, et al. 2021 ACC/AHA/SCAI guideline for coronary artery revascularization: a report of the American College of Cardiology/American Heart Association Joint Committee on Clinical Practice Guidelines. J Am Coll Cardiol. 2022;79:e21–9.
4. Bernat I, Aminian A, Pancholy S, Mamas MA, Gaudino M, Nolan J, et al. Best practices for the prevention of radial artery occlusion after transradial diagnostic angiography and intervention: an International Consensus Paper. JACC Cardiovasc Interv. 2019;12:2235–46.
5. Sgueglia GA, Di Giorgio A, Gaspardone A, Babunashvili A. Anatomic basis and physiological rationale of distal radial artery access for percutaneous coronary and endovascular procedures. JACC Cardiovasc Interv. 2018;11:2113–9.
6. Yoshimachi F, Ikari Y. Distal radial approach: a review on achieving a high success rate. Cardiovasc Interv Ther. 2021;36:30–8.
7. Sgueglia GA, Lee BK, Cho BR, Babunashvili A, Lee JB, Lee JW, et al. Distal radial access: consensus report of the first Korea-Europe transradial intervention meeting. JACC Cardiovasc Interv. 2021;14:892–906.
8. Sakai H, Ikeda S, Harada T, Yonashiro S, Ozumi K, Ohe H, et al. Limitations of successive transradial approach in the same arm: the Japanese experience. Catheter Cardiovasc Interv. 2001;54:204–8.
9. Abdelaal E, Molin P, Plourde G, Machaalany J, Bataille Y, Brousseau-Provencher C, et al. Successive transradial access for coronary procedures: experience of Quebec Heart-Lung Institute. Am Heart J. 2013;165:325–31.
10. Yoshimachi F, Kawamura Y, Nagamatsu H, Karasawa Y, Murotani N, Kasai S. Distal radial approach treating a left main lesion during hemostasis of the forearm radial artery on the same side in a case of unstable angina. J Cardiol Cases. 2021;25:52–4.
11. Colletti G, Aminian A, León Díaz V, Mitri K, Ungureanu C. Who's parked (again) in my spot?: Go distal! JACC Cardiovasc Interv. 2022;15:e195–6.
12. Yoshimachi F, Takagawa Y, Sakai K, Ikari Y. Simultaneous radial and distal radial access through a single hand in PCI for CTO—"BUSHI DO" (Bipoint Uni-lateral SHeathless catheter Insertion via Distal & prOximal radial artery) technique. PCR Online 2018. https://www.pcronline.com/Cases-resources-images/Images-interventional-cardiology/EuroIntervention-images/Simultaneous-radial-and-distal-radial-access-through-a-single-hand-in-PCI-for-CTO. Accessed 31 Jan 2023.
13. Sgueglia GA, Gioffrè G, Chiastra C, Di Giorgio A, Gaspardone A. First report of the one-point transradial two sheathless catheters insertion (OTRANTO) technique. JACC Cardiovasc Interv. 2020;13:e9–10.
14. Sgueglia GA, Santoliquido A, Gaspardone A, Di Giorgio A. First results of the Distal Radial Access Doppler study. JACC Cardiovasc Imaging. 2021;14:1281–3.
15. Pancholy SB, Bernat I, Bertrand OF, Patel TM. Prevention of radial artery occlusion after transradial catheterization: the PROPHET-II randomized trial. JACC Cardiovasc Interv. 2016;9:1992–9.
16. Cubero JM, Lombardo J, Pedrosa C, Diaz-Bejarano D, Sanchez B, Fernandez V, et al. Radial compression guided by mean artery pressure versus standard compression with a pneumatic device (RACOMAP). Catheter Cardiovasc Interv. 2009;73:467–72.
17. Mori S, Hirano K, Yamawaki M, Kobayashi N, Sakamoto Y, Tsutsumi M, et al. A comparative analysis between ultrasound-guided and conventional distal transradial access for coronary angiography and intervention. J Interv Cardiol. 2020;2020:7342732.

10 Troubleshooting Transradial Issues

Mauricio G. Cohen and Tejas Patel

10.1 Introduction

Transradial access (TRA) has become the preferred vascular access site for coronary and other angiographic procedures worldwide. Besides the need to develop skills to access the radial artery at the level of the wrist or the anatomical snuffbox by palpation or ultrasound guidance, operators need to be aware of a number of tips and tricks to deal with issues that may arise during TRA angiographic or interventional procedures. Operators acquire the necessary skills to deal with navigation issues, understand upper extremity vascular anatomy, and learn catheter manipulation for coronary engagement during the learning curve. In this chapter, we discuss the challenges the operator may encounter during transradial catheterization and describe tricks and tips to successfully navigate the upper extremity arterial system after vascular access.

M. G. Cohen (✉)
Interventional Cardiology, Cleveland Clinic Florida, Weston, FL, USA
e-mail: cohenm10@ccf.org

T. Patel
Apex Heart Institute, Ahmedabad, Gujarat, India

10.2 Mastering Transradial Access

The learning curve for conventional TRA was initially documented in a landmark study by Spaulding et al., who reported an initial access failure rate of more than 10%, which dramatically decreased to approximately 2% after the first 80 cases [1]. Subsequent studies have shown a steep decline in transradial access (TRA) procedural failure during the first 50 cases, after which the learning curve flattens. Ball and colleagues found that TRA PCI failure rates decreased from 7% to 2% ($p = 0.01$), with an associated reduction in contrast volume from 180 ± 79 to 168 ± 79 mL ($p = 0.05$) and fluoroscopy time from 15 ± 10 to 12 ± 9 min ($p = 0.02$) with increasing procedural volume among 28 operators [2]. An analysis of nearly 55,000 PCI procedures from the NCDR CathPCI database showed a significant reduction in contrast volume and fluoroscopy time after the first 30–50 procedures, despite increasing procedural and patient complexity [3]. During the learning curve, operators become familiar with the various hurdles that can arise when performing TRA.

10.3 Anatomical Variations

Rare anatomical anomalies may complicate catheter delivery to the aorta or increase the risk of adverse outcomes. These anomalies include tortuous radial configurations, stenoses, hypoplasia,

G. A. Sgueglia (ed.), *Distal Radial Access*, https://doi.org/10.1007/978-3-031-89925-6_10

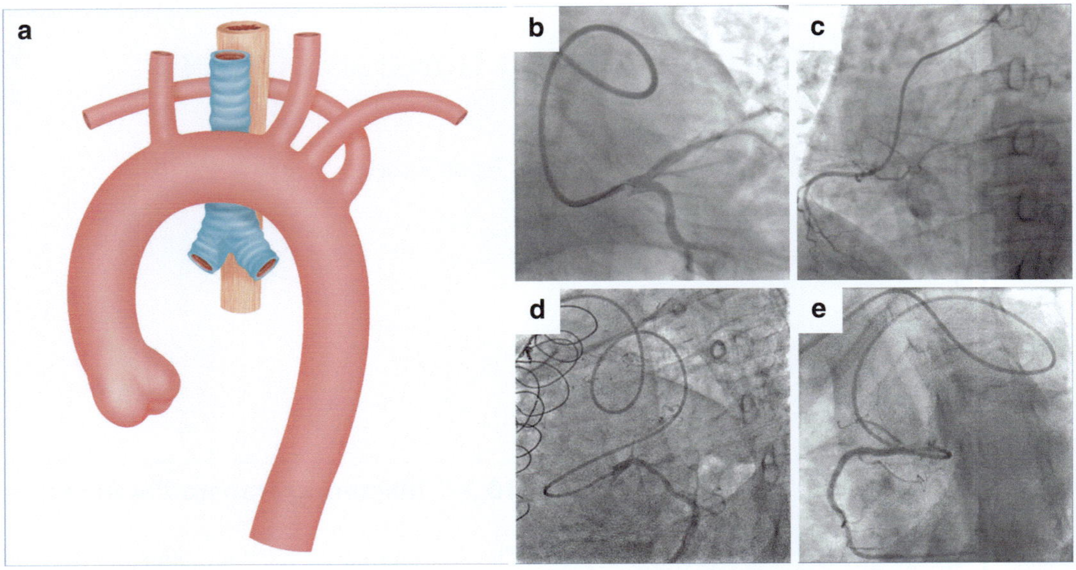

Fig. 10.1 (**a**) Anatomical relationship of the arteria lusoria to other anatomical structures in the thorax, with a retroesophageal trajectory and origin in the distal aortic arch. (**b–e**) Angiograms highlighting different configurations and navigation challenges that the operator faces in reaching the root of the aorta and selectively engaging the coronary arteries. (Adapted from Patel et al. [7])

radioulnar loops, anomalous right subclavian artery (arteria lusoria), and abnormal origin of the radial artery [4, 5]. Anatomical anomalies are present in approximately 15% of cases according to a series of 1540 TRA procedures [5]. Specifically, a high-origin radial artery at the level of the mid or upper humerus was found in 7% of cases, with a low failure rate of 4.6%, while a loop in the proximal radial artery was found in 2.3% of cases, with a high failure rate of 37.1%. Severe tortuosity was found in 2% of cases, and other miscellaneous anomalies were found in 2.5% of cases [5]. These anomalies are usually unilateral, and in cases of extreme tortuosity or angulated radial loops, vascular access crossover to the left radial artery is preferred to save time and prevent complications. Subclavian or brachiocephalic tortuosity occurs in approximately 10% of cases and is usually associated with advanced age, short stature, and a long history of hypertension. However, subclavian tortuosity is rarely a cause of procedural failure, as it can be easily overcome by the use of deep inspiration or supportive guidewires [6]. In rare cases (<1%), the right subclavian artery arises directly from the distal segment of the posterior aspect of the aortic arch and has a retroesophageal course toward the right upper extremity. This anomaly, known as arteria lusoria, may be associated with dysphagia but is mostly asymptomatic and presents a formidable challenge to catheter advancement from the subclavian artery to the ascending aorta, as shown in Fig. 10.1 [4].

10.4 Navigation of the Upper Extremity Arterial System

10.4.1 Guidewire Selection

After placement of the arterial sheath, operators advance their catheter of choice and a 0.035″ guidewire into the ascending aorta via the upper extremity arterial system. The type of guidewire used may vary between operators and local practices. J-tipped guidewires are preferred because they facilitate navigation by following the path of larger vessels and do not selectively enter small radial or brachial arterial branches. However, standard J-tipped guidewires have a

3-mm radius, which is much larger than the diameter of the radial artery and may cause vasospasm or failure to advance. Therefore, a smaller J-tipped guidewire (Glidewire Baby-J, Terumo; Silverway, Asahi; some version of Emerald, Cordis) with a 1.5-mm radius is better suited for navigating the upper extremity vasculature. Angled hydrophilic guidewires with stiff shafts are ideal for negotiating tortuous anatomy, particularly in the subclavian artery and brachiocephalic trunk, but require close fluoroscopic monitoring as they may inadvertently perforate small branches of the radial or brachial arteries. Since full anticoagulation is typically administered during transradial procedures, perforation of a small branch can result in significant hematoma formation.

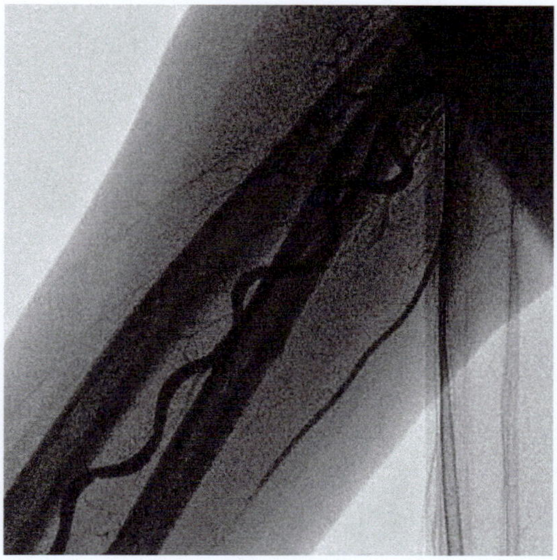

Fig. 10.2 Limited retrograde angiographic assessment of the radial artery demonstrating unusual tortuosity that can be easily negotiated with a guidewire

10.4.2 Techniques to Negotiate Anatomical Variations

In the presence of anatomical variations, the operator will face resistance to advancing guidewires or catheters and will be unable to reach the ascending aorta. An understanding of the normal vascular anatomy of this region is necessary to effectively address these issues (see also Chap. 3). In addition, the operator should be familiar with a variety of techniques for crossing peripheral vessels, catheter types, and guidewires. Due to the relatively small size of the upper extremity arterial system, devices should never be forced against resistance due to the risk of vessel injury, dissection, or reactive spasm. Instead, a limited retrograde angiographic assessment should be performed to identify a vascular anomaly or unusual tortuosity, plan a strategy, and prevent complications (Fig. 10.2). Once the anatomical challenge is understood, a catheter can be carefully advanced over the guidewire using a slow corkscrew motion under fluoroscopic guidance. Direct pushing of the catheter is not recommended as it may induce a reactive spasm. Spasm in a tortuous radial segment is a complex situation to manage. Repeated doses of a vasodilator cocktail may help work through a small-caliber radial artery and tortuous segments with or without spasm, as well as reduce the diameter of the catheter. Techniques such as balloon-assisted tracking (BAT), mother-and-child or Combo techniques, and good familiarity with the guidewires can help with effective navigation (see also Chap. 19) [8, 9].

The BAT technique can facilitate catheter passage through narrow or tortuous vessels (Fig. 10.3) [8]. An inflated coronary balloon is partially protruded through the distal end of a guiding or diagnostic catheter and inflated at low pressure between 3 and 6 atm. The recommended balloon diameter is 1.5 mm for 5-Fr diagnostic or guiding catheters and 2.0 mm for 6-Fr guiding catheters. A balloon length of 10 mm or 15 mm is sufficient. Once the balloon is partially protruded through the distal end of the catheter and inflated, the system is advanced as a unit over a soft-tipped 0.014″ coronary guidewire to allow smooth and atraumatic advancement through difficult vascular anatomy. Situations that may require BAT include very small–caliber radial arteries (less than 1.5 mm in diameter), tortuous radial or brachial arteries, severe and resistant radial spasm, atherosclerotic disease, complex loops, severe subclavian tortuosity, and subclavian stenosis.

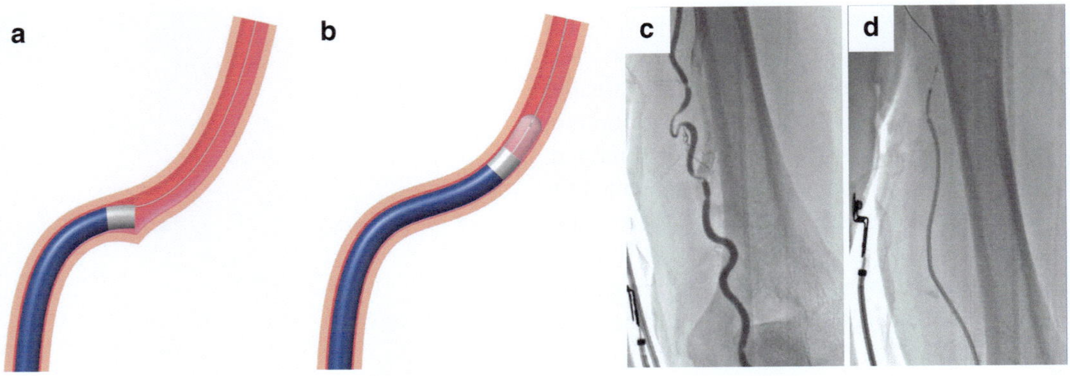

Fig. 10.3 (**a**) Guiding catheter proximal edge leading to razor effect in an artery tortuous segment that can cause injury or dissection. (**b**) Smooth tracking of a guide catheter over a balloon eliminates the razor effect in the artery tortuous segment. (**c**) Severe radial artery tortuosity. (**d**) Catheter advancement implementing the balloon-assisted tracking (BAT) technique. (Adapted from Patel et al. [8])

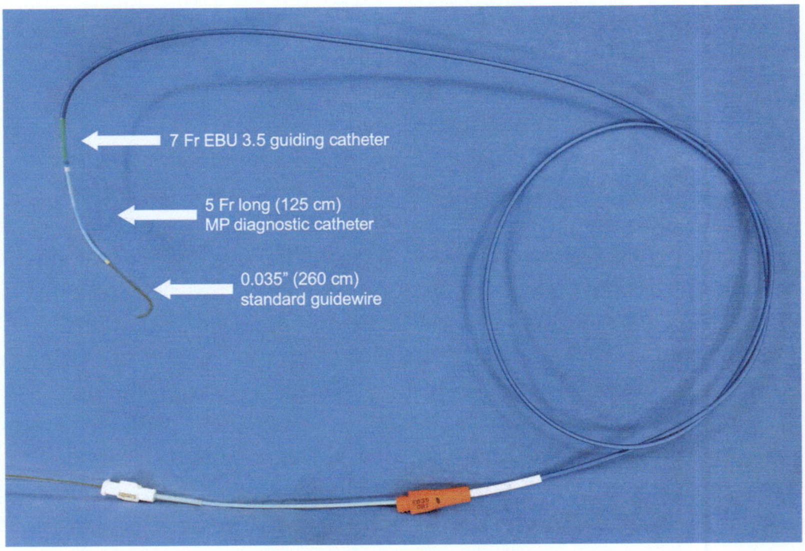

Fig. 10.4 The picture displays the assembly of catheters for a mother-and-child Combo configuration. A long 5-Fr multipurpose catheter is passed through a 7-Fr guiding catheter to allow a smooth transition between the 0.035-in. guidewire and the guiding catheter

The mother-and-child or Combo technique can also be used to advance a guiding catheter through complex vascular anatomy without significant trauma or local pain. It involves telescoping a long 125 cm 5-Fr multipurpose or JR4 catheter through a 6-Fr or 7-Fr guiding catheter to create a smooth transition between the guidewire and the guiding catheter, eliminating a leading edge that can be traumatic to the vessel (Fig. 10.4).

10.4.3 Tips and Tricks for Loops, Vascular Anomalies, and Other Challenges

10.4.3.1 Resistance to Instrument Advancement

Resistance to guidewire and/or catheter movement is most often interpreted as radial artery spasm. In most cases, what initially appears to be a radial spasm is actually an anatomical variation in the form of a tortuosity, loop, or severe curvature. Loops and curvatures are to be expected, and an operator must have a plan to work through this challenge. Loops can be simple or complex and come in a variety of common and unique configurations as shown in Fig. 10.5. To navigate radioulnar loops and tortuosity in the radial or brachial arteries, operators can use their preferred 0.014″ coronary guidewire along with a 4-Fr hydrophilic-coated Cobra or angled-tip catheter compatible with a 0.035-inch guidewire (Fig. 10.6a, b). If the guidewire crosses a loop, its tip should be parked as high as possible, typically in the high brachial, axillary or subclavian region, before advancing the catheter. As the catheter is advanced, the loop usually opens spontaneously (Fig. 10.6c), but there may be times when the catheter can be advanced over the guidewire through a 360° loop without changing its shape. If the catheter cannot be advanced through a loop, BAT can be attempted with a high success rate (Fig. 10.6d). However, if the patient experiences significant pain, the operator must consider switching to an alternative vascular access route.

It should be kept in mind that the guidewire can pass without resistance through a small accessory communicating vessel known as the "accessory radial artery" between the radioulnar

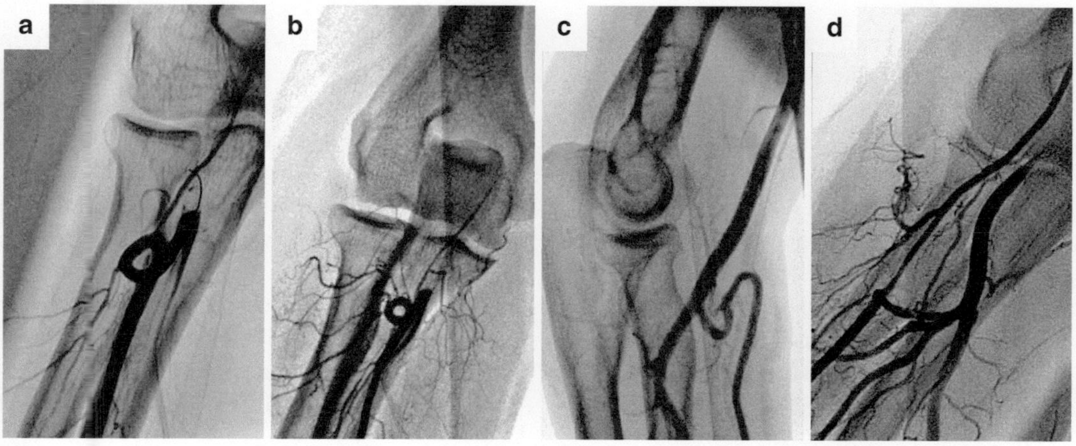

Fig. 10.5 Common radio-brachial loop configurations

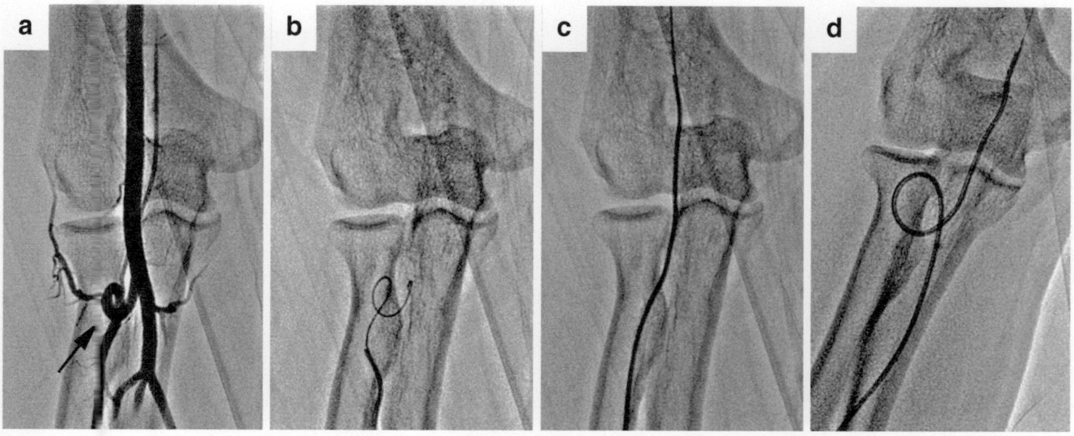

Fig. 10.6 (**a**) Negotiating a 360-degree radial artery loop with a small diameter. (**b**) A flexible J-tipped hydrophilic guidewire was used to cross the loop. (**c**) The loop was straightened by pulling back the entire assembly. (**d**) A 5-Fr guiding catheter was successfully negotiated through a complex 360-degree loop using the balloon-assisted tracking (BAT) technique

loop and the proximal brachial artery. Although the guidewire may appear to follow the expected path under fluoroscopy, the operator may encounter unusual resistance, and the patient may experience severe pain during catheter advancement due to spasms. If the operator recognizes this problem, he or she may choose to reduce the size of the catheter and repeat the dose of a spasmolytic cocktail. The BAT technique can be very useful when the radial artery diameter is very small. However, it should be noted that advancing the catheter into a very small artery carries a risk of dissection or perforation.

10.4.3.2 High Origin of the Radial Artery

A frequently occurring anomaly, high-origin radial artery from the proximal segment of the brachial artery (brachioradial artery), can pose additional challenges to the operator (Fig. 10.7a, b). Although diagnostic catheterization is feasible with minimal patient discomfort, ad hoc PCI can be more challenging due to unusual resistance when the leading edge of the guiding catheter reaches the angulated origin of the anomalous radial artery, causing vessel injury or perforation (Fig. 10.7c). In such situations, the BAT or mother-and-child techniques may be helpful.

An easy-to-follow algorithm for managing complex vascular anatomy in the upper extremity is outlined in Fig. 10.8.

10.4.3.3 Radial Artery Atherosclerosis

Radial artery atherosclerosis is rare and usually part of a generalized atherosclerotic process [7]. It is possible to successfully perform a diagnostic or interventional procedure in this situation (Fig. 10.9a). Atherosclerotic lesions in the radial artery resist the movement of a guidewire and/or catheter. If a limited radial angiogram reveals an atherosclerotic lesion, it is important to define its severity (mild to moderate or severe). If it is a mild obstruction, careful passage of the catheter through the affected segment under fluoroscopic guidance should allow the operator to perform and complete the procedure successfully. If there is a severe stenotic lesion, it is advisable to dilate the lesion with a coronary balloon and then work through the affected segment. In either situation, a repeat dose of an antispasmodic cocktail will facilitate catheter passage. The BAT technique should be implemented in difficult situations.

Radial artery calcification may be patchy or diffuse [7]. Patchy calcification offers little resistance to the passage of a guidewire and/or catheter. In fact, it can be easily crossed using standard

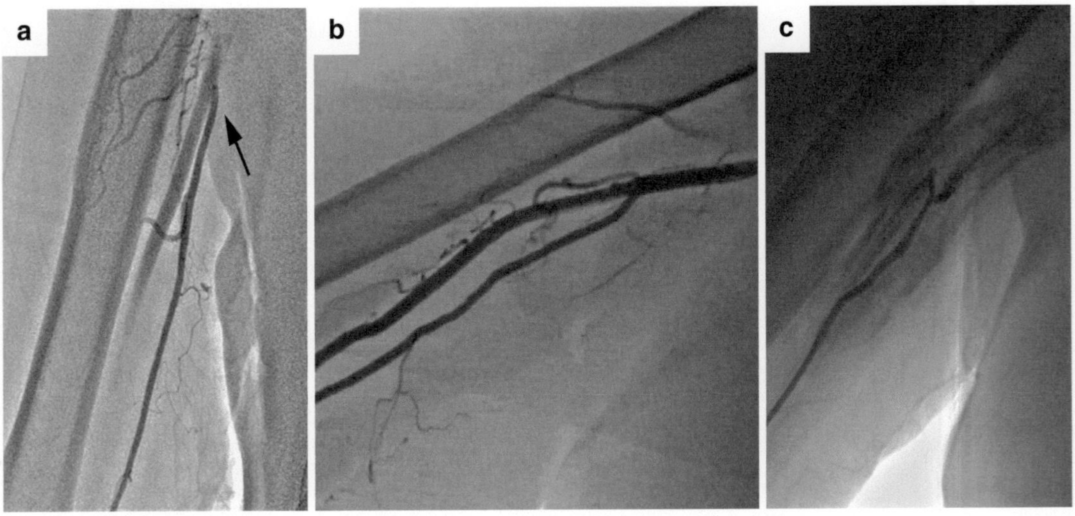

Fig. 10.7 (**a**, **b**) Examples of high-origin radial artery at the level of the proximal brachial artery. (**c**) Perforation and extravasation of contrast caused by forceful advancement of a guiding catheter causing injury

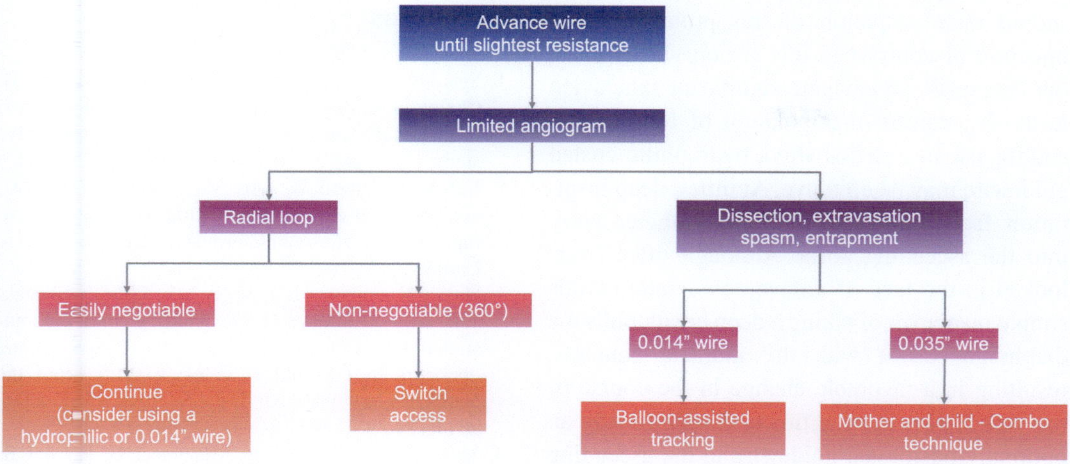

Fig. 10.8 Simple algorithm for negotiating complex upper extremity vascular anatomy

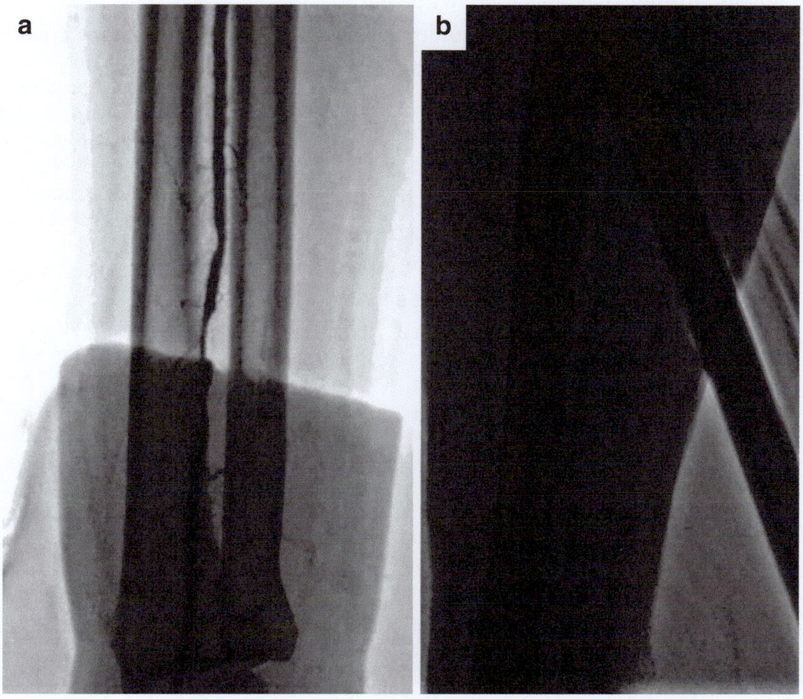

Fig. 10.9 (**a**) Severe radial artery atherosclerotic disease. (**b**) Heavy calcification of the forearm arteries

techniques. Diffuse calcification provides significant resistance to the passage of a guidewire and/or catheter (Fig. 10.9b). Instead of the standard push of the catheter over the guidewire, a slow corkscrew motion is recommended. This technique reduces friction in the affected segment. Once the segment is traversed by the initial portion of the catheter, the resistance disappears or decreases significantly, and the rest of the diagnostic or interventional procedure can be performed normally.

10.4.3.4 Tortuosity of Subclavian and Innominate Arteries

If a guidewire or catheter encounters resistance at the level of the shoulder, subclavian tortuosity may be the cause. Any resistance to movement of a standard 0.035″ guidewire and/or catheter should raise suspicion of this problem. Hand injection of contrast in this region will confirm the diagnosis. To navigate significant subclavian tortuosity, careful manipulation of the catheter and the use of a stiff-shafted, hydrophilic-coated guidewire may be effective. At times, deep inspiration facilitates guidewire and catheter entry into the ascending aorta. Although often overlooked in the face of unfavorable anatomy, this simple maneuver of taking a deep breath pulls the diaphragm down with the thoracic contents, resulting in a favorable change in the course of the vessel. However, at times, despite having an optimally positioned guidewire in the ascending aorta, catheter movement encounters severe resistance. At this point, instead of pushing the catheter further over the guidewire, pulling the catheter slightly back with the guidewire straightens the tortuosity, allowing smooth entry of the catheter into the ascending aorta [7]. The tortuous section usually straightens as the stiff part of the guidewire passes through. In the case of severe and complex stenosis, the BAT technique helps catheter entry in the ascending aorta. It is important to use fluoroscopic guidance while working through this region to prevent damage to the ostia of the carotid, vertebral, or internal mammary arteries [7, 10–12].

10.5 Conclusions

There are challenges to transradial catheterization procedures due to known anomalies and variations of the radial artery that occur in less than 10% of cases. Techniques to overcome these challenges are well described and require anatomical knowledge, dexterity, and finesse in guidewire and catheter manipulation. With experience, radial operators instinctively apply these techniques with great success and less than 2–3% crossover rates.

References

1. Spaulding C, Lefevre T, Funck F, Thebault B, Chauveau M, Ben Hamda K, et al. Left radial approach for coronary angiography: results of a prospective study. Catheter Cardiovasc Diagn. 1996;39:365–70.
2. Ball WT, Sharieff W, Jolly SS, Hong T, Kutryk MJ, Graham JJ, et al. Characterization of operator learning curve for transradial coronary interventions. Circ Cardiovasc Interv. 2011;4:336–41.
3. Hess CN, Peterson ED, Neely ML, Dai D, Hillegass WB, Krucoff MW, et al. The learning curve for transradial percutaneous coronary intervention among operators in the United States: a study from the National Cardiovascular Data Registry. Circulation. 2014;129:2277–86.
4. Valsecchi O, Vassileva A, Musumeci G, Rossini R, Tespili M, Guagliumi G, et al. Failure of transradial approach during coronary interventions: anatomic considerations. Catheter Cardiovasc Interv. 2006;67:870–8.
5. Lo TS, Nolan J, Fountzopoulos E, Behan M, Butler R, Hetherington SL, et al. Radial artery anomaly and its influence on transradial coronary procedural outcome. Heart. 2009;95:410–5.
6. Dehghani P, Mohammad A, Bajaj R, Hong T, Suen CM, Sharieff W, et al. Mechanism and predictors of failed transradial approach for percutaneous coronary interventions. JACC Cardiovasc Interv. 2009;2:1057–64.
7. Patel T, Shah S, Pancholy S, Deora S, Prajapati K, Coppola J, et al. Working through challenges of subclavian, innominate, and aortic arch regions during transradial approach. Catheter Cardiovasc Interv. 2014;84:224–35.
8. Patel T, Shah S, Pancholy S, Rao S, Bertrand OF, Kwan T. Balloon-assisted tracking: a must-know technique to overcome difficult anatomy during transradial approach. Catheter Cardiovasc Interv. 2014;83:211–20.
9. Patel T, Shah S, Pancholy S. "Combo" technique for the use of 7F guide catheter system during transradial approach. Catheter Cardiovasc Interv. 2015;86:1033–40.
10. Caputo RP, Tremmel JA, Rao S, Gilchrist IC, Pyne C, Pancholy S, et al. Transradial arterial access for coronary and peripheral procedures: executive summary by the Transradial Committee of the SCAI. Catheter Cardiovasc Interv. 2011;78:823–39.
11. Hamon M, Pristipino C, Di Mario C, Nolan J, Ludwig J, Tubaro M, et al. Consensus document on the radial approach in percutaneous cardiovascular interven-

tions: position paper by the European Association of Percutaneous Cardiovascular Interventions and Working Groups on Acute Cardiac Care** and Thrombosis of the European Society of Cardiology. EuroIntervention. 2013;8:1242–51.

12. Rao SV, Tremmel JA, Gilchrist IC, Shah PB, Gulati R, Shroff AR, et al. Best practices for transradial angiography and intervention: a consensus statement from the society for cardiovascular angiography and intervention's transradial working group. Catheter Cardiovasc Interv. 2014;83:228–36.

11 Hemostasis Methods

Bong-Ki Lee, Enrique A. Flores, and Samir B. Pancholy

11.1 Introduction

Vascular access is essential to any cardiovascular procedure. In addition, proper closure of the access site is essential to prevent potential complications and ensure positive outcomes [1]. The radial artery in the distal forearm lies on the flat surface of the radial bone, offering a predictable platform for applying direct compression for hemostatic purposes. After exiting the distal forearm, it courses inferiorly and laterally into the anatomical snuffbox before providing arterial supply to the thumb and forming the deep palmar arch. Distal radial access (DRA) in the anatomical snuffbox was proposed by Avtandil Babunashvili et al. in 2011, initially for the purpose of recanalization of an occluded radial artery [2], and has subsequently been shown to be a valid access site for cardiovascular procedures [3]. We here describe hemostatic strategies for patients undergoing DRA for percutaneous cardiovascular procedures.

B.-K. Lee
Division of Cardiology, Kangwon National University Hospital, Chuncheon, Republic of Korea

E. A. Flores
Georgia Heart Specialists, Conyers, GA, USA

S. B. Pancholy (✉)
The Wright Center for Graduate Medical Education, Scranton, PA, USA

11.2 Local Anatomy

Local anatomy actually favors hemostatic compression after DRA. Indeed, the sunken location of the radial artery in the anatomical snuffbox, combined with its complex bony floor, likely restricts the amount of pressure transmitted from the skin surface to the radial artery. At the same time, the relatively inelastic walls of the anatomical snuffbox allow sufficient compressive force to be transmitted to the puncture site for effective hemostasis without excessive compression and its negative consequences. Indeed, hemostasis plays an important role in the development of radial artery occlusion, and the opportunity to mitigate its relevance is a specific advantage of DRA (see also Chap. 4).

11.3 Distal Radial Access Hemostasis

In its distal course, the radial artery lies at the floor of the anatomical snuffbox, in a recessed position compared to the distal forearm. This makes the process of direct application of hemostatic compression different than when applied at the distal forearm puncture site. In addition, since the anatomical snuffbox is essentially at the level of the wrist, movement of the wrist will affect the local anatomy. For this reason, compression of a larger area covering the anatomical snuffbox may be more effective for successful hemostasis than

G. A. Sgueglia (ed.), *Distal Radial Access*, https://doi.org/10.1007/978-3-031-89925-6_11

focal compression and may also reduce the effort required to locate the exact focal point of compression.

When considering the appropriate pressure for compression, higher pressures are not more effective than modest pressures slightly above systolic blood pressure and may also cause pain at the site of hemostasis [4]. However, the strategy of compression at suprasystolic pressure for several minutes followed by compression at subsystolic pressure for a longer duration is potentially as useful as it has been shown to be when used with the FemoStop (Abbott) femoral access site compression system [5].

The efficacy of hemostatic compression at the anatomical snuffbox is highly effective and well tolerated. In a large multicenter randomized trial comparing DRA to conventional transradial access (TRA), the observed incidence of bleeding at the distal radial artery puncture site was not higher than that observed after conventional TRA [6]. In addition, a recent meta-analysis showed a lower incidence of major hematoma formation with DRA compared to conventional TRA [7].

11.4 Different Hemostasis Methods

Several strategies have been described in the literature, all essentially resulting in the direct application of pressure on the punctured artery.

11.4.1 Gauze and Bandaging

This is the basic and traditional method of hemostasis for vascular access sites. Figure 11.1 shows the method (Lee's bandaging) developed and primarily used by Dr. Bong-Ki Lee, one of the coauthors of this chapter. It involves the use of a block of gauze sponges placed over the puncture site, wrapped in an elastic bandage, and looped around the base of the thumb, allowing pressure to be applied to the puncture site and surrounding soft tissues with reasonable allowance for wrist movement without dislodgement (Fig. 11.1). Its main advantage is the stable three-point anchor mechanism, which provides consistent and reliable pressure and prevents the compression zone from deforming or dislodging with wrist movement [1]. Another advantage is that items such as gauze and elastic bandages are readily available. It is also likely to be the least expensive option, is generally very well tolerated by patients, and can even be performed quickly by experienced practitioners. When applying elastic bandages, the "joint to joint" concept should be considered to avoid discomfort and swelling of the hand due to the tourniquet effect [8]. Therefore, bandaging only the wrist should be avoided, and it is recommended that the entire thenar and hypothenar muscles be covered. Disadvantages include the need for a learning curve and the lack of visibility of the puncture site at the level of the skin and surrounding area, making it potentially difficult to detect puncture site bleeding and hematoma formation (Table 11.1).

11.4.2 Adjustable Bands

The HemoBand (HemoBand), a plastic strap with a locking mechanism, often used to achieve hemostasis after hemodialysis at the fistula site, can also be used at the distal radial puncture site. Since the HemoBand has a flat structure, a pledget is usually placed under it to apply vertical pressure at the puncture site with the circumferential force it provides. Typically, a cylindrical plastic structure, such as a needle cap wrapped in a 4 × 4-in. gauze sheet, is best suited for this purpose because its round shape increases its tolerability and its small diameter allows for relatively focused pressure application at the puncture site (Fig. 11.2). Its main drawback is that the relatively sharp edges of the HemoBand press against the skin of the hypothenar prominence, causing discomfort in some patients, and movement of the wrist may result in dislodgement of the entire assembly, requiring the patient to keep the forearm and hand immobile.

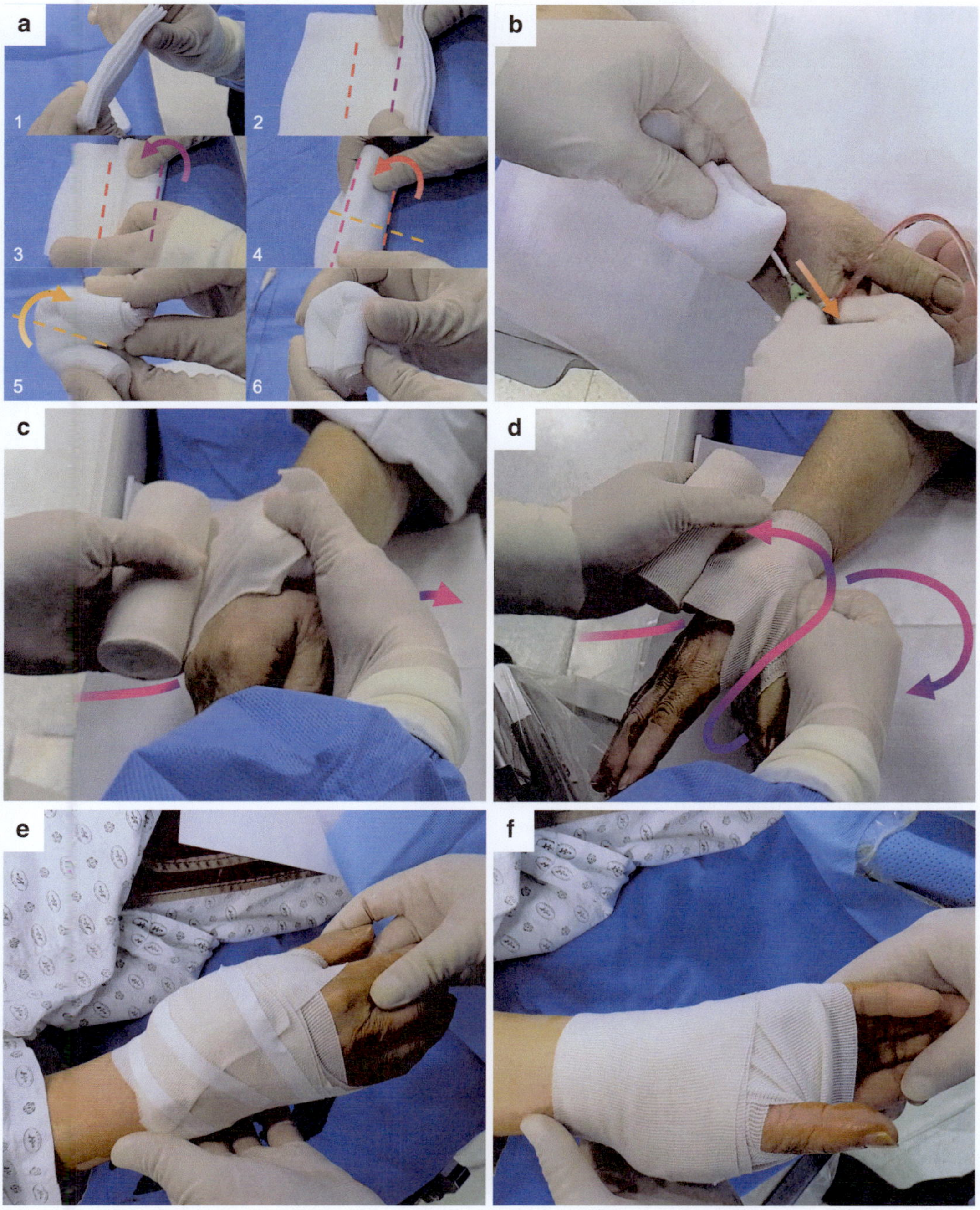

Fig. 11.1 Hemostatic method using an elastic bandage over a gauze block. (**a**) Prepare four layers of 4 × 4-in. dressing gauze (*1*), fold the layered gauze twice into three equal parts (*2–4*), and fold the folded gauze bundle in half to form a rectangular gauze block (*5–6*). (**b**) Remove the introducer sheath and compress the puncture site with the gauze block. (**c**) Using a 4-in.-wide elastic bandage, wrap the wrist twice starting from the gauze block in an ulnar direction. Tension should be modest, such as a 50% extension. Strong tension will cause pain and is not more effective. (**d**) When the bandage passes over the hypothenar muscle for the third time, pass the piece between the thumb and index finger. Then, use the gauze block as a pivot, and wrap around it. Repeat two more times, and wrap the wrist two more times. (**e**) After the cast is applied, the puncture site is safely and effectively compressed, while the hand is free to move. (**f**) The volar view shows balanced compression over the entire hand muscles, and it prevents hand swelling by avoiding the tourniquet effect. (Adapted from Lee et al. [1])

Table 11.1 Comparison of hemostasis methods for distal radial access

Method	Anchoring	Strengths	Weaknesses
Simple elastic bandaging	2 points	Readily available Low cost Easy to perform	Tourniquet effect Lack of visibility
Lee's bandaging	3 points	Readily available Stable compression Prevents hand swelling Low cost	Lack of visibility Learning curve
Simple encircling bands	2 points	Transparent Pressure adjustable	Tourniquet effect Dedicated for the wrist
PreludeSYNC DISTAL (Merit Medical)	3 points	Transparent Pressure adjustable Dedicated for distal radial access	Cost

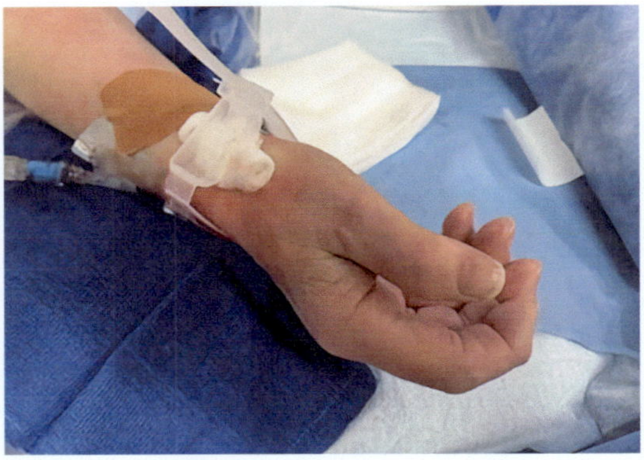

Fig. 11.2 HemoBand (HomeBand), a simple plastic and circular edge device, is used to apply circumferential pressure at the puncture site, with the use of a cylindrical plastic composed of a needle cap and gauze coating to focus the pressure at the puncture site

11.4.3 Conventional Hemostasis Devices

There are several hemostasis devices designed and used for conventional TRA such as TR Band (Terumo), Prelude SYNC (Merit Medical), or ZEPHYR (Cordis) that can be effectively used for hemostasis after DRA [9]. However, these devices were developed specifically for TRA and are not optimal for compression of the anatomical snuffbox, which has a different anatomy and is more complex than the wrist. For example, there are reports of using the TR Band (Terumo) for DRA with modifications such as removing [9] or modifying its hard plastic plate [10] (Fig. 11.3). However, when the plastic plate is removed, the band may tighten the wrist area, causing swelling of the hand due to the tourniquet effect [8], and when the plastic plate modification is applied, the procedure becomes cumbersome. Other compression devices, such as Vasc Band (Teleflex), also use air-filled bladder technology and can be used effectively for DRA hemostasis. Overall, the reliability of conventional hemostasis devices must be assessed on a case-by-case basis as there is no class effect.

11.4.4 Dedicated Hemostasis Devices

At least one dedicated device is commercially available that provides direct and focused compression of the distal radial puncture site. The design of this device, PreludeSYNC DISTAL (Merit Medical), is similar to the bandage applied around the thumb. The Velcro straps allow for proper application of the device to balance comfort and efficacy. The inflatable bladder-based compression creates a pressure point that applies focused pressure to the puncture site. Conforming material allows for some wrist mobility without major dislocation. The transparent material allows visualization of the puncture site and surrounding area (Fig. 11.4). It has been shown to be effective in a prospective study [11].

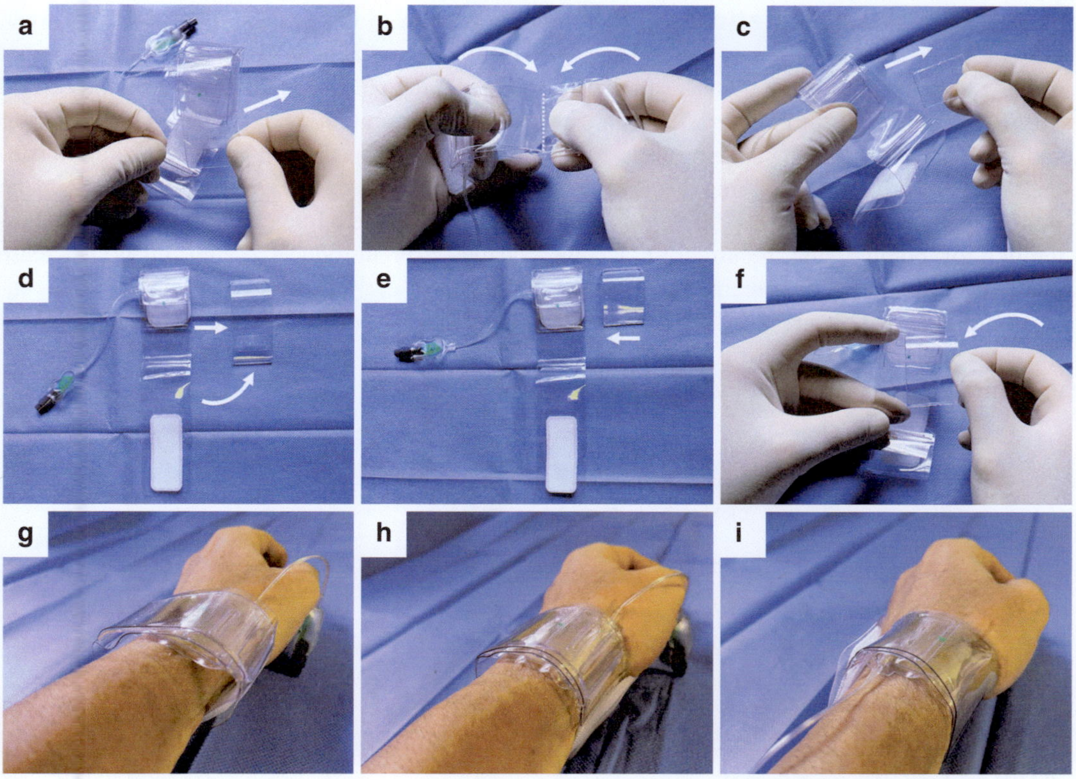

Fig. 11.3 Modification of the TR Band (Terumo) for hemostasis after distal radial access. (**a**) Removal of the TR Band hard plastic plate. (**b**) Modification of the TR Band by breaking the hard plastic plate. (**c**) Removal of the smallest portion of the divided hard plastic plate. (**d**) TR Band without its hard plastic plate. (**e**) and (**f**), Longer portion of the TR Band hard plastic plate divided after removal and subsequent reinsertion in its proper position. (**g**) Improper hemostasis with an unmodified TR Band. (**h**) Optimal distal radial access hemostasis with TR Band after removal of its hard plastic plate. (**i**) Optimal distal radial access hemostasis with TR Band after trimming its hard plastic plate

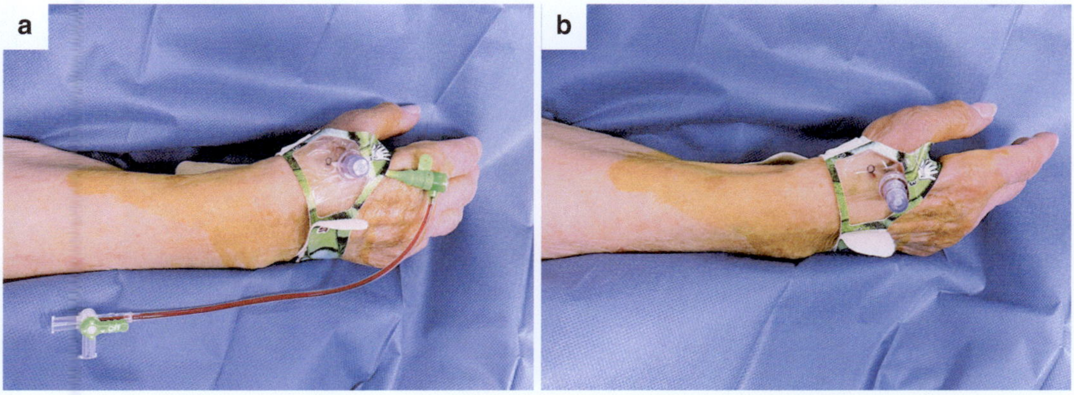

Fig. 11.4 The PreluydeSYND DISTAL (Merit Medical) distal radial access device. (**a**) Applied to the puncture site, the Velcro straps are approximated and wrapped around the thumb. (**b**) The transparent bladder is inflated to apply direct pressure to the puncture site

11.5 Hemostasis Duration

There is significant heterogeneity in the hemostasis times reported in the literature. Randomized controlled trials have shown hemostasis times ranging from 60 to 150 min [6, 12–16]. Intuitively, there should be no difference in the duration of compression required to achieve hemostasis between the forearm radial artery and the dorsal radial artery in the anatomical snuffbox, although mechanisms related to the anatomical differences mentioned above may play a role in the possible differences between the distal radial artery and the forearm radial artery. There has been an observed trend toward a shorter duration of compression required to achieve hemostasis with DRA compared to conventional TRA (Fig. 11.5), which needs to be further evaluated. Interestingly, the use of a thin-walled 5-Fr introducer sheath did not increase the rate of early hemostasis compared to a conventional 5-Fr introducer sheath in a randomized controlled trial of 352 patients [17].

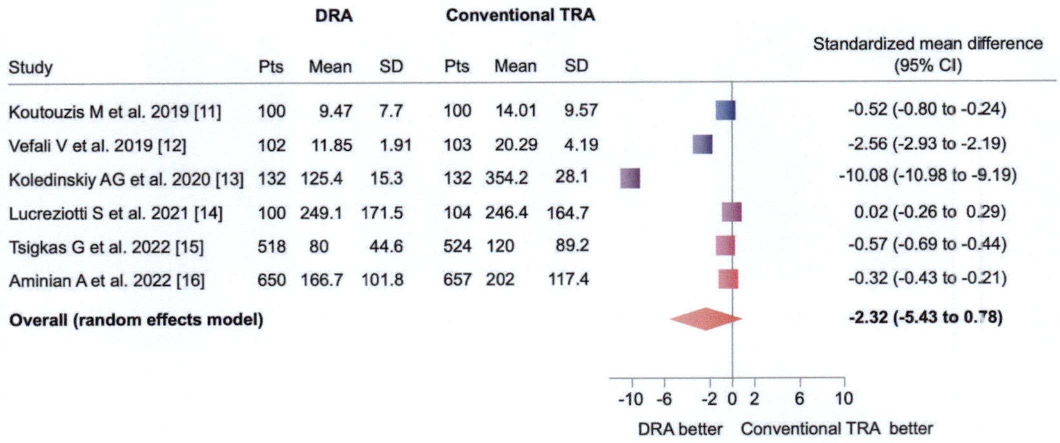

Fig. 11.5 Forest plot reporting trial-specific and summary standardized mean differences with 95% confidence interval for hemostasis duration. *CI* confidence interval, *Pts* patients, *SD* standard deviation

11.6 Patent Hemostasis

Given the sunken position of the distal radial artery in the anatomical snuffbox and a bony base that is not a flat platform, the application of direct pressure at the puncture site is likely to result in a lower probability of complete occlusion of the distal radial artery. Although plethysmographic confirmation of radial patency during compression is not reliable at this site, a recent report has demonstrated the effectiveness of using ultrasound visualization to guide hemostasis while maintaining patency. This involves the use of saline to inflate a bladder-based hemostasis device to allow ultrasound transmission [18]. In an attempt to maximize patency to preserve the access site for future access and to prevent potential sequelae, efforts to maximize preservation of radial artery flow during compression are expected to further reduce distal radial artery occlusion.

11.7 Ultrasound-Assisted Hemostasis

As described earlier, the firm floor created by the scaphoid and trapezium bones beneath the DRA allows for precise and effective hemostasis using a range of options, from a light pressure patch to a compression cuff.

11.7.1 Express Hemostasis

Express light pressure ultrasound–guided hemostasis can be achieved with a hemostatic patch in patients receiving or not receiving heparin, although a case can be made for avoiding routine use of heparin in selected DRA patients undergoing elective diagnostic coronary angiography. The advantages of this method are the short time to hemostasis and the ease of post-procedure care, as there is no need to deflate and remove a compression device. The use of vascular ultrasound to confirm adequate distal radial artery blood flow under the patch provides additional assurance that the radial artery is open and has adequate flow.

The goal of this personalized ultrasound-guided protocol is to simplify hemostasis and post-procedure recovery while virtually eliminating radial artery occlusion. This precision approach can improve patient satisfaction, facilitate post-catheterization care for the nursing staff, and expedite discharge.

Candidates for the express protocol include stable, elective coronary diagnostic patients with a sheath-to-artery ratio of <1.0 as measured by vascular ultrasound, procedures with short hydrophilic sheaths, and brief procedures with little catheter manipulation. These patients undergo a brief 5–10-min finger patch pressure hemostasis in the cardiac catheterization laboratory with vascular ultrasound visualization to confirm that the distal radial artery under the hemostatic patch is patent and free of thrombus. The distal radial artery under the hemostatic patch can be visualized with ultrasound when the topical patch is briefly immersed in sterile saline over the puncture site (Fig. 11.6). However, some patches dissolve when exposed to water, so vascular ultrasound imaging must be performed after several minutes of effective patch contact with the puncture site (Fig. 11.7).

11.7.2 Protocol for Express Hemostasis

1. A protocol is appropriate for stable outpatients undergoing elective diagnostic coronary angiography with 5- or 6-Fr sheaths and artery-to-sheath ratio >1.0.
2. Remove the arterial sheath 2–3 cm before placing the hemostatic patch over the sheath at the entry site; continue to pull the sheath while applying finger pressure on the patch to achieve hemostasis.
3. Reduce compression pressure until blood from the puncture site stains the patch to activate its hemostatic properties. The ideal image of a patch in the hand after pulling the sheath is a small ~5-mm-diameter red circle of blood

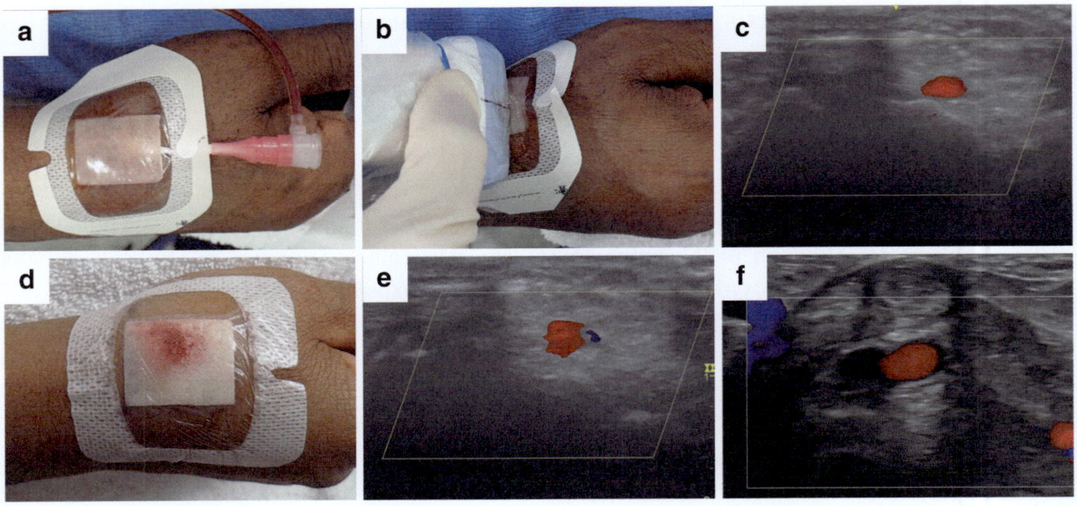

Fig. 11.6 Express hemostasis after distal radial access is achieved in 5 min with a vascular ultrasound probe pressed lightly over a D-Stat Dry Topical Hemostat (Teleflex) patch. (**a**) After flushing the side port of the sheath, a patch moistened with ~1 mL sterile saline is placed over the entry site and covered with a transparent film dressing (Tegarderm, 3 M). (**b**) The sheath is removed, and minimal controlled pressure is applied over the puncture site using either the ultrasound probe or the index finger to allow activation of the patch by contact with blood from the puncture site. (**c**) The distal radial artery flow (red) seen by color Doppler ultrasound under the patch shows little vessel wall deformation. (**d**) Successful hemostasis occurs after 5 min of combined probe and finger pressure. (**e**) The distal radial artery (red) is patent with good flow prior to discharge. (**f**) At a follow-up visit, the distal radial artery (red) is shown by color Doppler ultrasound to be open

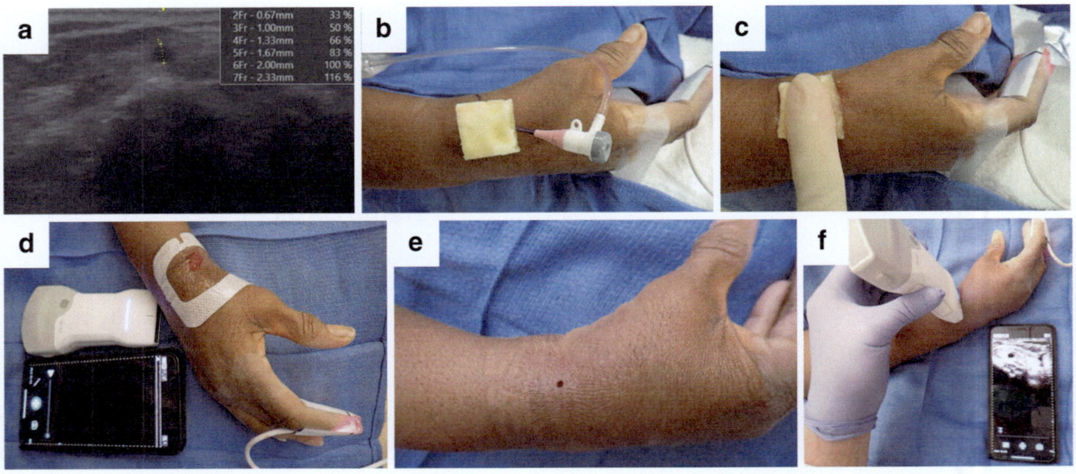

Fig. 11.7 Axiostat (Axio Biosolutions) patch pressure hemostasis achieved in 5 min in the cardiac catheterization laboratory after a diagnostic angiogram using 75 IU/kg of unfractionated heparin. (**a**) Patient selection for this protocol included the use of a 5-Fr catheter that occupied 83% of the vessel lumen. (**b**) The Axiostat patch is applied at the puncture site over the 5-Fr sheath at the trapezium. (**c**) Minimal finger pressure is applied for 5 min. (**d**) The Axiostat patch is removed after 5 min of contact, and the puncture site is covered with a transparent film dressing (Tegarderm, 3 M) and then with gel for ultrasound imaging to confirm radial artery patency. (**e**) Puncture site after ~1 h of observation. (**f**) Prior to discharge, vascular ultrasound confirmed patency of the distal and forearm radial artery; the total time spent for this express hemostasis case was ~10 min: 5 min of compression and 5 min of total ultrasound time

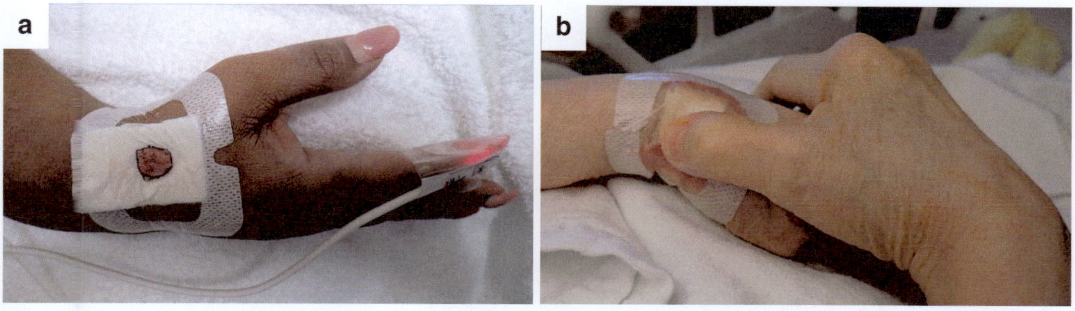

Fig. 11.8 (**a**) Patient hand after DRA express hemostasis with a ~5-mm circle of blood at the center of the patch, corresponding to the distal radial artery puncture site. (**b**) A fully awake patient holds the patch after ultrasound-guided express hemostasis while being transported to the recovery room after vessel patency was confirmed by vascular ultrasound; complete hemostasis was achieved in the catheterization laboratory

in the center of the patch at the DRA puncture site (Fig. 11.8a).

4. Once the blood spot has formed, outline the blood circle, and continue to apply pressure to prevent further blood staining. The appearance of new blood outside the circle signals the need for additional pressure.
5. The absence of blood in the patch at the time of hemostasis may indicate that the distal radial artery is occluded by a thrombus or vasospasm. Remove the patch, inspect the puncture site, and evaluate the distal and forearm radial artery with ultrasound imaging.
6. After 5 min of compression, assess distal radial artery patency with ultrasound either through a moist patch or with ultrasound gel applied to the skin. If thrombosis occurs, follow recommendations for prevention and treatment of radial artery occlusion [19].
7. If the patient is awake and stable, ask the patient to apply finger pressure to the patch site during transfer from the cath lab to the recovery area to prevent inadvertent bleeding (Fig. 11.8b).

11.7.3 Ultrasound Use in Conventional Hemostasis Protocols

The more traditional approach to hemostasis is with a compression cuff. Most devices require 12–16 cc of air in the cuff to achieve hemostasis of the radial artery at the wrist level, while compression of the distal radial artery requires only a fraction of this pressure, thus more easily achieving the "less is better" goal in hemostasis [20]. Interestingly, the conventional air-filled bladder cuff may miss the radial artery at the wrist level, and the artery may move out of the compression zone due to arm movement or adjacent intramuscular bleeding. Routine ultrasound imaging of the forearm and distal radial artery at the time of hemostasis can alert the operator to such misalignment and early hematoma formation, allowing immediate corrective actions to reduce bleeding. However, current air-filled hemostatic cuff systems do not allow ultrasound technology to image the underlying tissues. To overcome this limitation, filling the cuff with saline instead of air allows ultrasound waves to penetrate and directly visualize the arterial wall and blood flow at the time of hemostasis (Fig. 11.9). Ultrasound imaging helps minimize the risk of applying too much or too little pressure to the artery while balancing hemostasis with patency. This novel method of patent hemostasis may complement the currently accepted technique of using radial artery palpation along with oximetry plethysmography. Confirmation of uninterrupted arterial blood flow without bleeding and with minimal arterial wall collapse should help reduce radial artery occlusion.

Operators should conduct a follow-up patient evaluation soon after achieving hemostasis and before discharge to confirm the absence of bleed-

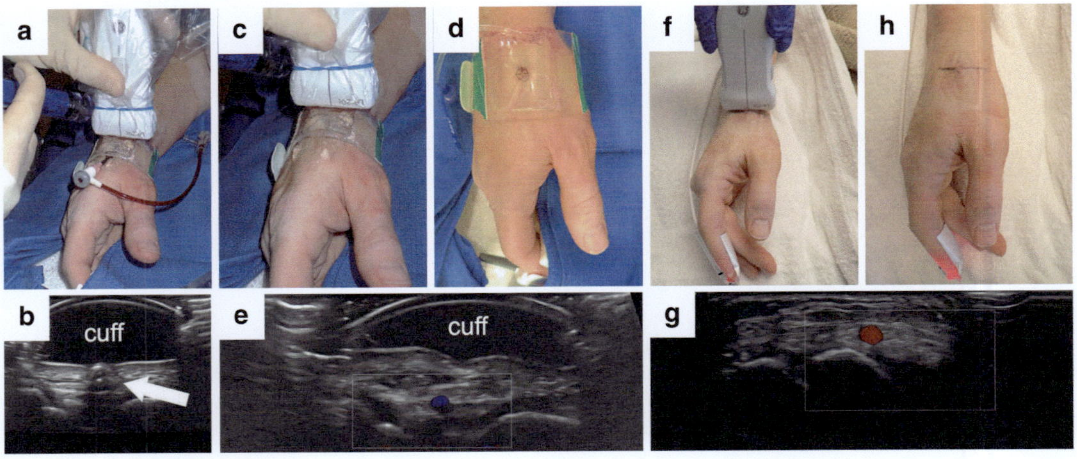

Fig. 11.9 Ultrasound-guided conventional patent hemostasis after outpatient percutaneous coronary procedure. (**a**) Conventional compression device is filled with 3 mL sterile saline and covered with gel to allow ultrasound visualization of the sheath in the distal radial artery. (**b**) The fluid-filled cuff is well centered around the 5-Fr sheath in the distal radial artery (arrow). (**c**) The centering line drawn on the transducer helps its proper placement. (**d**) The distal radial artery is patent over the trapezium during compression. (**e**) Hemostasis is effectively achieved. (**f**) Successful hemostasis. (**g**) Widely patent distal radial artery confirmed by vascular ultrasound before same-day discharge. (**h**) The patient hand after hemostasis is completed

ing and to exclude radial artery occlusion. Also, using vascular ultrasound helps establish a quality control program to monitor access-related complications, including radial artery occlusion.

References

1. Lee BK, Shin HY, Kim KH, Seo JH, Chun KJ, Ryu DJ, et al. Vascular access: the alpha and omega of cardiovascular intervention. J Cardiovasc Interv. 2023;2:170–86.
2. Babunashvili A, Dundua D. Recanalization and reuse of early occluded radial artery within 6 days after previous transradial diagnostic procedure. Catheter Cardiovasc Interv. 2011;77:530–6.
3. Kaledin AL, Kochanov IN, Seletskii SS, Arkharov IV, Burak TI, Kozlov KL. Peculiarities of arterial access in endovascular surgery in elderly patients. Adv Gerontol. 2014;27:115–9.
4. Chang K, Kim B, Shin J, Lim Y, Shin J, Lee Y, et al. Benefits of pressure-controlled hemostasis for transradial vascular access: a randomized controlled trial. Minerva Cardioangiol. 2020;68:34–41.
5. Schwartz BG, Burstein S, Economides C, Kloner RA, Shavelle DM, Mayeda GS. Review of vascular closure devices. J Invasive Cardiol. 2010;22:599–607.
6. Aminian A, Sgueglia GA, Wiemer M, Kefer J, Gasparini GL, Ruzsa Z, et al. Distal versus conventional radial access for coronary angiography and intervention: the DISCO RADIAL trial. JACC Cardiovasc Interv. 2022;15:1191–201.
7. Ferrante G, Condello F, Rao SV, Maurina M, Jolly S, Stefanini GG, et al. Distal vs conventional radial access for coronary angiography and/or intervention: a meta-analysis of randomized trials. JACC Cardiovasc Interv. 2022;15:2297–311.
8. Baxter H, Ballard K. Bandaging: a vital skill. Nurs Times. 2018;97:56–61.
9. Aoi S, Htun WW, Freeo S, Lee S, Kyaw H, Alfaro V, et al. Distal transradial artery access in the anatomical snuffbox for coronary angiography as an alternative access site for faster hemostasis. Catheter Cardiovasc Interv. 2019;94:651–7.
10. Martínez-Crespo J, Arroyo-Úcar E, Belda Cutillas JA, Benito Agüera I, González Ródenas L, Torres SF. TR Band modification for distal transradial access hemostasis. REC Interv Cardiol. 2020;2:157–60.
11. Lorena Malik J, Javed N, Naeem H. A comparative study of Terumo radial Band and PreludeSYNC hemostasis compression device after transradial coronary catheterization. Anatol J Cardiol. 2021;25:402–6.
12. Koutouzis M, Kontopodis E, Tassopoulos A, Tsiafoutis I, Katsanou K, Rigatou A, et al. Distal versus traditional radial approach for coronary angiography. Cardiovasc Revasc Med. 2019;20:678–80.
13. Vefalı V, Sarıçam E. The comparison of traditional radial access and novel distal radial access for cardiac catheterization. Cardiovasc Revasc Med. 2020;2:496–500.

14. Koledinskiy AG, Mikheeva YUV, Ogurtsov PP, Kurtasov DS, Vyazova NL. Hospital results of endovascular treatment of patients with acute coronary syndrome (ACS) through distal radial access. Eur Heart J. 2020;41(Suppl. 2):2498.
15. Lucreziotti S, Persampieri S, Gentile D, Barbieri L, Salerno-Uriarte D, Valli F, et al. Access-site hematoma in distal and conventional transradial access: a randomized trial. Minerva Cardiol Angiol. 2022;70:129–37.
16. Tsigkas G, Papageorgiou A, Moulias A, Kalogeropoulos AP, Papageorgopoulou C, Apostolos A, et al. Distal or traditional transradial access site for coronary procedures: a single-center, randomized study. JACC Cardiovasc Interv. 2022;15:22–32.
17. Tsigkas GG, Moulias AI, Spyropoulou PN, Almpanis GC, Stavrou K, Trigka-Vasilakopoulou AA, et al. Randomized comparison of Glidesheath Slender with conventional 5Fr arterial sheaths for coronary angiography through the distal radial artery. Minerva Cardiol Angiol. 2023;71:692–701.
18. Yamada T, Takahashi A, Mizuguchi Y, Hashimoto S, Hata T, Taniguchi N, Nakajima S, et al. A novel method for achieving patent hemostasis in patients undergoing percutaneous coronary intervention through the distal radial artery. Cath Lab Digest. 2018;26:60–3.
19. Bernat I, Aminian A, Pancholy S, Mamas M, Gaudino M, Nolan J, et al. Best practices for the prevention of radial artery occlusion after transradial diagnostic angiography and intervention: an International Consensus Paper. JACC Cardiovasc Interv. 2019;12:2235–46.
20. Pacchioni A, Mugnolo A, Sanz Sanchez J, Sgueglia GA, Pesarini G, Bellamoli M, et al. Radial artery occlusion after conventional and distal radial access: impact of preserved flow and time-to-hemostasis in a propensity-score matching analysis of 1163 patients. Catheter Cardiovasc Interv. 2022;99:827–35.

12 Prevention and Management of Complications

Aleksandr Kaledin and Andrea Pacchioni

12.1 Introduction

The increasing use of transradial access (TRA) for percutaneous coronary intervention (PCI) has improved patient comfort and safety but can still be associated with complications such as forearm radial artery occlusion (RAO) and hematoma, with the potential risk of compartment syndrome. To reduce TRA complications, efforts have focused on miniaturizing procedures and finding optimal puncture sites for easier and safer hemostasis.

Distal radial access (DRA) in the anatomical snuffbox or first metacarpal space is emerging as a viable solution. In fact, DRA has gained popularity in various interventional communities and has been shown to be safe and effective in a variety of percutaneous procedures [1–3]. However, concerns may still arise with DRA, especially in the presence of radial artery spasms or specific anatomical characteristics.

This chapter presents a systematic classification of access-related complications after DRA (Fig. 12.1). Each complication has its own unique incidence, prognosis, and management [4, 5]. Of note, radial artery spasm, which occurs in up to 34% of cases, is considered a paraphysiological response of the artery to a foreign stimulus rather than a complication, although it can still lead to complications in the access artery [4, 6].

A. Kaledin
Endovascular Surgery Department, Northwestern State Medical University named after I.I. Mechnikov, Saint-Petersburg, Russian Federation

A. Pacchioni (✉)
Division of Cardiology, Azienda Ospedaliera Universitaria Integrata Verona, Verona, Italy

G. A. Sgueglia (ed.), *Distal Radial Access*, https://doi.org/10.1007/978-3-031-89925-6_12

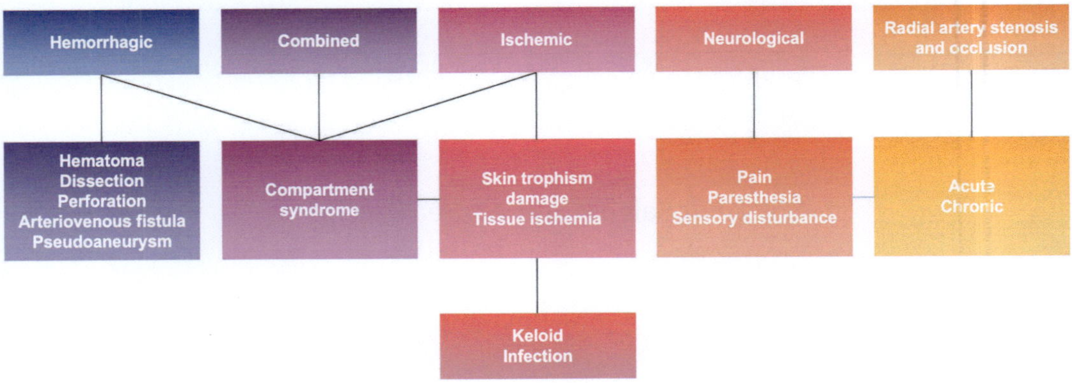

Fig. 12.1 Classification of radial access complications

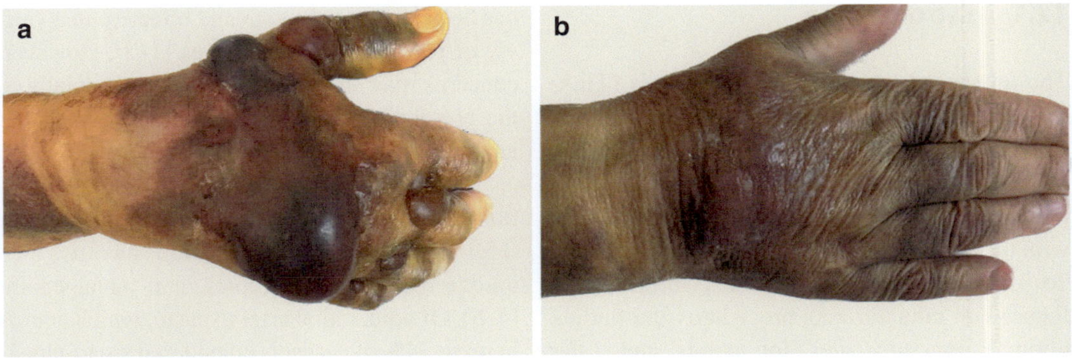

Fig. 12.2 Hand hematoma after distal radial access. (**a**) The first day after the procedure. (**b**) Fifteen days after the procedure

12.2 Hemorrhagic Complications

While the transition from transfemoral to TRA has reduced major hemorrhagic complications during endovascular procedures [7, 8], conventional TRA does not provide absolute protection against such problems [4, 9], and several studies show that both conventional TRA and DRA may lead to rare local hemorrhagic complications [10–13].

12.2.1 Hematoma

Hematoma is the most common local hemorrhagic complication of transradial procedures and is graded according to severity using the EASY scale [14]. A hematoma with an area of 15 cm^2 is considered significant (Fig. 12.2) [15]. Hematomas may result from factors such as ineffective hemostasis, perforation of the radial artery or its small branches, or repeated arterial puncture. The source of the hematoma may be either the puncture site or the forearm radial artery if damaged during the catheterization procedure.

Compartment syndrome, an extreme manifestation, can occur when an enlarging hematoma compresses tissue, resulting in secondary ischemia. Although DRA has a lower incidence of compartment syndrome compared to conventional TRA due to the unique anatomical structure of the hand, it cannot be completely excluded. Hematoma prevention involves optimizing radial artery puncture, ensuring effective hemostasis, and monitoring with ultrasound to assess local damage and determine the underlying cause. Conservative management is appropriate for small, uncomplicated hematomas and

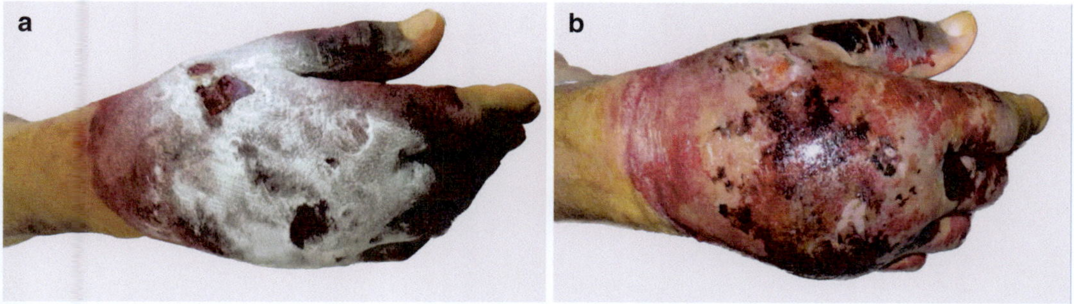

Fig. 12.3 (**a**) Conservative treatment of hand hematoma (streptocide powder) after distal radial access. (**b**) Scarring of the wound surface of the hand

includes tight bandaging of the hematoma area, administration of analgesics, and, if the hematoma is infected, use of antibiotics and antiseptics to treat the injury site prior to application of an aseptic dressing (Fig. 12.3). Larger hematomas may require ultrasound evaluation, and if the arterial wall is damaged, surgical intervention, either endovascular or open, may be required. Complicated hematomas associated with compartment syndrome require fasciotomy to decompress tissue, improve microcirculation, and reduce tissue ischemia. Compartment syndrome after DRA is most often due to injury to the forearm radial artery because the anatomic structures in the wrist tend to prevent hematoma extension from the hand to the forearm, emphasizing the need for hemostasis at the site of damage to the artery wall rather than at the puncture site.

12.2.2 Other Hemorrhagic Complications

Other types of hemorrhagic complications include dissection, arterial perforation, and pseudoaneurysm, which share a common mechanism involving varying degrees of mechanical damage to the arterial wall during instrument manipulation in the arterial lumen (Fig. 12.4). In particular, the introducer sheath may conceal immediate distal radial artery damage that may only become apparent after removal. In addition, the persistence of damage appears to correlate with its significance (Fig. 12.5).

12.2.2.1 Radial Artery Dissection

Dissection, often the result of instrument impact on the arterial wall or device-artery mismatch, generally responds well to conservative treatment. Unlike other local hemorrhagic complications, radial artery dissection lacks penetrating damage, limiting the spread of blood into surrounding tissue. Dissections vary in size, severity, and degree of restriction of blood flow. In DRA, dissections typically have a favorable prognosis due to the distal-to-proximal direction with antegrade blood flow pushing the flap back against the arterial wall. In addition, a "temporary stent" effect is exerted by the prolonged presence of the catheter/introducer sheath within the lumen, which promotes flap apposition to the arterial wall [15]. Persistent dissections can be managed with a pressure bandage and prolonged compression (Fig. 12.6). Retrograde flap dissections have a higher risk of thrombosis/occlusion (Fig. 12.7) and may require endovascular treatment. The absence of clinical symptoms often leads to incidental findings of dissection, which suggests an underreported incidence after endovascular procedures.

12.2.2.2 Radial Artery Perforation

Dissection and perforation of the radial artery wall are often related, with perforation rarely occurring without dissection. Wall perforation varies from angiographically invisible but detectable on intravascular imaging (Fig. 12.8) to pseudoaneurysm development. Clinical manifestations are usually obvious due to blood leakage into surrounding tissues, causing patient discomfort and hematoma. In

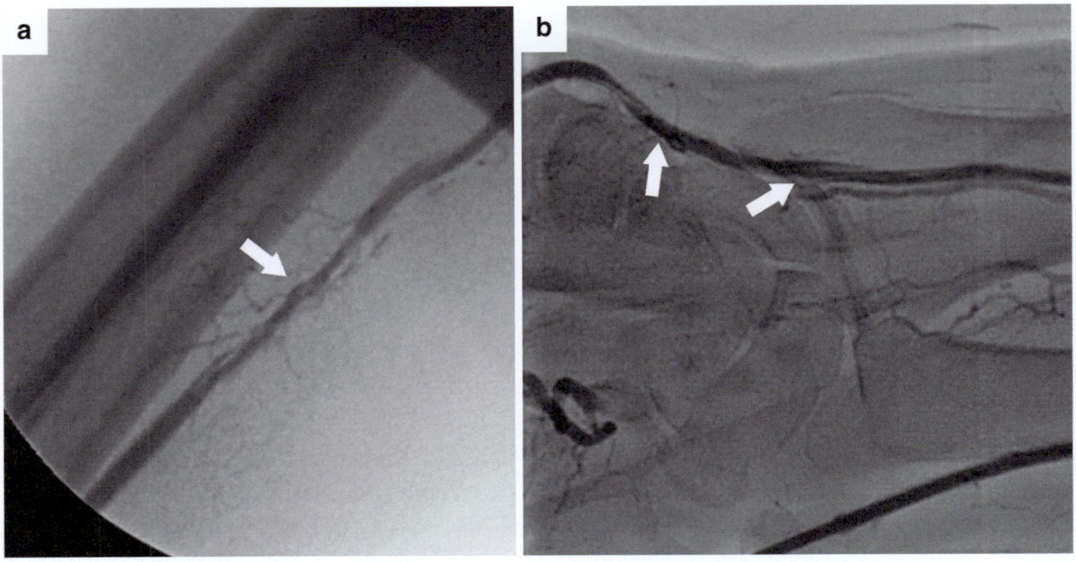

Fig. 12.4 (**a**) Dissection (arrow) of the medium segment of the radial artery. (**b**) Extended dissection of the radial artery on the rear of the wrist and in the anatomical snuffbox (arrows), after unsuccessful distal radial access and crossover to ulnar access

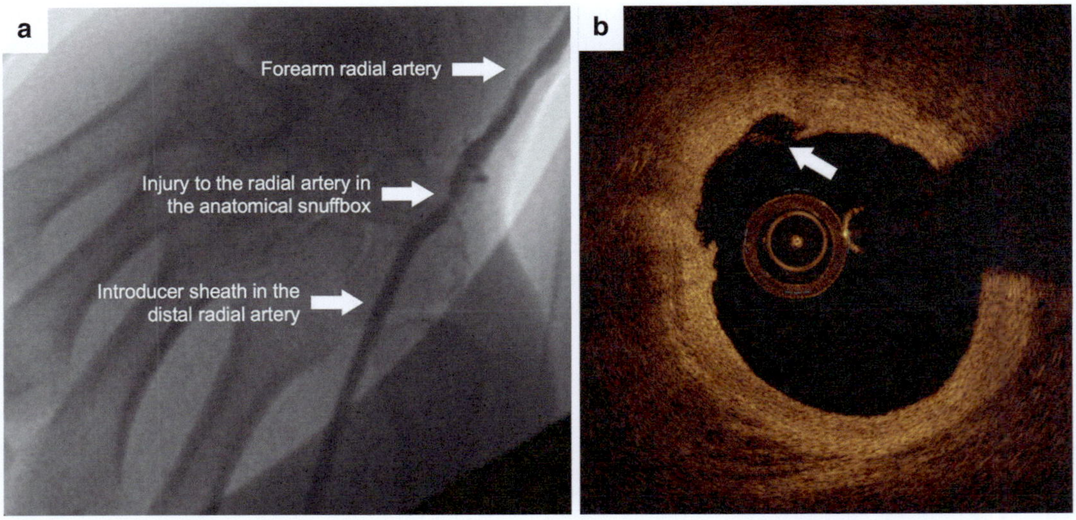

Fig. 12.5 (**a**) Angiography showing distal radial artery damage. (**b**) Optical coherence tomography of the radial artery in the anatomical snuffbox showing damage of the intima and partly of the medial layer (arrow)

addition, aggressive anticoagulation, antiplatelet therapy, or mechanical stress may worsen asymptomatic perforations into serious complications such as pseudoaneurysms or fistulas. Radial artery perforation, while relatively rare, requires a more aggressive approach because it involves all layers of the arterial wall. Treatment includes conservative measures such as ultrasound-guided external compression and pressure bandaging. If ineffective, surgical options are considered, including endovascular balloon angioplasty with angiographic guidance and external compression. If endovascular treatment fails, surgical repair becomes necessary.

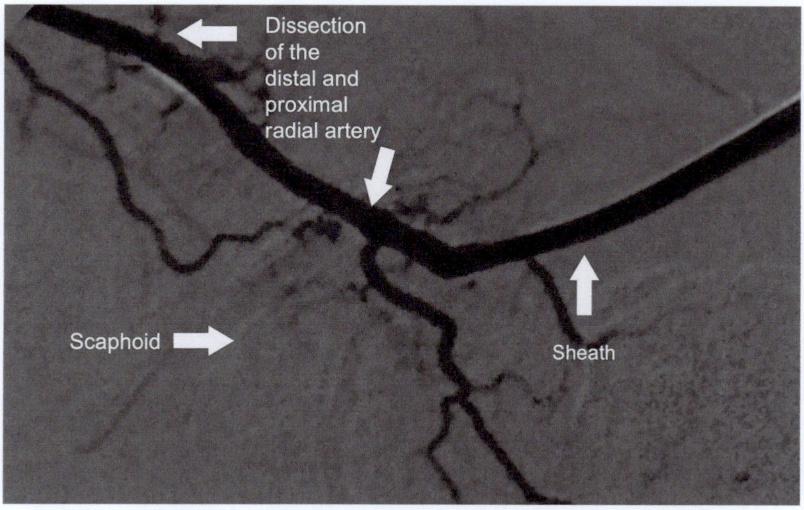

Fig. 12.6 Extended spiral dissection of the radial artery from the anatomical snuffbox to the distal forearm

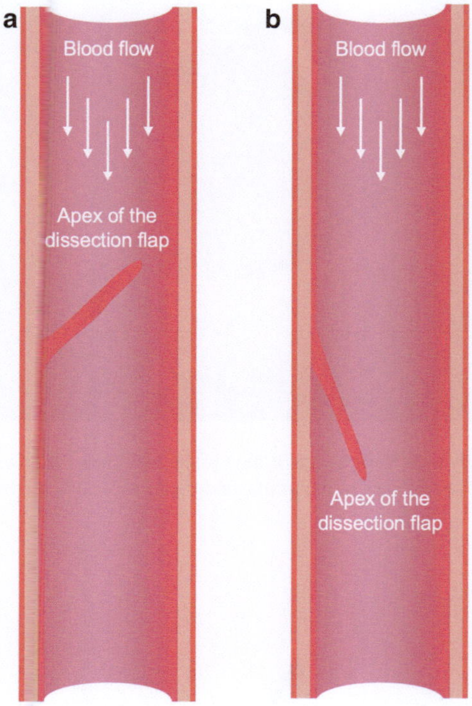

Fig. 12.7 (**a**) Retrograde flap dissection. (**b**) Antegrade flap dissection

12.2.2.3 Pseudoaneurysm

Pseudoaneurysms, which are rare in both conventional TRA and DRA, vary in size [11, 16]. Large pseudoaneurysms are identified visually and confirmed by ultrasound, whereas small pseudoaneurysms are often incidental and do not cause patient discomfort (Fig. 12.9). Incomplete hemostasis after radial artery puncture is the most common cause of pseudoaneurysm, with high-dose anticoagulants and antiplatelet agents as predisposing factors [17]. Pseudoaneurysms following radial artery catheterization in the anatomical snuffbox are typically small due to the artery's location on a bony base with limited soft tissue, which facilitates early detection and prevents their usual progression (Fig. 12.10).

Treatment options, ranging from conservative to surgical, depend on the size and severity of the pseudoaneurysm. Small pseudoaneurysms may respond well to external compression or tight bandaging. Larger ones may require endovascular techniques such as balloon occlusion, aneurysm embolization, or thrombin injection (Fig. 12.11). More radical surgical interventions include aneurysm excision, arterial plasty, or ligation.

12.2.2.4 Arteriovenous Fistula

Post-procedural arteriovenous fistula, which is often initially asymptomatic or with mild symptoms, may go undetected. In later stages, patients may notice swelling and pulsation of the hand and forearm veins. Visual inspection and ultrasound are the initial diagnostic tools (Fig. 12.12). Patients with fistulas may report a "buzzing" sound in the hand, indicating the fistula is approximately 3–4 weeks old. Angiography assesses the

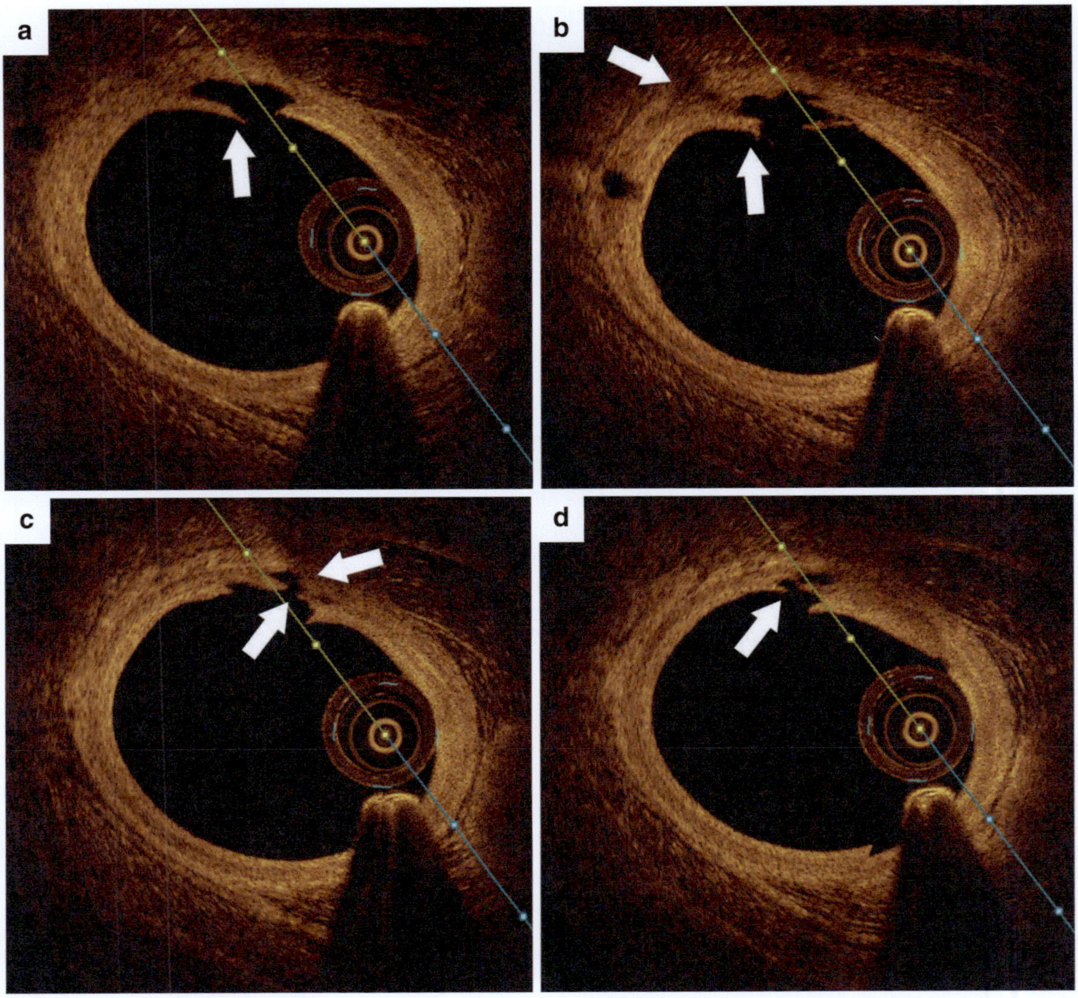

Fig. 12.8 Optical coherence tomography of the radial artery showing (**a**) damage to the intima and partly the medial layer (arrow), (**b**, **c**) damage to all layers of the artery with a site of perforation of the artery wall (arrows), and (**d**) damage to the intima and the medial layer (arrow)

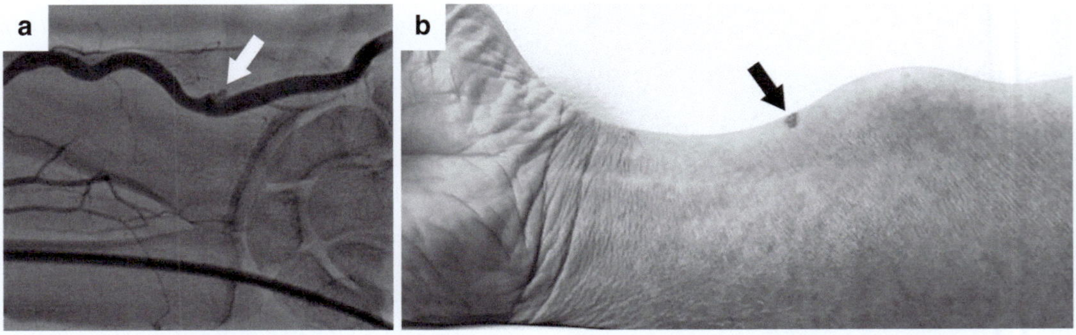

Fig. 12.9 (**a**) Angiography of the radial artery in the distal forearm showing a small pseudoaneurysm (arrow). (**b**) Forearm with a bulging large-size pseudoaneurysm of the radial artery, proximal to the puncture point (arrow)

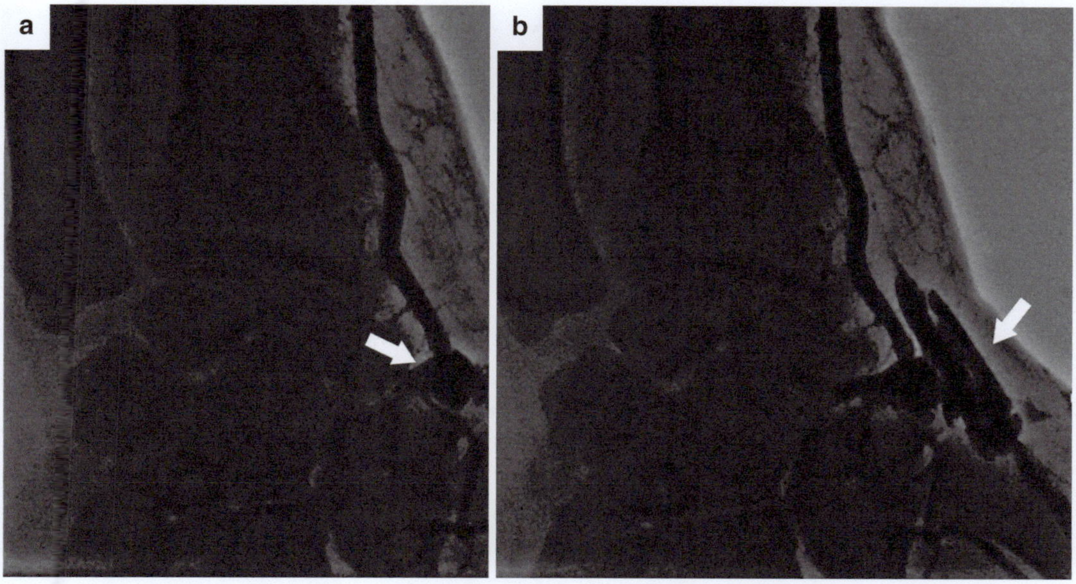

Fig. 12.10 (**a**) Angiography of the distal part of the radial artery showing a pseudoaneurysm in the anatomical snuffbox (arrow) and limited blood flow in the deep palmar arch. (**b**) Hematoma (arrow) at anatomical snuffbox radial artery puncture site after external compression

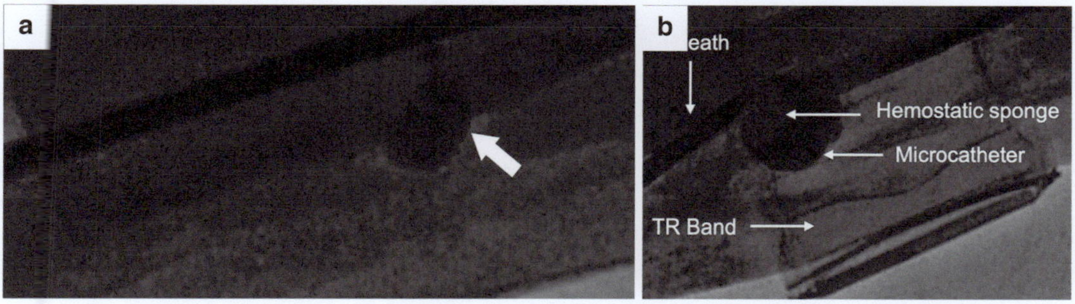

Fig 12.11 (**a**) Baseline angiography showing a large radial artery pseudoaneurysm (arrow). (**b**) Endovascular treatment with microcatheter, hemostatic sponge, and external compression with a TR Band compression devices

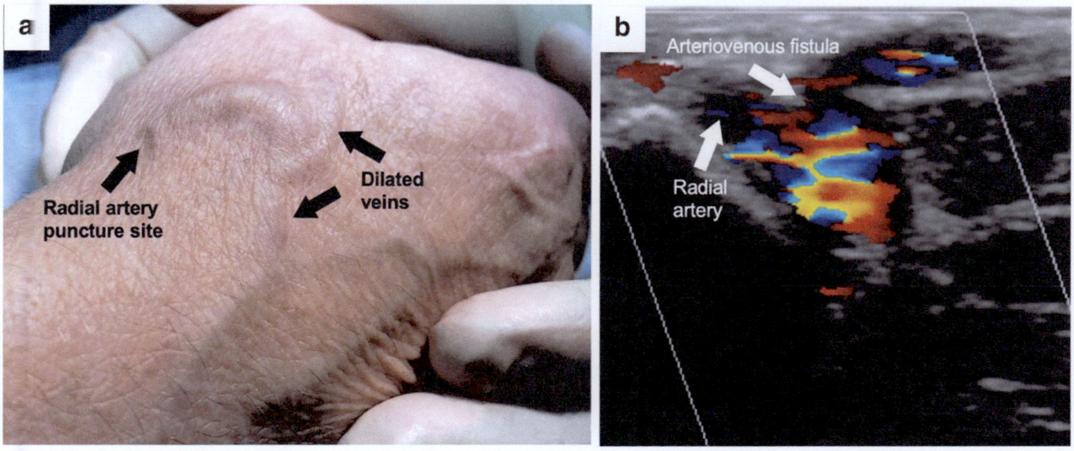

Fig. 12.12 (**a**) Swollen veins of the hand (arrows) suggesting arteriovenous fistula after distal radial access in the anatomical snuffbox. (**b**) Ultrasound findings

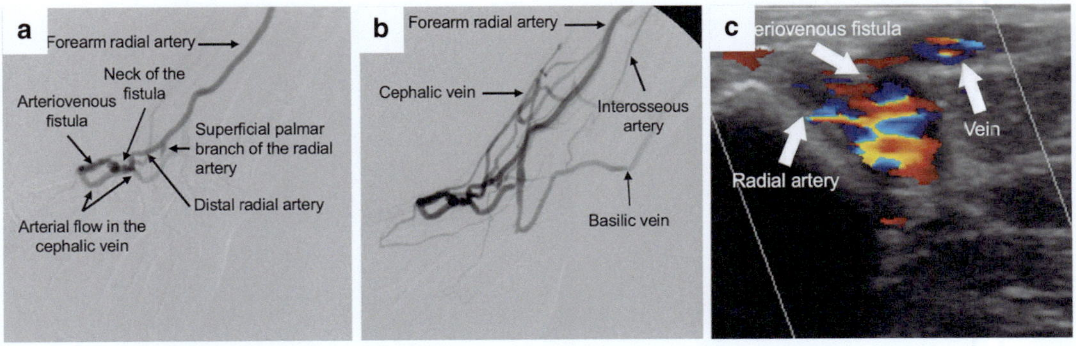

Fig. 12.13 (**a**, **b**) Post-procedural arteriovenous fistula in an anatomical snuffbox between the distal radial artery and superficial veins (there is no antegrade blood flow in the radial artery distal to the arteriovenous fistula). (**c**) Ultrasound findings

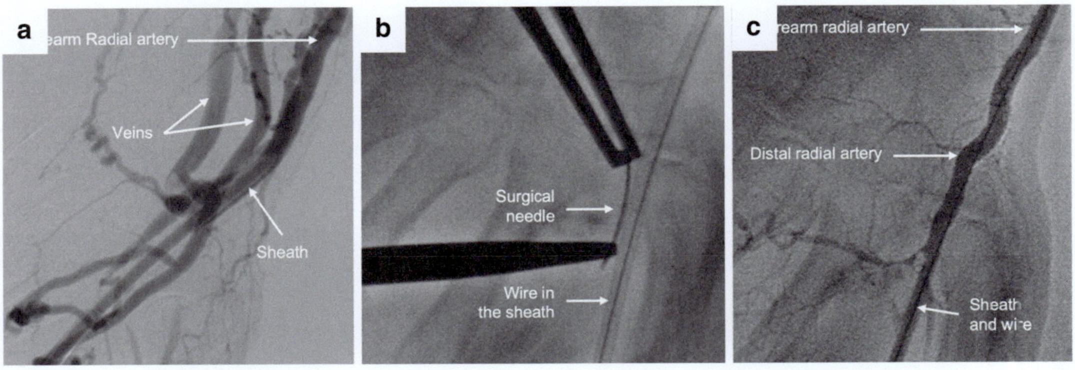

Fig. 12.14 (**a**) Angiography of the radial artery (the fistula is located under the sheath). (**b**) Percutaneous suturing of the arteriovenous fistula (the sheath is a marker for suture placement). (**c**) Control angiography of the radial artery showing disappearance of arterial blood shunting into the venous system

severity of the fistula and the presence of a neck (Fig. 12.13). If endovascular treatment fails, vascular surgery with partial radial artery resection, ligation, and excision is considered (Fig. 12.14) [18].

12.2.3 Preventing Hemorrhagic Complications of Radial Access

Hemorrhagic complications with radial access can occur not only at the puncture site, but also on the forearm if the artery is injured during catheter manipulation. To minimize hemorrhagic complications with radial access, consider the following precautions and best practices:

1. Educate patients about potential local complications and appropriate interventions.
2. Ensure adequate experience with DRA [10].
3. Evaluate hand conditions, and consider alternative approaches in the presence of deformities, motor or joint disorders, or skin changes (Fig. 12.15).
4. Avoid puncturing the distal radial artery if weak pulsation is observed without ultrasound guidance and choose an alternative puncture site.
5. Use ultrasound to assess artery characteristics, including diameter, topography, calcification, anomalies, and occlusions, before puncturing the distal radial artery [19–21].
6. Provide adequate anesthesia and spasm control; consider local anesthetic administration along the artery [22].

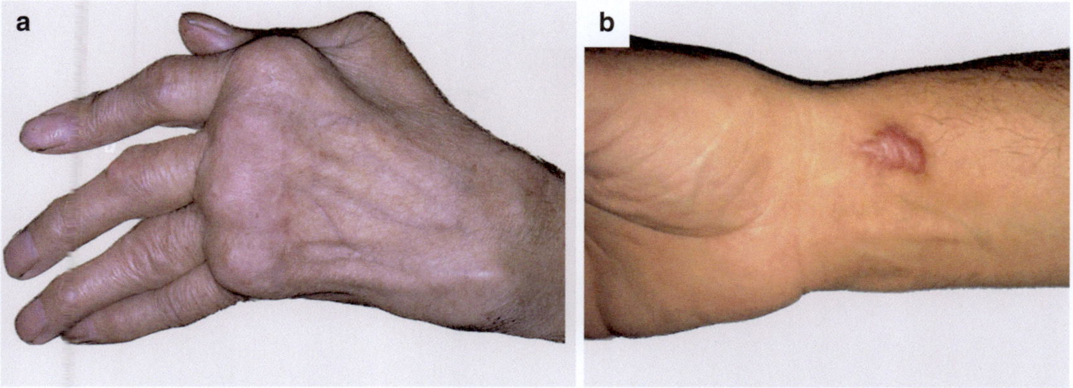

Fig. 12.15 (**a**) Deformation of the hand (ulnar deviation) in a patient with rheumatoid arthritis. (**b**) Keloid after conventional transradial access

7. Use ultrasound guidance for DRA [10, 19].
8. Aim to puncture only the anterior wall of the artery and provide adequate anticoagulation.
9. Use the lowest profile device that will allow the procedure to be successful, especially in tortuous anatomy where it is worth using an inflated balloon at the tip of the catheter (see also Chap. 10).
10. Avoid forceful manipulation of the catheter and wire, and perform immediate radial artery angiography if resistance is encountered.
11. Achieve complete hemostasis after sheath removal by monitoring blood flow with ultrasound [22].

12.3 Ischemic Complications

Ischemic complications after DRA are relatively rare, mainly due to certain peculiarities of the hand blood supply [23]. It is widely acknowledged that RAO is not the primary cause of ischemic complications [24]. Instead, hand ischemia may result from factors such as impaired arterial flow, hemostasis problems, or external compression in hemorrhagic complications (compartment syndrome). Although it is theoretically possible for wrist ischemia to develop in DRA, specific conditions must be met for this to occur:

1. RAO leads to distal embolization, resulting in occlusion of the digital arteries (Fig. 12.16) [25].
2. Absence or limitation of blood flow occurs through the ulnar and interosseous arteries.
3. Concomitant arm vascular pathologies include Raynaud's disease, vibration disease, Monckeberg's arteriosclerosis, atherosclerosis [26], vasculitis, arthritis, thrombosed hemodialysis fistulas, and fibrovascular dysplasia (Fig. 12.17) [27–29].
4. Contributing factors such as coagulopathy or infection (e.g., COVID-19) [30].
5. Impaired hemostasis (prolonged, tight bandaging) and unconsciousness of the patient.

Treatment involves identifying the source of the problem and restoring proper antegrade blood flow to the distal radial and digital arteries.

For thromboembolic occlusion, treatment options include conservative strategies with anticoagulants, thrombolytics, and antithrombotics or surgical intervention. Endovascular balloon angioplasty and embolectomy are used to remove the embolus. Surgical methods to resolve hand ischemia resulting from concomitant pathologies are diverse, ranging from arteriotomy, ligation, and artery excision with cephalic vein graft replacement to endoscopic thoracic sympathectomy [27, 28, 31].

To prevent ischemic complications, a multifaceted approach is recommended:

1. Identify comorbidities that may increase risk.
2. Consider alternative arterial access if appropriate.

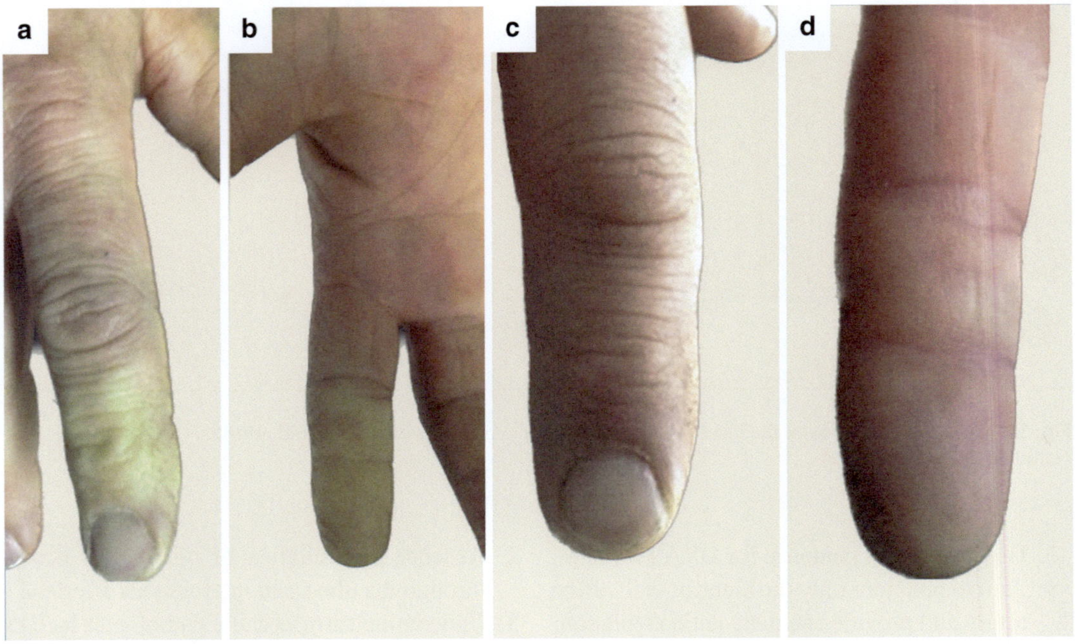

Fig. 12.16 (**a**–**d**) Embolic digital ischemia

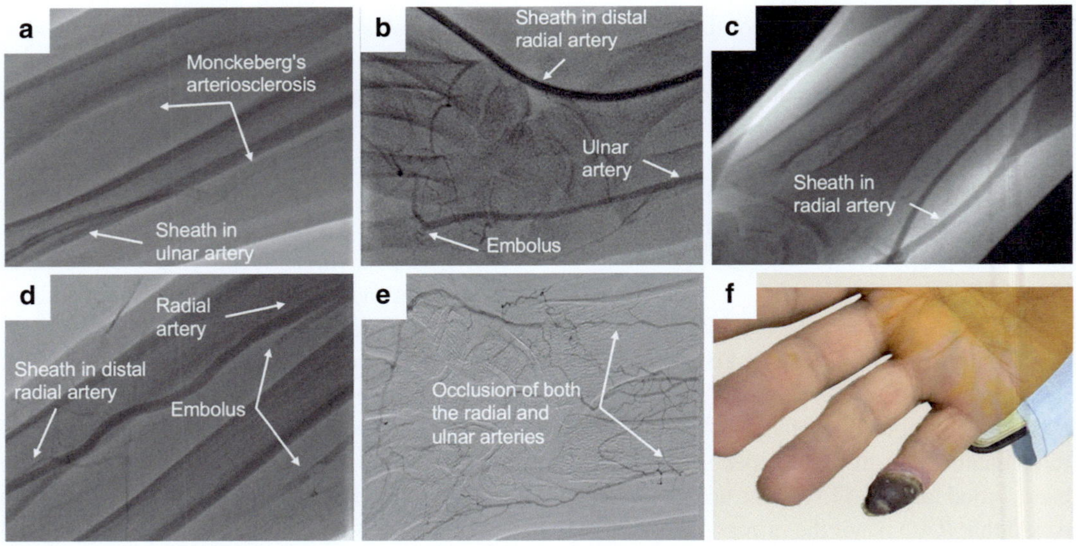

Fig. 12.17 Predictors of possible ischemic complications. (**a**) Monckeberg's arteriosclerosis of the radial and ulnar arteries. (**b**) Ulnar artery embolism with preserved blood flow in the deep palmar arch. (**c**) Limited blood flow in the ulnar and interosseous arteries. (**d**) Ulnar artery embolism with limited antegrade blood flow and occlusive embolus in the interosseous artery. (**e**) Occlusion of the radial and ulnar arteries (Monckeberg's arteriosclerosis) with filling of the deep palmar arch and the distal radial artery from the interosseous artery (limited blood flow to the fourth and fifth fingers). (**f**) Necrosis of the distal phalanx of the same patient's fifth finger

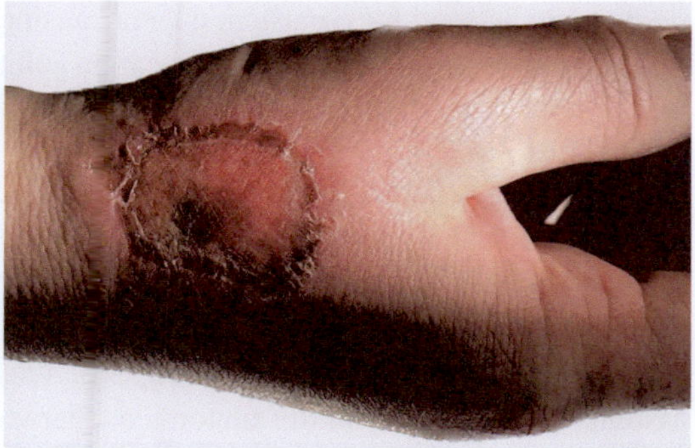

Fig. 12.18 Damaged skin surface 10 days after an excessively tight bandage was applied to the radial artery puncture site in the anatomical snuffbox

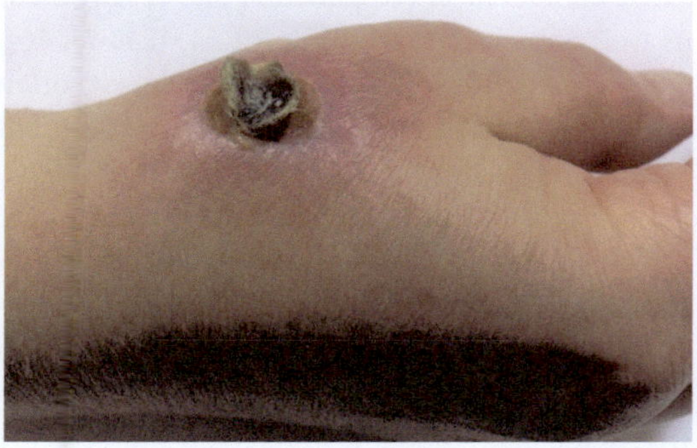

Fig. 12.19 Infected puncture site 12 days after removal of the procedure

3. Use ultrasound to monitor arterial patency in the first hours after device removal.
4. Ensure thorough control of hemostasis, and use plethysmography if necessary.

Improper hemostasis techniques, such as prolonged compression or the use of a bandage or hemostatic device that compresses the arterial puncture site, may result in local ischemia of the skin at the puncture site (Fig. 12.18). Ischemic skin lesions may occasionally induce infection around the radial artery puncture site (Fig. 12.19).

12.4 Pain, Paresthesia, and Impaired Sensitivity

These complications, collectively referred to as neuritis or neuropathy, often lack objective clinical manifestations and present primarily as subjective sensations. This variability in patient experience presents a challenge in addressing this adverse event, as each individual may perceive their sensations differently due to personal differences in perception and sensitivity thresholds.

The main questions raised by these complications are as follows:

1. The significance of the complication
2. The cause of the complication
3. The need for treatment, with considerations for approach and medication
4. The duration of tolerability if no treatment is required

While DRA does not eliminate access-related complications, it has the potential to reduce their incidence [32, 33], particularly those involving the superficial branch of the radial nerve (see also Chaps. 3 and 13) [34]. Mechanical or ischemic injury to the radial nerve may result from trauma, compression, hematoma, or violation of hemostasis techniques. Neuritis may result from prolonged mechanical compression of the radial nerve branches overlying the tendons of the hand finger muscles due to direct pressure or ischemic effects.

Impairment of blood flow to the nerve artery results in only relative ischemia as complete ischemia can only be achieved by removing or stretching the epineurium of the nerve [35]. Even without a blood supply, a completely ischemic nerve can function for some time, receiving oxygen by diffusion from neighboring tissues [36]. This is important in the context of DRA hemostasis, which is typically less prolonged than with conventional TRA [11, 13, 37–39]. Compression force also plays a critical role in radial nerve injury, with higher forces associated with increased risk [36]. Prolonged and intense compression can release lactate, which may contribute to ischemic pain. Chemical injury to the radial nerve is extremely rare and occurs only with intraneural drug administration.

Patients may report pain after distal radial artery catheterization, which is typically assessed using a visual analog scale [11, 33, 37]. It is important to distinguish between pain during instrument manipulation and persistent postprocedural pain. Inadequate local anesthesia or radial artery spasm may cause pain during manipulation, whereas persistent postprocedural pain (>1 day) may indicate underlying problems such as arteritis or infection. Predictors of postprocedural pain may include prolonged hemostasis, multiple puncture attempts, and small radial artery diameter [40]. Studies have linked pain and infectious complications to upper extremity dysfunction, affecting strength, sensation, coordination, and active range of motion [40, 41]. However, RAO does not appear to affect arm function [24].

Distal radial artery catheterization may also result in arm motor dysfunction, but this is not directly related to radial nerve injury because the superficial branch of the radial nerve has no motor branches. More likely, pain, inflammation, or infection at the puncture site may cause tissue swelling that limits hand function.

Therapeutic measures should prioritize hand immobilization, avoidance of movement, and conservative therapies such as anti-inflammatory medications, ultrasound, and physical therapy. Patients with extensive hematoma or swelling of the hand may require surgical treatment with decompression of the superficial branch of the radial nerve [42]. A minimally invasive technique called hydrodissection, which uses anesthetic or saline to separate the nerve from the surrounding tissue, may be used for persistent edema causing disabling pain in the wrist and radiocarpal joint [43, 44].

12.5 Radial Artery Occlusion

The original idea of DRA was to reduce or eliminate the occurrence of RAO [1–3, 32, 36]. This assumption was based on the anatomical characteristics of the radial artery of the wrist and forearm. However, time has shown that DRA does not completely eliminate this complication [11]. As with other local complications, RAO with DRA can occur at the puncture site (Fig. 12.20) as well as in the forearm (Fig. 12.21) [21, 45, 46].

Occlusion of the radial artery most often leaves the hand with compensated blood flow, but latent arterial insufficiency may occur [47, 48]. With occlusion of both forearm arteries, the effectiveness of compensatory mechanisms is reduced or hampered, potentially leading to ischemia in the arm and hand. In RAO, the formation of collateral circulation may provide an alternative to the main blood flow. Its main source is the anastomoses between the main arteries (radial, ulnar, and interosseous) and the palmar arches. If the existing anastomoses are not sufficient for the development of collateral circulation, neoangiogenesis is possible. However, the role of newly formed vessels in the process of compensating

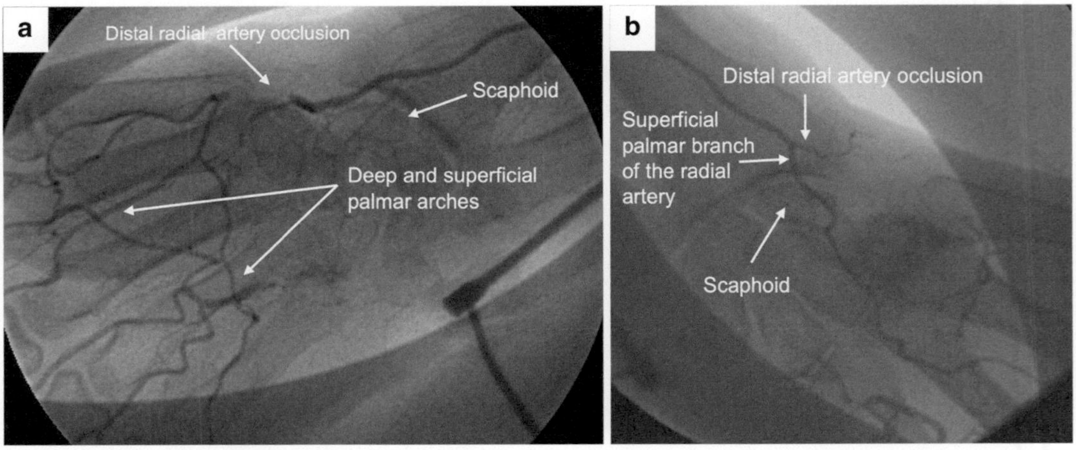

Fig. 12.20 Angiography of the forearm and the wrist in patients after distal radial access showing (**a**) distal radial artery occlusion in the backhand and (**b**) distal radial artery occlusion in the anatomical snuffbox

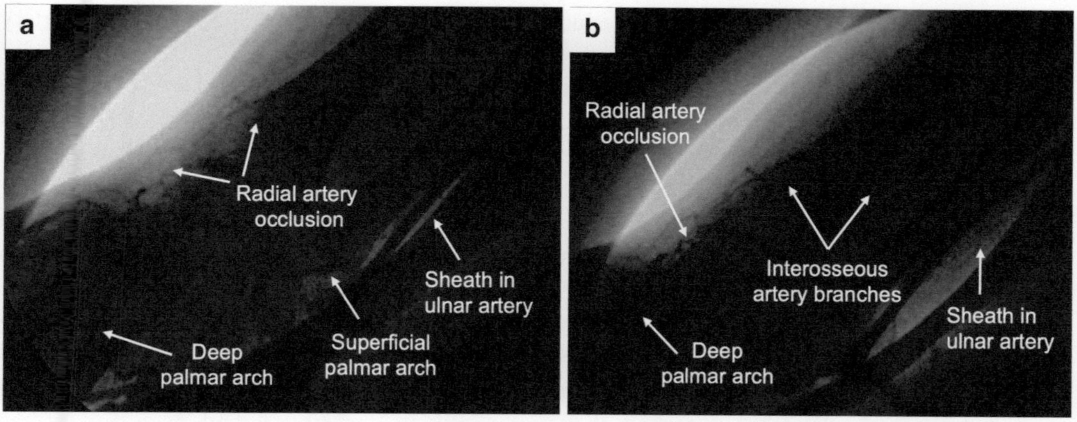

Fig. 12.21 Angiography of the forearm and the wrist showing distal radial artery occlusion extending to the forearm. (**a**) Late arterial filling. (**b**) Early arterial filling

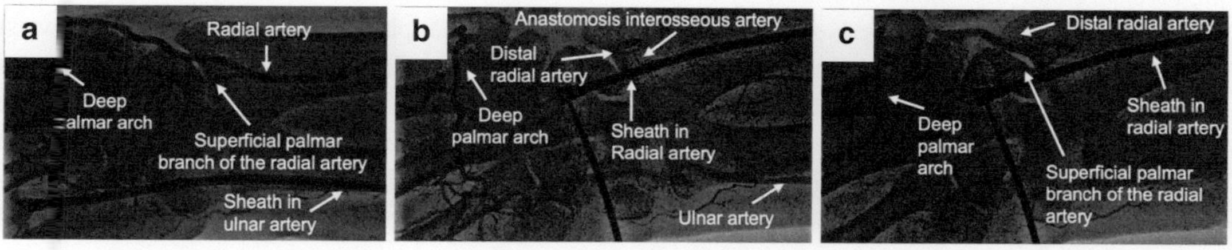

Fig. 12.22 (**a**) Baseline angiography of the radial artery during diagnostic coronary angiography. (**b**) Subsequent conventional transradial access shows collateralization due to anastomosis between the interosseous and radial arteries 1.5 h after forearm radial artery catheterization. (**c**) Preserved blood flow along the superficial palmar branch of the radial artery

for impaired blood flow is less significant, because the development of macroscopically visible collaterals after occlusion of the main arteries occurs only after 20–30 days [49].

The arterio-arterial anastomoses gradually expand to ensure that the ischemic zones are adequately supplied with blood in the early stages after RAO. This is achieved by incorporating the maximum number of anastomoses into the collateral blood flow in the affected area. The microcirculatory bed also undergoes significant compensatory changes, where arteriolo-arteriolar anastomoses turn into microvascular collaterals. After the main collaterals differentiate and stabilize, the changes in the microcirculatory bed gradually disappear, and hemodynamic conditions become similar to normal (Fig. 12.22) [49–51]. These described mechanisms explain why clinical manifestations are typically absent in cases of RAO.

12.5.1 Classification

To date, there is no classification that clearly distinguishes between acute/early and chronic/late RAO. Some investigators have suggested using coronary artery occlusion as a basis for classification. This approach seems plausible because the diameters of these arteries are comparable, and the time of radial artery catheterization and the time of removal of the introducer from the artery are known, potentially indicating the time of arterial thrombosis, if it occurs.

However, there are limitations to the use of coronary artery occlusion as a basis for classification. Not all cases of RAO occur within the first hours or days after introducer removal. For example, the Traditional ENtry point versus Distal puncturE of Radial Artery (TENDERA) trial reported cases of occlusion occurring 3 and 6 months after forearm radial artery catheterization, while the first 7 days after the procedure showed preservation of radial artery blood flow [11, 52]. Furthermore, the detection of acute radial artery thrombosis on the first day after catheterization does not necessarily guarantee progression to a chronic stage. Thus, a clear distinction between acute and chronic RAO based solely on the timing of occlusion may not be entirely reliable.

In certain cases, spontaneous lysis of the thrombus is possible, and compression of the ipsilateral ulnar artery may contribute to the recanalization of the thrombosed portion of the radial artery [53–55]. It is also important to note that radial artery thrombosis/occlusion often presents as an asymptomatic or mildly symptomatic condition [21, 33, 45]. Because of these differences, attempting a direct analogy between coronary artery occlusion and RAO is not entirely appropriate.

The use of the TASC II classification, which focuses primarily on the clinical manifestations of limb ischemia, is also inappropriate for the classification of RAO because it does not emphasize the timing of arterial occlusion [56].

Thus, these considerations strongly support the development of a separate classification specifically tailored to cases of forearm and hand artery occlusion.

12.5.2 Pathogenesis

The effectiveness of DRA as a panacea for RAO is not fully realized. Understanding this issue requires an examination of various factors, including a thorough analysis of the underlying causes and evolution of this complication.

Arterial occlusion is the result of several pathological processes, including media inflammation, tissue necrosis, endothelial dysfunction, smooth muscle layer damage, intimal hyperplasia, cell proliferation, collagen synthesis, adventitial neovascularization, and internal remodeling [57]. Mechanical damage to the arterial wall and hemostasis defects at the puncture site are important contributors to these processes. In particular, observations of recanalized RAOs have shown marked hyperplasia not only at the puncture site but also in the proximal portions of the artery (Fig. 12.23) [21].

However, the occurrence of RAO is not solely determined by arterial wall injury and hemostasis problems, as not all patients with such complications experience RAO. This suggests that individual variations in the body's response to mechanical stress on the arterial wall may play a significant role.

DRA offers the advantage of maintaining blood flow in the radial artery through the superficial palmar arch during hemostasis, reducing the risk of thrombosis and occlusion of the radial artery. However, certain anatomic features of the radial artery may counteract this advantage. These include the "low" take-off of the superficial palmar branch, either on the wrist or in the area of the wrist joint, or its hypoplasia or absence (Fig. 12.24). In cases where the superficial palmar branch is not functioning optimally, blood flow through the radial artery may be significantly slowed or even stopped during hemostasis, creating conditions susceptible to thrombosis and occlusion both at the puncture site and in the proximal portions of the artery. In addition, an inverted version of the radial artery anatomy may exist, with the bifurcation of the radial artery and the superficial palmar branch located "high" on the forearm. This configuration makes the conventional radial approach more similar to the DRA, as blood flow remains along the radial artery and superficial palmar arch during hemostasis (Fig. 12.25).

Several conditions may contribute to RAO, which are briefly reviewed and summarized here:

1. Anomalies and variations in the anatomy of the radial artery
   - Small radial artery diameter or mismatch between device size and radial artery diameter
   - High radial artery bifurcation
   - Tortuosity of the radial artery
2. Radial artery spasm
3. Mediacalcinosis
4. Trauma of the radial artery wall
5. Insufficient anticoagulation
6. Inappropriate hemostasis techniques

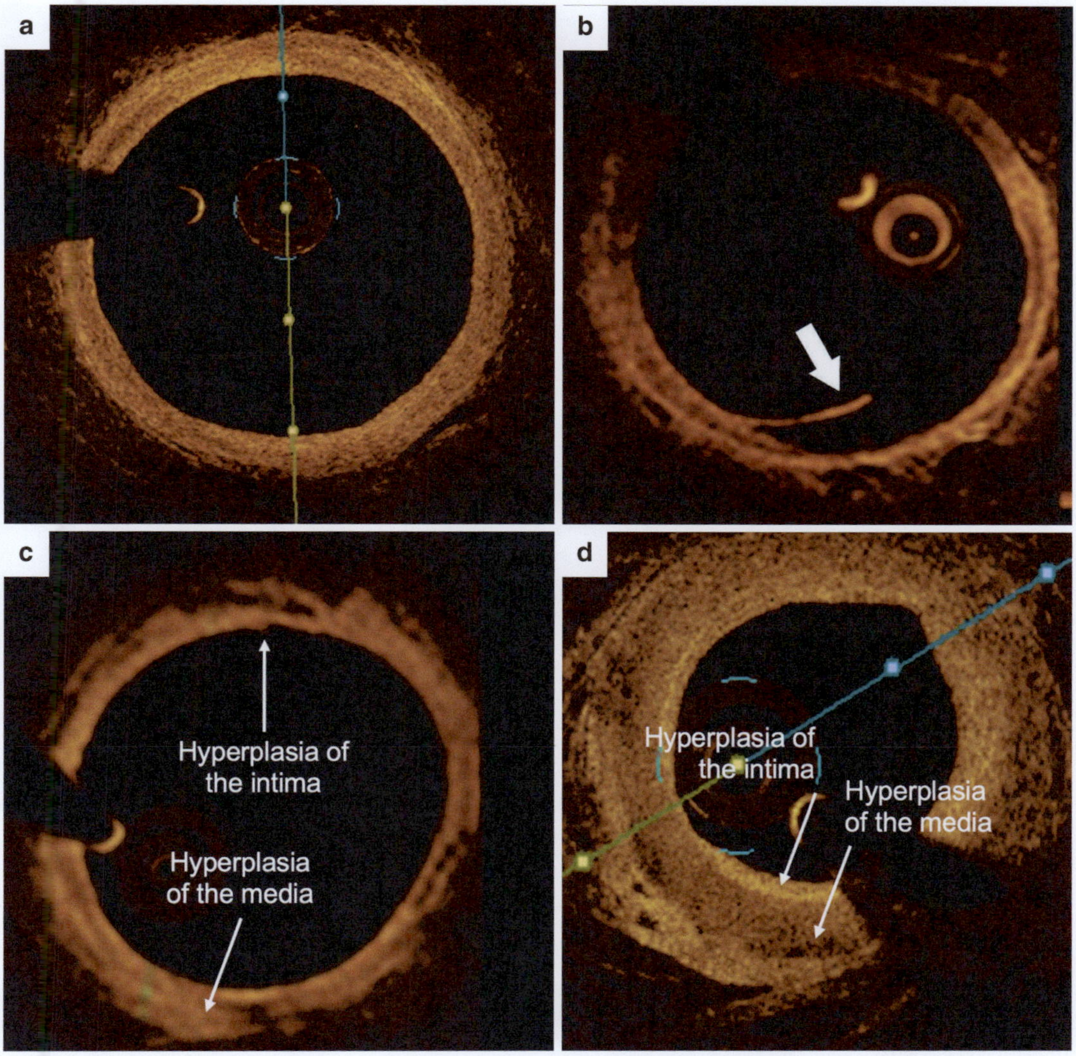

Fig. 12.23 Optical coherence tomography imaging of the radial artery (**a**) at baseline before any procedure, showing (**b**) an intimal flap (arrow) after a percutaneous coronary procedure has been performed and (**c**, **d**) hyperplasia of the intima and the media at a subsequent catheterization

12.5.2.1 Anomalies and Variations in the Anatomy of the Radial Artery

Variations and peculiarities in the anatomy of the radial artery are relatively common, occurring in approximately 20% of cases [58, 59]. Each of these factors, alone or in combination, can increase the likelihood of RAO (Fig. 12.26).

These predictors contribute significantly to the occurrence of RAO, especially when combined with various forms of arterial wall damage (as discussed previously).

12.5.2.2 Radial Artery Spasm

As mentioned previously, radial artery spasm is a physiological response to mechanical stress during transradial access and occurs in approximately 30% of procedures [4]. The unique anatomy of the radial artery, characterized by a significant muscular component and a high density of α_1-adrenergic receptors, makes it particularly susceptible to spasm [60]. Vasospasm can lead to pain, difficulty with instrument manipulation, and an increased risk of endothelial or deeper arterial layer damage, potentially activat-

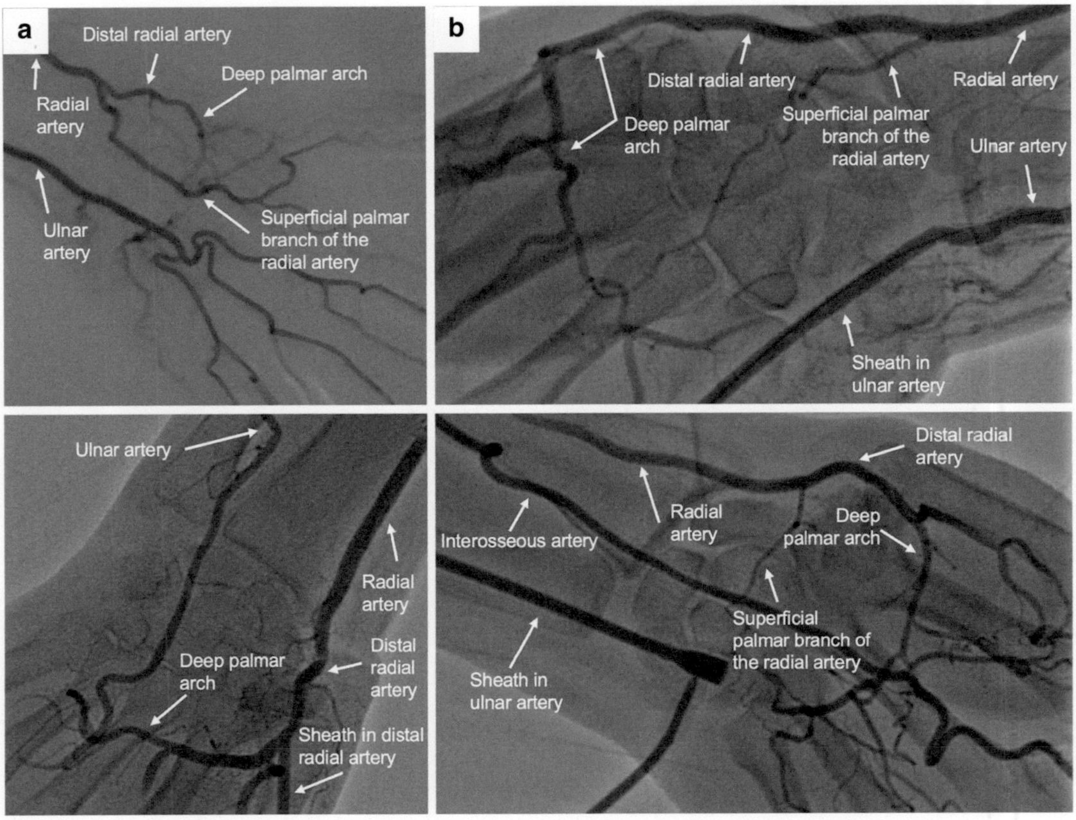

Fig. 12.24 Angiography of the forearm and the wrist showing (**a**, **b**) classical anatomical outline. (**c**) Variant anatomy without the superficial palmar branch of the radial artery. (**d**) Variant anatomy with "low" take-off of the superficial palmar branch of the radial artery

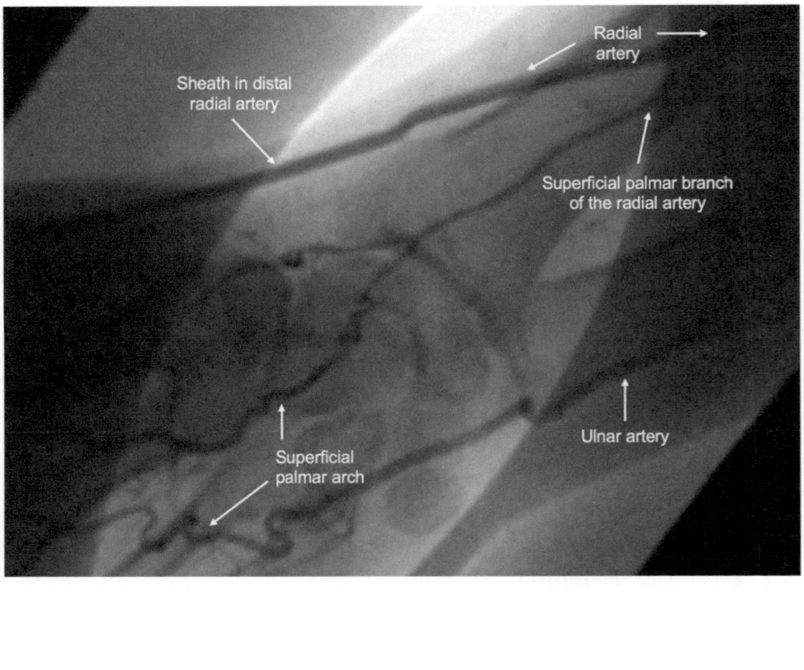

Fig. 12.25 Angiography of the forearm and the wrist showing variant anatomy with "high" take-off of the superficial palmar branch of the radial artery

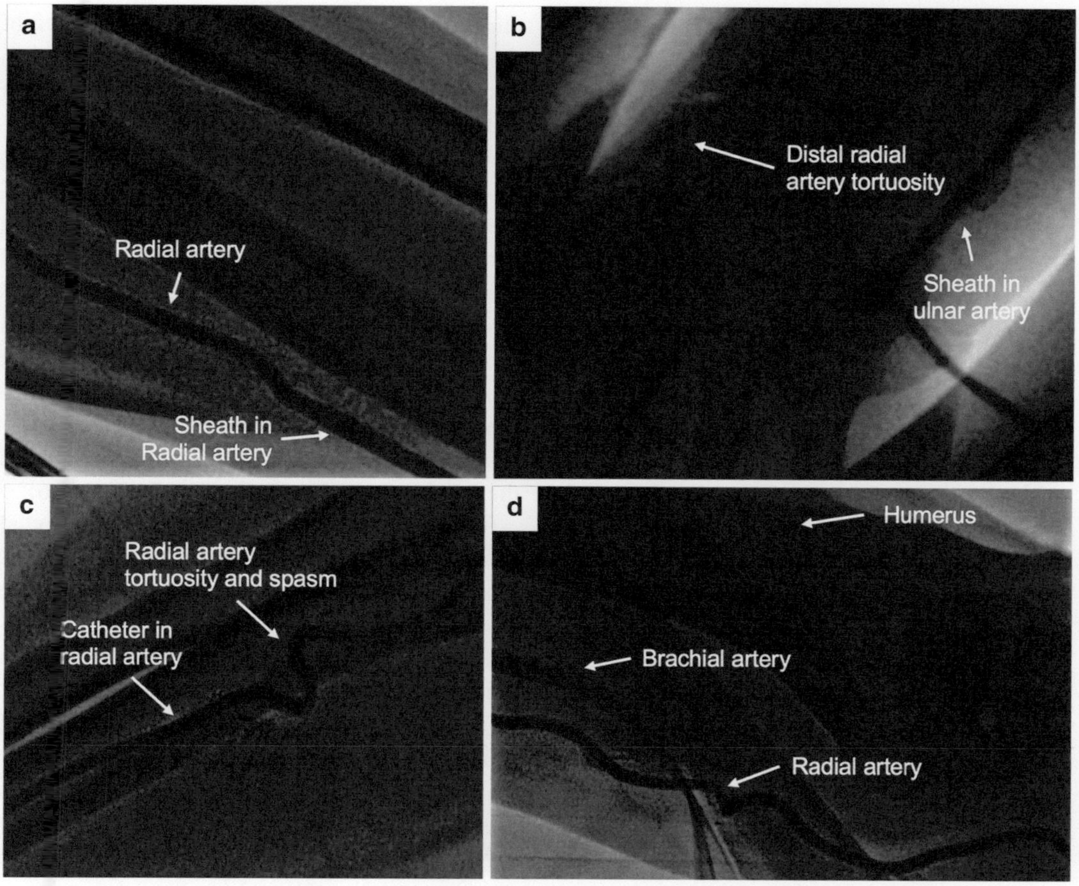

Fig. 12.26 Angiography of the forearm and the wrist showing (**a**) forearm radial artery smaller than the introducer sheath. (**b**) Tortuosity of the distal radial artery. (**c**) Tortuosity of the forearm radial artery. (**d**) High bifurcation (from the middle of the brachial artery) and tortuosity of the radial artery

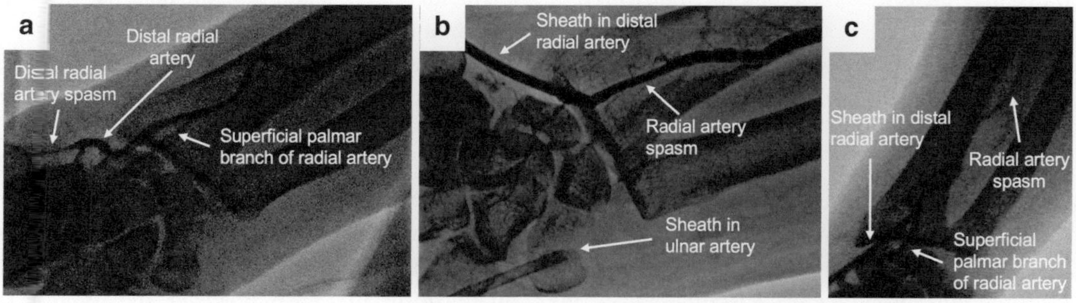

Fig. 12.27 Angiography of the forearm and the wrist showing (**a**) distal radial artery spasm after unsuccessful catheterization, (**b**) spasm of the distal and forearm radial artery, and (**c**) forearm radial artery spasm

ing the coagulation cascade and leading to RAO. In addition, patient discomfort caused by spasm reduces the chances of successful catheterization of the artery. Radial artery spasm can occur in both the forearm and distal portions (Fig. 12.27).

Currently, there is no clear definition of the severity of vasospasm [60]. While an objective method to quantify spasm using a 23-cm introducer has been described [61], it is rarely used in daily practice where shorter radial introducers are more common and affect less the risk of radial artery spasm. Efforts have been made to develop a scale to assess patient discomfort and operator technical difficulty in order to predict and prevent spasm. This scale includes anatomical anomalies found in more than 10% of patients [58, 59, 62], which increase the likelihood of spasm by a factor of 5, as well as small radial artery diameter, repeated diagnostic and/or guiding catheter changes, and pain [61, 63]. However, this scale has not been widely implemented in endovascular practice. Patel et al. proposed a classification of radial artery spasm, from mild to very severe, based on patients' subjective assessment of pain and/or discomfort along the radial artery during and/or immediately after the procedure [64]. However, the weakness of this classification is the subjectivity of the patient's perception and the lack of objective data. In addition, it characterizes spasm that has already occurred rather than predicting its occurrence, which is essential for operators to anticipate and prevent in emergency situations. It should be noted that spasm and damaged walls of the radial artery are related phenomena; spasm can cause damage to the arterial wall, and conversely, damaged arterial walls can cause spasm. Regardless of which of these processes is the primary cause, the end result is a high probability of RAO.

Anticipating vasospasm during transradial catheterization is challenging [65] and requires preventive measures, including the following:

1. Reviewing the anatomical characteristics and determining the size (small diameter) of the radial artery
2. Adequate analgesia at the catheterization site
3. Minimizing (if necessary) manipulation with a (hydrophilic) instrument in the lumen of the radial artery
4. Providing prophylactic vasodilators in the radial artery lumen after catheterization.
5. Use of non-drug methods of radial artery vasodilation

Attitudes toward pharmacologic prevention of radial artery spasm in the endovascular community vary, with some advocating the mandatory use of vasodilators and others rejecting their use altogether. This discrepancy is due to the lack of clear guidelines or recommendations for the routine use of vasodilators, as well as variations in drug administration among operators [66].

Currently, verapamil and nitroglycerin solution, either alone or in combination, are considered optimal vasodilators. The efficacy of a vasodilator is not only determined by the type of drug, but also by the appropriate dosage. Studies have shown that verapamil at a dose of at least 5 mg is highly effective, reducing the incidence of radial artery spasm to as low as 4%. The combination of nitroglycerin and verapamil in appropriate doses also shows promising results, with the incidence of spasm not exceeding 9% [66].

Research on the relationship between radial artery spasm and its potential to cause occlusion is mixed. Some studies found no association, while others, such as the TENDERA trial, reported a significant reduction in the incidence of RAO with the use of radial artery vasodilators [11].

In addition to pharmacological prevention and relief of vasospasm, there are alternative methods to address this issue. One such method is pressure-mediated dilatation of the radial artery [67], which involves the rapid injection of 10 mL of saline solution (10 mL/s) through the introducer (Fig. 12.28). This approach is thought to provide a dual mechanism of action, combining drug-induced and pressure-induced dilation of the radial artery. In addition, the pharmacological vasodilating effect is likely to be prolonged.

Another technique is flow-mediated dilation, which involves compressing the brachial artery for 10 minutes before puncturing the radial artery, followed by decompression, resulting in radial artery dilation [68]. Both methods have a similar mechanism of action in which fluid or blood flow exerts a "shock" effect on the artery, causing it to dilate. In the first case, however, the solution is injected directly into the radial artery under high pressure through a previously placed introducer, causing dilation. In the second case, the artery is first dilated, and then, catheterization is performed.

In addition, thermal methods of vasospasm relief involve the application of a thermal compress to the forearm or wrist [69].

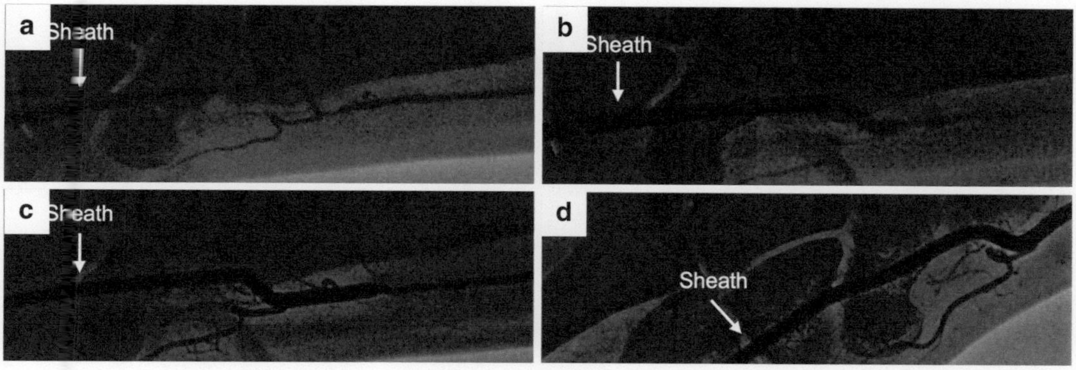

Fig. 12.28 Angiography of the forearm and the wrist showing (**a**) diffuse radial artery spasm at baseline. (**b–d**) Successive phases of arterial dilation by high-pressure saline solution injection

12.5.2.3 Mediacalcinosis

Medial calcification of the radial artery presents challenges for catheterization and manipulation within its lumen and represents a significant predictor of RAO. The medial layer of the arterial wall is composed of smooth muscle cells and elastic fibers with numerous fenestrations in the inner elastic layer, making it susceptible to atheromatous plaque formation. Medial calcification occurs primarily along the elastic plate, resulting in progressive compaction of the elastic layer of the arterial wall (Fig. 12.29).

This condition, known as medial Monckeberg's sclerosis, is common in patients with diabetes mellitus and chronic kidney disease. Typically, medial calcification does not cause arterial luminal obstruction [70], but in its advanced stages, it can lead to occlusion of the radial and ulnar arteries [71]. Such damage may occur due to intimal rupture and exposure of the local endothelial cell layer and/or media dissection. As a result, the anti-inflammatory and antithrombotic functions of the endothelium, which provides endogenous vasodilating and antithrombotic substances, are disrupted, leading to intimal hyperplasia [72]. The combined hyperplasia of the intima and medial layer, together with diffuse calcinosis, may lead to occlusion of the arterial lumen.

It is noteworthy that mediacalcinosis predominantly affects the radial artery of the forearm, sparing the distal radial artery and the interosseous artery, which remain relatively intact or minimally damaged. This aspect warrants further investigation as it has received limited attention in research. The preservation of the integrity of the distal radial artery makes it suitable for use as an access artery during endovascular procedures and for recanalization of RAO (Fig. 12.30). However, it is important to recognize that the patency of the radial artery may be restored only for a short period of time after recanalization.

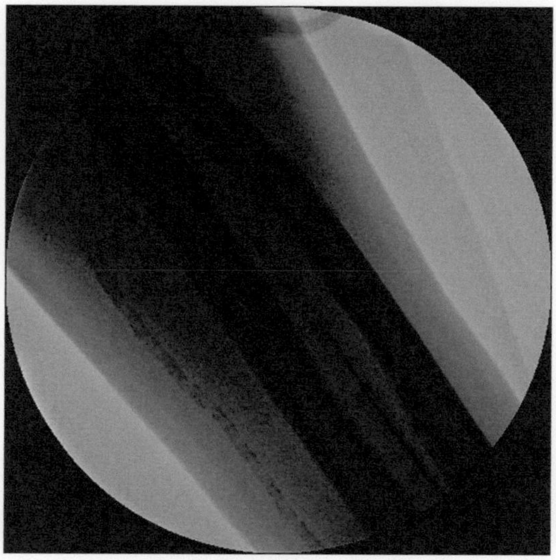

Fig. 12.29 Mediacalcinosis of the radial and ulnar arteries in a patient with severe chronic kidney disease

12.5.2.4 Mechanical Damage to the Radial Artery

Trauma to the radial artery wall, as discussed above, increases the risk of RAO. In this regard, it is important to consider another factor that pre-

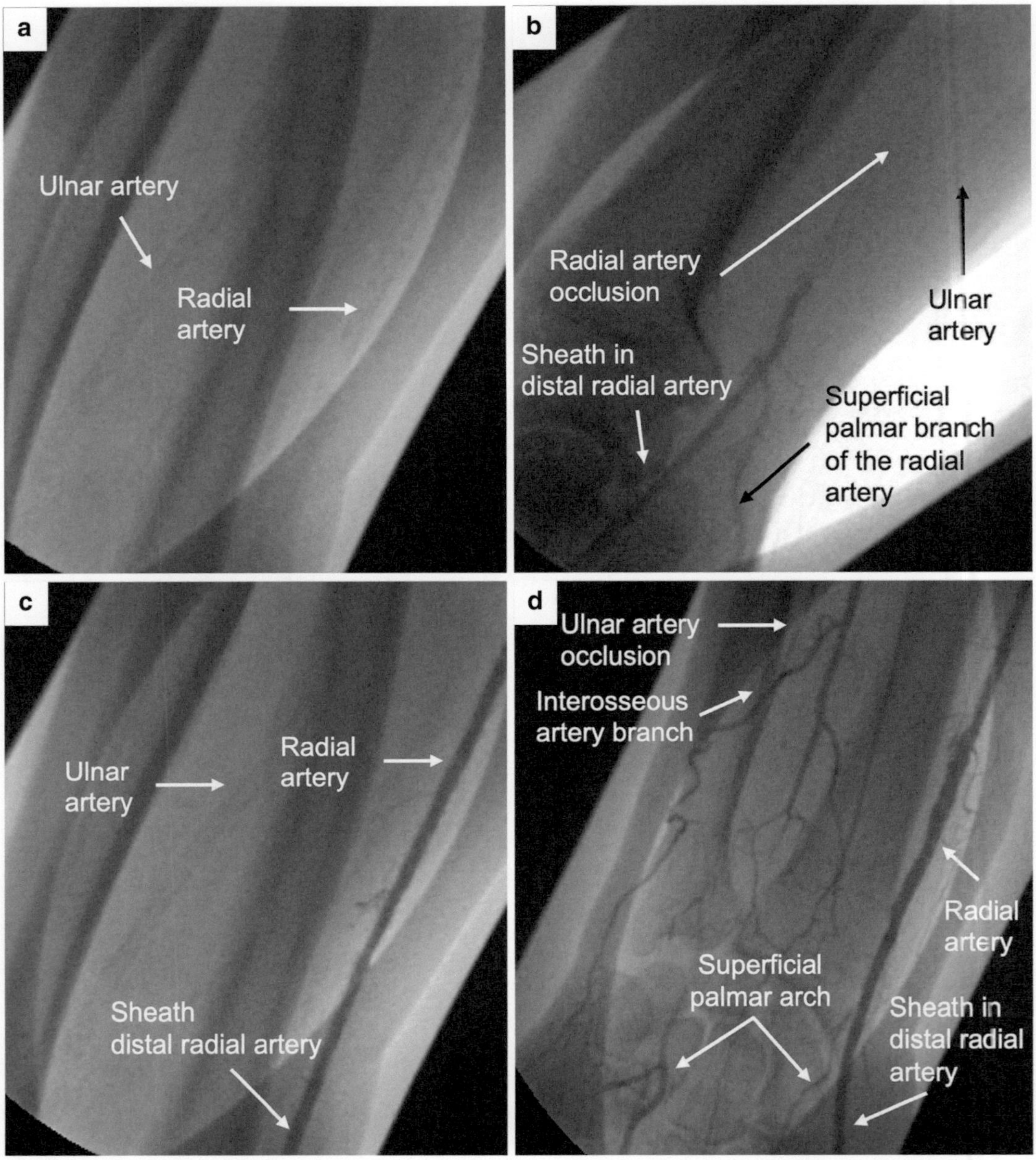

Fig. 12.30 (**a**) Fluoroscopy showing calcification of the forearm radial and ulnar arteries. (**b**) Angiography of the forearm showing occlusion of the forearm radial artery with preserved flow in its superficial palmar branch. (**c**) After retrograde recanalization of the radial artery. (**d**) Activated interosseous artery anastomoses

disposes to occlusion: repeated cannulation of the radial artery. Frequent puncture and catheterization of the artery can lead to the development of intimal hyperplasia and an increase in intimal media thickness. These changes contribute to adverse remodeling of the arterial wall, further increasing the likelihood of RAO [73–75]. In addition, numerous catheter exchanges can significantly contribute to RAO [76].

12.5.2.5 Anticoagulation

Proper procedural anticoagulation is a critical preventive measure against RAO. Unfractionated heparin (UFH) is the preferred choice for most operators, with approximately 92% using it. However, there is considerable variation in the dose and method of administration [77]. While meta-analyses have confirmed the efficacy of high-dose UFH, several questions remain:

1. Determine the optimal and effective dosage of UFH.
2. Evaluate the risk-benefit ratio of RAO versus local hemorrhagic complications.
3. Assess anticoagulant efficacy using coagulation testing after initiation of UFH.
4. Identify and evaluate potential risks and interactions associated with the concomitant use of parenteral anticoagulants, oral anticoagulants, and antiplatelet agents.
5. Consider the use of UFH in conjunction with long-term dual antiplatelet therapy or IIb/IIIa blockers.

In a meta-analysis, UFH at a dose of 5000 IU reduced the risk of RAO compared with lower doses but also increased the risk of hematoma and prolonged radial artery compression time [78].

In a study comparing the risk of RAO and the activated clotting time (ACT) index with the use of UFH, a paradoxical effect was observed [79]. A significant increase in the ACT index (>250 s) correlated with a higher frequency of RAO due to the need for longer hemostasis time, which in turn negatively affects radial artery patency. In contrast, the TENDERA study reported no significant difference in the risk of RAO based on UFH dose (50 IU/kg vs. >50 IU/kg) [11]. In still another study, patients receiving intravenous UFH had a significantly lower incidence of RAO than those receiving warfarin therapy, despite adequate anticoagulation [80].

In addition, low molecular weight heparin (LMWH) has been shown to prevent the risk of RAO. LMWH provides a more stable and predictable level of anticoagulation than UFH and eliminates the need for regular monitoring of anticoagulation levels [81]. However, the potential advantages of LMWH over other anticoagulants need to be confirmed by randomized trials.

12.5.2.6 Hemostasis Techniques

Radial artery hemostasis should have two main goals: preventing hemorrhagic complications at the puncture site and maintaining blood flow through the radial artery. Compression during radial artery hemostasis is a major factor contributing to the interruption of blood flow and may serve as a predictor of RAO [82]. The concept of "patent hemostasis" has been developed to maintain blood flow at the puncture site during hemostasis with the idea that it may reduce the incidence of RAO (Fig. 12.31). There is substantial evidence that this approach reduces the risk of RAO [83]. However, despite its efficacy, the adoption of patent hemostasis in clinical practice has been limited.

In the TENDERA trial, patients who underwent bandaging had lower rates of RAO than those who underwent patent hemostasis [11]. There is potential to use patent hemostasis for DRA to prevent RAO. Hemostasis devices for DRA have become available, and their mechanism of action is similar to that of devices for conventional TRA hemostasis. Attempt to apply patent hemostasis to the distal radial artery reduced the risk of RAO [83]. Using hemostatic devices with patent hemostasis for both DRA and conventional TRA may allow a more objective comparison between the two approaches.

Another promising method to prevent RAO during hemostasis is compression of the ipsilateral ulnar artery [54]. This compression increases blood flow through the radial artery in patients with conventional TRA, thereby reducing the risk of RAO [55]. However, it also increases blood flow through the interosseous arteries, leading to the formation of collaterals and anastomoses that offset the effects of increased radial artery flow. This raises the question of the optimal compression time of the ulnar artery and whether it is necessary to compress the ulnar artery when patent hemostasis is used, since blood flow through the radial artery can be regulated by the degree of compression.

Compression of the ipsilateral ulnar artery may be of interest in patients with "early" post-catheterization radial artery thrombosis and in those who have undergone radial artery recanali-

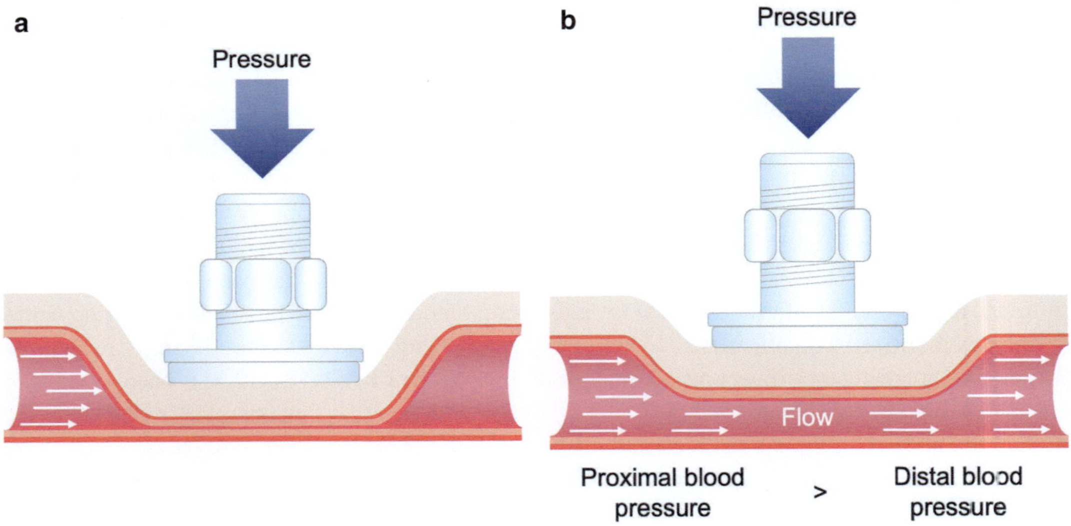

Fig. 12.31 (**a**) Occlusive hemostasis: external compression of the puncture site exceeds the blood pressure in the vessel, occluding the vessel lumen with complete cessation of blood flow. (**b**) Hemostasis with preserved blood flow (patent hemostasis): the blood pressure proximal to the hemostasis site is greater than the blood pressure distal to the compression site

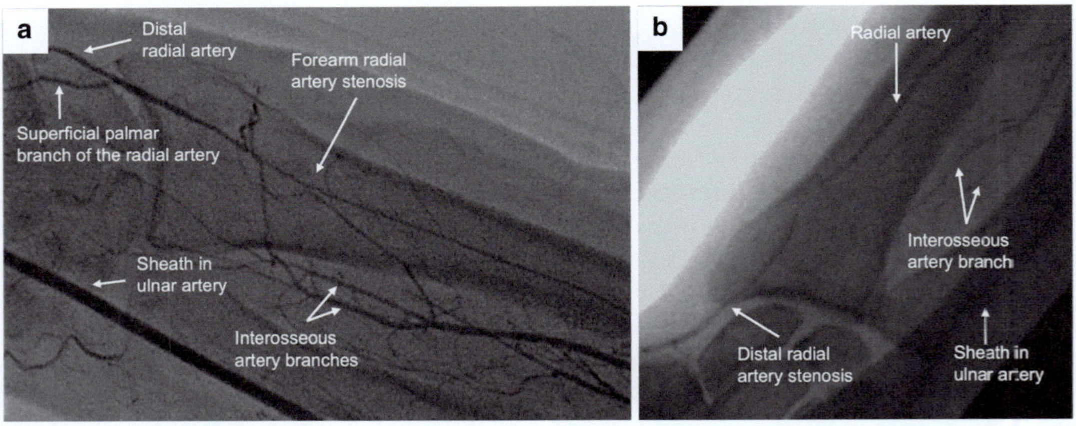

Fig. 12.32 Angiography of the forearm and the wrist showing (**a**) forearm radial artery stenosis in 2.5 months after distal radial access in an anatomical snuffbox and (**b**) stenosis of the distal and forearm radial artery, 1 month after distal radial access to the anatomical snuffbox

zation. However, there are currently no studies on these specific issues or on the use of ipsilateral ulnar artery compression with DRA.

Damage to the radial artery can manifest not only as occlusion but also as stenosis, which can occur in both the forearm and distal portions of the radial artery (Fig. 12.32). With stenosis, the pulsation of the radial artery remains, but its use as an access artery becomes problematic. Differentiating between long-term recanalized thrombosis and radial artery stenosis can be challenging, and intravascular imaging may be helpful in this regard. However, identifying the cause of radial artery lumen injury in such cases may be of more academic interest than practical significance.

12.5.3 Treatment of Radial Artery Occlusion

Occlusion of the radial artery with DRA may occur at the puncture site, in the forearm, or throughout the radial artery (Fig. 12.33). The goal of the treatment of RAO is to recanalize the artery to restore its lumen for potential future use. Recanalization can be performed either by the retrograde method using DRA at the beginning of the endovascular procedure or by the antegrade method using the ipsilateral ulnar artery, which can be performed either before or after the endovascular procedure (Fig. 12.34) [21, 84, 85].

For forearm and distal RAO, antegrade recanalization through the ipsilateral ulnar artery is preferred when access to the radial artery of the hand is difficult or impossible (Figs. 12.35 and 12.36).

The need for radial artery recanalization should be carefully evaluated. Recanalization may not be advisable for a radial artery with a small diameter, tortuosity, or calcification, as these factors may adversely affect its patency. Therefore, it is best to avoid recanalization if other viable access arteries are available.

Regarding the timing of treatment, early radial artery thrombosis recanalization is technically

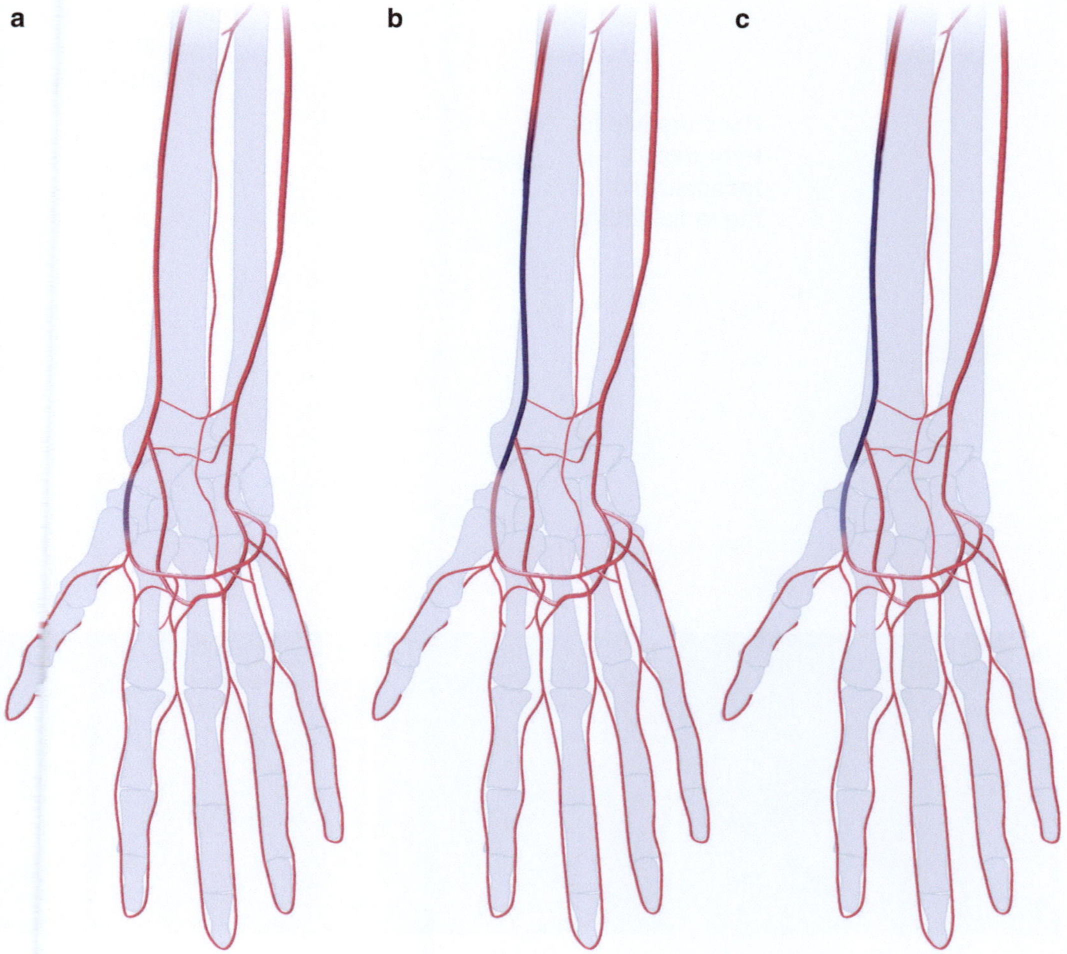

Fig. 12.33 Schematic representation of (**a**) occlusion of the distal radial artery, (**b**) occlusion of the forearm radial artery, and (**c**) occlusion of both the distal and forearm radial artery

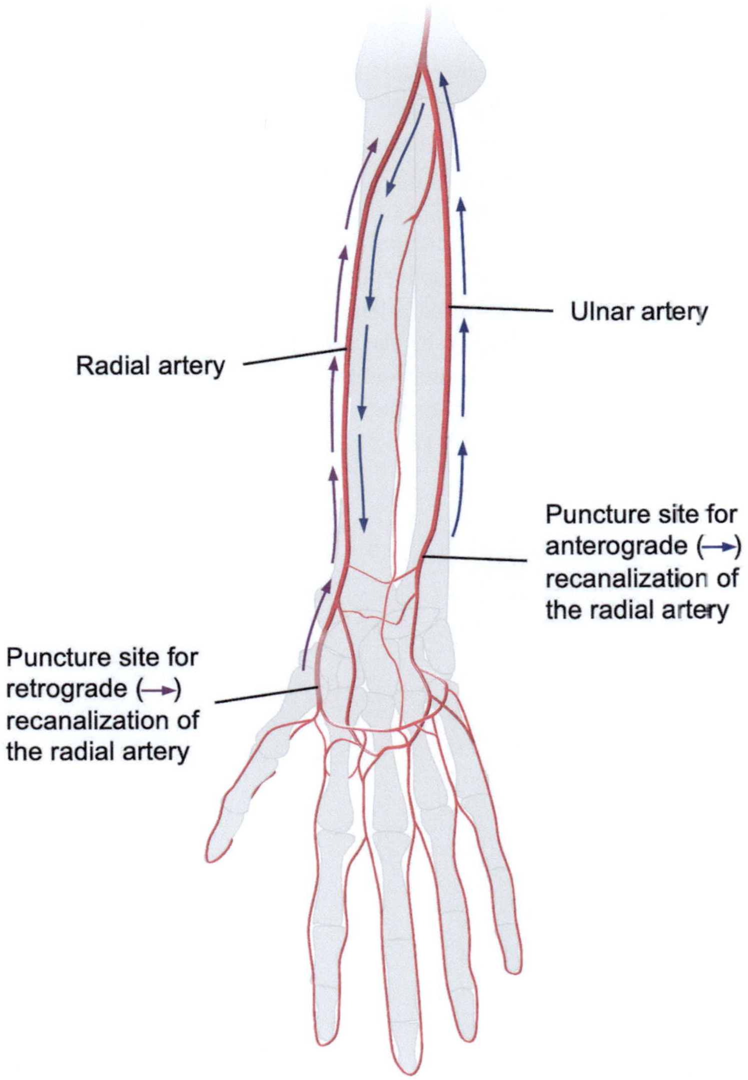

Fig. 12.34 Retrograde recanalization of the radial artery and antegrade recanalization of the radial artery

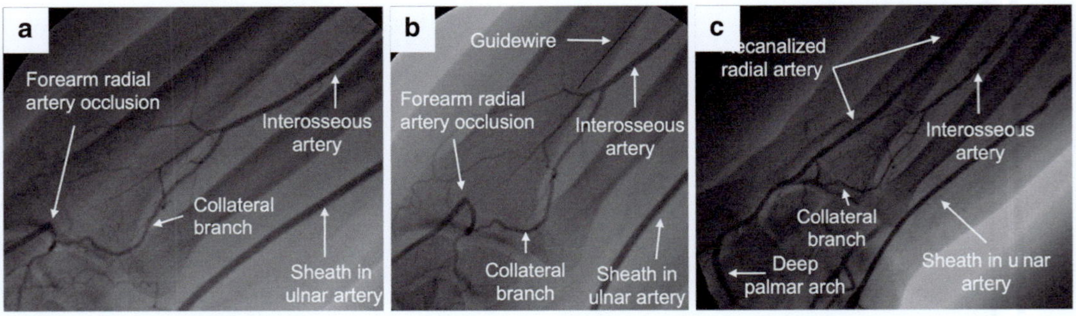

Fig. 12.35 Antegrade recanalization of the forearm radial artery through the ipsilateral ulnar access. (**a**) Baseline angiography showing occlusion of the forearm radial artery with collateral filling of the distal forearm artery from the interosseous artery. (**b**) Coronary guidewire through the occlusion. (**c**) Final angiography after balloon angioplasty

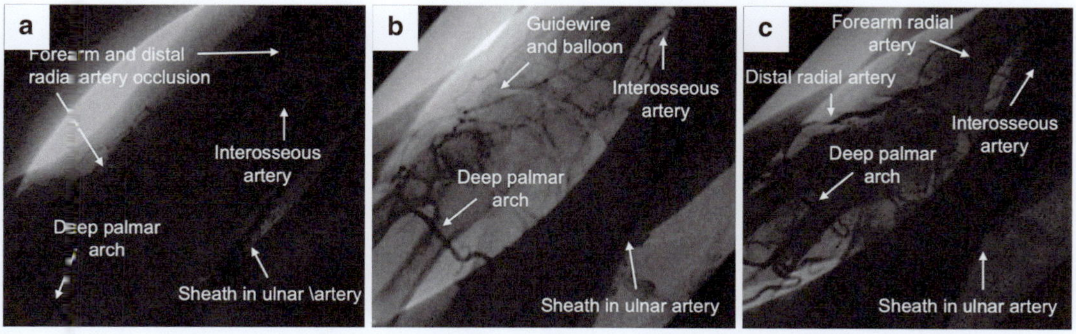

Fig. 12.36 Antegrade recanalization of the forearm and distal radial artery through the ipsilateral ulnar access. (**a**) Baseline angiography showing occlusion of the radial artery with collateral filling from the interosseous artery. (**b**) Coronary guidewire and balloon through the occlusion. (**c**) Final angiography after balloon angioplasty of the radial artery

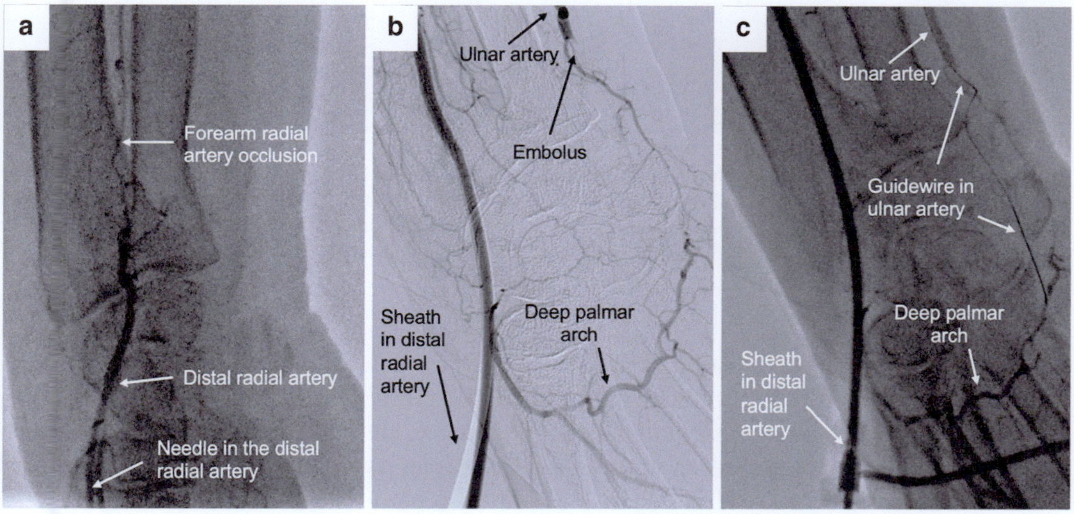

Fig. 12.37 Retrograde recanalization of forearm radial artery through distal radial access. (**a**) Baseline angiography 4 weeks after conventional transradial access. (**b**) Embolization in the distal forearm ulnar artery. (**c**) Coronary guidewire through the embolic occlusion of the ulnar artery into the superficial palmar arch

easier but carries a higher risk of embolic complications. Retrograde recanalization offers some advantages, such as the prolonged presence of a guiding catheter during the procedure, but may still carry a risk of embolization to other arteries (Fig. 12.37) [15, 21]. Antegrade recanalization, however, has a positive outcome in most cases with minimal risk of embolization, but residual "near wall" thrombosis may require further intervention with "peripheral" balloons (Fig. 12.38).

Long-term RAO with a hard cap and multiple collaterals presents a greater challenge to recanalization, and the ability to restore the lumen of the artery in such cases is limited. However, when recanalization is successful, the occurrence of embolic complications is less frequent.

Differentiating chronic RAO artery from recanalized thrombosis can be difficult, and intravascular imaging may be helpful in certain cases.

When comparing antegrade and retrograde methods for the recanalization of long-standing occlusions, retrograde methods have a higher success rate [21]. However, antegrade recanaliza-

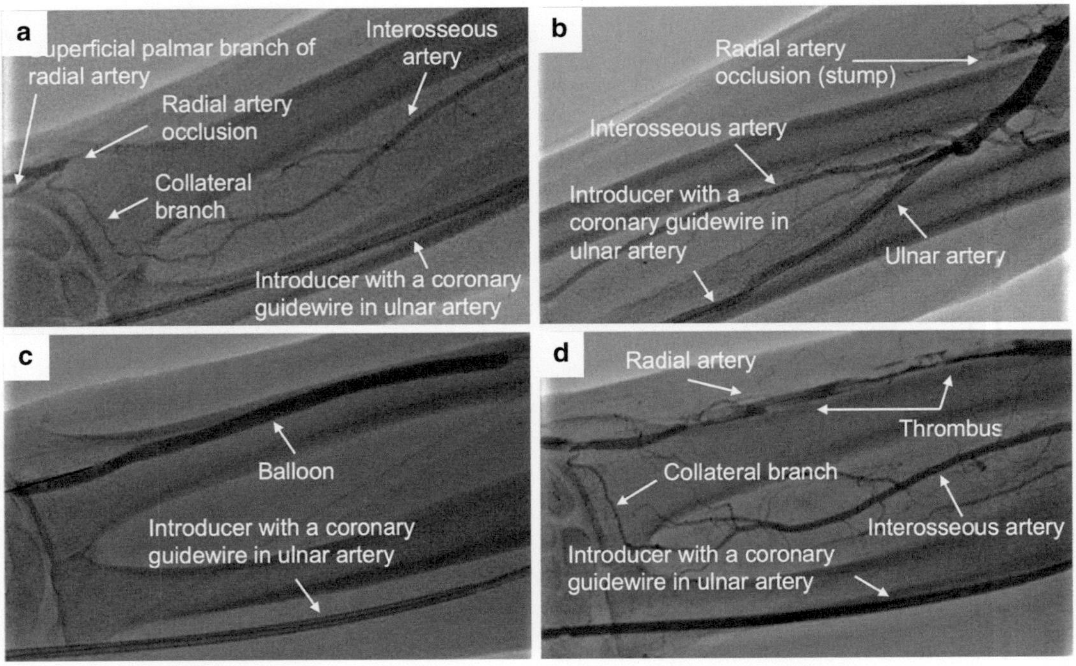

Fig. 12.38 Antegrade recanalization of the forearm radial artery through the ipsilateral ulnar access. (**a**, **b**) Baseline angiography 4 weeks after conventional transradial access showing occlusion of the radial artery with collateral filling from the interosseous artery. (**c**) Balloon angioplasty of the thrombotic occlusion. (**d**) Residual "near-wall" thrombosis in the forearm radial artery after balloon angioplasty

tion has several advantages. In antegrade recanalization, hemostasis is not performed on the radial artery but on the ulnar artery after the procedure, which promotes better blood flow in the recanalized radial artery and reduces the risk of reocclusion. Also, retrograde recanalization with unknown anatomy may present unexpected challenges and increase the risk of reocclusion, especially in cases with anatomical variations (Fig. 12.39) [21].

Similar to chronic total coronary occlusions, the success of treatment for chronic radial artery occlusions depends on specific characteristics such as the presence of a stump, collateral branches, calcification, extent of occlusion, and radial artery tortuosity. Occlusions with these characteristics without clinical symptoms do not require treatment.

As the field advances, a better understanding of the efficacy and appropriate approaches to recanalization will contribute to improved outcomes and patient care. Recanalization of radial artery occlusions.

1. Gives priority to the preservation of the radial artery
2. Requires operator experience and careful planning
3. May cause patient discomfort, necessitating appropriate pain management
4. Lacks extensive research, limiting objective evaluation
5. Benefits from ongoing technological advances and further research in distal access

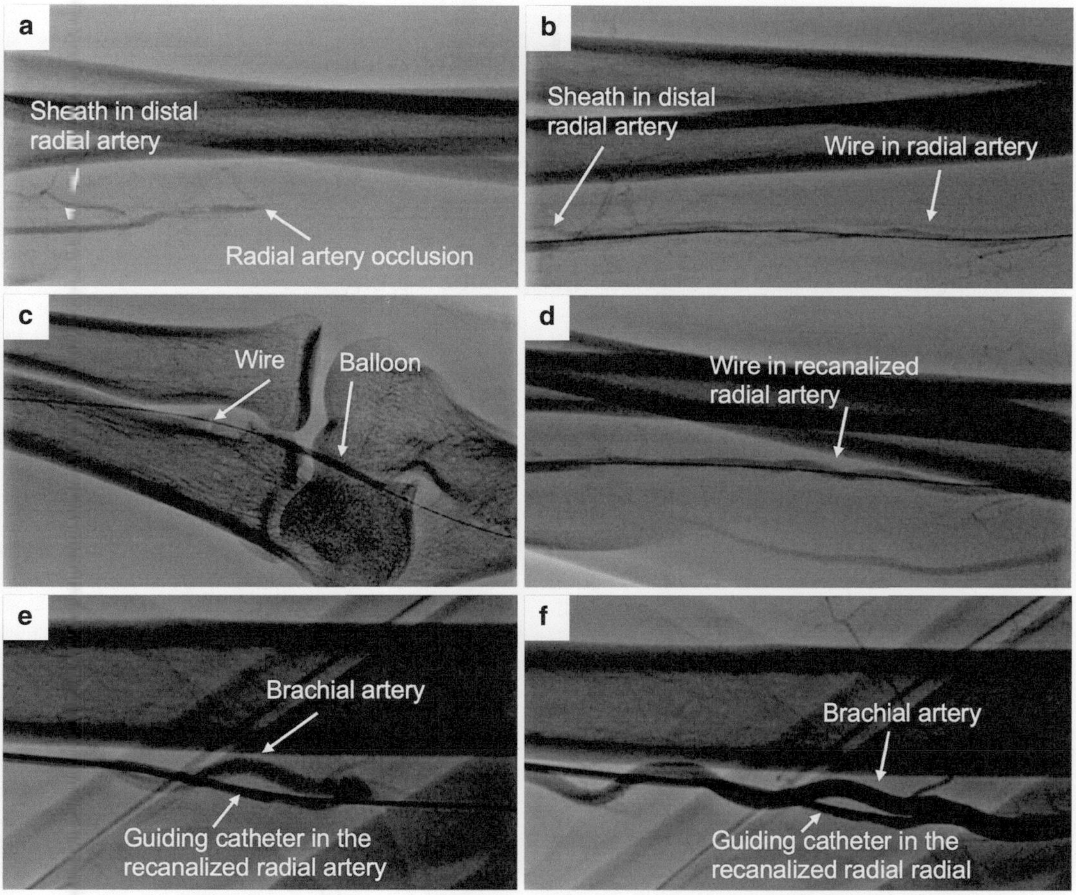

Fig. 12.39 Retrograde recanalization of the forearm radial artery through distal radial access. (**a**) Baseline angiography. (**b**) Coronary guidewire through the occlusion. (**c**) Balloon angioplasty of the thrombotic occlusion. (**d**) Restoration of blood flow in the forearm radial artery. (**e**, **f**) Final angiographies showing the divergence of the radial artery in the middle part of the brachial artery

12.6 Conclusions

This chapter on the prevention and treatment of complications associated with DRA provides valuable insight into the potential of the radial artery and its distal segment. However, it is important to recognize that there are still many unanswered questions in this field. Medicine is an ever-evolving science, and the exploration of the potential of the radial artery continues to advance.

The radial artery era, sparked by the pioneering work of Lucien Campeau and Ferdinand Kiemeneij, has revolutionized the use of access arteries and pushed the boundaries of what can be achieved [86, 87]. The adoption of DRA into routine clinical practice has gained momentum, opening new avenues for endovascular interventions.

References

1. Kaledin AL, Kochanov IN, Seletskii SS, Arkharov IV, Burak T, Kozlov KL. Peculiarities of arterial access in endovascular surgery in elderly patients. Adv Gerontol. 2014;27:115–9.
2. Kiemeneij F. Left distal transradial access in the anatomical snuffbox for coronary angiography (ldTRA) and interventions (ldTRI). EuroIntervention. 2017;13:851–7.

3. Roghani-Dehkordi F, Hashemifard O, Sadeghi M, Mansouri R, Akbarzadeh M, Dehghani A, et al. Distal accesses in the hand (two novel techniques) for percutaneous coronary angiography and intervention. ARYA Atheroscler. 2018;14:95–100.
4. Coghill EM, Johnson T, Morris RE, Megson IL, Leslie SJ. Radial artery access site complications during cardiac procedures, clinical implications and potential solutions: the role of nitric oxide. World J Cardiol. 2020;12:26–34.
5. Korotkikh AV, Babunashvili AM, Kazantsev AN, Annaev ZS. Distal radial access: is there a clinical benefit? Cardiol Rev. 2024;32:110–113.
6. He GW, Yang CQ. Characteristics of adrenoceptors in the human radial artery: clinical implications. J Thorac Cardiovasc Surg. 1998;115:1136–41.
7. Hamon M, Pristipino C, Di Mario C, Nolan J, Ludwig J, Tubaro M, et al. Consensus document on the radial approach in percutaneous cardiovascular interventions: position paper by the European Association of Percutaneous Cardiovascular Interventions and Working Groups on Acute Cardiac Care and Thrombosis of the European Society of Cardiology. EuroIntervention. 2013;8:1242–51.
8. Ferrante G, Rao SV, Juni P, Da Costa BR, Reimers B, Condorelli G, et al. Radial versus femoral access for coronary interventions across the entire spectrum of patients with coronary artery disease: a meta-analysis of randomized trials. JACC Cardiovasc Interv. 2016;9:1419–34.
9. Zhang J, Liu C, Tian B, Lin X. Success rate, efficacy and complications of the transradial artery approach to percutaneous coronary intervention for coronary heart disease. Int J Clin Exp Med. 2017;10:12571–6.
10. Sgueglia GA, Lee BK, Cho BR, Babunashvili A, Lee JB, Lee JW, et al. Distal radial access: consensus report of the first Korea-Europe transradial intervention meeting. JACC Cardiovasc Interv. 2021;14:892–906.
11. Korotkikh A, Babunashvili A, Kaledin AL, Akhramovich RV, Derkach VV, Portnov RM, et al. Analysis of intermediate results of a comparative multicenter randomized TENDERA study investigating the distal radial access. Novosti Khirurgii. 2021;29:285–95.
12. Kaledin AL, Kochanov IN, Ardeev VN, Burak TY, Seletskyi SS, Golovchanskyi PO, et al. Proximal and distal radial access for endovascular interventions in patients with ACS. Int J Interv Cardioangiol. 2021;67:10–25.
13. Daralammouri Y, Nazzal Z, Mosleh YS, Abdulhaq HK, Khayyat ZY, Hamshary YE, et al. Distal radial artery access in comparison to forearm radial artery access for cardiac catheterization: a randomized controlled trial (DARFORA trial). J Interv Cardiol. 2022;2022:7698583.
14. Bertrand OF, De Larochelliere R, Rodes-Cabau J, Proulx G, Gleeton O, Nguyen CM, et al. A randomized study comparing same-day home discharge and abciximab bolus only to overnight hospitalization and abciximab bolus and infusion after transradial coronary stent implantation. Circulation. 2006;114:2636–43.
15. Babunashvili AM, Kartashov DS. Guidelines for the use of radial access in interventional angiocardiology. Moscow: Publishing House of the Association of Construction Universities; 2017.
16. Yamamoto Y, Kudo T, Igari K, Toyofuku T, Inoue Y. Radial artery aneurysm in the anatomical snuff box: a case report and literature review. Int J Surg Case Rep. 2016;27:44–7.
17. Zegri I, Garcia-Touchard A, Cuenca S, Oteo JF, Fernandez-Diaz JA, Goicolea J. Radial artery pseudoaneurysm following cardiac catheterization: clinical features and nonsurgical treatment results. Rev Esp Cardiol. 2015;68:349–51.
18. Dehghani P, Culig J, Patel D, Kraushaar G, Schulte P. Arteriovenous fistula as a complication of transradial coronary angiography: a case report. J Med Case Rep. 2013;7:21.
19. Hadjivassiliou A, Kiemeneij F, Nathan S, Klass D. Ultrasound-guided access to the distal radial artery at the anatomical snuffbox for catheter-based vascular interventions: a technical guide. EuroIntervention. 2021;16:1342–8.
20. Chugh SK, Chugh Y, Chugh S. How to tackle complications in radial procedures: tip and tricks. Indian Heart J. 2015;67:275–81.
21. Kaledin AL, Kochanov IN, Podmetin PS, Seletskiy SS, Ardeev VN, Garin YY. Recanalization of the post-catheterization occlusion in the radial artery. Curiosity or necessity. Int J Interv Cardioangiol. 2018;54:20–33.
22. Shroff AR, Gulati R, Drachman DE, Feldman DN, Gilchrist IC, Kaul P, et al. SCAI expert consensus statement update on best practices for transradial angiography and intervention. Catheter Cardiovasc Interv. 2020;95:245–52.
23. Sgueglia GA, Di Giorgio A, Gaspardone A, Babunashvili A. Anatomic basis and physiological rationale of distal radial artery access for percutaneous coronary and endovascular procedures. JACC Cardiovasc Interv. 2018;11:2113–9.
24. Sciahbasi A, Rigattieri S, Sarandrea A, Cera M, Di Russo C, Fedele S, et al. Radial artery occlusion and hand strength after percutaneous coronary procedures: results of the HANGAR study. Catheter Cardiovasc Interv. 2016;87:868–74.
25. Pacchioni A, Sanz Sanchez J, Gasparini GL. Digital ischemia after snuffbox radial approach. JACC Cardiovasc Interv. 2020;13:2940–2.
26. Longo GM, Friedman AC, Hollins RR, Buresh CJ, Baxter BT. Distal radial artery lesion as a source of digital emboli. J Vasc Surg. 1998;28:710–4.
27. Kamiya C, Kitaoka T, Yamamoto K, Matsumoto H, Deguchi J, Sato O. Acute palmer digital artery occlusion treated using endoscopic ablation of the thoracic sympathetic. Ann Vasc Dis. 2010;3:77–80.

28. Alejandro G, Adolfo FG, Hugo TA. Digital embolization from a thrombosed aneurysmal hemodialysis arteriovenous fistula. Nefrologia. 2021;41:593–4.
29. Khatri VP, Gaulin JC, Amin AK. Fibromuscular dysplasia of distal radial and ulnar arteries: uncommon cause of digital ischemia. Ann Plast Surg. 1994;33:652–5.
30. Schultz K, Wolf JM. Digital ischemia in COVID-19 patients: case report. J Hand Surg Am. 2020;45:518–22.
31. McNamara MG, Butler TE, Sanders WE, Pederson WC. Ischaemia of the index finger and thumb secondary to thrombosis of the radial artery in the anatomical snuffbox. J Hand Surg Br. 1998;23:28–32.
32. Amin R, Singha CK, Banerjee SK, Hoque H, Mahbub S, Hoque M, et al. Comparison of distal transradial in the anatomical snuffbox versus conventional transradial access for coronary angiography and intervention – an experience in 100 cases. Univ Heart J. 2017;13:40–5.
33. Sgueglia GA, Hassan A, Harb S, Ford TJ, Koliastasis L, Milkas A, et al. International hand function study following distal radial access: the RATATOUILLE study. JACC Cardiovasc Interv. 2022;15:1205–15.
34. Robson AJ, See MS, Ellis H. Applied anatomy of the superficial branch of the radial nerve. Clin Anat. 2008;21:38–45.
35. Richards RL. Ischaemic lesions of peripheral nerves: a review. J Neurol Neurosurg Psychiatry. 1951;14:76–87.
36. Bentley FH, Schlapp W. The effects of pressure on conduction in peripheral nerve. J Physiol. 1943;102:72–82.
37. Li F, Shi GW, Yu XL, Song RX, Xiao JQ, Huang HM, et al. Safety and efficacy of coronary angiography and percutaneous coronary intervention via distal transradial artery access in the anatomical snuffbox: a single-centre prospective cohort study using a propensity score method. BMC Cardiovasc Disord. 2022;22:74.
38. Langer C, Prog R. Arterial accesses in coronary angiography and intervention—review with a focus on prognostic relevance. Rev Cardiovasc Med. 2022;23:331.
39. Horak D, Bernat I, Jirous S, Slezak D, Rokyta R. Distal radial access and postprocedural ultrasound evaluation of proximal and distal radial artery. Cardiovasc Interv Ther. 2022;37:710–6.
40. Zwaan EM, Koopman AG, Holtzer CA, Zijlstra F, Ritt MJ, Amoroso G, et al. Revealing the impact of local access-site complications and upper extremity dysfunction post transradial percutaneous coronary procedures. Neth Heart J. 2015;23:514–24.
41. Dharma S, Kedev S, Patel T, Gilchrist IC, Rao SV. The predictors of post-procedural arm pain after transradial approach in 1706 patients underwent transradial catheterization. Cardiovasc Revasc Med. 2019;20:674–7.
42. Bolster MA, Bakker XR. Radial tunnel syndrome: emphasis on the superficial branch of the radial nerve. J Hand Surg Eur. 2009;34:343–7.
43. Hill EJR, Patterson JMM, Yee A, Crock LW, Mackinnon SE. What is operative? Conceptualizing neuralgia: neuroma, compression neuropathy, painful hyperalgesia, and phantom nerve pain. J Hand Surg Glob Online. 2023;5:126–32.
44. Thaper A, Miller ME. Ultrasound-guided hydrodissection is a safe and effective nonsurgical treatment for superficial radial sensory neuropathy. J Ultrasound Med. 2019;38:3359–61.
45. Sharma AK, Razi MM, Prakash N, Sharma A, Sarraf S, Sinha S, et al. A comparative assessment of Dorsal radial artery access versus classical radial artery access for percutaneous coronary angiography-a randomized control trial (DORA trial). Indian Heart J. 2020;72:435–41.
46. Akhramovich RV, Semitko SP, Azarov AV, Melnichenko IS, Analeev AI, Chernyisheva IE, et al. Radial artery occlusion after primary percutaneous coronary interventions performed using different radial approaches. Patologiya krovoobrashcheniya i kardiokhirurgiya. 2020;24:33–42.
47. Sultanov DD, Karimov TN. Revascularization in distal lesions of upper extremities arteries. Vestnik Avitsenny. 2012;2:167–73.
48. Karimov TN, Sultanov DD, Hodzhaev FM. Direct and indirect methods of revascularization in distal lesions of upper extremities arteries. Vestnik Tadzhikskogo natsional'nogo universiteta. Seriya estestvennykh nauk. 2014;1:231–8.
49. Gayvoronskiy IV. Collateral circulation: past, present, future. Meditsina XXI Vek. 2006;3:32–8.
50. Prives MG, Lysenkov VI, Bushkevich VI. Anatomiya cheloveka. 12th ed. Saint-Petersburg: SPbMAPO; 2010.
51. Kalinin RE, Suchkov IA, Mjavanadze ND, Mustafaeva RM. Anatomical variations in upper limb arteries. Vestnik Avitsenny. 2017;19:113–9.
52. Korotkikh A, Babunashvili A, Kaledin A, Akhramovich R, Derkach V, Portnov R, et al. Distal radiation access as an alternative to conventional radial access for coronary angiography and percutaneous coronary interventions (according to TENDERA trial). Curr Probl Cardiol. 2023;48:101546.
53. Ognerubov DV, Provatorov SI, Merkulov EV, Tereshchenko AS, Samko AN. Radial artery occlusion after interventional procedures performed through the radial access. Predictors, strategy to reduce frequency. The Sib J Clin Exp Med. 2018;33:9–16.
54. Bernat I, Bertrand OF, Rokyta R, Kacer M, Pesek J, Koza J, et al. Efficacy and safety of transient ulnar artery compression to recanalize acute radial artery occlusion after transradial catheterization. Am J Cardiol. 2011;107:1698–701.
55. Pancholy SB, Bernat I, Bertrand OF, Patel TM. Prevention of radial artery occlusion after transradial catheterization: the PROPHET-II randomized trial. JACC Cardiovasc Interv. 2016;9:1992–9.
56. Norgren L, Hiatt WR, Dormandy JA, Nehler MR, Harris KA, Fowkes FG, et al. Inter-society consensus for the management of peripheral arterial disease

(TASC II). Eur J Vasc Endovasc Surg. 2007;33(Suppl 1):S1–75.
57. Staniloae CS, Mody KP, Sanghvi K, Mindrescu C, Coppola JT, Antonescu CR, et al. Histopathologic changes of the radial artery wall secondary to transradial catheterization. Vasc Health Risk Manag. 2009;5:527–32.
58. Vandana R, Suresh NM, Lakshmiprabha R, Pai VP. Variation in course and branching pattern of brachial artery. Anatomica Karnataka. 2012;6:42–8.
59. Gupta C, Palimar V, Murlimanju BV, Shetti VR. A morphological study of variations in the origin and course of radial artery. Res J Pharm Biol Chem Sci. 2012;3:333–40.
60. Ruiz-Salmeron RJ, Mora R, Velez-Gimon M, Ortiz J, Fernandez C, Vidal B, et al. Radial artery spasm in transradial cardiac catheterization. Assessment of factors related to its occurrence, and of its consequences during follow-up. Rev Esp Cardiol. 2005;58:504–11.
61. Kiemeneij F, Vajifdar BU, Eccleshall SC, Laarman G, Slagboom T, van der Wieken R. Measurement of radial artery spasm using an automatic pullback device. Catheter Cardiovasc Interv. 2001;54:437–41.
62. Lo TS, Nolan J, Fountzopoulos E, Behan M, Butler R, Hetherington SL, et al. Radial artery anomaly and its influence on transradial coronary procedural outcome. Heart. 2009;95:410–5.
63. Saito S, Ikei H, Hosokawa G, Tanaka S. Influence of the ratio between radial artery inner diameter and sheath outer diameter on radial artery flow after transradial coronary intervention. Catheter Cardiovasc Interv. 1999;46:173–8.
64. Patel T, Shah S, Pancholy S, Radadiya R, Deora S, Vyas C, et al. Working through complexities of radial and brachial vasculature during transradial approach. Catheter Cardiovasc Interv. 2014;83:1074–88.
65. Sandoval Y, Bell MR, Gulati R. Transradial artery access complications. Circ Cardiovasc Interv. 2019;12:e007386.
66. Kwok CS, Rashid M, Fraser D, Nolan J, Mamas M. Intra-arterial vasodilators to prevent radial artery spasm: a systematic review and pooled analysis of clinical studies. Cardiovasc Revasc Med. 2015;16:484–90.
67. Collet C, Corral JM, Cavalcante R, Tateishi H, Belzarez O, Ribamar Costa J, et al. Pressure-mediated versus pharmacologic treatment of radial artery spasm during cardiac catheterisation: a randomised pilot study. EuroIntervention. 2017;12:e2212–8.
68. Ying L, Xu K, Gong X, Liu X, Fan Y, Zhao H, et al. Flow-mediated dilatation to relieve puncture-induced radial artery spasm: a pilot study. Cardiol J. 2018;25:1–6.
69. Barcin C, Kursaklioglu H, Kose S, Amasyali B, Isik E. Resistant radial artery spasm during coronary angiography via radial approach responded to local warm compress. Anadolu Kardiyol Derg. 2010;10:90–1.
70. Rocha-Singh KJ, Zeller T, Jaff MR. Peripheral arterial calcification: prevalence, mechanism, detection, and clinical implications. Catheter Cardiovasc Interv. 2014;83:E212–20.
71. Wang J, Yi C, Zhang J. Study on influencing factors of radial artery occlusion after repeated right radial artery coronary intervention. Contrast Media Mol Imaging. 2022;2022:9624339.
72. Mitchell A, Fujisawa T, Mills NL, Brittan M, Newby DE, Cruden NLM. Endothelial progenitor cell biology and vascular recovery following transradial cardiac catheterization. J Am Heart Assoc. 2017;6:e006610.
73. Yonetsu T, Kakuta T, Lee T, Takayama K, Kakita K, Iwamoto T, et al. Assessment of acute injuries and chronic intimal thickening of the radial artery after transradial coronary intervention by optical coherence tomography. Eur Heart J. 2010;31:1608–15.
74. Wakeyama T, Ogawa H, Iida H, Takaki A, Iwami T, Mochizuki M, et al. Intima-media thickening of the radial artery after transradial intervention. An intravascular ultrasound study. J Am Coll Cardiol. 2003;41:1109–14.
75. Sakai H, Ikeda S, Harada T, Yonashiro S, Ozumi K, Ohe H, et al. Limitations of successive transradial approach in the same arm: the Japanese experience. Catheter Cardiovasc Interv. 2001;54:204–8.
76. Sadaka MA, Etman W, Ahmed W, Kandil S, Eltahan S. Incidence and predictors of radial artery occlusion after transradial coronary catheterization. Egypt Heart J. 2019;71:12.
77. Bossard M, Lavi S, Rao SV, Cohen DJ, Cantor WJ, Bainey KR, et al. Heparin use for diagnostic cardiac catheterization with a radial artery approach: an international survey of practice patterns. Catheter Cardiovasc Interv. 2018;92:854–9.
78. Dahal K, Sharma S, Yousuf A, Lee J, Azrin M, Jimenez E, et al. A comparison of standard versus low dose heparin on access-related complications after coronary angiography through radial access: a meta-analysis of randomized controlled trials. Cardiovasc Revasc Med. 2018;19(5 Pt B):575–9.
79. Pacchioni A, Ferro J, Pesarini G, Mantovani R, Mugnolo A, Bellamoli M, et al. The activated clotting time paradox: relationship between activated clotting time and occlusion of the radial artery when used as vascular access for percutaneous coronary procedures. Circ Cardiovasc Interv. 2019;12:e008045.
80. Pancholy SB, Ahmed I, Bertrand OF, Patel T. Frequency of radial artery occlusion after transradial access in patients receiving warfarin therapy and undergoing coronary angiography. Am J Cardiol. 2014;113:211–4.
81. Feray H, Izgi C, Cetiner D, Men EE, Saltan Y, Baltay A, et al. Effectiveness of enoxaparin for prevention of radial artery occlusion after transradial cardiac catheterization. J Thromb Thrombolysis. 2010;29:322–5.
82. Sanmartin M, Gomez M, Rumoroso JR, Sadaba M, Martinez M, Baz JA, et al. Interruption of blood flow during compression and radial artery occlusion after transradial catheterization. Catheter Cardiovasc Interv. 2007;70:185–9.

83. Paccagnioni A, Mugnolo A, Sanz Sanchez J, Sgueglia GA, Pesarini G, Bellamoli M, et al. Radial artery occlusion after conventional and distal radial access: impact of preserved flow and time-to-hemostasis in a propensity-score matching analysis of 1163 patients. Catheter Cardiovasc Interv. 2022;99:827–35.
84. Babunashvili A, Dundua D. Recanalization and reuse of early occluded radial artery within 6 days after previous transradial diagnostic procedure. Catheter Cardiovasc Interv. 2011;77:530–6.
85. Valsecchi O, Nardin M, Vassileva A, Bernelli C. Transulnar recanalization of a chronic radial artery occlusion. Cardiovasc Revasc Med. 2017;18:504–6.
86. Campeau L. Percutaneous radial artery approach for coronary angiography. Catheter Cardiovasc Diagn. 1989;16:3–7.
87. Kiemeneij F, Laarman GJ. Percutaneous transradial artery approach for coronary stent implantation. Catheter Cardiovasc Diagn. 1993;30:173–8.

Part III

Safety and Efficacy

13 Hand Function

Christian F. Said, Sudhir Rathore, and Tom J. Ford

13.1 Background

Distal radial access (DRA) via the anatomical snuffbox or dorsum of the hand is gaining popularity as the standard vascular access for many interventional cardiologists and radiologists due to several advantages over conventional transradial access (TRA) and transfemoral access (TFA). In addition to improved ergonomics for both patient and operator, a significant benefit of DRA is a reduction in radial artery occlusion (RAO) compared to TRA [1, 2]. The more distal puncture in DRA in a compact space over the scaphoid and trapezium bones has theoretical advantages that may reduce hematoma and bleeding, resulting in a lower incidence of hand dysfunction.

13.2 Hand Function

The hand is a sophisticated and specialized part of the body with a complex anatomy that enables it to perform a range of challenging tasks. These require complex combinations of intricate movements and finely controlled force production with constant sensory feedback. As such, there is an intimate relationship between the various soft tissue structures and the bones. Injury to any one component can significantly alter the overall function of the hand, which is associated with a reduction in patient quality of life [3]. In addition, post-procedural access site pain can be particularly troublesome in patients with affective disorders, including depression, which are independently associated with chronic pain syndromes. This, in turn, can lead to cyclical feedback with structural and functional changes in brain structures with associated detrimental effects on hand function [4].

Hand function is complex but can be defined as the ability to use the hand in daily activities. The clinical assessment of hand function remains multifaceted, challenging, and controversial. Hand function depends not only on the anatomical integrity, sensation, coordination, strength, and dexterity of various components of the hand, but also on other sensory organs. For example, hand function is highly dependent on visual acuity, depth perception, and accommodation. In addition, an individual's gender, age, and level of motivation are known to affect the level of hand function. There is still no single gold standard for assessing hand function, but rather the assessment depends on multimodal approach composed of a range of activities exmaining sensory and motor function [5, 6].

C. F. Said · T. J. Ford (✉)
Gosford Hospital, Gosford, NSW, Australia
e-mail: tom.ford@health.nsw.gov.au

S. Rathore
Frimley Health NHS Foundation Trust,
Camberley, Surrey, UK

G. A. Sgueglia (ed.), *Distal Radial Access*, https://doi.org/10.1007/978-3-031-89925-6_13

13.3 Potential Mechanisms of Hand Dysfunction After Radial Access

Despite the widespread use of TRA for increasingly complex procedures in patients, hand dysfunction remains a rare complication. A large meta-analysis of more than 3800 patients reported sensory dysfunction in less than 2% of patients and motor dysfunction in less than 0.3% of patients [7].

The flexor carpi radialis and flexor pollicis longus tendons, the median and superficial radial nerves, and the radial artery run at the level of the wrist. Functional deficits may result from direct damage to these structures during radial artery cannulation. There is also the possibility of extrinsic compression of these structures due to hematoma or pseudoaneurysm formation of the radial artery, which may result in transient or permanent ischemia of the nerve supply to the hand. There are isolated case reports describing sensory deficits or motor dysfunction of the small hand muscles due to this mechanism [8–10].

Endothelial dysfunction, intimal hyperplasia, and medial dissections resulting in radial artery stenosis or RAO are well-documented complications associated with TRA [11–13]. Notably, RAO is often asymptomatic and rarely causes ischemia due to the robust collateral blood supply to the hand from the ulnar and anterior interosseous arteries [7, 11–15]. The Hand Grip Test After Transradial Percutaneous Coronary Procedures (HANGAR) study [16] demonstrated no significant difference in grip, thumb pinch, and index finger pinch tests compared to baseline at a median follow-up of more than 80 days. Occasionally, RAO has been associated with abnormal hand sensation compared to the contralateral hand [17]. Mechanistically, this is unlikely to be due to RAO, but rather to injury to the superficial radial nerve at the time of the procedure or during post-procedural compression with a hemostatic device [17]. Ultrasound-guided radial access has been shown to improve the success and efficiency of radial artery canulation, and routine use may reduce the rate of RAO [18].

Hand function
Capacity of the hand in everyday activities

Vascular injury
Ecchymoses/hematoma
Radial artery occlusion

Muscle/tendon damage
Thumb abduction
Extension of the first MCP joint
Hand abduction
Wrist extension

Sensory dysfunction
Paresthesia of dorsal thumb (possibly including dorsal index and long fingers)

Fig. 13.1 Potential etiology of injury and hand dysfunction associated with distal radial access. *MCP* metacarpophalangeal

Potential mechanisms of injury and hand dysfunction associated with distal radial access are summarized in Fig. 13.1.

13.4 Prospective Study of Distal Radial Access on Hand Function

DRA is a relatively new approach for coronary angiography and percutaneous coronary intervention (PCI), especially when compared to conventional TRA and TFA. The largest study to date evaluating hand function after DRA, the International Hand Function Study Following Distal Radial Access (RATATOUILLE), demonstrated no impairment of hand function after DRA at up to 12 months post procedure. This conclusion was based on a comprehensive and repeated multidimensional evaluation incorporating both subjective and objective measures. Additionally DRA is associated with the lowest reported pain response to percutaneous arterial

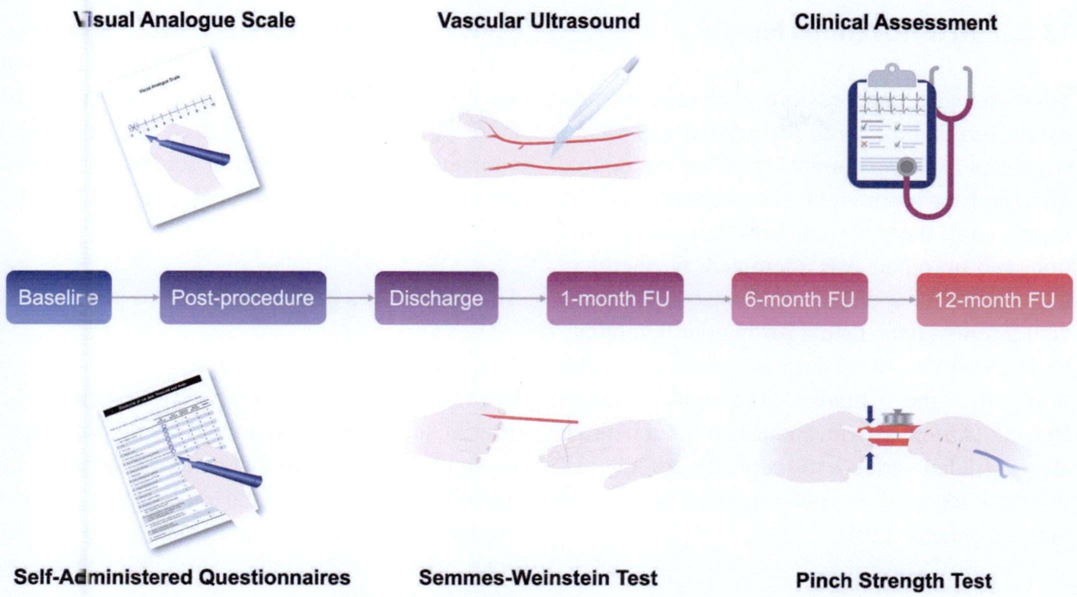

Fig. 13.2 Multimodality assessment of hand function in the RATATOUILLE study

access [19]. These results confirm the findings of other smaller studies evaluating DRA [20, 21].

RATATOUILLE was an international, multicenter, prospective cohort study that performed a comprehensive evaluation of hand function in 313 patients undergoing DRA for coronary angiography or PCI. Multimodality assessment of hand function was performed at baseline and at follow-up using several well-validated tools, including self-reported questionnaires (Disabilities of the Arm, Shoulder, and Hand (DASH) and Levine-Katz) and tests of pain, sensation, strength, and functional status (Fig. 13.2).

13.5 Anatomical Considerations for Potential Injury Associated with Distal Radial Access

13.5.1 Arterial Supply

The arterial supply to the hand is so robust that guidelines no longer recommned the routine use of the Allen or Barbeau test to assist in procedural access route decisions [22]. Furthermore, international guidelines unanimously support a radial-first approach for all coronary angiography and PCI [22, 23]. A significant advantage of DRA above TRA is the reduced rate of Radial Artery Occlusion (ROA) due to continued raidal artery blood flow via wrist and hand arterial anastomoses [2, 24]. The rate of RAO after conventional TRA has been reported as high as 30% [25, 26] compared to <1% ROA with DRA in the RATATOUILLE [19] study. Although RAO often does not affect hand function [16, 27], it may necessitate the use of an alternative access site in future procedures, namely, the contralateral radial or femoral artery.

13.5.2 Veins and Lymphatics

The cephalic vein passes through the anatomical snuffbox before terminating as part of the dorsal venous network of the hand. The vascular consequences of venous injury to the cephalic vein or the associated lymphatics in the anatomical snuffbox are identical to those associated with intravenous cannulation, namely, ecchymosis, and will not be discussed further.

13.5.3 Arteriovenous Fistula

There remains the possibility of arteriovenous fistula formation if both the arterial and venous structures in the anatomical snuffbox are injured. This has been reported in one case study [28], but in this case, there was no impact on hand function, and no repair was attempted. Furthermore, the creation of a distal radial artery to cephalic vein arteriovenous fistula for regular hemodialysis is a well-described surgical procedure in addition to the more commonly created Brescia-Cimino arteriovenous fistula for hemodialysis (radial artery to cephalic vein), with minimal reported impact on hand function in dialysis patients [29].

13.5.4 Skin and Connective Tissue

Current literature does not suggest any difference in rates of skin infection or irritation between DRA and conventional TRA.

13.5.5 Tendons and Muscles

The anatomical snuffbox is a depression in the dorsum of the hand. It is bordered medially by the tendons of the extensor pollicis longus and laterally by the tendons of the extensor pollicis brevis and abductor pollicis longus. The base of the snuffbox is formed by the tendons of the extensor carpi radialis longus and extensor carpi radialis brevis along with the carpal bones. The base of the first metacarpal can be palpated distally, and the styloid process of the radius can be palpated proximally.

Injury to any of the structures within the anatomical snuffbox, especially the tendons, can potentially affect hand function (especially activities requiring a pinch grip). Tendinitis or trauma (e.g., from a needle, sheath, or hematoma) can impair the ability of the muscles to transmit adequate force to their respective joints or cause pain. The likelihood of this occurring is low because these structures are easily palpable and therefore easily avoided during the procedure. Advantageously, the distal radial artery runs along the bottom of the snuffbox away from many of these structures, making it easy to locate and puncture. To date, no clinical study has reported any decrease in muscle strength after DRA [19].

13.5.6 Bones and Joints

The floor of the anatomical snuffbox is formed by the scaphoid and trapezium carpal bones. The arterial supply to the scaphoid is unique in that much of the blood supply (80%) comes from the dorsal branch of the distal radial artery, which provides retrograde intraosseous supply to the bone, while a volar branch supplies the remainder (Fig. 13.3) [30].

A scaphoid fracture can disrupt its dominant retrograde intraosseous blood supply, potentially leading to avascular necrosis (Preiser's disease) [31, 32]. Scaphoid necrosis is an undesirable clinical outcome that can result in pain and swelling around the anatomical scaphoid, along with loss of strength and reduced range of motion of the wrist [33, 34]. However, because the distal radial artery puncture site lies proximal to the dorsal scaphoid branch—and the dorsal division of the anterior interosseous system provides a

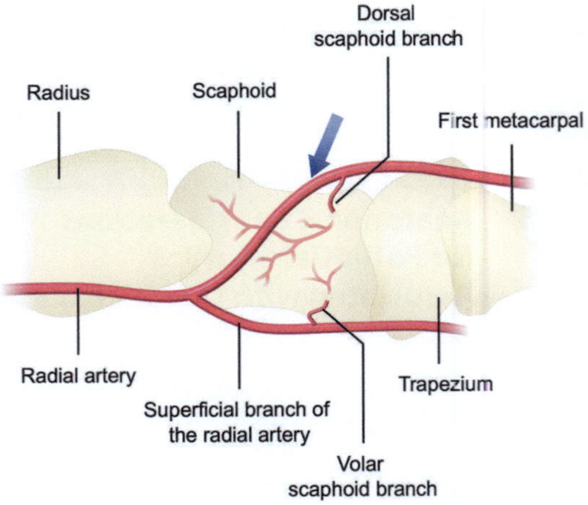

Fig. 13.3 Schematic scaphoid blood supply. (Adapted from Pettrone et al. [30]). The arrow shows a typical distal radial artery puncture site

secondary arterial supply—distal radial puncture does not typically affect scaphoid perfusion [31] (Fig. 13.3). Scaphoid necrosis has never been reported as a complication of DRA.

13.5.7 Sensory Nerves

By the time the radial nerve reaches the anatomical snuffbox, it has already divided into its terminal branches, the superficial branch of the radial nerve (also known as the superficial radial nerve), which is itself composed of a medial and a lateral branch (Fig. 13.4). These innervate the dorsum of the index and middle fingers, a portion of the radial aspect of the fourth finger, the ulnar aspect of the dorsum of the thumb, the radial aspect of the thumb, and the dorsal surface of the base of the thumb. Injury to the superficial branch of the radial nerve (Wartenberg's syndrome) may affect somatosensory function in these areas, yet no study has shown loss of somatosensory or hand function at follow-up after DRA or conventional TRA compared to baseline [11, 19].

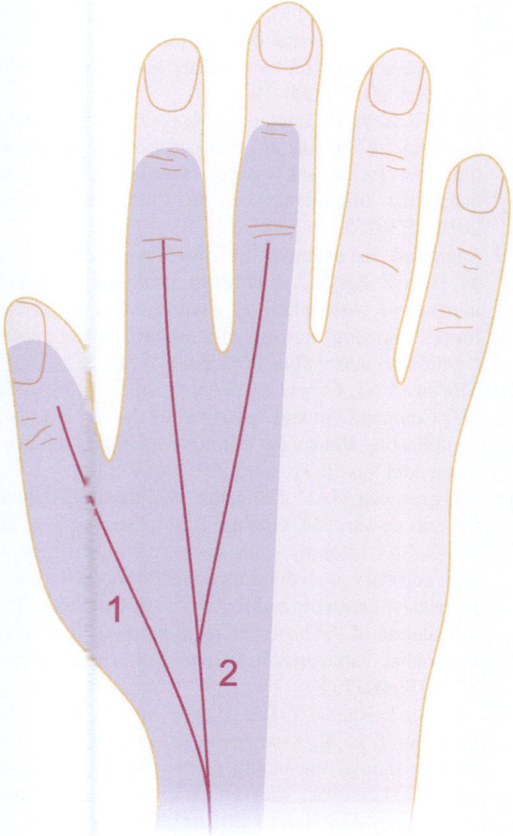

Fig. 13.4 Sensory innervation of the lateral (1) and medial (2) branches of the superficial radial nerve

13.6 Risk Factors for Hand Dysfunction

To date, there is a paucity of literature describing risk factors for hand dysfunction after DRA. However, it would be reasonable to consider potential influences such as female gender [35, 36], shorter height, smoking status, hypertension, family history of cardiovascular disease, and a history of osteoarthritis of the upper extremity [36].

13.7 Treatment Considerations

In rare cases where patients experience hand dysfunction following DRA or conventional TRA procedures, the majority of symptoms resolve without long-term clinical sequelae [7, 35]. Literature regarding the treatment and outcomes of hand dysfunction following transradial access has historically been produced in the conventional TRA setting.

The ARCUS study [36] was a multicenter, prospective cohort study that provided insight into upper extremity dysfunction following conventional TRA and subsequent management. More than 500 consecutive patients admitted for PCI were followed for up to 6 months using a strict multimodality criterion to assess upper extremity dysfunction. In an ARCUS sub-study [37], pain was found as the most commonly reported reason for referral to a hand clinic.

The most common symptoms requiring treatment were preexisting or latent carpal tunnel syndrome and osteoarthritis exacerbated by the procedure, possibly due to local edema or immobilization. Carpal tunnel syndrome was diagnosed in 18 patients (five of whom had unilateral carpal tunnel syndrome in the intervention arm).

The majority of these patients were successfully treated with a combination of carpal tunnel release, local injections, and hand therapy. Also, 15 patients were diagnosed with osteoarthritis, typically treated conservatively, and half had worsening of preexisting upper extremity osteoarthritis. Tendinitis was diagnosed in only three of 294 patients (1%) and successfully treated with immobilization therapy.

Hand grip training after conventional TRA has been shown to aid in the recovery of radial artery vasodilator and vasoconstrictor function and may minimize complications and impact on hand function [38]. The potential impact on hand function is significantly reduced with DRA, but if it does occur, treatment modalities may include early referral to a hand clinic, hand physiotherapy, simple analgesics and nonsteroidal anti-inflammatory drugs, steroid injection, decompression treatment, and, in rare cases, surgery.

13.8 Conclusions

Hand dysfunction manifest as hand stiffness, muscle weakness, and nonspecific sensory disturbances remains a rare complication of conventional TRA for coronary angiography and PCI and is very rare after DRA. DRA is increasingly becoming a safer alternative to TRA, offering several additional benefits due to a more distal puncture site, reduced hand immobilization time, and lower rates of radial artery occlusion. All of these factors may reduce the potential for hand dysfunction. Potential risk factors for developing hand dysfunction may include female gender, smoking, hypertension, family history of cardiovascular disease, and a history of osteoarthritis of the upper extremity. When hand dysfunction occurs, referral for physical therapy with consultation to a subspecialist hand clinic may be considered. Fortunately, symptoms of hand dysfunction usually resolve with conservative treatment and time.

References

1. Ferrante G, Condello F, Rao SV, Maurina M, Jolly S, Stefanini GG, et al. Distal vs conventional radial access for coronary angiography and/or intervention: a meta-analysis of randomized trials. JACC Cardiovasc Interv. 2022;15:2297–311.
2. Eid-Lidt G, Rivera Rodriguez A, Jimenez Castellanos J, Farjat Pasos JI, Estrada Lopez KE, Gaspar J. Distal radial artery approach to prevent radial artery occlusion trial. JACC Cardiovasc Interv. 2021;14:378–85.
3. Pathmanathan C, Deveza LA, Robbins SR, Duong V, Venkatesha V, Hunter DJ. Determinants of quality of life and hand function among people with hand osteoarthritis. Int J Rheum Dis. 2022;25:1408–15.
4. Yang S, Chang MC. Chronic pain: structural and functional changes in brain structures and associated negative affective states. Int J Mol Sci. 2019;20:3130.
5. MacDermid J, Solomon G, Valdes K. ASHT clinical assessment recommendations. 3rd ed. Mount Laurel: American Society of Hand Therapists; 2015.
6. Duruöz MT. Assessment of hand function. In: Duruöz MT, editor. Hand function – a practical guide to assessment. 2nd ed. Cham: Springer Nature; 2019. p. 43–53.
7. Ul Haq MA, Rashid M, Kwok CS, Wong CW, Nolan J, Mamas MA. Hand dysfunction after transradial artery catheterization for coronary procedures. World J Cardiol. 2017;9:609–19.
8. Araki T, Itaya H, Yamamoto M. Acute compartment syndrome of the forearm that occurred after transradial intervention and was not caused by bleeding or hematoma formation. Catheter Cardiovasc Interv. 2010;75:362–5.
9. Sugimoto A, Iwamoto J, Tsumuraya N, Nagaoka M, Ikari Y. Acute compartment syndrome occurring in forearm with relatively small amount of hematoma following transradial coronary intervention. Cardiovasc Interv Ther. 2016;31:147–50.
10. Mouawad NJ, Capers Q, Allen C, James I, Haurani MJ. Complete "in situ" avulsion of the radial artery complicating transradial coronary rotational atherectomy. Ann Vasc Surg. 2015;29(123):e7–11.
11. van Leeuwen MAH, Hollander MR, van der Heijden DJ, van de Ven PM, Opmeer KHM, Taverne Y, et al. The ACRA anatomy study (assessment of disability after coronary procedures using radial access): a comprehensive anatomic and functional assessment of the vasculature of the hand and relation to outcome after transradial catheterization. Circ Cardiovasc Interv. 2017;10:e005753.
12. Yonetsu T, Kakuta T, Lee T, Takayama K, Kakita K, Iwamoto T, et al. Assessment of acute injuries and chronic intimal thickening of the radial artery after transradial coronary intervention by optical coherence tomography. Eur Heart J. 2010;31:1608–15.

13. Dawson EA, Rathore S, Cable NT, Wright DJ, Morris JL, Green DJ. Impact of introducer sheath coating on endothelial function in humans after transradial coronary procedures. Circ Cardiovasc Interv. 2010;3:148–56.
14. Mamas MA, Fraser DG, Ratib K, Fath-Ordoubadi F, El-Omar M, Nolan J, et al. Minimising radial injury: prevention is better than cure. EuroIntervention. 2014;10:824–32.
15. Agostoni P, Zuffi A, Biondi-Zoccai G. Pushing wrist access to the limit: homolateral right ulnar artery approach for primary percutaneous coronary intervention after right radial failure due to radial loop. Catheter Cardiovasc Interv. 2011;78:894–7.
16. Sciahbasi A, Rigattieri S, Sarandrea A, Cera M, Di Russo C, Fedele S, et al. Radial artery occlusion and hand strength after percutaneous coronary procedures: results of the HANGAR study. Catheter Cardiovasc Interv. 2016;87:868–74.
17. van der Heijden DJ, van Leeuwen MAH, Ritt MJPF, Dapper MML, Boer K, Teerenstra S, et al. Hand sensibility after transradial arterial access: an observational study in patients with and without radial artery occlusion. J Vasc Interv Radiol. 2019;30:1832–9.
18. Seto AH, Roberts JS, Abu-Fadel MS, Czak SJ, Latif F, Jain SP, et al. Real-time ultrasound guidance facilitates transradial access. JACC Cardiovasc Interv. 2015;8:283–91.
19. Sgueglia GA, Hassan A, Harb S, Ford TJ, Koliastasis L, Milkas A, et al. International hand function study following distal radial access: The RATATOUILLE study. JACC Cardiovasc Interv. 2022;15:1205–15.
20. Bhambhani A, Pandey S, Nadamani AN, Tyagi K. An observational comparison of distal radial and traditional radial approaches for coronary angiography. J Saudi Heart Assoc. 2020;32:17–24.
21. Hammami R, Zouari F, Ben Abdessalem MA, Sassi A, Ellouze T, Bahloul A, et al. Distal radial approach versus conventional radial approach: a comparative study of feasibility and safety. Libyan J Med. 2021;16:1830600.
22. Mason PJ, Shah B, Tamis-Holland JE, Bittl JA, Cohen MG, Safirstein J, et al. An update on radial artery access and best practices for transradial coronary angiography and intervention in acute coronary syndrome: a scientific statement from The American Heart Association. Circ Cardiovasc Interv. 2018;11:e000035.
23. Shroff AR, Gulati R, Drachman DE, Feldman DN, Gilchrist IC, Kaul P, et al. SCAI expert consensus statement update on best practices for transradial angiography and intervention. Catheter Cardiovasc Interv. 2020;95:245–52.
24. Tsigkas G, Papageorgiou A, Moulias A, Kalogeropoulos AP, Papageorgopoulou C, Apostolos A, et al. Distal or traditional transradial access site for coronary procedures: a single-center, randomized study. JACC Cardiovasc Interv. 2022;15:22–32.
25. Sadaka MA, Etman W, Ahmed W, Kandil S, Eltahan S. Incidence and predictors of radial artery occlusion after transradial coronary catheterization. Egypt Heart J. 2019;71:12.
26. Sandoval Y, Bell MR, Gulati R. Transradial artery access complications. Circ Cardiovasc Interv. 2019;12:e007386.
27. Avdikos G, Karatasakis A, Tsoumeleas A, Lazaris E, Ziakas A, Koutouzis M. Radial artery occlusion after transradial coronary catheterization. Cardiovasc Diagn Ther. 2017;7:305–16.
28. Shah SR, Kiemeneij F, Khuddus MA. Distal arteriovenous fistula formation after percutaneous coronary intervention: an old complication of a new access site. Catheter Cardiovasc Interv. 2021;97:278–81.
29. Maharaj D, Ramdass MJ, Baksh R, Oladiran A, Budhoo E. Distal-to-snuffbox arteriovenous fistula. Int J Angiol. 2018;27:227–31.
30. Pettrone S, Bridgeman J, Trumble TE. Volar wedge grafting for scaphoid nonunions. In: Slutsky DJ, editor. Principles and practice of wrist surgery. Philadelphia: Saunders; 2010. p. 249.
31. Gelberman RH, Menon J. The vascularity of the scaphoid bone. J Hand Surg Am. 1980;5:508–13.
32. Sendher R, Ladd AL. The scaphoid. Orthop Clin North Am. 2013;44:107–20.
33. Herbert TJ, Lanzetta M. Idiopathic avascular necrosis of the scaphoid. J Hand Surg Br. 1994;19:174–82.
34. Claessen F, Schol I, Kolovich GP, Ring D. Avascular Necrosis of the Scaphoid Preiser Disease. Arch Bone Jt Surg. 2020;8:94–8.
35. Harvey JA, Kim S, Ireson ME, Gulati R, Bell MR, Moran SL. Acute upper-limb complications following radial artery catheterization for coronary angiography. J Hand Surg Am. 2020;45(655):e1–5.
36. Zwaan EM, Cheung ES, Ijsselmuiden AJJ, Holtzer CAJ, Schreuders TAR, Kofflard MJM, et al. Upper extremity function following transradial percutaneous coronary intervention: results of the ARCUS trial. J Interv Cardiol. 2022;2022:6858962.
37. Cheung ES, Zwaan EM, Schreuders TAR, Kofflard MJM, Coert JH, Alings M, et al. Treatment and management of upper extremity dysfunction following transradial percutaneous coronary intervention: a prospective cohort study. Hand. 2022;19:154–62.
38. Dawson EA, Alkarmi A, Thijssen DH, Rathore S, Marsman DE, Cable NT, et al. Low-flow mediated constriction is endothelium-dependent effects of exercise training after radial artery catheterization. Circ Cardiovasc Interv. 2012;5:713–9.

Radiation Exposure

14

Alessandro Sciahbasi and Mladen I. Vidovich

14.1 Introduction

Over the last decade, the increased ability to perform more complex percutaneous coronary interventions (PCIs) has been associated with longer procedures and a progressive increase in radiation dose to both patients and operators. In particular, PCI is one of the procedures with higher radiation exposure in interventional cardiology [1], and increased radiation doses could be associated with deterministic (long-term risk of cancer induction) and stochastic (skin lesions, cataracts) risks. In a previous study [2], an increased risk of brain and neck tumors was observed among physicians performing interventional procedures, and operators should keep radiation exposure to a level that is "As Low As Reasonably Achievable" (ALARA principle). Consequently, awareness of the risks of radiation exposure and dose reduction are important issues during PCI, as confirmed by statements from international medical societies [3, 4].

A. Sciahbasi (✉)
Interventional Cardiology, Sandro Pertini Hospital, Rome, Italy

M. I. Vidovich
Jesse Brown Veterans Affairs Medical Center, University of Illinois at Chicago, Chicago, IL, USA

14.2 How to Measure Radiation Exposure?

The simplest indicator of radiation exposure is fluoroscopy time, which is the total time fluoroscopy was used during the procedure. However, this is a weak indicator of radiation exposure that does not take into account many procedural variables (patient body mass index, tube angulation, cineangiography time, etc.) and should not be considered a good and effective measure of the radiation dose absorbed by the patient or operator [5]. In contrast, patient radiation doses can be better estimated by measuring air kerma (AK) and dose area product (DAP), which are regularly recorded in all current angiographic machines. AK is the amount of energy released per unit mass at a reference point in the air (generally located 15 cm from the isocenter). AK correlates well with the patient's peak skin dose and can be used to estimate the risk of skin lesions. In contrast, DAP, the product of AK and the x-ray field is a measure of the global dose received by the patient and is a good marker of long-term deterministic risk.

AK and DAP are currently used to assess patient exposure and, indirectly, operator exposure, although the correlation with operator dose is weak. In fact, the positioning of the operator as well as the correct use of the suspended leaded screen or the use of additional protective drapes can expose the operators to different radiation doses for the same DAP values [6]. Consequently,

G. A. Sgueglia (ed.), *Distal Radial Access*, https://doi.org/10.1007/978-3-031-89925-6_14

the correct system for operators to measure radiation dose is the use of dedicated wearable dosimeters that accurately evaluate exposure independently of DAP and AK.

14.3 Radiation Dose According to Vascular Access

A key element of radiation exposure is the vascular access for diagnostic coronary procedures and PCI: in particular, a previous large meta-analysis that included studies with small numbers of patients and operators and with limited experience with transradial access (TRA) showed a slight but significant increase in radiation exposure with TRA compared to femoral access. Subsequently, the large RAD-MATRIX trial [7], performed in more than 7000 patients by skilled radial operators, confirmed a higher radiation exposure with TRA compared to the femoral approach for both patients and operators [8]. There are several possible explanations for the increased radiation dose with TRA: slightly longer fluoroscopy times, the positioning of the operator (closer to the patient), and the need to manipulate the catheters more frequently during the procedure.

The absolute increase in DAP values for patients with radial rather than femoral access is limited (5.6 Gy*cm^2 in the RAD-MATRIX trial) and very small when expressed in terms of patient effective dose (1.12 mSv). The operator's exposure was almost twice as high with the radial than with the femoral access, and we should keep in mind that interventional cardiologists perform thousands of procedures in their lifetime, with the potential for a cumulative effect.

Another aspect to consider in vascular access is the side-arm effect (right vs. left approach). The right TRA is usually preferred because it is more comfortable for the operator who is on the right side of the patient, whereas the left approach requires the operator to bend over the patient to gain vascular access and manipulate the catheters, increasing discomfort for operators of short stature or those with back problems. However, the left approach may be advantageous compared to the right approach in terms of radiation exposure: many different studies and meta-analyses have shown that the left TRA is associated with lower radiation exposure for both patient and operator compared to the right approach [9–12]. In particular, in the TALENT trial, which included more than 1400 patients [9], the left TRA was associated with significantly shorter fluoroscopy time (149 s, interquartile range [IQR] 95–270) and DAP (10.7 Gy*cm^2, IQR 6–20.5) compared with the right approach (168 s, IQR 110–277, p = 0.0025 and 12.1 Gy*cm^2, IQR 7–23.8, p = 0.004, respectively).

14.4 Radiation Exposure in Distal Radial Access

The effect of distal radial access (DRA) on radiation dose is controversial, with a general perception of possible increased radiation exposure due to more catheter manipulation and longer fluoroscopy times [13]. In the majority of studies [14–20], DRA is associated with an increase in patient radiation exposure in terms of DAP and AK (Table 14.1), but radiation dose to the operator has not been evaluated. The increased patient dose is probably due to the longer fluoroscopy times in procedures performed by operators not familiar with this approach. In fact, in the largest randomized trial, which included more than 1300 patients and compared DRA with conventional TRA, no differences in DAP and AK were found: AK was 1222 ± 2846 mGy with DRA vs. 1298 ± 3143 mGy with TRA, p = 0.70 [17].

A limitation of the studies evaluating radiation exposure in DRA is the lack of data on side effects (left vs. right) and very limited data on operator exposure. In a series of 180 consecutive procedures performed at our center (90 DRA and 90 TRA), there was no difference in operator radiation dose comparing DRA vs. TRA (5.6 μSv, IQR 1.8–13.5 vs. 5.7 μSv, IQR 2–12, p = 0.84) (unpublished data).

Based on the available data, an intriguing hypothesis is that the left DRA approach could be used to take advantage of the reduced radiation exposure found with left radial access without

Table 14.1 Radiation doses in studies comparing distal radial access with conventional transradial access

Trial	Year	Design	Number of procedures	DRA-DAP (Gy*cm^2)	TRA-DAP (Gy*cm^2)	*p*	DRA-AK (mGy)	TRA-AK (mGy)	*p*
Coughlan et al. [14]	2018	Observational	94	5033±2740[a]	4826±2796[a]	0.72			
Bhambhani et al. [15]	2020	Observational	200	17.8 ± 8	16.5 ± 6	0.38	298 ± 124	273 ± 99	0.30
Tsigkas et al. [16]	2021	Randomized	1042	327[a]	289[a]	0.02			
Aminian et al. [17]	2021	Randomized	1307				1298 ± 3143	1222 ± 2846	0.70
Rivera K et al. [18]	2022	Observational	182	32	32	0.47			
Ghose et al. [19]	2022	Observational	108	39	44	0.56			
Achim et al. [20]	2022	Observational	337	1	1.5	0.018			

[a]Gy/cm^2

AK air kerma, *DAP* dose area product, *DRA* distal radial access, *TRA* conventional transradial access

compromising operator comfort (as the instrumented arm is placed on the patient's abdomen, allowing the operator standing on the right side of the patient without the need to bend over). This idea has been tested in the prospective observational RADIANT-II study (NCT04403815), which has just completed enrollment, and in the randomized DOSE study (NCT 04023838). Preliminary data from RADIANT-II confirmed a potential role for the left DRA compared to the right TRA in reducing the operator's thorax dose: the dose was significantly lower with left DRA compared to right radial access (6.9 μS, IQR 3–18 vs. 17 μS, IQR 7–31, $p < 0.0001$). After propensity matching, left DRA reduced effectively thorax dose compared to right radial access (12 μS, 95% confidence interval [CI] 9–14 vs. 20 μS, 95% CI 15–26, $p = 0.029$), and at regression analysis, left DRA remained an independent predictor of reduced radiation exposure [21].

14.5 How to Improve Operator Radiation Protection?

As mentioned above, radial access is associated with higher radiation exposure for patients and operators. For patients, according to the RAD-MATRIX results, the risk is very limited (one possible cancer case per almost 35,714 procedures), and this risk could be considered acceptable considering that radial instead of femoral access can avoid one death per 166 procedures [8]. On the other hand, the operator does not benefit from the radial approach and is chronically exposed to this possible increase in radiation dose. Therefore, it is necessary for radial operators to use adjunctive protective devices to reduce their exposure, and a simple method is to use adjunctive protective drapes placed on the patient's abdomen [22]. With the use of these drapes, the operator's radiation exposure is even lower than the exposure during transfemoral procedures [23]. These drapes could be easily used even in the case of left DRA (Fig. 14.1) and are effective for the first operator as well as for all the staff involved during the procedure (e.g., nurse or technician) [24].

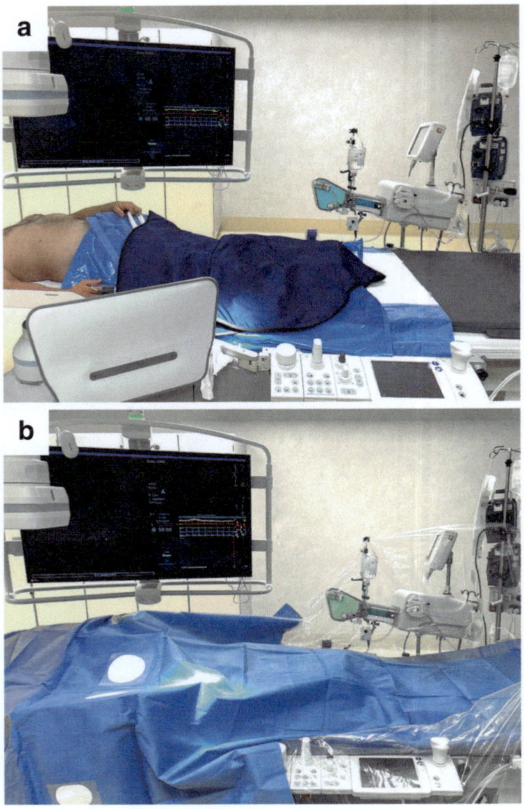

Fig. 14.1 (**a**) During patient preparation, adjunctive protective drapes are placed on the patient's pelvic region. (**b**) These drapes are subsequently covered with the sterile sheet without discomfort for the patient or the operator

There are several approaches to reducing radiation exposure during cardiac catheterization. Contemporary angiographic systems have significantly reduced radiation doses through the use of image noise reduction technologies. Reductions as high as 45% are achievable and are particularly attractive for radial access, which is inherently associated with higher overall radiation doses [25]. In addition to special drapes [26], various floor- or ceiling-mounted systems have been developed to protect the operator (e.g., Zero-Gravity or Rampart) [27, 28]. Since these systems provide universal radiation protection, it is expected that the level of protection provided would be equivalent for DRA. It should be noted that the suspended lead suit systems (Zero-Gravity, CFI Medical), at least in part, reduce the operator's ability to move during the procedure and may be difficult to use during left TRAI/left DRA procedures due to the need to lean over the patient. On the other hand, the more recent innovation (M1128 system, Rampart), a floor-mounted system, allows the operator to perform procedures without wearing a lead, which is a significant ergonomic advantage.

As mentioned above, the operator's choice of access site does have an impact on radiation, with left radial access generally associated with slightly lower doses than right radial access. However, most operators worldwide choose the right radial approach due to its mostly unfavorable ergonomic aspects [29].

An often overlooked aspect of radiation dose during radial access is the interaction between table height and operator height. Shorter operators receive more radiation than taller operators due to the relationship between table height and radiation dose [30]. Due to ergonomic concerns, operators choose a lower table height for left radial access and may receive higher doses as a result.

Finally, robotic angiography and percutaneous coronary intervention completely eliminate radiation exposure to the operator [31]. It should be noted, however, that while the operator is protected from radiation during the procedure, the technologist loading the equipment onto the robotic device and the nursing staff remain exposed to radiation. It remains to be determined whether the physician's trade-off of radiation over ergonomics holds true for DRA.

Patient preferences have been studied to determine whether patients value radiation dose over access site choice (radial vs. femoral), bleeding reduction, or length of hospital stay. A crowd-sourcing study demonstrated that patients placed the greatest value on length of hospital stay and less value on access site choice or radiation dose [32].

14.6 Conclusions

While radial access has provided an exceptional reduction in access site complications and access-related bleeding, tremendous improvements in patient comfort, and streamlined early/same-day discharge, the small but consistent increase in radiation dose to the operator and staff remains an ongoing challenge. While left radial access is generally associated with slightly lower doses, most operators worldwide perform right radial access for ergonomic reasons. Distal radial access offers improved operator ergonomics and patient positioning comfort but may have other radiation dose implications. Dedicated and randomized studies, such as the RADIANT-II trial, will help us fully understand these differences. Improvements in angiography laboratory equipment and radiation shielding technology remain an urgent need to protect operators from radiation exposure during their careers.

References

1. Sciahbasi A, Ferrante G, Fischetti D, Miklin DJ, Sarandrea A, Schirripa V, et al. Radiation dose among different cardiac and vascular invasive procedures: the RODEO study. Int J Cardiol. 2017;240:92–6.
2. Roguin A, Goldstein J, Bar O, Goldstein JA. Brain and neck tumors among physicians performing interventional procedures. Am J Cardiol. 2013;111:1368–72.
3. Hirshfeld JW Jr, Ferrari VA, Bengel FM, Bergersen L, Chambers CE, Einstein AJ, et al. 2018 ACC/HRS/NASCI/SCAI/SCCT expert consensus document on optimal use of ionizing radiation in cardiovascular imaging: best practices for safety and effectiveness: a report of the American College of Cardiology Task Force on Expert Consensus Decision Pathways. J Am Coll Cardiol. 2018;71:e283–351.
4. Sciahbasi A, Piccaluga E, Andreassi MG, Trianni A, Rosi A, Sarandrea A, et al. SICI-GISE position paper: enhancing radiation safety in the catheterization laboratory. G Ital Cardiol. 2019;20:14S–28S.
5. Skripochnik E, Loh SA. Fluoroscopy time is not accurate as a surrogate for radiation exposure. Vascular. 2017;25:466–71.
6. Sciahbasi A, Frigoli E, Sarandrea A, Calabrò P, Rubartelli P, Cortese B, et al. Determinants of radiation dose during right transradial access: insights from the RAD-MATRIX study. Am Heart J. 2018;196:113–8.
7. Sciahbasi A, Calabrò P, Sarandrea A, Rigattieri S, Tomassini F, Sardella G, et al. Randomized comparison of operator radiation exposure comparing transradial and transfemoral approach for percutaneous coronary procedures: rationale and design of the minimizing adverse haemorrhagic events by TRansradial access site and systemic implementation of angioX – RAdiation Dose study (RAD-MATRIX). Cardiovasc Revasc Med. 2014;15:209–13.

8. Sciahbasi A, Frigoli E, Sarandrea A, Rothenbühler M, Calabrò P, Lupi A, et al. Radiation exposure and vascular access in acute coronary syndromes: the RAD-matrix trial. J Am Coll Cardiol. 2017;69:2530–7.
9. Sciahbasi A, Romagnoli E, Burzotta F, Trani C, Sarandrea A, Summaria F, et al. Transradial approach (left vs right) and procedural times during percutaneous coronary procedures: TALENT study. Am Heart J. 2011;161:172–9.
10. Dominici M, Diletti R, Milici C, Bock C, Placanica A, D'Alessandro G, et al. Operator exposure to x-ray in left and right radial access during percutaneous coronary procedures: OPERA randomized study. Heart. 2013;99:480–4.
11. Biondi-Zoccai G, Sciahbasi A, Bodí V, Fernández-Portales J, Kanei Y, Romagnoli E, et al. Right versus left radial artery access for coronary procedures: an international collaborative systematic review and meta-analysis including 5 randomized trials and 3210 patients. Int J Cardiol. 2013;166:621–6.
12. Kado H, Patel AM, Suryadevara S, Zenni MM, Box LC, Angiolillo DJ, et al. Operator radiation exposure and physical discomfort during a right versus left radial approach for coronary interventions: a randomized evaluation. JACC Cardiovasc Interv. 2014;7:810–6.
13. Apostolos A, Vasilagkos G, Tsigkas G. Could radiation exposure be the Achilles' heel of distal transradial access? Indian Heart J. 2022;74:338–9.
14. Coughlan JJ, Zebrauskaite A, Arnous S. Left distal transradial access facilitates earlier discharge post coronary angiography. J Interv Cardiol. 2018;31:964–8.
15. Bhambhani A, Pandey S, Nadamani AN, Tyagi K. An observational comparison of distal radial and traditional radial approaches for coronary angiography. J Saudi Heart Assoc. 2020;32:17–24.
16. Tsigkas G, Papageorgiou A, Moulias A, Kalogeropoulos AP, Papageorgopoulou C, Apostolos A, et al. Distal or traditional transradial access site for coronary procedures: a single-center, randomized study. JACC Cardiovasc Interv. 2022;15:22–32.
17. Aminian A, Sgueglia GA, Wiemer M, Kefer J, Gasparini GL, Ruzsa Z, et al. Distal versus conventional radial access for coronary angiography and intervention: the DISCO RADIAL trial. JACC Cardiovasc Interv. 2022;15:1191–201.
18. Rivera K, Fernández-Rodríguez D, Casanova-Sandoval J, Barriuso I, Zielonka M, Pueyo-Balsells N, et al. Comparison between the right and left distal radial access for patients undergoing coronary procedures: a propensity score matching analysis. J Interv Cardiol. 2022;2022:7932114.
19. Ghose T, Kachru R, Dey J, Khan WU, Sud R, Jabeen S, et al. Safety and feasibility of ultrasound-guided access for coronary interventions through distal left radial route. J Interv Cardiol. 2022;2022:2141524.
20. Achim A, Szigethy T, Olajos D, Molnár L, Papp R, Bárczi G, et al. Switching from proximal to distal radial artery access for coronary chronic Total occlusion recanalization. Front Cardiovasc Med. 2022;9:895457.
21. Pacchioni A, Sciahbasi A, Tumscitz C, Mugnolo A, Calcagno S, Sgueglia GA, et al. Reduction of radiation exposure using left distal radial access for coronary procedures the RADIANT II study. G Ital Cardiol. 2021;22:e32.
22. Sciahbasi A, Rigattieri S, Sarandrea A, Cera M, Di Russo C, Fedele S, et al. Radiation dose absorbed by operators during transradial percutaneous coronary procedures comparing different protective drapes: the RADIATION study. EuroIntervention. 2017;12:e2253–61.
23. Sciahbasi A, Rigattieri S, Sarandrea A, Cera M, Di Russo C, Fedele S, et al. Determinants of operator radiation exposure during percutaneous coronary procedures. Am Heart J. 2017;187:10–8.
24. Sciahbasi A, Sarandrea A, Rigattieri S, Patrizi R, Cera M, Di Russo C, et al. Staff radiation dose during percutaneous coronary procedures role of adjunctive protective drapes. Cardiovasc Revasc Med. 2018;19:755–8.
25. Gunja A, Pandey Y, Xie H, Wolska BM, Shroff AR, Ardati AK, et al. Image noise reduction technology reduces radiation in a radial-first cardiac catheterization laboratory. Cardiovasc Revasc Med. 2017;18:197–201.
26. Ertel A, Nadelson J, Shroff AR, Sweis R, Ferrera D, Vidovich MI. Radiation dose reduction during radial cardiac catheterization: evaluation of a dedicated radial angiography absorption shielding drape. ISRN Cardiol. 2012;2012:769167.
27. Scott H, Gallagher S, Abbott W, Talboys M. Assessment of occupational dose reduction with the use of a floor mounted mobile lead radiation protection shield. J Radiol Prot. 2022;42:033501.
28. Salcido-Rios J, McNamara DA, VanOosterhout S, VanLoo L, Redmond M, Parker JL, et al. Suspended lead suit and physician radiation doses during coronary angiography. Catheter Cardiovasc Interv. 2022;99:981–8.
29. Vidovich MI, Khan AA, Xie H, Shroff AR. Radiation safety and vascular access: attitudes among cardiologists worldwide. Cardiovasc Revasc Med. 2015;16:109–15.
30. Pancholy SB, Payne M, Pancholy PS, Patel GA, Patel S, Shah SC, et al. Association between distance from the radiation source and radiation exposure: a phantom-based study. Catheter Cardiovasc Interv. 2021;97:E810–6.
31. Swaminathan RV, Rao SV. Robotic-assisted transradial diagnostic coronary angiography. Catheter Cardiovasc Interv. 2018;92:54–7.
32. Ross J, Vidovich MI. Relative importance of attribute preferences for radial vs. femoral arterial access: a crowdsourcing study of healthy online-recruited volunteers. Catheter Cardiovasc Interv. 2019;93:1237–43.

15 Evidence from Clinical Registries

Karsten Schenke and Jin Bae Lee

15.1 Introduction

The first reports on distal radial access (DRA) by Avtandil Babunashvili [1] and Aleksandr Kaledin [2] inspired Ferdinand Kiemeneij [3] to publish a technical overview in a small registry of 70 patients in whom he performed a coronary angiography via the left DRA and produced a corresponding YouTube video. This paper turned out to be the most frequently downloaded paper of EuroIntervention in 2017, inspiring investigators around the world to learn DRA and to collect and publish their experiences. In this chapter, we take a look at a selection of these registries.

15.2 The Early Safety and Feasibility Studies

Shortly after the EuroIntervention paper by Kiemeneij [3], cardiologists from around the world adopted this new technique and began to collect and publish registry data. Mostly, cannulation success, crossover rates, and safety endpoints were analyzed. Table 15.1 provides an overview of these registries [4–24], most of which report datasets between 50 and 200 patients. The results were very positive with a cannulation success rate of well over 90% and a crossover rate of less than 10%. This seems to be comparable to the 7% procedural failure rate reported in TRA trials, such as the RIVAL trial [25].

Some of the registries also reported the rate of RAO (radial artery occlusion), which was considered to be one of the major advantages of DRA over conventional transradial access (TRA). In the registries that reported on forearm RAO, the rate was 1% or less and, for RAO in the snuffbox region, 2% or less, suggesting support for the concept that the preservation of flow in the forearm radial artery and lack of local wall trauma reduces the RAO rate. The RAO rate for TRA has been reported to be approximately 5% [26–28].

Regarding the safety endpoints reported in these registries, there have been no major concerns with mostly minor bleeding or hematoma, which are inherent risks of any type of arterial puncture.

K. Schenke (✉)
Agaplesion Bethesda Krankenhaus Bergedorf, Hamburg, Germany

J. B. Lee
Department of Cardiology, Daegu Catholic University Medical Center, Daegu, Republic of Korea

G. A. Sgueglia (ed.), *Distal Radial Access*, https://doi.org/10.1007/978-3-031-89925-6_15

Table 15.1 Overview of early feasibility studies on distal radial access

Study	Year	Country	Design	Number of DRA patients	Access success	Access time (min)	Right DRA	RAO	Complications
Kiemeneij [3]	2017	The Netherlands	Prospective	70	89%	NA	0%	1%	Ecchymosis 1% Bleeding 1%
Amin et al. [4]	2017	Bangladesh	Prospective	50	98%	1.2	100%	0%	None
Andrade et al. [5]	2018	Brazil	Prospective	61	95%	NA	0%	0%	None
Barros de Toledo et al. [6]	2018	Brazil	Prospective	151	94%	2.3 ± 0.4	87%	0%	Hematoma 0.7%
Coughlan et al. [7]	2018	Ireland	Prospective	47	100%	NA	0%	0%	None
Gajurel et al. [8]	2018	Nepal	Prospective	82	98%	1.2 ± 0.9	100%	0%	None
Lee et al. [9]	2018	South Korea	Prospective	200	96%	3.0 ± 2.8	0%	0%	Hematoma 7.4% Dissection 0.5%
Roghani-Dehkordi et al. [10]	2018	Iran	Prospective	235	94%	NA	NA	1.4%	Ecchymosis 5.1%
Soydan et al. [11]	2018	Turkey	Prospective	54	100%	1.2 ± 0.9	0%	0%	None
Valsecchi et al. [12]	2018	Italy	Prospective	52	90%	NA	85%	NA	NA
Al-Azizi et al. [13]	2019	USA	Retrospective	61	98%	4.32	0%	0%	None
Aoi et al. [14]	2019	USA	Retrospective	202	99%	7.3 ± 5.7	88%	0%	Hematoma 3.5%
Aqel et al. [15]	2019	Jordan	Retrospective	200	98%	1.4 ± 0.6	95%	0%	None
El Tahaan et al. [16]	2019	Egypt	Prospective	50	92%	10.6 ± 2.2	44%	6%	Bleeding 4%
Yu et al. [17]	2019	China	Retrospective	92	96%	2.3 ± 1.8	96%	0%	Hematoma 3.2%
Bhambhani et al. [18]	2020	India	Prospective	100	78%	4.1 ± 2.9	100%	0%	None
Escutia-Cuevas et al. [19]	2020	Mexico	Prospective	100	100%	6.36	74%	0%	Hematoma 12%
Maskey et al. [20]	2020	Nepal	Prospective	128	100%	NA	75%	0%	Swelling 2.3%
Roghani-Dehkordi et al. [21]	2020	Iran	Prospective	70	89%	4.8 ± 0.5	NA	2%	1.8%
Ziakas et al. [22]	2020	Greece	Prospective	49	90%	3.9 ± 4.1	100%	0%	Hematoma 14.2% Bleeding 4.1%
Mokbel et al. [23]	2021	Romania	Prospective	57	89%	1.1 ± 0.5	100%	0%	Hematoma 3.5%
Tsigkas et al. [24]	2021	Greece	Prospective	167	91%	1.5 ± 0.5	100%	3.2%	Arteriovenous fistula 3.2%

DRA distal radial access, *RAO* radial artery occlusion

15.3 Larger All-Comers Cohorts

These early registries demonstrating the feasibility and safety of DRA have led to the design of the randomized trials discussed in Chap. 16 and to the collection of larger real-world all-comers registries discussed here (Table 15.2). In general, they have focused on success rate, RAO rate, hemostasis time, and safety issues. They were designed to lay the groundwork for the adoption of DRA as a routine, primary access route for coronary procedures.

The Very Distal Transradial Approach (VITRO) study prospectively screened 320 consecutive patients scheduled for coronary angiography (CAG) or percutaneous coronary intervention (PCI) via DRA [29]. In 102 (32%) patients, the distal radial artery pulse was absent or too weak, and thus, conventional TRA was attempted instead of DRA. This finding was similar to the screening failures in the Kiemeneij paper [3], where only two-thirds of patients screened by palpation were considered suitable for DRA puncture. The cannulation success rate in the 218 patients with a DRA puncture attempt was 96% (9/218). In 14 additional patients, the wire could not be advanced to the aorta, also resulting in crossover. Thus, the crossover rate in this study was 11% (23/218), with the main alternative being conventional TRA (n = 21). No major complications were observed in this study.

The inteRnATional hAnd funcTiOn stUdy following dIstaL radiaL accEs (RATATOUILLE) study was an investigator-driven, prospective, multicenter, international, cohort study designed to assess hand function after DRA coronary angiography or percutaneous coronary intervention [30]. Overall, 313 patients were enrolled to undergo repeated multimodality assessments of hand function. Clinical evaluation and vascular ultrasound to check for distal and forearm RAO were also performed at baseline and during the follow-up. Access-related adverse events included 19 harmless bleedings, and three patients showed RAO following DRA at the longest follow-up (forearm and distal RAO, n = 2; isolated distal RAO, n = 1).

The TwitteR Initiated registry for coronary ANgiography in Germany via distaL radial access (TRIANGLE) registry was a German multicenter registry designed to further elucidate DRA as the standard of care, looking at success rates, RAO rates, and complications, while also investigating a possible difference between distal dorsal and true anatomical snuffbox access sites that are separated by the extensor pollicis longus tendon [31]. Overall, DRA was attempted in 327 patients.

The puncture success rate was 95% and was similar between left and right punctures, with no difference seen between anatomical snuffbox and distal dorsal puncture sites. The only difference that was statistically significant was the puncture time between anatomical snuffbox (81 s) and distal dorsal (99 s) and left-side DRA (109 s) and right-side DRA (84 s). This is consistent with the findings of Rivera et al., who reported a comparable puncture success rate, but a faster puncture time for right-side access compared to left-side access in a prospective registry of 382 patients that were included in a propensity score matching analysis [39]. In the TRIANGLE registry, routine ultrasound follow-up within 2 days of the procedure revealed three distal RAOs at the puncture site and two forearm RAOs, all of which were asymptomatic. No major complications were noted.

Oliveira et al. reported a prospective all-comers registry of 435 consecutive patients from Brazil [32]. The presence of any pulse in the anatomical snuffbox region was the eligibility criterion for DRA puncture. The indications for CAG or PCI were largely (49%) acute coronary syndromes (ACS) with a significant proportion (15%) of ST-elevation myocardial infarction (STEMI). The cannulation success rate was very high at 98.6%. Ultrasound was not used for guidance in this registry. One reason for the high success rate may be that all procedures were performed by two experienced interventionalists. The overall crossover rate was 3% (13/435). The standard sheath size was 6 Fr (97.6%), and 229 PCIs were performed. No major adverse cardiac events (MACE) were observed, and all patients

Table 15.2 Overview of larger all-comers registries on distal radial access

Study	Year	Country	Number of DRA patients	Age (years)	Men	Right DRA	Access success	Access time (s)	PCI
Wretowski et al. VITRO [29]	2019	Poland	218	68 ± 11	65.1%	23.4%	89.4%	NA	36.2%
Sgueglia et al. RATATOUILLE [30]	2022	International	313	66 ± 1o	70.3%	46.0%	97.1%	42 (26–80)	38.3%
Schenke et al. TRIANGLE [31]	2021	Germany	327	69 ± 12	68.8%	77.7%	95.2%	89 ± 79	48.3%
Oliveira et al. [32]	2019	Brazil	435	62 ± 10	66.0%	63%	98.6%	NA	52.6%
Achim et al. [33]	2021	Hungary	1240	66 ± 12	66.9%	89.4%	97.5%	89 ± 70	77.9%
Bompotis et al. [34]	2022	Greece	2034	66 (58–74)	71.8%	0.05%	90.1%	NA	26.3%
Oliveira et al. DISTRACTION [35]	2022	Brazil	3683	63 ± 14	66.1%	91.1%	97.5%	NA	60.4%
Ikuta et al. [36]	2023	Japan	3610	71 ± 10	89.9%	79.8%	90.4%	NA	23.6%
Lee et al. KODRA [37]	2024	South Korea	4977	66 ± 12	67.6%	40%	94.4%	105 (65–180)	32.3%
Roh et al. [38]	2021	South Korea	1000	66 ± 11	73.3%	5.5%	95.2%	118 (81–203)	37.2%

DRA distal radial access, *PCI* percutaneous coronary intervention, *RAO* radial artery occlusion

had a palpable pulse in the distal and proximal radial artery segments after the procedure.

Achim et al. prospectively collected the data from 1240 coronary ($n = 918$) and peripheral ($n = 322$) procedures carried out via DRA in a multicenter registry from Hungary [33]. Overall, the puncture success rate was 97.4%, with only 33 cases (2.58%) requiring crossover to another access site. All punctures were performed under ultrasound guidance, and the puncture time was short with a mean of 1.2 min. In this study, a novice DRA operator needed only 15 successful punctures to achieve a rate comparable to an experienced interventionalist with the difference in puncture time and number of puncture attempts remaining. During follow-up, all radial arteries were assessed for RAO by ultrasound. The reported RAO rate was 0.7%, further supporting the reduction of RAO with DRA. Complications included a small number of asymptomatic dissections (0.4%) which resolved spontaneously. No major bleeding or hematoma was reported.

Bomzotis et al. evaluated 2034 consecutive patients with left DRA as the standard approach [34]. The right-side puncture was chosen in 42 patients because of left-hand dominance, and 15 patients were excluded for anatomical or other reasons. Thus, left-side DRA was ultimately performed in 1977 cases. The access-related failure rate was reported to be 9.9% ($n = 196$). The distal radial artery could not be punctured in 43 (22%) of failed cases, and the wire could not be advanced in 147 (75%) cases. They also report on the learning curve and observed a failure rate of 20% in the first 200 cases, decreasing to less than 10% in the next 200 cases.

Also of note, similar to most other publications, the authors of this registry observed that female sex was associated with access failure. Women had a 75.2% higher risk of access failure (95% CI 28.9–138, $p < 0.001$). However, after adjustment for height, this difference was no longer significant (adjusted hazard ratio 1.29, 95% CI 0.89–1.87, $p = 0.18$).

The DIStal TRAnsradial access as default approach for Coronary angiography and interventIONs (DISTRACTION) registry prospectively enrolled 3683 consecutive patients undergoing coronary procedures via DRA [35]. This large real-world all-comers study included all types of stable and acute indications, as well as patients with complex coronary interventions, including rotational atherectomy, cardiogenic shock, and chronic total occlusion (CTO). Also, STEMI was the indication in 22.9% of cases. The reported conversion rate of 2.5% was very low and confirms that DRA can be used as a standard approach for all coronary procedures and with larger sheath sizes. A 7-Fr sheath was used in 30 cases.

There was one case of radial artery pseudoaneurysm after right-side DRA that was successfully treated with ultrasound-guided compression and one case of radial artery wire perforation that was sealed with the guiding catheter.

Ikuta et al. conducted a study involving 3610 patients undergoing coronary procedures via DRA to identify predictors of DRA success and access site complications [36]. The success rate for DRA was 90.4%, while the rate of access site complications was 7.7%. Positive predictors of DRA success included PCI and ultrasound-guided access, whereas low body weight and dual antiplatelet therapy were negative predictors. Conversely, low body weight, peripheral arterial disease, dual antiplatelet therapy, anticoagulant therapy, and PCI were associated with a higher risk of access site complications. Ultrasound-guided puncture was the strongest predictor of successful DRA without access site complications (odds ratio 1.72, 95% confidence interval 1.4–2.1, $p < 0.01$).

The Korean Distal Radial Access (KODRA) registry published by Lee et al. is the largest study on DRA to date and provides an exceptionally comprehensive dataset on current DRA practices [37]. It included 4977 of 5712 screened patients indicated for coronary procedures via DRA who were prospectively enrolled in 14 Korean hospitals. As the registry provided valuable insights into operators' reluctance to use DRA, weak distal radial pulse (39.3%), peripheral arterial disease (12.9%), and acute myocardial infarction (11.2%) emerged as the most common reasons for not attempting DRA. The overall success rate of DRA was 94.4%, with crossovers primarily to ipsilateral conventional TRA, preserving the initial upper extremity vascular access strategy. The incidence of forearm radial artery occlusion (RAO) was 0.2% at discharge and increased to 0.8% at 1 month. These real-world results are consistent with those seen in randomized controlled trials, with similar rates of crossover, successful PCI completion, and RAO. In addition to demonstrating the reproducibility of randomized trial results in routine practice, the detailed data on patient and procedural factors allowed for robust analysis, identifying weak distal radial pulse and limited operator experience as the only independent predictors of puncture failure.

To elucidate the learning curve required to master DRA, Roh et al. retrospectively collected data on 1000 patients who underwent DRA by a single interventional cardiologist [38]. The primary endpoint was the success rate per 100 cases. The distal puncture was successful in 952 patients; in almost half of the failed cases, the puncture was unsuccessful (2.7%), and in other cases, it was not possible to advance the wire (2.1%). Of note, none of the 1000 cases in this cohort required conversion to transfemoral access (TFA). All 48 cases were converted to ipsi- or contralateral TRA.

In this study, a compression bandage was used for hemostasis. The duration of hemostasis was 144.6 ± 91.3 min for CAG (n = 580) and 217.3 ± 121.3 min for PCI (n = 372). There was no forearm or distal radial artery occlusion during hospitalization. Puncture-related local numbness was observed in two cases (0.2%) and local hematoma in 29 cases (3.0%).

15.4 Subgroup Registries

15.4.1 ST-Elevation Myocardial Infarction

Very rapid coronary access and therapy are of paramount importance in patients with STEMI. Any new approach must be suitable in this setting and must not prolong the door-to-balloon time. To evaluate this subgroup, Lee et al. compared left-side DRA with TRA and TFA in a retrospective registry of 109 patients with STEMI [40]. After excluding patients with cardiogenic shock that were treated with extracorporeal membrane oxygenation (ECMO), 94 patients were analyzed. The majority were treated via DRA (n = 42) and 26 patients each via TRA and TFA. Crossover was required in seven patients in the DRA group with five puncture failures and two cases of severe spasm. These patients were punctured via TFA. No crossover was observed in the TRA and TFA groups.

The puncture time was similar in the groups with a successful puncture (DRA 116 s, conventional TRA 101 s, TFA 129 s, $p > 0.05$), while the puncture time was obviously longer in patients requiring crossover. However, the puncture time was acceptable in all patients, requiring less than 5 min. While the patients in the conventional TRA and DRA groups had no major complications, one patient in the TFA group required transfusion and vascular surgery, again highlighting the advantage of radial access over TFA.

One reason for the relatively low cannulation success rate in the DRA group discussed in the manuscript was the fact that three of the participating interventional cardiologists had no prior experience with DRA. For highly experienced operators who have overcome the learning curve, the success rate improves to a rate comparable to conventional TRA, making it a true alternative for acute coronary syndrome and STEMI patients.

In another Korean multicenter registry of STEMI patients, Kim et al. included 138 patients treated with DRA [41]. In this study, all participating cardiologists were experienced in DRA, resulting in a puncture success rate of 93% (128/138). In the previously discussed study by Lee et al. [40], the success rate was 84%, so a learning curve of 100 punctures in stable patients is advisable before treating STEMI patients in order to achieve a satisfactory puncture success rate of over 90%.

There was no control group in this study to compare DRA and TRA success rates or puncture times. The mean puncture time was 2.7 min, and in 95% of patients, the puncture time was less than 5 min. Minor access-related complications were reported in four cases, three small hematomas, and one case of local numbness that resolved within 3 months.

15.4.2 Chronic Total Occlusion

The first report on the feasibility of using larger-size guiding catheters for CTO PCI through a 7-Fr thin-walled sheath via left DRA was published by Gasparini et al. [42]. They included 41 patients and achieved a puncture success rate of 83%. In three cases, the distal radial pulse was too weak or absent, and in four cases, the wire could not be advanced. Technical success was achieved in 90% of the patients. Ultrasound follow-up revealed no cases of forearm RAO and no other complications.

Lin et al. published a registry of 298 patients undergoing CTO PCI to evaluate the feasibility and safety of DRA for this challenging coronary procedure, which often requires larger guiding catheters and dual coronary access [43]. Left DRA was successfully performed in 286 patients (access success rate 96.5%) and right DRA in 133 patients (97.7%). Bilateral DRA was performed in 107 patients. A 7-Fr guiding catheter with a 7-in-6-Fr thin-walled sheath was used in 18.5% of cases and a 6-in-5-Fr thin-walled sheath in the remaining cases. Mild ecchymosis was observed in nine patients, and more severe access-related complications occurred in two cases. One case was severe forearm bleeding requiring transfusion after perforation of a branch of the brachial artery, and another case was an arteriovenous fistula that resolved after 9 months of follow-up. Distal RAO was observed in two cases, but no forearm RAO was detected

In a multicenter study from Hungary, Achim et al. compared 337 CTO procedures via conventional TRA ($n = 257$) and via DRA ($n = 80$) [44]. As the standard access route in the participating centers was changed from conventional TRA to DRA, the conventional TRA CTO procedures performed before the change were compared with the DRA CTO procedures performed after the change.

To further improve the comparison of the two groups, propensity score matching was performed, and after matching, no significant differences were observed in procedural success (86% with DRA vs. 88% with conventional TRA, $p = 1$) and clinical success (84% with DRA vs. 78% with conventional TRA, $p = 0.664$). The RAO rate was higher in the conventional TRA cohort (2.72%) than in the DRA cohort (1.25%), although this difference did not reach statistical significance. Short-term complications and long-term follow-up for MACE were similar in both groups.

This study comparing conventional TRA and DRA for CTO PCI underscores the feasibility of using DRA even in complex procedures. As these patients have a high likelihood of repeat percutaneous coronary procedures, preserving the radial artery for future access seems to be a particularly relevant goal.

15.4.3 Small Patients and Small Vessels

Vascular access is more challenging in smaller vessels, and the radial artery in the snuffbox region is 10% smaller than at the wrist and even smaller in patients with a low body mass index (BMI) [45]. To investigate the feasibility of DRA in this cohort, Li et al. published a study comparing patients with a body mass index (BMI) of less than 18.5 kg/m^2 who underwent a CAG or a PCI via DRA (29 patients) and conventional TRA (38 patients) [46]. The mean BMI was 17.5 and was similar in both groups. Overall puncture success and puncture time were reported. The success rate was similar in both groups (96.6% in DRA vs. 97.4% in conventional TRA). Puncture time was significantly shorter in conventional TRA (72 s in DRA. vs. 60 s in conventional TRA, $p < 0.003$) with a higher success rate on the first puncture attempt (51.7% in DRA vs. 81.6% in conventional TRA, $p < 0.020$). The main advantage of DRA remained, however, as the incidence of RAO was significantly lower in the DRA group than in the

TRA group (4.0% vs. 33.3%, $p < 0.007$), with no significant differences in other complications. This stark difference in RAO can possibly be attributed to the longer compression time in TRA vs. DRA (mean: 6h vs 4h respectively).

The distal radial versus transradial access in small transradial arteries (D.A.T.A-S.T.A.R) study compared DRA with conventional TRA in patients with a radial artery size of less than 2.1 mm [47]. The mean forearm radial artery diameter in this study was 1.6 mm. A total of 545 patients were enrolled, of whom 328 underwent a coronary procedure via conventional TRA and 209 via DRA without ultrasound puncture guidance. The puncture success rate in the DRA cohort was significantly lower than in the conventional TRA group (79.5% vs. 98.5%, $p < 0.001$), but after excluding patients with a poorly palpable pulse in the anatomical snuffbox, the puncture success rate was 88.7% vs. 98.5%, making the puncture success rate more acceptable. As in most other studies, the puncture time was significantly shorter in the conventional TRA group (1 min) than in the DRA group (2.1 min, $p < 0.001$). Interestingly, and in contrast to most other studies, the RAO rate at ultrasound follow-up was similar in both groups on day 1 (2.4% in both groups) and was almost unchanged on day 30.

15.4.4 Repeated Puncture

A significant proportion of patients with coronary artery disease have extensive multivessel disease requiring repeat coronary procedures. Yamada et al. performed a retrospective analysis of 2406 coronary procedures [48]. Within this cohort, repeat coronary angiography via DRA was attempted in 419 cases and analyzed for success and safety. The successful cannulation rate was 94.3% for the second consecutive procedure ($n = 419$) and decreased to a still acceptable rate of 89.6% for the third ($n = 121$) and fourth ($n = 22$) punctures. The reason for puncture failure was distal RAO in nine patients, arterial stenosis in 19 patients, and two puncture failures in patent vessels.

15.4.5 Bypass Patients

One of the advantages of DRA for the patient is the ergonomic benefit of placing the arm in a natural position with the back of the hand facing up, eliminating the need to supinate the hand. When performing left radial access, placing the patient's left hand over the groin also makes DRA more ergonomic for the operator. This advantage makes left DRA very attractive, especially in patients with a history of previous coronary artery bypass grafting (CABG) with a left internal mammary artery (LIMA) graft. Oliviera et al. published a report of 111 consecutive post-CABG patients who underwent a coronary procedure via left DRA [49]. Successful sheath insertion was achieved in all patients, while five patients (4.5%) required access site crossover to complete the procedure. There were no adverse events or complications reported.

15.4.6 Dialysis

The creation of an arteriovenous fistula (AVF) via the radial artery is a standard procedure in patients undergoing hemodialysis. And because RAO is a complication of TRA that would preclude this shunt creation, many interventional cardiologists prefer to use TFA over TRA in patients with advanced or end-stage renal disease. Yokota et al. collected the data of 117 consecutive patients on hemodialysis who underwent a coronary procedure with an attempt to puncture the distal radial artery [50]. The puncture success rate was 90.5% (106/117), and the radial artery was evaluated for RAO by ultrasound. Five (4.7%) patients had distal RAO, and three (2.8%) patients had forearm RAO. All patients with forearm RAO were females with small (<1.8 mm) radial artery diameter. This RAO rate is higher than in most other studies of DRA, but patients on hemodialysis generally have a higher complication rate, especially after TFA [51], and also have a reported RAO rate of >6% after conventional TRA [52].

Shima et al. compared 2402 non-hemodialysis patients with 98 hemodialysis patients from their catheterization laboratory who underwent coronary angiography or intervention via DRA [53]. They evaluated success and complication rates (especially bleeding). The procedural success rates were similar (p = 0.61), and the bleeding rates were not statistically different (p = 0.41). In one case in the hemodialysis group, RAO was diagnosed after prolonged hemostasis (7 h) due to bleeding. The non-hemodialysis group was not evaluated by ultrasound for this complication, so no comparison was possible.

15.4.7 Larger Sheaths

The distal radial artery is approximately 10% smaller than the radial artery at the conventional forearm puncture site [33, 54], which naturally leads to caution in the use of larger sheath sizes that are often required for complex coronary interventions such as rotational atherectomy or CTO procedures. Zong et al. published a retrospective registry of 102 patients who underwent PCI via DRA using a thin-walled 7-Fr sheath with the same outer diameter as a standard 6-Fr sheath [55]. All patients had their forearm radial artery and distal radial artery diameters measured before and after the procedure. The mean diameters in this study were 2.62 mm and 2.17 mm, respectively, making both vessels smaller than the outer diameter of the thin-walled 7-Fr sheath used (2.72 mm). Puncture and sheath placement were successful in 90.2% (92/102). Local hematoma was observed in 5% of the patients, one case of arteriovenous fistula and two cases of spasm were also reported. Ultrasound follow-up revealed two cases of forearm RAO and three cases of distal RAO, all asymptomatic.

15.5 Hemostasis and Complication

Sheath brand and size, choice and doses of vasodilators, doses of unfractionated heparin and hemostasis approach used, and observed access site complications varied widely in the larger all-comers registries (Table 15.3) [29–39]. A hydrophilic coated thin-walled sheath was used in most registries, and the most commonly used sheath size was 6 Fr (range 4 Fr to 8.5 Fr).

After sheath insertion, a vasodilator agent (nitroglycerin and/or verapamil) was injected into the sheath, with some registries escalating to intravenous morphine or sedatives for prolonged and increasing pain. A dose of 2000–5000 IU of unfractionated heparin (UFH) was administered in all patients undergoing coronary angiography and was typically higher in PCI cases. Hemostasis after DRA was achieved with a hemostatic band or special radial compression devices.

Regarding access site complications, the registries report a radial artery occlusion rate of 0–1%, and hematoma occurred in less than 5.1%. Puncture-related local numbness was observed in 0–0.2%, and dissection was observed in less than 0.4% [29–36, 39]. There were very rare local access site complications with very few cases of pseudoaneurysm and radial artery perforation.

Table 15.3 Selected procedural data of larger all-comers registries on distal radial access

Study	Year	Sheath	Sheath size	Spasmolytic regimen	Heparin	Hemostasis	Access site complication
Wretowski et al. VITRO [29]	2019	Radifocus Introducer II (Terumo) Prelude Radial (Merit Medical)	6 Fr	NTG 0.1–0.2 mg	5000 U	Io (Comed)	Minor bleeding 0.5%
Sgueglia et al. RATATOUILLE [30]	2022	NA	4–7 Fr	NTG 0.2 mg Verapamil 5 mg	Weight-adjusted dose	NA	BARC 1 bleeding 4.8% BARC 2 bleeding 1.3% RAO 1%
Schenke et al. TRIANGLE [31]	2021	Glidesheath Slender (Terumo)	4–7 Fr	NTG 0.2–0.3 mg Morphine IV	2000–5000 U	TR Band (Terumo) SafeGuard (Merit Medical)	Hematoma 5.1% RAO 0.9%
Oliveira et al. [32]	2019	Radifocus Introducer II (Terumo)	5–7 Fr	NTG 0.2 mg	5000 U	TR Band (Terumo)	No access site complication
Achim et al. [33]	2021	Glidesheath Slender (Terumo)	5–8.5 Fr	NTG 0.2 mg Morphine IV	2000 U	StatSeal (Biolife) Compression bandage	Hematoma 0.3% RAO 0.4% Artery dissection 0.4%
Bompotis et al. [34]	2022	PreludeEase (Merit Medical)	4–7 Fr	NTG 0.2 mg	5000 U	NA	RAO 0.2% Numbness or pain 0.1%
Oliveira et al. DISTRACTION [35]	2022	Radifocus Introducer II (Terumo) Glidesheath slender (Terumo)	4–7 Fr	NTG 0.2 mg	50 U/kg	TR band (Terumo) PreludeSYNC (Merit Medical) Seal-One (Vygon)	Pseudoaneurysm 0.03% Radial artery perforation 0.03%
Ikuta et al. [36]	2023	Glidesheath Slender (Terumo)	4–6 Fr	NA	NA	Compression bandage	Minor bleeding 7.3% Pseudoaneurysm 0.46%
Lee et al. KODRA [37]	2024	NA	4–7 Fr	Per institution protocol	Per institution protocol	Per institution protocol	RAO 0.2% Hematoma 3.6% Radial artery perforation 0.1%
Roh et al. [38]	2021	Radifocus Introducer II (Terumo) Prelude Radial (Merit Medical)	4–7 Fr	NTG 0.2 mg Verapamil 2.5 mg	3000 U	Compression bandage	Hematoma 3% Numbness 0.2%

NTG nitroglycerine, *RAO* radial artery occlusion

15.6 Conclusion

In recent years, a large number of real-world registries have been published on the use of DRA for all types of coronary procedures in stable and acute settings, including complex procedures. Collectively, they represent well over 10,000 patient records and confirm the feasibility and safety of DRA for coronary angiography and interventions.

In this chapter, we have presented data from registries that have evaluated DRA as the standard of care in all-comers situations with little or no preselection. In general, cannulation and procedural success rates have been very satisfactory, with puncture success rates greater than 95%, procedural success rates greater than 90%, and puncture and procedural times comparable to the current gold standard, which is conventional TRA via the forearm radial artery.

A typical complication of TRA is chronic, asymptomatic RAO, and one of the major advantages of DRA reported in early studies was a lower rate of this complication due to the lack of vessel wall trauma, shorter compression time, and preservation of blood flow during post-procedural compression at the puncture site.

Several of the studies presented here have evaluated the radial artery for patency after the procedure. Due to differences in anticoagulation regimens, expertise, and hemostasis techniques, there is some variability in this endpoint across studies. However, most studies that have systematically evaluated this endpoint have found a RAO rate of <1%, but some have seen rates as high as 3% in certain subgroups, such as patients on hemodialysis or after the use of larger sheaths. However, it is safe to assume that DRA results in a lower RAO rate than TRA, which is certainly beneficial for patients who may require future use of the radial artery for medical purposes (multivessel coronary artery disease, end-stage renal disease).

All studies presented here have reported their complications to ensure that DRA is not only feasible but also safe. None of them have a concerning number of bleedings or neurological or vascular complications, and in those studies that have a control group, the incidence of complications is similar.

References

1. Kaledin AL, Kochanov IN, Seletskiĭ SS, Arkharov IV, Burak TI, Kozlov KL. Peculiarities of arterial access in endovascular surgery in elderly patients. Adv Gerontol. 2014;27:115–9.
2. Babunashvili A, Dundua D. Recanalization and reuse of early occluded radial artery within 6 days after previous transradial diagnostic procedure. Catheter Cardiovasc Interv. 2011;77:530–6.
3. Kiemeneij F. Left distal transradial access in the anatomical snuffbox for coronary angiography (ldTRA) and interventions (ldTRI). EuroIntervention. 2017;13:851–7.
4. Amin R, Singha CK, Banerjee SK, Hoque H, Mahabub S, Hoque M, et al. Comparison of distal transradial in the anatomical snuffbox versus conventional transradial access for coronary angiography and intervention – an experience in 100 cases. Univ Heart J. 2017;13:40–5.
5. Andrade PB, Tebet MA, Rinaldi FS, Bienert IR, Barbosa RA, Esteves VC, et al. Initial experience with left distal transradial access for invasive coronary procedures. J Transcat Intervent. 2018;26:1–5.
6. Barros de Toledo JF, Gubolino LA, Teixeirense PT, Bragalha AM, Zotarelli Filho IJ. Diagnostic and interventional coronary procedures by the distal radial artery in the anatomical SnuffBox: a real world analysis. J Cardiovasc Dis Diagn. 2018;6:1000337.
7. Coughlan JJ, Zebrauskaite A, Arnous S, Kiernan TJ. Left distal trans-radial access facilitates earlier discharge post-coronary angiography. J Interv Cardiol. 2018;31:964–8.
8. Gajurel RM, Sahi R, Shrestha H, Thapa S, Khanal R. Initial experience on anatomical snuff box approach for coronary angiogram & percutaneous coronary intervention in a tertiary care center Nepal. World J Cardiovasc Dis. 2018;8:578–87.
9. Lee JW, Park SW, Son JW, Ahn SG, Lee SH. Real-world experience of the left distal transradial approach for coronary angiography and percutaneous coronary intervention: a prospective observational study (LeDRA). EuroIntervention. 2018;14:e995–1003.
10. Roghani-Dehkordi F, Hashemifard O, Sadeghi M, Mansouri R, Akbarzadeh M, Dehghani A, et al. Distal accesses in the hand (two novel techniques) for percutaneous coronary angiography and intervention. ARYA Atheroscler. 2018;14:95–100.
11. Soydan E, Akın M. Coronary angiography using the left distal radial approach – an alternative site to

conventional radial coronary angiography. Anatol J Cardiol. 2018;19:243–8.
12. Valsecchi O, Vassileva A, Cereda AF, Canova P, Satogami K, Fiocca L, et al. Early clinical experience with right and left distal transradial access in the anatomical snuffbox in 52 consecutive patients. Invasive Cardiol. 2018;30:218–23.
13. Al-Azizi KM, Grewal V, Gobeil K, Maqsood K, Haider A, Mohani A, et al. The left distal transradial artery access for coronary angiography and intervention: a US experience. Cardiovasc Revasc Med. 2019;20:786–9.
14. Aoi S, Htun WW, Freeo S, Lee S, Kyaw H, Alfaro V, et al. Distal transradial artery access in the anatomical snuffbox for coronary angiography as an alternative access site for faster hemostasis. Catheter Cardiovasc Interv. 2019;94:651–7.
15. Aqel R, Alzughayyar TZ, Misk RA. Radial: time to go distal. Cardiol Cardiovasc Med. 2019;3:432–7.
16. El Tahaan MH, Hamid IA, Samad AA. Immediate outcomes of trans radial approach versus anatomical snuff box access for coronary procedures. Egypt J Hosp Med. 2019;76:4099–105.
17. Yu W, Hu P, Wang S, Yao L, Wang H, Dou L, et al. Distal radial artery access in the anatomical snuffbox for coronary angiography and intervention: a single center experience. Medicine. 2020;99:1–5.
18. Bhambhani A, Pandey S, Nadamani AN, Tyagi K. An observational comparison of distal radial and traditional radial approaches for coronary angiography. J Saudi Heart Assoc. 2020;32:17–24.
19. Escutia-Cuevas HH, Alcántara-Meléndez MA, Torres-Sánchez J, Muratalla-González R, Jiménez-Valverde AS, Zaragoza-Rodríguez G, et al. Distal transradial access for coronary angiography and percutaneous coronary intervention: an observational study in a Latin-American center. Cardiovasc Metab Sci. 2020;31:9–16.
20. Maskey A, Timalsena BK, Aslam S, Pandey R, Roka M, Bhandari S, et al. Feasibility and safety of distal radial artery access in anatomical snuffbox for coronary angiography and coronary intervention. J Nepal Health Res Counc. 2020;18:259–62.
21. Roghani-Dehkordi F, Riazi A, Shafie D, Khosravi A, Sadeghi M, Vakhshoori M, et al. Trans-snuff box approach as a new access site for coronary angiography and angioplasty versus trans-radial approach in terms of feasibility, safety, and complications. ARYA Atheroscler. 2020;16:263–8.
22. Ziakas A, Koutouzis M, Didagelos M, Tsiafoutis I, Kouparanis A, Gossios T, et al. Right arm distal transradial (snuffbox) access for coronary catheterization: initial experience. Hell J Cardiol. 2020;61:106–9.
23. Mokbel M, Florescu N, Sinecsu CJ. Distal trans-radial approach for coronary angiography and percutaneous coronary interventions – single-centre experience. Acta Medica Transilvanica. 2021;26:13–6.
24. Tsigkas G, Moulias A, Papageorgiou A, Ntouvas I, Grapsas N, Despotopoulos S, et al. Transradial access through the anatomical snuffbox: results of a feasibility study. Hell J Cardiol. 2021;62:201–5.
25. Jolly SS, Yusuf S, Cairns J, Niemelä K, Xavier D, Widimsky P, et al. Radial versus femoral access for coronary angiography and intervention in patients with acute coronary syndromes (RIVAL): a randomised, parallel group, multicentre trial. Lancet. 2011;377:1409–20.
26. Avdikos G, Karatasakis A, Tsoumeleas A, Lazaris E, Ziakas A, Koutouzis M. Radial artery occlusion after transradial coronary catheterization. Cardiovasc Diagn Ther. 2017;7:305–16.
27. Sciahbasi A, Rigattieri S, Sarandrea A, Cera M, Di Russo C, Fedele S, et al. Radial artery occlusion and hand strength after percutaneous coronary procedures: results of the HANGAR study. Catheter Cardiovasc Interv. 2016;87:868–74.
28. Zankl AR, Andrassy M, Volz C, Ivandic B, Krumsdorf U, Katus HA, et al. Radial artery thrombosis following transradial coronary angiography: incidence and rationale for treatment of symptomatic patients with low-molecular-weight heparins. Clin Res Cardiol. 2010;99:841–7.
29. Wretowski D, Krakowian M, Łabyk A, Pruszczyk P, Roik M. Very distal transradial approach (VITRO) for coronary interventions. Adv Interv Cardiol. 2019;15:42–5.
30. Sgueglia GA, Hassan A, Harb S, Ford TJ, Koliastasis L, Milkas A, et al. International hand function study following distal radial access: the RATATOUILLE study. JACC Cardiovasc Interv. 2022;15:1205–15.
31. Schenke K, Viertel A, Joghetaei N, Prog R, Matthiesen T, Ohm S, et al. Distal transradial access for coronary angiography and interventions in everyday practice: data from the TRIANGLE registry (TwitteR initiated registry for coronary ANgiography in Germany via distaL radial accEss). Cardiol Ther. 2021;10:241–53.
32. Oliveira MDP, Navarro EC, Kiemeneij F. Distal transradial access as default approach for coronary angiography and interventions. Cardiovasc Diagn Ther. 2019;9:513–9.
33. Achim A, Kákonyi K, Jambrik Z, Nagy F, Tóth J, Sasi V, et al. Distal radial artery access for coronary and peripheral procedures: a multicenter experience. J Clin Med. 2021;10:5974.
34. Bompotis GC, Giannopoulos G, Karakanas AI, Meletidou M, Vrachatis D, Lazaridis I, et al. Left distal radial artery access for coronary angiography and interventions: a 12-month all-comers study. J Invasive Cardiol. 2022;34:E505–9.
35. Oliveira MD, Navarro EC, Caixeta A. Distal transradial access for coronary procedures: a prospective cohort of 3,683 all-comers patients from the DISTRACTION registry. Cardiovasc Diagn Ther. 2022;12:208–19.
36. Ikuta A, Kubo S, Osakada K, Takamatsu M, Takahashi K, Ohya M, et al. Predictors of success and puncture site complications in the distal radial approach. Heart Vessel. 2023;38:147–56.

37. Lee JW, Kim Y, Lee BK, Yoo SY, Lee SY, Kim CJ, et al. Distal radial access for coronary procedures in a large prospective multicenter registry: the KODRA trial. JACC Cardiovasc Interv. 2024;17:329–40.
38. Roh JW, Kim Y, Lee OH, Im E, Cho DK, Choi D, et al. The learning curve of the distal radial access for coronary intervention. Sci Rep. 2021;11:13217.
39. Rivera K, Fernández-Rodríguez D, Casanova-Sandoval J, Barriuso I, Zielonka M, Pueyo-Balsells N, et al. Comparison between the right and left distal radial access for patients undergoing coronary procedures: a propensity score matching analysis. J Interv Cardiol. 2022;2022:7932114.
40. Lee OH, Kim Y, Son NH, Roh JW, Im E, Cho DK, et al. Comparison of distal radial, proximal radial, and femoral access in patients with ST-elevation myocardial infarction. J Clin Med. 2021;10:3438.
41. Kim Y, Lee JW, Lee SY, Bae JW, Lee SJ, Jeong MH, et al. Feasibility of primary percutaneous coronary intervention via the distal radial approach in patients with ST-elevation myocardial infarction. Korean J Intern Med. 2021;36(Suppl 1):S53–61.
42. Gasparini GL, Garbo R, Gagnor A, Oreglia J, Mazzarotto P. First prospective multicentre experience with left distal transradial approach for coronary chronic total occlusion interventions using a 7 Fr Glidesheath slender. EuroIntervention. 2019;15:126–8.
43. Lin CJ, Lee WC, Lee CH, Chung WJ, Hsueh SK, Chen CJ, Yang CH, et al. Feasibility and safety of chronic total occlusion percutaneous coronary intervention via distal transradial access. Front Cardiovasc Med. 2021;8:673858.
44. Achim A, Szigethy T, Olajos D, Molnár L, Papp R, Bérczi G, et al. Switching from proximal to distal radial artery access for coronary chronic total occlusion recanalization. Front Cardiovasc Med. 2022;9:895457.
45. Kim Y, Ahn Y, Kim MC, Sim DS, Hong YJ, Kim JH, et al. Gender differences in the distal radial artery diameter for the snuffbox approach. Cardiol J. 2018;25:639–41.
46. Li LM, Zhang LY, Huang HM, Chen T, Li F, Shi GW, et al. Efficacy and safety of coronary intervention via distal transradial access (dTRA) in patients with low body mass index. J Interv Cardiol. 2022;2022:1901139.
47. Chugh Y, Kanaparthy NS, Piplani S, Chugh S, Shroff A, Vidovich M, et al. Comparison of distal radial access versus standard transradial access in patients with smaller diameter radial arteries (the distal radial versus transradial access in small transradial arteries study: D.A.T.A – S.T.A.R study). Indian Heart J. 2021;73:26–34.
48. Yamada T, Washimi S, Hashimoto S, Taniguchi N, Nakajima S, Hata T, et al. Feasibility and safety of the successive use of distal transradial access for coronary angiography and intervention in the same arm. Catheter Cardiovasc Interv. 2021;98:E796–801.
49. Oliveira MDP, Navarro EC, Caixeta A. Distal transradial access for post-CABG coronary and surgical grafts angiography and interventions. Indian Heart J. 2021;73:440–5.
50. Yokota S, Shishido K, Tobita K, Hayashi T, Miyashita H, Yokoyama H, et al. Distal transradial access for cardiac catheterization in patients undergoing hemodialysis. J Invasive Cardiol. 2022;34:E627–32.
51. Hayashi T, Shishido K, Yokota S, Miyashita H, Mashimo Y, Yokoyama H, et al. Impact of bleeding events after percutaneous coronary intervention in patients on hemodialysis. Heart Vessel. 2020;35:1323–30.
52. Kuno T, Hirano K, Imaeda S, Hashimoto K, Ryuzaki T, Saito T, et al. A transradial approach of cardiac catheterization for patients on dialysis. J Invasive Cardiol. 2018;30:212–7.
53. Shima Y, Kubo S, Ikuta A, Ohya M, Tada T, Tanaka H, et al. Feasibility and safety of coronary catheterization with the distal radial approach for hemodialysis patients. J Cardiol. 2022;80:162–6.
54. Mizuguchi Y, Izumikawa T, Hashimoto S, Yamada T, Taniguchi N, Nakajima S, et al. Efficacy and safety of the distal transradial approach in coronary angiography and percutaneous coronary intervention: a Japanese multicenter experience. Cardiovasc Interv Ther. 2020;35:162–7.
55. Zong B, Liu Y, Han B, Feng CG. Safety and feasibility of a 7F thin-walled sheath via distal transradial artery access for complex coronary intervention. Front Cardiovasc Med. 2022;9:959197.

16 Evidence from Randomized Controlled Trials

Adel Aminian and Shigeru Saito

16.1 Introduction

The past two decades have seen tremendous advances in the practice of interventional cardiology that have revolutionized our approach to the treatment of many cardiac diseases. Among these major advances, the advantages of transradial over transfemoral access (TFA) have been supported by a strong body of clinical evidence from large observational registries and multicenter randomized controlled trials (RCTs) [1–3], which have established TRA as the recommended first-line vascular access for percutaneous coronary interventions in both European and US guidelines, regardless of clinical presentation [4, 5].

Over the past 5 years, distal radial access (DRA) has emerged as an attractive alternative vascular access due to numerous potential advantages over conventional TRA, such as improved procedural ergonomics and patient comfort, easier and safer hemostasis, and, most importantly, a physiological basis for reducing forearm radial artery occlusion (RAO). Following early reported experiences from pioneers and a small single-operator registry by Kiemeneij in 2017 [6–9], DRA has spread widely via social media in the new connected world in which many clinicians now find themselves, leading to questions about the impact of instant access to a wealth of information as a surrogate for well-designed scientific papers [10, 11].

Meanwhile, numerous multinational observational registries have demonstrated the feasibility and safety of DRA in a variety of clinical settings, highlighting in particular a consistently low rate of forearm RAO and shorter time to hemostasis.

In addition to observational registries, the amount of evidence in this field has rapidly increased with the publication of several recent RCTs comparing DRA with conventional TRA for coronary interventions, providing a wealth of data to further evaluate the benefits and limitations of this new technique. The aim of this chapter is to provide a comprehensive review of RCTs comparing DRA with conventional TRA.

This chapter will focus primarily on the comparison between the two vascular access sites in terms of forearm RAO, access site crossover, radial artery spasm (RAS), and hemostasis time.

16.2 Overview of Randomized Trials Comparing Distal Radial Access and Conventional Transradial Access

From August 2019 to November 2022, a total of 11 RCTs involving 5559 patients were published as full papers [12–22]. An overview of these RCTs

A. Aminian (✉)
Department of Cardiology, Centre Hospitalier Universitaire de Charleroi, Charleroi, Belgium

S. Saito
Department of Cardiology, Shonan Kamakura General Hospital, Kanagawa, Japan

G. A. Sgueglia (ed.), *Distal Radial Access*, https://doi.org/10.1007/978-3-031-89925-6_16

Table 16.1 Overview of randomized controlled trials comparing distal radial access with conventional transradial access

Trial	Year	Enrolling sites	Number of patients	Country	Primary outcome	Clinical presentation
Koutouzis et al. [12]	2019	2	200	Greece	Access crossover	CCS
Vefali et al. [3]	2019	1	205	Turkey	Not prespecified	CCS
Lu et al. [14]	2020	1	80	China	Not prespecified	CCS
Lin et al. [15]	2020	1	900	China	Access success	CCS/ACS
Sharma et al. DORA [16]	2020	3	970	India	Not prespecified	NA
Eid-Lidt et al. DAPRAO [17]	2021	1	242	Mexico	Rate of forearm RAO at 24 h assessed by vascular ultrasound	CCS
Lucreziotti et al. [18]	2021	1	204	Italy	EASY grade ≥ 2 hematoma	CCS/ACS[a]
Tsigkas et al. ANGIE [19]	2022	1	1042	Greece	Forearm RAO at 60 days	CCS/ACS[a]
Aminian et al. DISCO RADIAL [20]	2022	16	1307	Europe/ Japan	Forearm RAO at discharge assessed by vascular ultrasound	CCS/ACS[a]
Daralammouri et al. DARFORA [21]	2022	1	209	Palestine	Access success	CCS/ACS[a]
Wang et al. [22]	2022	1	200	China	Forearm RAO at discharge assessed by vascular ultrasound	STEMI

ACS acute coronary syndrome, *CCS* chronic coronary syndrome, *NA* not available, *RAO* radial artery occlusion, *STEMI* ST-elevation myocardial infarction

[a]STEMI patients excluded

is shown in Table 16.1. Only three studies were multicenter RCTs, one 2-center [12], one 3-center [16], and 1 large multicenter RCT with 16 centers (15 centers in Europe and 1 center in Japan) [20]. Coronary angiography alone was performed in two trials [12, 14], while percutaneous coronary intervention (PCI) was performed in a variable proportion of patients ranging from 24% to 100% in nine trials. Clinical presentation was reported in all but one study [16]. Chronic coronary syndrome (CCS) alone was present in four trials [12–14, 16], a combination of CCS and acute coronary syndrome (ACS) in five trials [15, 18–21], while one trial included only patients with ST-elevation myocardial infarction (STEMI) [22].

16.3 Impact of Distal Radial Access on Forearm Radial Artery Occlusion

Assessment of RAO rates was reported in all but two trials [13, 18], with four RCTs having forearm RAO as the primary outcome measure [17, 19, 20, 22]. Rates of forearm RAO in DRA and TRA groups are shown in Fig. 16.1. The overall results of these trials are quite variable, with forearm RAO ranging from 0.2% to 13% after conventional TRA and from 0% to 5% after DRA. The average rates of forearm RAO are 5.6% after TRA (146 events/2602 patients) and 1.6% after DRA (42 events/2602 patients).

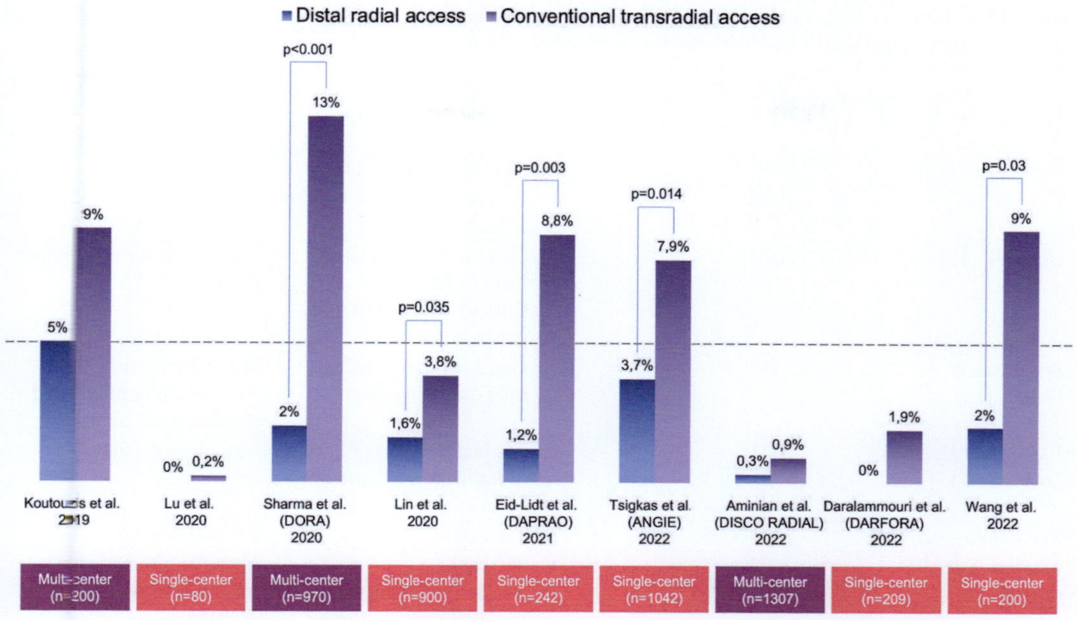

Fig. 16.1 Rates of forearm radial artery occlusion in randomized clinical trials comparing distal radial access and conventional transradial access. Only significant p values are reported. The dotted line outlines the radial artery occlusion threshold recommended by the international consensus paper on the best practices for the prevention of radial artery occlusion after transradial diagnostic angiography and intervention [29]

These results suggest a reduced risk of forearm RAO with DRA and support the physiological and anatomical advantage of puncturing the radial artery distal to the superficial anastomotic palmar arch, thereby avoiding flow interruption and retrograde thrombus formation in the forearm radial artery [23, 24].

Nevertheless, some limitations of the current studies need to be highlighted. These include a single-center design in most trials and a high rate of RAO after conventional TRA in several studies, which is in contrast to recent randomized trials evaluating different preventive strategies after conventional TRA, showing an average RAO rate of less than 5% [25–27]. In fact, several known modifiable and non-modifiable factors have been associated with an increased risk of developing early RAO [28].

A recent international consensus document summarized the best practice recommendations for the prevention of RAO [29]. These include reduction of sheath outer diameter, adequate procedural anticoagulation, non-occlusive hemostasis, and a minimal pressure strategy with a short hemostasis time (≤120 min).

The timing of RAO assessment and hemostasis methods in recent RCTs comparing DRA and TRA are shown in Table 16.2. There was a high heterogeneity of hemostasis methods in the conventional TRA arm, most of which were not specifically aimed at RAO prevention. In addition, manual compression was used to achieve hemostasis in some studies. The mean hemostasis time was not reported in the Distal Radial Approach to Prevent Radial Artery Occlusion (DAPRAO) trial, and four trials reported hemostasis time ≥ 120 min in the conventional TRA arm.

The lack of specific preventive strategies against RAO in some of these trials may be a possible explanation for the observed high pooled rate of RAO in the conventional TRA arm, which is above the threshold of <5% identified as an in-hospital quality measure to be achieved for all TRA programs [29]. Moreover, these high rates of RAO in the conventional arm may have magnified the preventive effect of DRA on the risk of RAO.

Table 16.2 Hemostasis methods and timing of radial artery occlusion assessment in randomized controlled trials comparing distal radial access with conventional transradial access

Trial	Year	Hemostasis methods	Timing of RAO assessment
Koutouzis et al. [12]	2019	Manual compression	Vascular ultrasound after successful hemostasis
Vefali et al. [13]	2019	Manual compression	NA
Lu et al. [14]	2020	Compressive dressing with a small gauze plug	Vascular ultrasound during hospitalization
Lin et al. [15]	2020	Commercial hemostatic band in TRA Compressive bandage with gauze in DRA	Vascular ultrasound before discharge
Sharma et al. DORA [16]	2020	Gauze wrapped with a tight elastic bandage	Manual palpation after 12 h; vascular ultrasound if radial pulse absent
Eid-Lidt et al. DAPRAO [17]	2021	TR-band in TRA "Modified" TR-band in DRA	Vascular ultrasound at 24 h
Lucreziotti et al. [18]	2021	TR-band	Manual palpation
Tsigkas et al. ANGIE [19]	2022	TR-band Plastic strip if TR-band not fitting the snuffbox area	Vascular ultrasound at a median follow-up of 46 days
Aminian et al. DISCO RADIAL [20]	2022	Various hemostatic devices (TR-band, safeguard) in both DRA and TRA and manual compression in DRA	Vascular ultrasound at hospital discharge
Daralammouri et al. DARFORA [21]	2022	TR-band in TRA Safeguard in DRA	Vascular ultrasound at 24 h
Wang et al. [22]	2022	Radial compression device (air power, Shenzhen, China)	Vascular ultrasound before hospital discharge

DRA distal radial access, *RAO* radial artery occlusion, *TRA* conventional transradial access

In support of this hypothesis, the Distal vs. Conventional Radial Access (DISCO RADIAL) trial was the first large-scale multicenter RCT comparing DRA and TRA but with systematic implementation of the best practice recommendations to reduce RAO after conventional TRA [20]. Such an approach resulted in effective patent hemostasis in 94.4% of cases, resulting in an intention-to-treat RAO rate of 0.91% in the conventional arm compared to a RAO rate of 0.31% in the DRA arm. The difference was not statistically significant ($p = 0.29$), possibly due to the reduced statistical power of the study as a result of a considerably lower than expected incidence of RAO in both groups. Indeed, it is noteworthy that the incidence of forearm RAO in the conventional TRA arm of DISCO RADIAL is among the lowest ever reported for a multicenter TRA trial, which strongly supports the implementation of the best preventive strategies as a standard approach in all TRA programs. All centers participating in DISCO RADIAL also had a high level of expertise in TRA and RAO prevention strategies. Notably, DISCO RADIAL was a unique industry-sponsored RCT evaluating a technique rather than an interventional device. Future studies are needed to determine whether such strict adherence to the best preventive practices can be replicated in real-world settings.

Overall, the results of the RCTs show consistent and extremely low rates of forearm RAO with the use of DRA, which appears to be independent of the hemostasis techniques used. These results therefore support DRA as a single, simple (requiring fewer nursing resources), and highly effective strategy to prevent forearm RAO. However, the results of DISCO RADIAL also remind us that the best preventive strategies against RAO should be better implemented in centers using only conventional TRA.

16.4 Technical Aspects and Crossover with Distal Radial Access

The distal radial artery has a smaller diameter than the forearm radial artery (0.3 mm smaller on average), with a more angulated and tortuous course, contributing to technically more difficult puncture and vascular access [30].

The rates of access site crossover in the DRA and TRA arms of ten RCTs are shown in Fig. 16.2. As with RAO rates, there is a large heterogeneity in reported crossover rates, ranging from 0% to 8.7% for TRA and from 2% to 34% for DRA. The average rates of access site crossover are 4% for TRA (92 events/2324 patients) and 12% for DRA (276 events/2305 patients).

The observed higher risk of access site crossover in the DRA arm of current RCTs highlights one of the major remaining limitations of DRA. Previous meta-analyses have also described longer time to successful radial puncture and sheath insertion, as well as more puncture attempts when using DRA, all of which indicate a more challenging vascular access, even when performed by experienced operators [31, 32]. However, in a recent meta-analysis of six published RCTs, the observed difference in cannulation time was less than 1 min (mean difference 0.68 min, 95% CI 0.17–1.18), which is unlikely to have a significant impact on overall procedure time [33].

In case of DRA or TRA failure, crossover access sites were described in seven RCTs and are shown in Table 16.3. Overall, the vast majority of access site crossovers in DRA failure occurred to the ipsilateral conventional TRA, with conversion to TFA observed in only 11% of cases (12/105 patients), allowing all the clinical benefits associated with the use of the wrist access to be maintained. In contrast, in patients with conventional TRA failure, crossover to TFA occurred in as many as 45% of cases (24/53 patients).

However, unlike conventional TRA, the learning curve required to achieve proficiency with DRA has not been well defined. In a prespecified

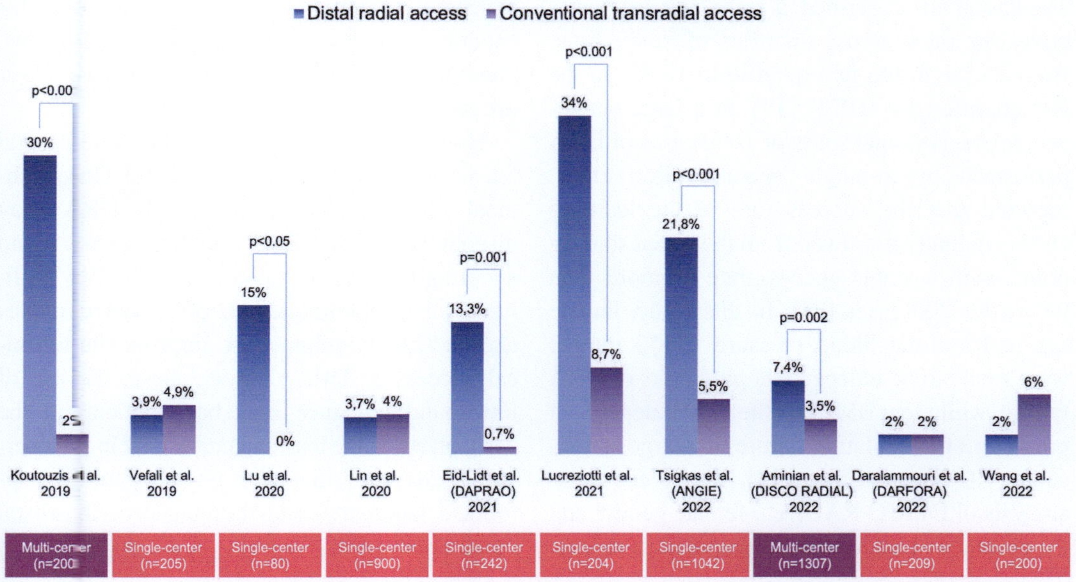

Fig. 16.2 Rates of access site crossover in randomized clinical trials comparing distal radial access and conventional transradial access. Only significant *p* values are reported

Table 16.3 Access site crossover and crossover sites in randomized controlled trials comparing distal radial access with conventional transradial access

Trial	Year	DRA		TRA	
		Number of crossovers	Crossover site	Number of crossovers	Crossover site
Koutouzis et al. [12]	2019	30	Ipsilateral TRA = 30 (100%)	2	Contralateral TRA = 2 (100%)
Vefali et al. [13]	2019	15	TRA = 5 (100%)	4	Femoral = 4 (100%)
Lin et al. [15]	2020	18	TRA = 10 (55%) Femoral = 8 (45%)	15	DRA = 6 (40%) Femoral = 9 (60%)
Eid-Lidt et al. DAPRAO [17]	2021	19	Contralateral TRA = 19 (100%)	1	Contralateral TRA = 1 (100%)
Aminian et al. DISCO RADIAL [20]	2022	48	Ipsilateral TRA = 30 (62.5%) Contralateral TRA = 2 (4.2%) Contralateral DRA = 3 (6.2%) Ulnar/brachial = 1 (2.1%) Femoral = 12 (25%)	23	Contralateral TRA = 9 (39%) Ipsilateral DRA = 1 (4.4%) Ulnar/brachial = 3 (13.2%) Femoral = 10 (43.4%)
Daralammouri et al. DARFORA [21]	2022	2	Contralateral TRA = 2 (100%)	2	Contralateral TRA = 2 (100%)
Wang et al. [22]	2022	2	TRA = 2 (100%	6	DRA = 4 (66%) Femoral = 1 (17%) Ulnar/brachial = 1 (17%)

DRA distal radial access, *TRA* conventional transradial access

analysis of the Anatomical sNuffbox for Coronary anGiography and IntervEntions (ANGIE) trial, Tsigkas et al. described a trend toward lower crossover rates across quartiles of study time, from 26.2% in the first quartile to 16.4% in the last quartile ($p = 0.073$) [19]. In a large single-center observational study of 1000 cases of DRA performed by a single operator, Roh et al. reported that the success rate of the learning curve gradually improved from the initial starting point, with a stable success rate of more than 94% after 200 cases [34]. In this study, female sex and systolic blood pressure < 120 mmHg were found to be independent predictors of DRA failure, while low BMI was the only independent predictor of cannulation failure in a large single-center RCT from China [15]. In a recent sub-analysis of DISCO RADIAL, female gender and the presence of RAS were independent predictors of access site crossover [35]. As with all new techniques, the learning curve for DRA is expected to improve over time with operator experience, reducing the number of punctures, puncture duration, and ultimately the access failure rate [21].

However, despite the potential benefits and feasibility of DRA over conventional TRA, technical challenges associated with DRA may discourage experienced radial operators from adopting this new vascular approach. This highlights the need to implement effective techniques and dedicated equipment to improve the technical success of DRA. Among these, the use of ultrasound guidance may be beneficial in the early phase of the learning curve to help the operator become familiar with the surrounding anatomical landmarks and the course of the distal radial artery [36].

16.5 Impact of Distal Radial Access on the Occurrence of Radial Artery Spasm and Procedural Outcomes

The incidence of RAS in DRA and conventional TRA has been described in seven RCTs and is shown in Fig. 16.3.

In the large multicenter DISCO RADIAL study, DRA was associated with a twofold higher risk of RAS (5.4% vs. 2.7%, $p = 0.015$) (20), while in a smaller single-center study by Lucreziotti et al., the risk of RAS was found to be higher with TRA (44% vs. 21%, $p < 0.01$), with unusually high RAS rates reported in both arms [18]. The remaining five studies reported low rates of RAS with no significant difference.

These mixed results are partly explained by differences between studies in endpoint definitions and rigorous assessment of RAS. In addition, a large meta-analysis of trials published before March 2022 did not show an increased risk of RAS with DRA [33]. Also, although the risk of RAS was slightly but significantly higher with DRA in the DISCO RADIAL trial, there was no significant difference in self-reported pain scores at the end of the procedure, providing some reassurance against a more painful experience with DRA.

Regarding other procedural outcomes, several meta-analyses of RCTs have shown no significant differences in procedure time, fluoroscopy time, and contrast volume, with a high technical success rate for successful DRA [31–33].

Overall, the current level of evidence from RCTs suggests that procedural outcomes do not appear to be affected by the use of DRA. However, the profile of patients enrolled in current RCTs is not fully representative of real-world complexity.

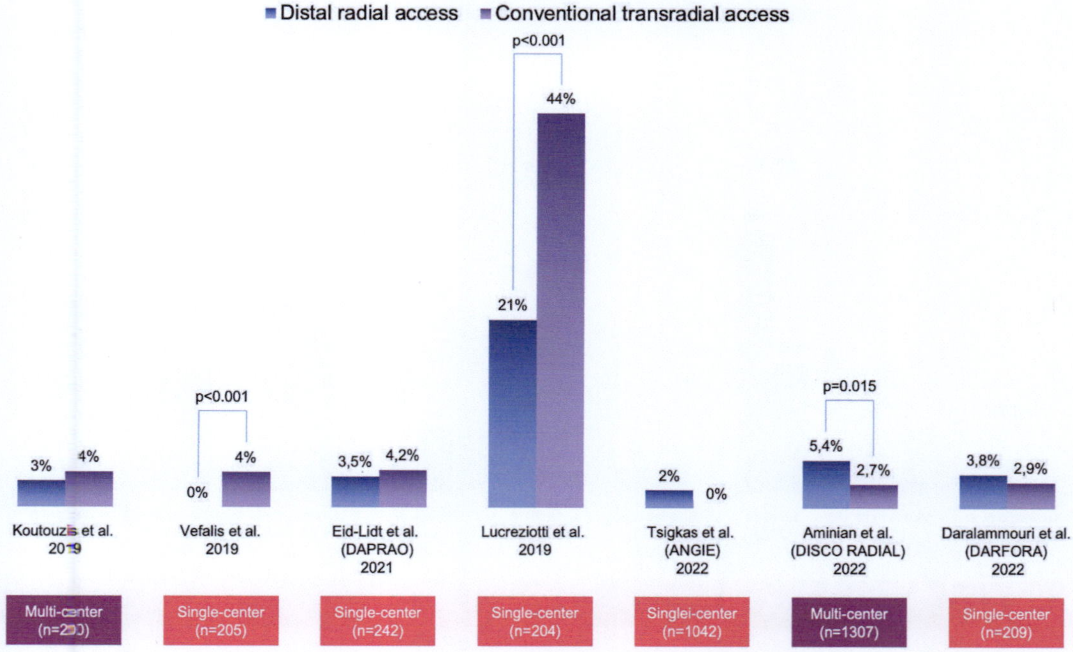

Fig. 16.3 Rates of radial artery spasm in randomized clinical trials comparing distal radial access and conventional transradial access. Only significant *p* values are reported

16.6 Post-procedural Care Following Distal Radial Access

Compared to the forearm radial artery, the distal radial artery at the level of the anatomical snuffbox has a more superficial location and its course just over the surface formed by the scaphoid and trapezium carpal bones, with the potential for an easier, safer, and faster hemostasis process [23, 30].

Comparisons between hemostasis times after DRA and conventional TRA were evaluated in nine published RCTs and are shown in Fig. 16.4. All but one study showed a consistent and significant reduction in mean hemostasis times after DRA.

As shown in Table 16.2, there was a high heterogeneity in hemostasis techniques after DRA, which included either the standard technique used for conventional TRA or another hemostasis technique for DRA (e.g., compression device, elastic bandage). Manual compression alone was used in three RCTs and resulted in extremely short mean hemostasis times for DRA, ranging from 10 to 28 min [12, 13, 15].

The safer aspect of the hemostasis process after DRA was highlighted in a recent meta-analysis of RCTs, where DRA was associated with a lower risk of EASY grade ≥ 2 hematoma and a similarly low rate of vascular complications [32, 37, 38]. These benefits may be attributed to the shorter course of the access wire and introducer sheath in the forearm vasculature with DRA.

Overall, the ease and safety of the hemostasis process represents one of the most attractive advantages of DRA, with the potential to significantly improve the Cathlab workflow by reducing the nursing care required during the hemostasis process, thereby facilitating the implementation of same-day discharge programs.

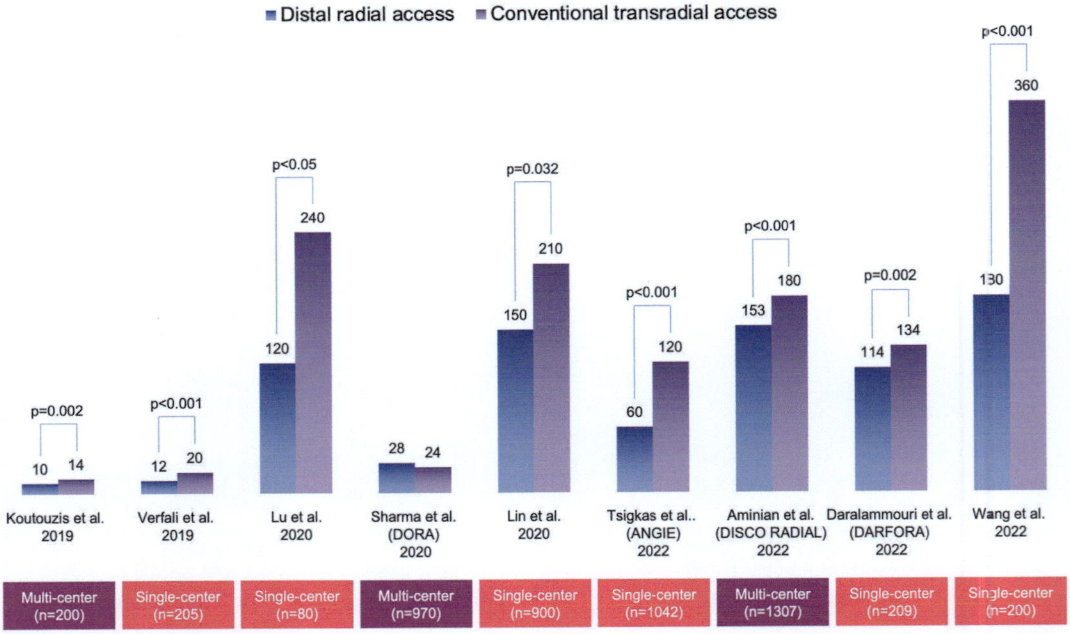

Fig. 16.4 Mean hemostasis time (min) in randomized clinical trials comparing distal radial access and conventional transradial access. Only significant *p* values are reported

16.7 Remaining Gaps of Evidence from Randomized Trials

With the exception of DISCO RADIAL, most of the RCTs included in this review were small- to medium-sized single-center studies, which limit the generalizability of the results. There was also a high variability in study design, endpoint definitions, and patient populations included.

Several more complex populations for DRA, such as women and ACS patients, are underrepresented in currently published RCTs. Only one small single-center study included patients with STEMI exclusively [22]. Whether the systematic use of DRA in the setting of primary PCI for STEMI may lead to delayed revascularization should be addressed by an appropriately powered multicenter RCT.

Finally, the predictors of DRA failure are poorly understood. It is anticipated that upfront identification of patients at high risk of DRA failure may allow operators to anticipate and/or overcome technical difficulties and ultimately improve DRA success rates.

Well-designed ongoing and future RCTs of DRA will play a critical role in providing an objective assessment of the benefits and limitations of this relatively new vascular access.

16.8 Conclusions

Evidence from currently published RCTs comparing DRA and conventional TRA shows that DRA is associated with a lower risk of forearm RAO, particularly when effective RAO prevention strategies are not used in the conventional TRA arm.

In addition, DRA is technically more challenging with a variable but consistently higher risk of access site crossover, although without a significant impact on procedural outcomes once DRA is successfully achieved.

Finally, DRA is associated with a safer and easier post-procedural course, including shorter hemostasis times and lower rates of significant local bleeding.

References

1. Ratib K, Mamas MA, Anderson SG, Bhatia G, Routledge H, De Belder M, et al. Access site practice and procedural outcomes in relation to clinical presentation in 439,947 patients undergoing percutaneous coronary intervention in the United Kingdom. JACC Cardiovasc Interv. 2015;8(1 Pt A):20–9.
2. Ferrante G, Rao SV, Jüni P, Da Costa BR, Reimers B, Condorelli G, et al. Radial versus femoral access for coronary interventions across the entire spectrum of patients with coronary artery disease: a meta-analysis of randomized trials. JACC Cardiovasc Interv. 2016;9:1419–34.
3. Valgimigli M, Frigoli E, Leonardi S, Vranckx P, Rothenbühler M, Tebaldi M, et al. Radial versus femoral access and bivalirudin versus unfractionated heparin in invasively managed patients with acute coronary syndrome (MATRIX): final 1-year results of a multicentre, randomised controlled trial. Lancet. 2018;392:835–48.
4. Neumann FJ, Sousa-Uva M, Ahlsson A, Alfonso F, Banning AP, Benedetto U, et al. 2018 ESC/EACTS guidelines on myocardial revascularization. Eur Heart J. 2019;40:87–165.
5. Lawton JS, Tamis-Holland JE, Bangalore S, Bates ER, Beckie TM, Bischoff JM, et al. 2021 ACC/AHA/SCAI guideline for coronary artery revascularization: a report of the American College of Cardiology/American Heart Association Joint Committee on clinical practice guidelines. J Am Coll Cardiol. 2022;79:e21–9.
6. Kaledin AL, Kochanov IN, Seletskiĭ SS, Arkharov IV, Burak TIA, Kozlov KL. Peculiarities of arterial access in endovascular surgery in elderly patients. Adv Gerontol. 2014;27:115–9.
7. Roghani-Dehkordi F, Hashemifard O, Sadeghi M, Mansouri R, Akbarzadeh M, Dehghani A, et al. Distal accesses in the hand (two novel techniques) for percutaneous coronary angiography and intervention. ARYA Atheroscler. 2018;14:95–100.
8. Babunashvili A, Dundua D. Recanalization and reuse of early occluded radial artery within 6 days after previous transradial diagnostic procedure. Catheter Cardiovasc Interv. 2011;77:530–6.
9. Kiemeneij F. Left distal transradial access in the anatomical snuffbox for coronary angiography (ldTRA) and interventions (ldTRI). EuroIntervention. 2017;13:851–7.
10. Serruys PW, Onuma Y. Twitterature: will social media have an impact on scientific journals? EuroIntervention. 2018;14:e962–4.
11. Capodanno D. Twitterature. EuroIntervention. 2018;14:e959–61.
12. Koutouzis M, Kontopodis E, Tassopoulos A, Tsiafoutis I, Katsanou K, Rigatou A, et al. Distal versus traditional radial approach for coronary angiography. Cardiovasc Revasc Med. 2019;20:678–80.

13. Vefalı V, Sarıçam E. The comparison of traditional radial access and novel distal radial access for cardiac catheterization. Cardiovasc Revasc Med. 2020;21:496–500.
14. Lu H, Wu D, Chen X. Comparison of distal transradial access in anatomic snuffbox versus transradial access for coronary angiography. Heart Surg Forum. 2020;23:E407–10.
15. Lin Y, Sun X, Chen R, Liu H, Pang X, Chen J, et al. Feasibility and safety of the distal transradial artery for coronary diagnostic or interventional catheterization. J Interv Cardiol. 2020;2020:4794838.
16. Sharma AK, Razi MM, Prakash N, Sharma A, Sarraf S, Sinha S, et al. A comparative assessment of dorsal radial artery access versus classical radial artery access for percutaneous coronary angiography-a randomized control trial (DORA trial). Indian Heart J. 2020;72:435–41.
17. Eid-Lidt G, Rivera Rodríguez A, Jimenez Castellanos J, Farjat Pasos JI, Estrada Lopez KE, Gaspar J. Distal radial artery approach to prevent radial artery occlusion trial. JACC Cardiovasc Interv. 2021;14:378–85.
18. Lucreziotti S, Persampieri S, Gentile D, Barbieri L, Salerno-Uriarte D, Valli F, et al. Access-site hematoma in distal and conventional transradial access: a randomized trial. Minerva Cardiol Angiol. 2021;70:129–37.
19. Tsigkas G, Papageorgiou A, Moulias A, Kalogeropoulos AP, Papageorgopoulou C, Apostolos A, et al. Distal or traditional transradial access site for coronary procedures: a single-center, randomized study. JACC Cardiovasc Interv. 2022;15:22–32.
20. Aminian A, Sgueglia GA, Wiemer M, Kefer J, Gasparini GL, Ruzsa Z, et al. Distal versus conventional radial access for coronary angiography and intervention: the DISCO RADIAL trial. JACC Cardiovasc Interv. 2022;15:1191–201.
21. Daralammouri Y, Nazzal Z, Mosleh YS, Abdulhaq HK, Khayyat ZY, Hamshary YE, et al. Distal radial artery access in comparison to forearm radial artery access for cardiac catheterization: a randomized controlled trial (DARFORA trial). J Interv Cardiol. 2022;2022:7698583.
22. Wang Y, Liu Z, Wu Y, Li Z, Wang Y, Wang S, et al. Early prevention of radial artery occlusion via distal transradial access for primary percutaneous coronary intervention. Front Cardiovasc Med. 2022;9:1071575.
23. Sgueglia GA, Di Giorgio A, Gaspardone A, Babunashvili A. Anatomic basis and physiological rationale of distal radial artery access for percutaneous coronary and endovascular procedures. JACC Cardiovasc Interv. 2018;11:2113–9.
24. Sgueglia GA, Santoliquido A, Gaspardone A, Di Giorgio A. First results of the distal radial access Doppler study. JACC Cardiovasc Imaging. 2002;14:1281–3.
25. Pancholy SB, Bernat I, Bertrand OF, Patel TM. Prevention of radial artery occlusion after transradial catheterization: the PROPHET-II randomized trial. JACC Cardiovasc Interv. 2016;9:1992–9.
26. Aminian A, Saito S, Takahashi A, Bernat I, Jobe RL, Kajiya T, et al. Comparison of a new slender 6 Fr sheath with a standard 5 Fr sheath for transradial coronary angiography and intervention: RAP and BEAT (radial artery patency and bleeding, efficacy, adverse event), a randomised multicentre trial. EuroIntervention. 2017;13:e549–56.
27. Dangoisse V, Guédès A, Chenu P, Hanet C, Albert C, Robin V, et al. Usefulness of a gentle and short hemostasis using the transradial band device after transradial access for percutaneous coronary angiography and interventions to reduce the radial artery occlusion rate (from the prospective and randomized CRASOC I II, and III studies). Am J Cardiol. 2017;120:374–9.
28. Mamas MA, Fraser DG, Ratib K, Fath-Ordoubadi F, El-Omar M, Nolan J, et al. Minimising radial injury: prevention is better than cure. EuroIntervention. 2014;10:824–32.
29. Bernat I, Aminian A, Pancholy S, Mamas M, Gaudino M, Nolan J, et al. Best practices for the prevention of radial artery occlusion after transradial diagnostic angiography and intervention: an international consensus paper. JACC Cardiovasc Interv. 2019;12:2235–46.
30. Sgueglia GA, Lee BK, Cho BR, Babunashvili A, Lee JB, Lee JW, et al. Distal radial access: consensus report of the first Korea-Europe Transradial intervention meeting. JACC Cardiovasc Interv. 2021;14:892–906.
31. Mhanna M, Beran A, Nazir S, Al-Abdouh A, Barbarawi M, Sajdeya O, et al. Outcomes of distal versus conventional transradial access for coronary angiography and intervention: an updated systematic review and meta-analysis. Int J Cardiol. 2021;344:47–53.
32. Ferrante G, Condello F, Rao SV, Maurina M, Jolly S, Stefanini GG, et al. Distal vs conventional radial access for coronary angiography and/or intervention: a meta-analysis of randomized trials. JACC Cardiovasc Interv. 2022;15:2297–311.
33. Talha KM, Waqar E, Ashley KE, Cohen MG, Lemor A, McMullan MR, et al. Distal trans-radial access compared to conventional trans-radial access in coronary interventions: a meta-analysis. Crit Pathw Cardiol. 2022;21:176–8.
34. Roh JW, Kim Y, Lee OH, Im E, Cho DK, Choi D, et al. The learning curve of the distal radial access for coronary intervention. Sci Rep. 2021;11:13217.

35. Aminian A, Sgueglia GA, Wiemer M, Kefer J, Gasparini GL, Ruzsa Z, et al. TCT-591 predictors of cross-over for distal radial access: insights from the DISCO RADIAL study. J Am Coll Cardiol. 2022;80(12 Supplement):B243.
36. Zuin M, Turchetta S, Drudi A, Gasparetto M, Rubin L, Rigatelli G. Ultrasound-guided distal transradial access for cardiac catheterization: technical notes for the interventionalist. Catheter Cardiovasc Interv. 2023;101:67–71.
37. Bertrand OF, Larose E, Rodés-Cabau J, Gleeton O, Taillon I, Roy L, et al. Incidence, predictors, and clinical impact of bleeding after transradial coronary stenting and maximal antiplatelet therapy. Am Heart J. 2009;157:164–9.
38. Bertrand OF. Acute forearm muscle swelling post transradial catheterization and compartment syndrome: prevention is better than treatment. Catheter Cardiovasc Interv. 2010;75:366–8.

Part IV

Advanced Applications

17 Acute Coronary Syndrome

Grigorios Tsigkas, Anastasios Apostolos, and Marco Valgimigli

17.1 Introduction

Acute coronary syndrome (ACS), either manifested as ST-elevation myocardial infarction (STEMI) or non-ST-elevation acute coronary syndrome (NSTE-ACS), is the most severe form of coronary heart disease, causing more than 1.8 million deaths per year [1]. Therefore, timely diagnosis and optimal management are required to reduce the burden of ACS.

Despite recent advances in coronary computed tomography angiography, coronary angiography remains the gold standard for assessing coronary anatomy and flow in the acute setting [2]. Arterial access is a prerequisite for performing coronary angiography. Transradial arterial access (TRA) has been established as the first-line access site for coronary angiography and percutaneous coronary intervention (PCI) because it has been shown to prevent major bleeding, blood transfusion, and vascular injury requiring surgery and improve mortality.

In addition, TRA is associated with shorter hospital stay and improved patient satisfaction and quality of life. The RadIal Vs femorAL access for coronary intervention (RIVAL) trial showed that both TRA and TFA were safe and effective for performing PCI in ACS patients; however, TRA was associated with fewer vascular complications [3, 4]. The Minimizing Adverse Haemorrhagic Events by Transradial Access Site and Systemic Implementation of AngioX (MATRIX) trial showed that TRA was associated with lower rates of net adverse clinical events compared with TFA access in patients with ACS during a 1-year follow-up [5]. Thus, guidelines from the European Society of Cardiology (ESC) and the American Heart Association/American College of Cardiology recommend the radial approach for NSTE-ACS and STEMI when performed by experienced operators with a class I recommendation and level of evidence A [2, 6, 7]. These recommendations have recently been reinforced by an individual patient data meta-analysis including a total of 21,600 patients (10,775 TRA, 10,825 TFA) from seven randomized clinical trials (RCTs), showing that TRA is associated with lower all-cause mortality and major bleeding at 30 days compared with TFA [8].

G. Tsigkas (✉)
Faculty of Medicine, Department of Cardiology, University of Patras, University Hospital of Patras, Patras, Greece
e-mail: gregtsig@upatras.gr

A. Apostolos
Faculty of Medicine, Department of Cardiology, University of Patras, University Hospital of Patras, Patras, Greece

First Department of Cardiology, Medical School, National and Kapodistrian University of Athens, Hippocration General Hospital of Athens, Athens, Greece

M. Valgimigli
Cardiocentro Ticino Institute and Università della Svizzera Italiana (USI), Lugano, Switzerland
e-mail: marco.valgimigli@eoc.ch

G. A. Sgueglia (ed.), *Distal Radial Access*, https://doi.org/10.1007/978-3-031-89925-6_17

Transulnar artery access has been studied as an alternative strategy to TRA for using forearm arteries for cardiac catheterization. A higher crossover rate and more punctures were observed with transulnar access compared to TRA [9, 10]. Nevertheless, the incidence of arterial occlusion was comparable between the two main forearm arteries [11].

Recently, an alternative approach included catheterization of the distal part of the radial artery through the anatomical snuffbox. Distal radial access (DRA) is increasingly becoming part of daily clinical practice, both in the acute and stable setting [12]. The aim of our chapter is to review the existing literature to tackle the evidence surrounding DRA approach in ACS, to focus on different clinical situations, and to highlight which are the next steps required for the advancement of DRA.

17.2 First Reports

Ferdinand Kiemeneij was the first to promote the concept of vascular access through the anatomical snuffbox [13]. He reported the first 70 cases of left DRA in selected cases with a crossover rate of 11% and no radial artery occlusion (RAO) in 50 patients who underwent radial artery vascular ultrasound evaluation. A significant proportion of patients (33%) were catheterized for ACS. Six of them were diagnosed with STEMI and the other with NSTE-ACS [13]. Numerous studies following this first report included patients with ACS; however, data on this patient category remained scarce [14–18]. Lee and colleagues from a tertiary center in South Korea conducted the first medium-size prospective study of 136 patients with ACS, of whom 17, 40, and 69 had STEMI, NSTEMI, and UA, respectively [19].

In the first semester of 2019, a Brazilian registry enrolled 435 consecutive patients who underwent coronary angiography through DRA, including 66 with STEMI, 102 with NSTE-ACS, and 43 with UA [20]. Four patients were in cardiogenic shock, and all were successfully catheterized through the right DRA (Fig. 17.1). The overall crossover rate was only 3%.

To our knowledge, Soydan and Akin were the first to publish results focusing on patients undergoing DRA for STEMI [21]. In their retrospective observational cohort study, 30 consecutive patients undergoing primary PCI through the left DRA were analyzed. All procedures were successfully performed with a low puncture time (37.4 s).

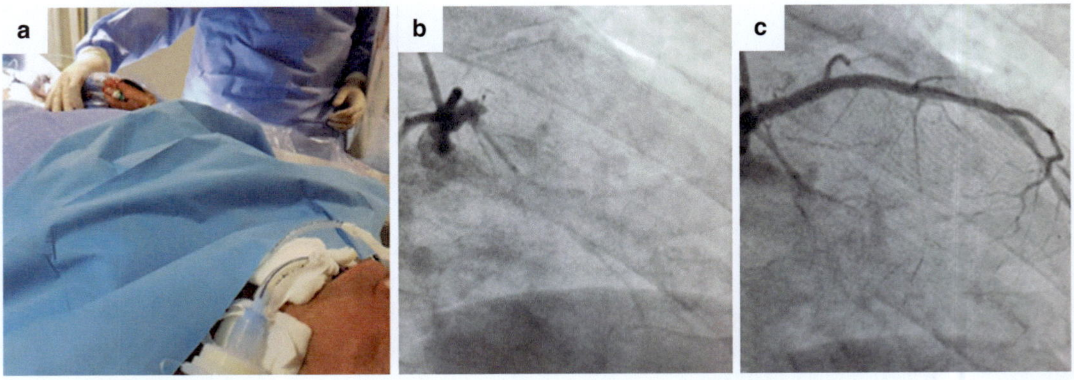

Fig. 17.1 Distal radial access in cardiogenic shock. (**a**) A 66-year-old intubated patient with anterior ST-elevation myocardial infarction and cardiogenic shock is catheterized through distal radial access. (**b**) Coronary angiography reveals total occlusion of the proximal segment of the left anterior descending artery. (**c**) Percutaneous coronary intervention is successfully completed with total recanalization of the left anterior descending artery through distal radial access, without local or systemic complications

Furthermore, Kim et al. reported a medium-sized cohort of patients with STEMI undergoing urgent coronary angiography and primary PCI [18]. A total of 138 patients were retrospectively reviewed; the success rate of DRA was 92.8%, and PCI was successfully completed in all patients. The three participating operators preferred left DRA (80.5%) and 6 Fr catheters (97.7%). Implantation of at least two stents or PCI to more than one vessel was performed in 36 and 20 patients, respectively. Almost half of the patients required thrombus aspiration, which was successfully performed in all patients. Local hematoma (EASY type I) was observed in only three patients (2.3%). Yamada et al. studied 116 patients having undergone PCI (STEMI: 77, NSTE-ACS: 39) and showed very low incidence of access-site complications within indicated revascularization time [22].

Oliveira and Caixeta reported the largest series of STEMI patients undergoing urgent coronary angiography and primary PCI though DRA. Of the 849 patients with STEMI and DRA, only 17 (2%) required crossover to another access site due to failure of sheath wire insertion. However, the authors did not record data on time to access or procedure time and patient selection [23, 24]. Xu et al. compared retrospectively patients diagnosed with ACS having undergone PCI via DRA and TRA and were followed for 1-3 years after PCI. After performing propensity score matching, they concluded that all-cause, cardiovascular mortality, major cardiac adverse events and unplanned revascularization were not significantly different between the two groups. [25].

17.3 Randomized Controlled Trials

The first RCT including only patients with ACS was performed by Koledinskiy et al. and presented at the 2020 Congress of the ESC [26]. They included 264 patients who underwent PCI in a high-volume center in Russia between 2018 and 2019. A total of 160 patients were diagnosed with UA and the remainder with either STEMI or NSTE-ACS. While the mean puncture time was higher in DRA compared to conventional TRA (125.1 ± 11.9 versus 58.8 ± 8.2 s), the total procedure time was comparable between the two arms (30.5 ± 7.1 versus 29.4 ± 4.6 min). Hemostasis time and local complications (hematoma, radial artery spasm, RAO) were significantly reduced with DRA. Major adverse cardiovascular events during hospitalization were similar between the two arms.

Recently, Wang et al. performed a single-center RCT comparing the two approaches in STEMI patients. They found that DRA was associated with a lower incidence of RAO (2.0 vs. 9.0%, p = 0.030), shorter hemostasis time [3.1 (2.7–3.3) vs. 6.2 (5.9–6.4) h, $p < 0.001$], and fewer hematomas >5 cm (0 vs. 6.0%, $p = 0.029$). Access rate and door-to-wire time were comparable between arms, while puncture time was significantly longer in the DRA group [2.4 (1.7–4.2) vs. 1.7 (1.4–2.3) min, $p < 0.001$] [27]. Distal radial access to prevent radial artery occlusion for STEMI patients (RAPID III) was a randomized trial comparing the incidence of RAO between DRA and TRA 24 h after primary PCI in patients with STEMI. Five hundred and twenty patients (mean age: 61.3 ± 13.0 years; 81% male) with STEMI were randomized. The incidence of RAO was significantly lower in the DRA group than that in the TRA group (1.9% vs. 8.5%, p = 0.001). The crossover rate was 5.4% in both groups. The median time taken for sheath insertion was longer using DRA (133 s vs. 114 s, p = 0.009), whereas the mean hemostasis time was shorter (209 ± 71 min vs. 372 ± 70 min, p < 0.001) in DRA group. However, it did not provide any date about the total amount of time required for angiography and PCI [28].

Actually, some RCTs did not provide data on patients' indication for catheterization [29–31], while Sharma et al. included only patients with chronic stable angina [32].

To our knowledge, all remaining RCTs enrolled patients with both ACS and chronic coronary syndromes. Lin et al. enrolled 900 patients between 2019 and 2020 in a single-center study conducted in China. Two hundred twenty-six patients suffered from ACS and were catheterized by DRA. The authors concluded that STEMI

(48 patients, 10.67%) was not a risk factor for DRA failure (OR = 2.54, $p = 0.180$) according to logistic multivariable analysis [33].

The DARFORA study included mainly patients with NSTE-ACS (172 patients, 82.3%) and showed that DRA was associated with shorter procedure, fluoroscopy and hemostasis time, equivalent success rate, and longer puncture duration compared to conventional TRA. Despite the lack of any subgroup or multivariable analysis, the large proportion of patients with NSTE-ACS shows that DRA could be considered safe and feasible in this clinical setting [34].

The single-center Anatomical sNuffbox for Coronary anGiography and IntervEntions (ANGIE) trial included a total of 338 patients (32.4%) with NSTE-ACS, whereas STEMI was an exclusion criterion. DRA was associated with a lower rate of forearm RAO, shorter time to hemostasis, higher crossover rate and dose area product, and longer procedure time compared with conventional TRA [35, 36].

DISCO RADIAL, the largest RCT of DRA to date, included 197 patients (15.1%) with NSTE-ACS and supported that DRA was associated with faster hemostasis but higher crossover rate [37, 38]. Similar to the ANGIE trial, DISCO RADIAL did not provide specific data on patients with NSTE-ACS undergoing coronary angiography and/or PCI via DRA.

17.4 Meta-analyses

Numerous systematic reviews and meta-analyses have been performed, but the majority of them did not provide adequate data regarding DRA in patients with ACS [39–46]. Only Mhanna et al. pointed out that only 3 of the 12 studies included in their meta-analysis enrolled patients with ACS, suggesting that the overall results of the meta-analysis may not be applicable in such a population [47]. The only dedicated meta-analysis for patients undergoing emergency coronary angiography included four studies and 543 patients and showed that DRA was superior to TRA regarding RAO and hemostasis time, with comparable rates of periprocedural complications [48]. The largest meta-analysis to date, which pooled data from RCTs only, found no association between RAO incidence and ACS indication. However, the authors expressed skepticism about the use of DRA in patients with ACS due to the increased number of puncture attempts, prolonged sheath insertion time, and lack of adequate literature in this population [49].

17.5 Remaining Issues and Future Perspectives

In recent years, DRA to perform coronary angiography with or without PCI has gained increasing acceptance in clinical practice. Despite the high quality of the existing literature (large registries, RCTs, and meta-analyses), data on ACS patients remain limited (Table 17.1), with few studies enrolling exclusively ACS patients and no dedicated aggregate data or individual patient meta-analyses on ACS patients [50].

ACS patients differ from CCS patients in many ways, including a higher ischemic and bleeding risk. Therefore, periprocedural times should be shortened, and bleeding events should be avoided. While DRA is associated with a faster hemostasis time and has the potential to further reduce local bleeding complications compared to conventional TRA, the increased access time may be a major drawback in these patients. In our opinion, the first attempt at DRA in ACS is reasonable given the positive experience with this access site in the literature and across multiple centers and operators. However, if the first attempt fails, it seems prudent to quickly switch to conventional TRA to minimize delays in diagnosis and treatment (Fig. 17.2).

Two RCTs are currently underway in STEMI setting. The Comparison of Distal Transradial

Table 17.1 Summary of the studies assessing distal radial access in patients with acute coronary syndromes

Study	Year	Design	DRA (n)	DRA and ACS (n)	STEMI (n)	NSTEMI (n)	UA (n)	Comments
Kiemeneij et al. [13]	2017	Observational	70	23	6	17	NA	The first report of DRA in ACS patients
Oliveira et al. [20]	2019	Observational	435	211	66	102	43	Right DRA successfully performed in four patients with cardiogenic shock
Soydan and Akin [2[illegible]]	2020	Observational	30	30	30	0	0	Left DRA primary PCI successful in all patients
Kim et al. [18]	2021	Observational	128	128	128	0	0	DRA successful in 128/138 patients and DRA primary PCI was completed in all patients
Koledinskiy et al. [25]	2020	Randomized controlled trial	132	132	NA	NA	NA	DRA did not increase procedure time, reduced significantly local complications, and was comparable with TRA regarding major complications
Lin et al. [33]	2020	Randomized controlled trial	450	226	48	178	0	STEMI was not a significant risk factor for DRA failure after multivariable logistic analysis
Tsigkas et al. [35]	2022	Randomized controlled trial	518	164	0	98	66	First randomized controlled trial including more than 1000 patients
Aminian et al. [37]	2022	Randomized controlled trial	650	91	0	44	47	Largest randomized controlled trial comparing DRA with TRA
Wang et al. [27]	2022	Randomized controlled trial	200	200	200	0	0	Unique randomized controlled trial comparing DRA with TRA in patients with STEMI
Mhanna et al. [47]	2021	Systematic review and meta-analysis	1634	NA	NA	NA	NA	Only 3 of the 12 included studies reported patients with ACS; authors support that the overall results may not be applicable in the ACS population

ACS acute coronary syndrome, *DRA* distal transradial artery, *NA* not available, NSTEMI non-ST-elevation myocardial infraction, *PCI* percutaneous coronary intervention, *STEMI* ST-elevation myocardial infraction, *TRA* conventional transradial access, *UA* unstable angina

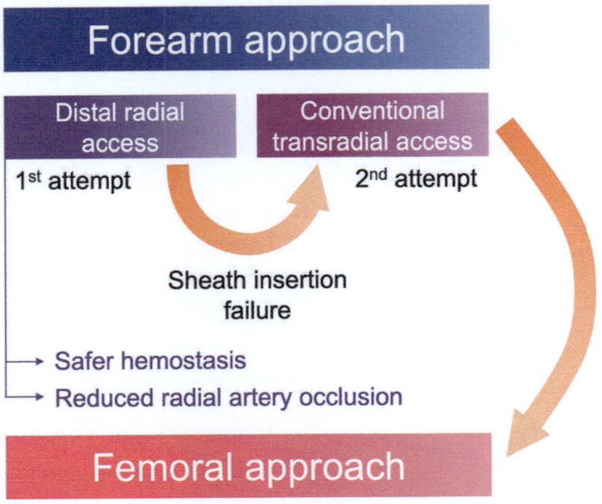

Fig. 17.2 Proposed approach for catheterization of patients with acute coronary syndrome

Access and Transradial Access for Primary Percutaneous Coronary Intervention in STEMI Patients (RESERVE, NCT04861389) trial is a single-center RCT that started in 2021 and plans to enroll 414 STEMI patients. Its primary endpoint is the incidence of RAO during hospitalization. The Distal Versus Conventional Transradial Artery Access for Coronary Catheterization in Patients With ST-elevation Myocardial Infraction (DR-STEMI, NCT05605288) trial is an international RCT that started in 2024, plans to enroll 578 participants with STEMI and is about to be completed in 2025. Its primary outcome will be needle-to-balloon time. By estimating and comparing the time from the first puncture to balloon inflation, DR-STEMI could shed some additional light on DRA in STEMI. Further studies to assess the learning curve of DRA and whether radiation exposure is not increased compared to TRA are critical.

17.6 Conclusions

The forearm approach should be preferred for access site in patients with ACS when performed by experienced operators. Conventional TRA has shown conclusive evidence of superiority over TFA, not only in terms of local vascular complications and bleeding but also in terms of outcomes. Nowadays, DRA is prominently emerging as a valid alternative to conventional TRA to further optimize hemostasis time and reduce RAO. However, its overall efficacy compared with TRA remains to be established in ACS patients, where delays in diagnosis and treatment may be associated with poorer outcomes.

References

1. Cardiovascular disease in Europe. 2016: an epidemiological update. Eur Heart J. 2016:3182–3.
2. Collet JP, Thiele H, Barbato E, Barthélémy O, Bauersachs J, Bhatt DL, et al. 2020 ESC guidelines for the management of acute coronary syndromes in patients presenting without persistent ST-segment elevation. Eur Heart J. 2021;42:1289–367.
3. Tsigkas G, Papanikolaou A, Apostolos A, Kramvis A, Timpilis F, Latta A, et al. Preventing and Managing Radial Artery Occlusion following Transradial Procedures: Strategies and Considerations. J Cardiovasc Dev Dis. 2023;10:283.
4. Jolly SS, Yusuf S, Cairns J, Niemelä K, Xavier D, Widimsky P, et al. Radial versus femoral access for coronary angiography and intervention in patients with acute coronary syndromes (RIVAL): a randomised, parallel group, multicentre trial. Lancet. 2011;377:1409–20.
5. Valgimigli M, Frigoli E, Leonardi S, Vranckx P, Rothenbühler M, Tebaldi M, et al. Radial versus femoral access and bivalirudin versus unfractionated heparin in invasively managed patients with acute coronary syndrome (MATRIX): final 1-year results of a multicentre, randomised controlled trial. Lancet. 2018;392:835–48.
6. Ibanez B, James S, Agewall S, Antunes MJ, Bucciarelli-Ducci C, Bueno H, et al. 2017 ESC guidelines for the management of acute myocardial infarction in patients presenting with ST-segment elevation: the task force for the management of acute myocardial infarction in patients presenting with ST-segment elevation of the European Society of Cardiology (ESC). Eur Heart J. 2018;39:119–77.
7. Lawton JS, Tamis-Holland JE, Bangalore S, Bates ER, Beckie TM, Bischoff JM, et al. 2021 ACC/AHA/SCAI guideline for coronary artery revascularization: a report of the American College of Cardiology/American Heart Association Joint committee on clinical practice guidelines. Circulation. 2022;145:e18–114.
8. Gargiulo G, Giacoppo D, Jolly SS, Cairns J, Le May M, Bernat I, et al. Effects on mortality and major bleeding of radial versus femoral artery access for coronary angiography or percutaneous coronary intervention: meta-analysis of individual patient data from

7 multicenter randomized clinical trials. Circulation. 2022;146:1329–43.
9. Hahalis G, Tsigkas G, Xanthopoulou I, Deftereos S, Ziakas A, Raisakis K, et al. Transulnar compared with transradial artery approach as a default strategy for coronary procedures: a randomized trial. The Transulnar or Transradial instead of coronary Transfemoral Angiographies Study (the AURA of ARTEMIS Study). Circ Cardiovasc Interv. 2013;6:252–61.
10. Dahal K, Rijal J, Lee J, Korr KS, Azrin M. Transulnar versus transradial access for coronary angiography or percutaneous coronary intervention: a meta-analysis of randomized controlled trials. Catheter Cardiovasc Interv. 2016;87:857–65.
11. Hahalis G, Aznaouridis K, Tsigkas G, Davlouros P, Xanthopoulou I, Koutsogiannis N, et al. Radial artery and ulnar artery occlusions following coronary procedures and the impact of anticoagulation: ARTEMIS (radial and ulnar ARTEry occlusion meta-AnalysIS) systematic review and meta-analysis. J Am Heart Assoc. 2017;6:e005430.
12. Tsigkas G, Moulias A, Papageorgiou A, Ntouvas I, Grapsas N, Despotopoulos S, Apostolos A, Papanikolaou A, Smaili K, Vasilagkos G, Davlouros P, Hahalis G. Transradial access through the anatomical snuffbox: Results of a feasibility study. Hellenic J Cardiol. 2021;62:201–5.
13. Kiemeneij F. Left distal transradial access in the anatomical snuffbox for coronary angiography (ldTRA) and interventions (ldTRI). EuroIntervention. 2017;13:851–7.
14. Soydan E, Akın M. Coronary angiography using the left distal radial approach – an alternative site to conventional radial coronary angiography. Anatol J Cardiol. 2018;19:243–8.
15. Valsecchi O, Vassileva A, Cereda AF, Canova P, Satogami K, Fiocca L, et al. Early clinical experience with right and left distal transradial access in the anatomical snuffbox in 52 consecutive patients. J Invasive Cardiol. 2018;30:218–23.
16. Amin MR, Singha CK, Banerjee SK, Hoque H, Mahabub SM, Hoque M, et al. Comparison of distal transradial in the anatomical snuff-box versus conventional transradial access for coronary angiography and intervention – an experience in 100 cases. Univ Heart J. 2018;13:40–5.
17. Al-Azizi KM, Grewal V, Gobeil K, Maqsood K, Haider A, Mohani A, et al. The left distal transradial artery access for coronary angiography and intervention: a US experience. Cardiovasc Revasc Med. 2019;20:786–9.
18. Kim Y, Lee JW, Lee SY, Bae JW, Lee SJ, Jeong MH, et al. Feasibility of primary percutaneous coronary intervention via the distal radial approach in patients with ST-elevation myocardial infarction. Korean J Intern Med. 2021;36(Suppl 1):S53–61.
19. Lee JW, Park SW, Son JW, Ahn SG, Lee SH. Real-world experience of the left distal transradial approach for coronary angiography and percutaneous coronary intervention: a prospective observational study (LeDRA). EuroIntervention. 2018;14:e995–1003.
20. Oliveira MDP, Navarro EC, Kiemeneij F. Distal transradial access as default approach for coronary angiography and interventions. Cardiovasc Diagn Ther. 2019;9:513–9.
21. Soydan E, Akın M. Left distal radial artery access site in primary percutaneous coronary intervention: is it safe? Balkan Med J. 2020;37:276–80.
22. Yamada T, Matsubara Y, Washimi S, Hashimoto S, Hata T, Taniguchi N, et al. Vascular Complications of Percutaneous Coronary Intervention Via Distal Radial Artery Approach in Patients With Acute Myocardial Infarction With and Without STSegment Elevation. J Invasive Cardiol. 2022;34:E259–E265.
23. Oliveira MD, Caixeta A. Distal transradial access for primary PCI in ST-segment elevation myocardial infarction. JACC Cardiovasc Interv. 2022;15:794–5.
24. Tsigkas G, Papageorgiou A, Moulias A, Apostolos A, Kalogeropoulos AP, Davlouros P. Reply: distal transradial access for primary PCI in ST-segment elevation myocardial infarction. JACC Cardiovasc Interv. 2022;15:795–6.
25. Xu L, Lu W, Shi G, Li W, Xiao J, Yang A, et al. Comparison of long-term prognoses of percutaneous coronary intervention via distal transradial and conventional transradial access for acute coronary syndrome. Hellenic J Cardiol. 2025;83:28–37.
26. Koledinskiy AG, Mikheeva YUV, Ogurtsov PP, Kurtasov DS, Vyazova NL. Hospital results of endovascular treatment of patients with Acute Coronary Syndrome (ACS) through distal radial access. Eur Heart J. 2020;41(Suppl 2):2498.
27. Wang Y, Liu Z, Wu Y, Li Z, Wang Y, Wang S, et al. Early prevention of radial artery occlusion via distal transradial access for primary percutaneous coronary intervention. Front Cardiovasc Med. 2022;9:1071575.
28. Li Z, Wang Y, Song J, Wang S, Wang Y, Wu Y, et al. Distal radial access to prevent radial artery occlusion for STEMI patients (RAPID III): a randomized controlled trial. BMC Med. 2025;23:173.
29. Koutouzis M, Kontopodis E, Tassopoulos A, Tsiafoutis I, Katsanou K, Rigatou A, et al. Distal versus traditional radial approach for coronary angiography. Cardiovasc Revasc Med. 2019;20:678–80.
30. Vefalı V, Sarıçam E. The comparison of traditional radial access and novel distal radial access for cardiac catheterization. Cardiovasc Revasc Med. 2020;21:496–500.
31. Eid-Lidt G, Rivera Rodríguez A, Jimenez Castellanos J, Farjat Pasos JI, Estrada López KE, Gaspar J. Distal radial artery approach to prevent

radial artery occlusion trial. JACC Cardiovasc Interv. 2021;14:378–85.
32. Sharma AK, Razi MM, Prakash N, Sharma A, Sarraf S, Sinha S, et al. A comparative assessment of Dorsal radial artery access versus classical radial artery access for percutaneous coronary angiography-a randomized control trial (DORA trial). Indian Heart J. 2020;72:435–41.
33. Lin Y, Sun X, Chen R, Liu H, Pang X, Chen J, et al. Feasibility and safety of the distal transradial artery for coronary diagnostic or interventional catheterization. J Interv Cardiol. 2020;2020:4794838.
34. Daralammouri Y, Nazzal Z, Mosleh YS, Abdulhaq HK, Khayyat ZY, Hamshary YE, et al. Distal radial artery access in comparison to forearm radial artery access for cardiac catheterization: a randomized controlled trial (DARFORA trial). J Interv Cardiol. 2022;2022:7698583.
35. Tsigkas G, Papageorgiou A, Moulias A, Kalogeropoulos AP, Papageorgopoulou C, Apostolos A, et al. Distal or traditional Transradial access site for coronary procedures: a single-center, randomized study. JACC Cardiovasc Interv. 2022;15:22–32.
36. Valgimigli M, Landi A. Distal transradial access for coronary procedures: old certainties, novel challenges, and future horizons. JACC Cardiovasc Interv. 2022;15:33–8.
37. Aminian A, Sgueglia GA, Wiemer M, Kefer J, Gasparini GL, Ruzsa Z, et al. Distal versus conventional radial access for coronary angiography and intervention: the DISCO RADIAL trial. JACC Cardiovasc Interv. 2022;15:1191–201.
38. Tsigkas G, Apostolos A, Davlouros P. Less is more, but not always: distal transradial access for radial artery occlusion prevention. JACC Cardiovasc Interv. 2022;15:1202–4.
39. Hamandi M, Saad M, Hasan R, Megaly M, Abbott JD, Dib C, et al. Distal versus conventional transradial artery access for coronary angiography and intervention: a meta-analysis. Cardiovasc Revasc Med. 2020;21:1209–13.
40. Cao J, Cai H, Liu W, Zhu H, Cao G. Safety and effectiveness of coronary angiography or intervention through the distal radial access: a meta-analysis. J Interv Cardiol. 2021;2021:4371744.
41. Liang C, Han Q, Jia Y, Fan C, Qin G. Distal Transradial access in anatomical snuffbox for coronary angiography and intervention: an updated meta-analysis. J Interv Cardiol. 2021;2021:7099044.
42. Rigatelli G, Zuin M, Daggubati R, Vassilev D, Zuliani G, Nguyen T, et al. Distal snuffbox versus conventional radial artery access: an updated systematic review and meta-analysis. J Vasc Access. 2022;23:653–9.
43. Elbadawi A, Elgendy IY, Jia X, Hamed M, Shnoda M, Eid M, et al. Meta-analysis of randomized trials comparing distal transradial versus conventional transradial approach for coronary procedures. Am J Cardiol. 2022;173:147–9.
44. Prasad RM, Pandrangi P, Pandrangi G, Yoo H, Salazar AM, Ukponmwan E, et al. Meta-analysis comparing distal radial artery approach versus traditional for coronary procedures. Am J Cardiol. 2022;164:52–6.
45. Sattar Y, Talib U, Faisaluddin M, Song D, Lak HM, Laghari A, et al. Meta-analysis comparing distal radial versus traditional radial percutaneous coronary intervention or angiography. Am J Cardiol. 2022;170:31–9.
46. Isath A, Elson D, Kayani W, Wang Z, Sharma S, Naidu SS, et al. A meta-analysis of traditional radial access and distal radial access in transradial access for percutaneous coronary procedures. Cardiovasc Revasc Med. 2023;46:21–6.
47. Mhanna M, Beran A, Nazir S, Al-Abdouh A, Barbarawi M, Sajdeya O, et al. Outcomes of distal versus conventional transradial access for coronary angiography and intervention: an updated systematic review and meta-analysis. Int J Cardiol. 2021;344:47–53.
48. Bittar V, Trevisan T, Clemente MRC, Pontes G, Felix N, Gomes WF. Distal versus traditional radial access in patients undergoing emergency coronary angiography or percutaneous coronary intervention: a systematic review and meta-analysis. Coron Artery Dis. 2025;36:18–27.
49. Ferrante G, Condello F, Rao SV, Maurina M, Jolly S, Stefanini GG, et al. Distal vs conventional radial access for coronary angiography and/or intervention: a meta-analysis of randomized trials. JACC Cardiovasc Interv. 2022;15:2297–311.
50. Apostolos A, Vasilagkos G, Tsigkas G. Distal Transradial Access in Acute Coronary Syndromes: Should We Give the First Try? JACC Cardiovasc Interv. 2023;16:238–239.

Slender Approach

18

Giovanni Amoroso and Takashi Matsukage

18.1 Definition and Rationale

The first successful worldwide implementation of the transradial accesss (TRA) for percutaneous coronary intervention (PCI) was performed at the Onze Lieve Vrouwe Gasthuis Hospital in Amsterdam in the early 1990s [1]. Since then, TRA has been shown to have significant clinical advantages over the traditional transfemoral approach, including a reduction in bleeding complications and mortality. As a result, it has been recognized as the preferred method in European and North American guidelines [2, 3].

The femoral artery could easily accommodate larger introducers and guiding catheters, as its internal diameter ranges from 5 to 7 mm. The radial artery, on the other hand, has a much smaller internal diameter, typically around 2.5 mm. In addition, 5–10% of individuals are born with a hypoplastic radial artery, which is less than 2 mm in diameter [4]. Factors that increase the likelihood of having a small radial artery include Asian ancestry, older age, and female sex.

When looking at the internal diameter of the radial artery, a significant proportion (20%) of patients undergoing intervention have a radial artery smaller than a 6 French introducer [5] (Fig. 18.1a). A mismatch between the inner diameter of the radial artery and the outer diameter of the introducer, resulting in a ratio of less than 1, can lead to several complications, including endothelial disruption, arterial spasm, patient pain and discomfort, potential procedural failure, and radial artery occlusion [6].

Radial artery occlusion (RAO) is considered the major drawback of TRA. Although not life-threatening, RAO can lead to a variety of symptoms and deficits, including numbness, pain, loss of strength, and hand ischemia, known as upper extremity dysfunction (UED). In addition, even in the absence of symptoms, RAO may prevent a repeat procedure through the same arterial access in the future [7].

To avoid RAO and ensure successful TRA for all patients, it is important to reduce the size of introducers and devices to fit any radial artery and eliminate the mismatch between arterial and introducer diameters. This would allow TRA to be performed in patients with small radial anatomy while minimizing RAO in patients with normal caliber radial arteries by reducing entry hole, vessel trauma, hemostasis time, and local endothelial dysfunction [8].

Downsizing TRA procedures is commonly referred to as "Slender." The term was introduced by a group of Japanese colleagues who formed the Slender Club Japan more than a decade ago to

G. Amoroso (✉)
Department of Cardiology, OLVG Hospital, Amsterdam, The Netherlands
e-mail: g.amoroso@olvg.nl

T. Matsukage
Department of Cardiology, Shonan Oiso Hospital, Oiso, Japan

G. A. Sgueglia (ed.), *Distal Radial Access*, https://doi.org/10.1007/978-3-031-89925-6_18

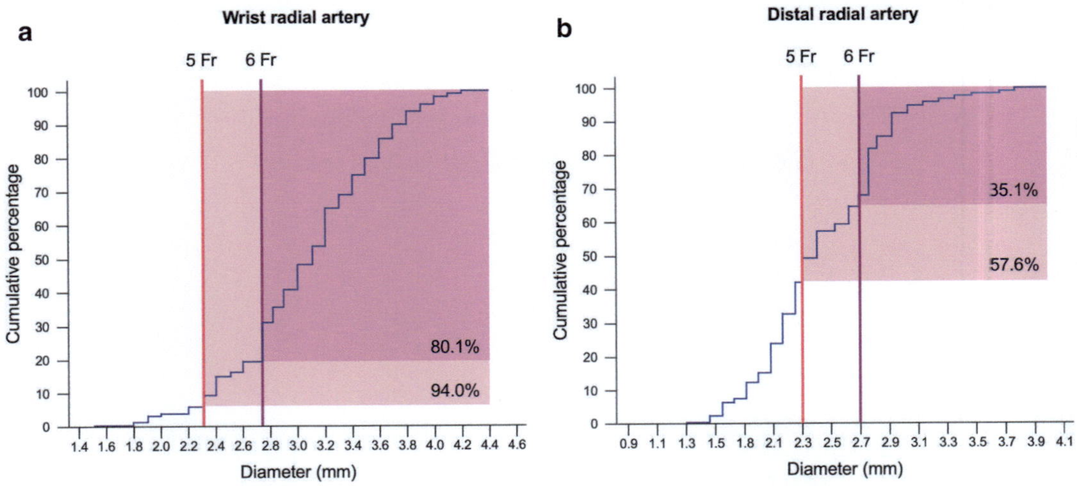

Fig. 18.1 Main introducer sheath diameters and frequency distribution diameter of (**a**) the radial artery at the wrist level and (**b**) the distal radial artery. By switching from a 6 Fr to a 5 Fr introducer sheath, the percentage of patients with an arterial/introducer mismatch decreases from approximately 20 to 5% for conventional transradial access and from 65% to 40% for distal radial access

promote the development of downsized materials and techniques [9]. Specifically, Slender PCI refers to cases where the introducer is smaller than 6 Fr, which is traditionally considered the standard size. To achieve this, Slender interventionalists often use specialized devices such as balloons and stents. In general, any procedure that seeks to reduce radial artery trauma, patient discomfort, and clinical complications can be considered a Slender PCI. In recent years, the "Slender" philosophy has spread from Japan to Europe, where a Slender Club Europe has been established [10].

Despite the clear clinical benefits, adoption of a Slender approach in interventional cardiology has been slow, even in countries where the smaller diameter of the radial artery could be an incentive. One reason is that Slender products often require more advanced technological development and are therefore more expensive and less available than standard products. In addition, operators may face a steep learning curve when using Slender devices and techniques, which may discourage inexperienced or low-volume operators from starting Slender programs.

Furthermore, some physicians may not consider the clinical benefits of Slender TRA, such as reduced RAO and incidence of UED, to be important enough to outweigh the additional cost and effort required to adopt this new technique. This perception is likely one of the main reasons why the Slender approach has not yet achieved mainstream status in interventional cardiology.

The recent popularity of distal radial access (DRA) as an alternative or replacement for conventional TRA has rekindled interest in the Slender technique [11]. The distal radial artery is approximately one-fifth smaller than the forearm radial artery [12], and with a mean diameter of approximately 2.1 mm, the use of a conventional 6 Fr introducer seems problematic in most patients. Slender techniques would also be very useful to navigate the upper limb vasculature, especially against the more tortuous bends of the distal radial artery.

18.2 Five French Percutaneous Coronary Intervention

The easiest way to perform a Slender PCI is to downsize from a 6 Fr to a 5 Fr introducer. However, it is important to note that when reporting the size of an introducer, the inner diameter is generally used, whereas for a guiding catheter, the outer diameter is generally used. Therefore, it is common to refer to 6 Fr and 5 Fr introducers, although the correct terminology would be 6 Fr-compatible and 5 Fr-compatible introducers. This makes the compatibility between the outer diameter of the introducer and the (distal) radial artery less obvious.

One French is one-third of a millimeter, so 6 French is approximately 2 mm and 5 French is 1.67 mm. When determining the outer diameter of an introducer, which is the measure of its interaction with the artery, the wall thickness should also be considered. Conventional 6 Fr introducers have an outer diameter of 2.62 to 2.81 mm, depending on the manufacturer. Conventional 5 Fr introducers range in outer diameter from 2.29 to 2.50 mm (Fig. 18.2).

Downsizing from 6 Fr to 5 Fr introducers results in a 20% reduction in outer diameter and a 40% reduction in cross-sectional area. While these changes may seem trivial to some, it is important to remember that the distribution curve of distal radial artery diameters is steepest between 2.1 and 2.8 mm. This means that downsizing from 6 Fr to 5 Fr introducers would halve the likelihood of arterial/introducer mismatch (approximately from% 70 to 40%) and allow the majority of patients (both male and female) to undergo DRA without complications (Fig. 18.1b).

Research has shown that the use of 5 Fr guiding catheters in conventional TRA can significantly reduce the incidence of RAO from 5.9% to 1.1% without compromising procedural success (92.9–95.4%) [8]. More recent studies using 5 Fr and DRA have reported an incidence of RAO approaching 0% [12].

A 5 Fr guiding catheter not only creates a smaller entry site but also respects the physiological laminar flow in the radial artery, especially through smaller vessels, better than larger catheters. It also maintains distal perfusion and preserves endothelial function, which is likely to prevent puncture site thrombosis [13]. Procedures based on the use of 5 Fr are also associated with less contrast use, shorter hemostasis time, and shorter hospital stay [14, 15], which are additional advantages of the Slender approach.

Coronary interventions with smaller guiding catheters are said to present three major technical challenges: reduced catheter support, reduced vessel opacification, and device incompatibility.

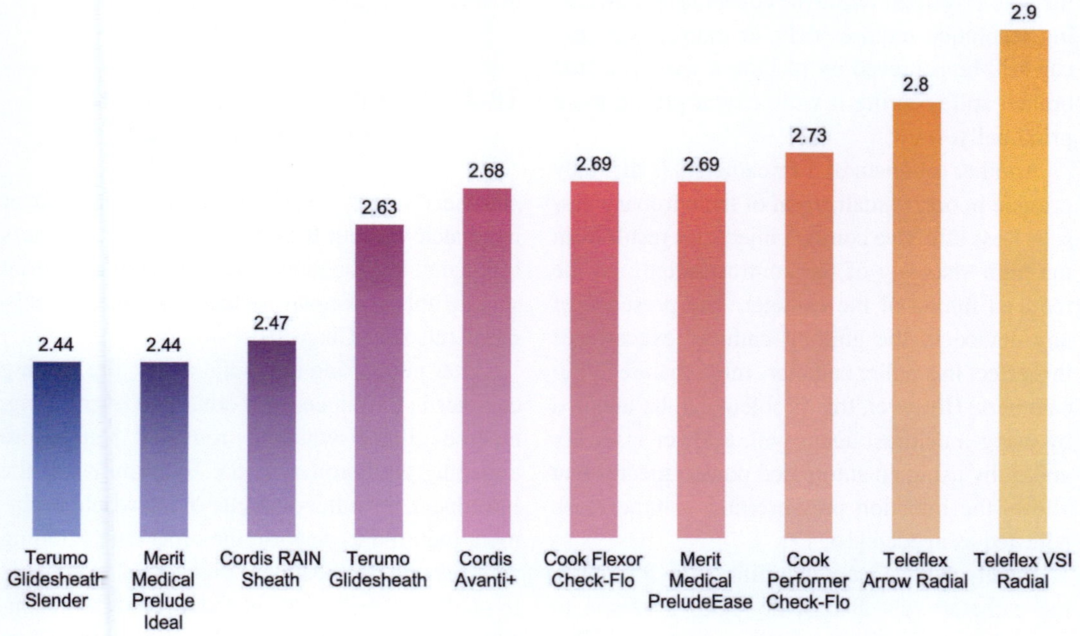

Fig. 18.2 Outer diameters of different 6 Fr introducers: the range can vary from 2.45 to 2.9 mm

One of the challenges is indeed that 5 Fr guiding catheters have less passive catheter support than larger catheters, even in the more aggressive shapes such as Extra Back-Up or Amplatz curves. This is because the shaft of the guiding catheter becomes less rigid and more flexible as the size decreases.

The limitations of passive support can be overcome by carefully advancing the guiding catheter a few centimeters into the coronary artery while pulling on the wire or balloon (so-called deep intubation). Care must be taken to avoid coronary dissections caused by interaction between the vessel wall and the tip of the guiding catheter. It is not recommended to advance the guiding catheter on the coronary wire alone nor to perform this maneuver with 6 Fr guiding catheters. Deep intubation improves stability and provides "active" support that is comparable to or exceeds the "passive" support provided by larger, more rigid catheters and in fact provides the same benefits as a guiding catheter extension system. Deep intubation is not the only technique to increase support with 5 Fr guiding catheters. With the anchoring technique, we intend to keep an additional balloon inflated in a side branch while treating the main vessel to give stability to the whole system. While the conventional anchoring technique requires 6 Fr or more, anchoring can still be achieved by placing a wire in a side branch and securing it with a stent placed more proximally.

Another criticism of 5 Fr catheters is that they provide poorer visualization of the coronary vessels. Less effective contrast injections result from the high viscosity of the contrast agent and the reduced lumen of the catheter. The presence of any device in the guiding catheter exacerbates this effect in smaller catheters more than in larger catheters. However, this problem can be avoided by using a contrast agent with a lower viscosity and/or by using an automated power injector that allows the injection pressure and volume to be adjusted as needed [16, 17].

Finally, device incompatibility with 5 Fr guiding catheters has historically been a reason to avoid downsizing from 6 Fr to smaller sizes. This was certainly true for earlier coronary devices such as stents, balloons, and imaging catheters, which required the use of at least 6 Fr guiding catheters. In recent years, however, most conventional devices have been improved for use with 5 Fr guiding catheters. This is largely due to manufacturers' efforts to both reduce the profile of devices and increase the inner diameter of 5 Fr guiding catheters to the current standard of 0.058″. The result of these iterations is that most modern PCI procedures can now be successfully performed with 5 Fr catheters. Only a few exceptions remain, particularly in complex procedures such as chronic total occlusions, vein graft interventions, left main procedures, complex bifurcations, and heavily calcified lesions, where larger guiding catheters may be recommended to allow for the simultaneous use of multiple devices or the use of specialized devices.

The risk of arterial/introducer mismatch would be even less likely with catheters smaller than 5 Fr. Coronary angiography can be successfully performed with 4F and in selected cases even with 3 Fr diagnostic catheters. This minimizes radial artery trauma and the incidence of RAO. However, excluding diagnostic procedures, the range of coronary interventions that can be performed with 4 Fr systems is still quite limited and should be reserved for highly selected cases [18].

18.3 Sheathless Percutaneous Coronary Intervention

Another way to avoid radial artery/introducer mismatch without the need for smaller catheters is to cannulate the radial artery without an arterial sheath: this is known as the "sheathless" technique (also see Chap. 19).

After puncturing the radial artery, the guiding catheter is introduced and advanced over a long, tapered dilator, which is removed just before engaging the coronary ostia. By eliminating the introducer, the outer diameter of the whole equipment required to perform the procedure (guiding catheter only in sheathless procedures in contrast to guiding catheter plus introducer sheath in conventional procedures) is reduced by almost two French (i.e., the thickness of the introducer).

Therefore, a 5 Fr sheathless procedure is often referred to as a "virtual" 3 Fr procedure (Fig. 18.3): "virtual" indicates the size of the combination guiding catheter plus introducer sheath that would have an entry hole of the same diameter in the radial artery. Sheathless 6 Fr and 7 Fr PCI procedures allow for a significant reduction in distal radial artery trauma without having to deal with a limited internal lumen diameter and have been used successfully in various settings [19].

Due to the lack of an introducer, catheter exchange, if required, is always more difficult. On the other hand, navigation of sheathless catheters throughout the arm vasculature is smoother than with conventional catheters. This is because the tapered profile of the entire device (wire, dilator, and guide catheter) can prevent the tip of the guide catheter from scratching along the inner vessel wall, known as the "razor" effect (Fig. 18.4). This is more common in tortuous or small anatomy, such as DRA. The razor effect, along with arterial/introducer mismatch, has been implicated in radial artery trauma and its recurrence.

From a pragmatic point of view, sheathless 6 Fr is probably the most efficient application of this concept in daily practice, as it allows for a

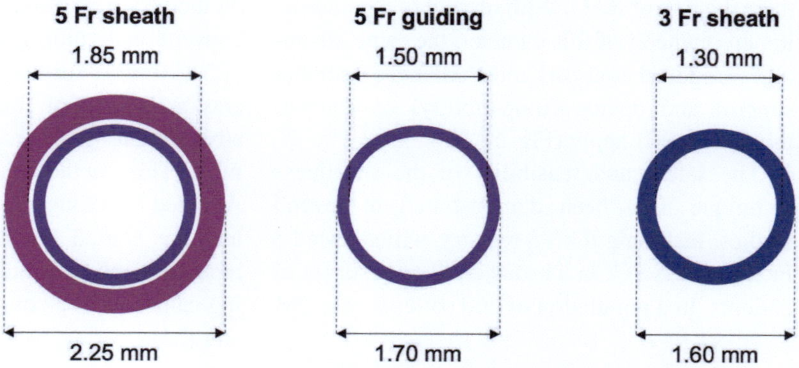

Fig. 18.3 Sheathless 5 Fr ("virtual" 3F) guiding catheter has approximately the same external diameter (1.7 mm) as a 3F introducer sheath

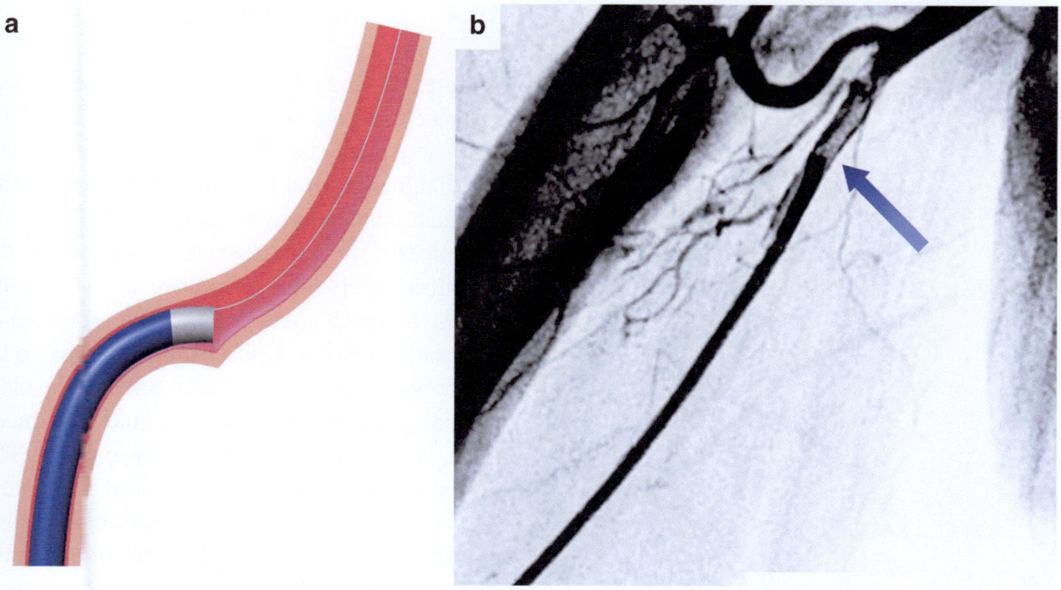

Fig. 18.4 So-called "razor" effect. (**a**) The tip of the guiding catheter scrapes on the arterial wall, (**b**) causing a dissection of the radial artery

reduction in vascular invasiveness without significant issues with device compatibility and therefore changes to the standard procedure [20]. Sheathless 7 Fr could still be used in selected cases, possibly after verification (by vascular ultrasound) of sufficient distal radial artery diameter. Finally, sheathless 5 Fr allows for the maximum reduction of vascular trauma and may be required for very small anatomy [21, 22].

The outer diameter of a sheathless 5 Fr guiding catheter is 1.75 mm, which is compatible with virtually any distal radial artery. Proper hemostasis can often be achieved in less than 1 h after sheathless 5 Fr PCI and without aggressive compression, which is also important to minimize the risk of RAO. With respect to the internal lumen diameter of this catheter, the same advantages (reduced contrast) and challenges (catheter support and device compatibility) of conventional 5 Fr PCI apply (Fig. 18.5).

The safety and feasibility of the sheathless technique have been demonstrated in several studies, including the V3 registry, which tested 5 Fr sheathless PCI in a broad and larger subset of patients. In a population of 260 patients with 361 lesions, this registry reported a procedural success rate of 99.2% with only two failures, both in chronic total occlusion (CTO) procedures. In addition, no adverse events were reported, and the incidence of radial RAO was 0.4% [23]. Furthermore, in a series of 127 patients treated with the latest generation of sheathless guiding catheters, the incidence of RAO was 0% for the 6F and 2.7% for the 7F catheters [24].

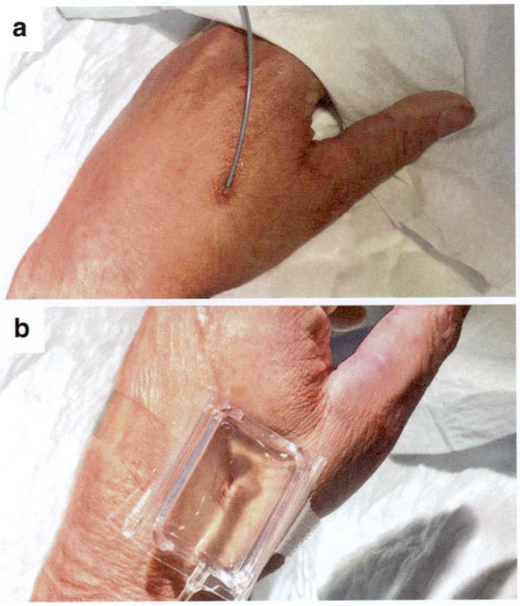

Fig. 18.5 (**a**) "Virtual" 3F PCI performed via distal radial access: the guiding is introduced directly into the vessel after puncture and (**b**) hemostasis achieved by TR Band (Terumo) compression (8 cc of air, 1 h)

Sheathless PCI kits typically consist of a tapered dilator a few centimeters longer than the guiding catheter, a guiding catheter compatible with the dilator, and in some cases a puncture kit. These kits are traditionally made by Japanese manufacturers (Medikit, Asahi). A homemade method for performing sheathless PCI is to use a conventional guiding catheter and inflate a small (1.5–2.0 mm) coronary balloon at its tip, which acts as a kind of dilator, and then insert and advance the guiding catheter onto a coronary wire. This method is known as the Balloon-Assisted Tracking (BAT) technique. In Europe and the United States, a universal dilator has recently become available that allows any guiding catheter to be converted to a sheathless catheter [25].

18.4 Slender Introducers

A more practical option to reduce arterial/inducer mismatch are the so-called "Slender" introducers. These newly developed arterial sheaths have a wall thickness of 0.12 mm, which is much thinner than conventional sheaths (0.20–0.30 mm). This means that the "actual" diameter of the introducer and guide combined is reduced by almost 1 French size, resulting in a reduction in vascular invasiveness. For example, a procedure performed with a 6 Fr guiding catheter, the most common size in daily practice, could be reduced to the invasiveness of a 5 Fr guiding catheter. The availability of Slender introducers in 5, 6, and 7 Fr sizes means that even very small distal radial arteries can be accessed (5 Fr) and complex procedures (7 Fr) can be performed via DRA, at least in selected patients [26].

The first Slender introducer on the market was the Glidesheath Slender (Terumo). The 6 Fr Glidesheath Slender has the same inner diameter as other 6 Fr introducers, but its outer diameter has been reduced to 2.45 mm, which is approximately 0.3 mm smaller than the average outer diameter of previous sheaths (2.74 mm) (Fig. 18.6). The introducer is available in a variety of puncture kits and lengths, all of which are similar to previous products, and both puncture techniques, the "trough-trough" technique and the "anterior wall" technique), can be performed. The color of the hub closest to the insertion valve, as well as the head of the dilator, is green, which is the international standard color for 6 Fr, to emphasize its lumen compatibility. The color of the part closest to the tip side is gray, which is the international standard color for 5 Fr, to emphasize its insertion profile. Accordingly, the 5 Fr version has a gray/red color combination, and the 7 Fr version has an orange/green color combination. These products have been available in Japan since April 2014 and in Europe and worldwide a few years later.

In the first single-center prospective study of 114 consecutive patients, including 35 patients undergoing PCI, manipulation was successful in 113 patients (99.1%). Minor hematoma at the puncture site was observed in six patients (5.2%). Symptomatic radial artery spasm and RAO occurred in five patients (4.4%) and one patient (0.8%), respectively. However, vascular ultrasound follow-up at 1 month after the procedure showed that the radial artery was patent in all patients except the patient with RAO mentioned above [27, 28].

The RAP and BEAT study, which randomized approximately 2000 patients to either a 6 Fr Slender or a 5F conventional introducer, found that the feasibility and safety of the 6 Fr Slender introducers were excellent. However, the incidence of RAO wasn't better than that of conventional 5 Fr introducers (3.4% vs. 1.7%), despite the fact that the outer diameter was almost similar [29].

Furthermore, in the larger DISCO RADIAL trial, in which 1307 patients were randomized to either conventional TRA or DRA, all using 6 Fr Slender introducers, the incidence of RAO was extremely low with DRA (0.3%), but not significantly different from conventional TRA (0.9%) [30]. Finally, when the 6 Fr Glidesheath Slender

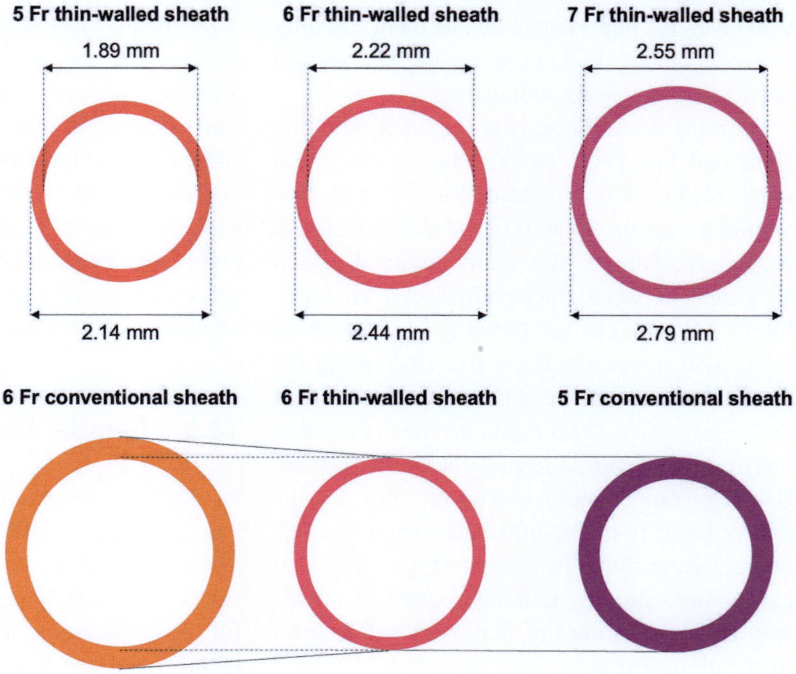

Fig. 18.6 Comparison of the inner and outer diameters of Glidesheath Slender (Terumo, Japan) vs. conventional introducer sheaths. For the 6 Fr sheath, the luminal diameter does not change, but the outer diameter is reduced to 2.44 mm, which is approximately 0.3 mm smaller than the average outer diameter (2.74 mm) of a conventional sheath

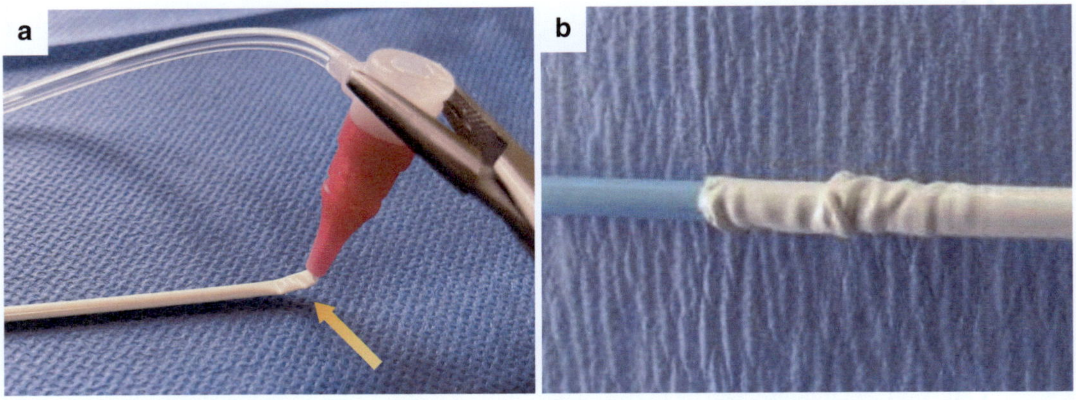

Fig. 18.7 (**a**) Kinking of a Glidesheath Slender introducer; this tends to occur at the junction of the shaft and hub and (**b**) wrinkling as a result of friction during sheath insertion

was compared to a 6.5 Fr sheathless guiding catheter with a similar outer diameter, the sheathless technique showed slightly better results in terms of both RAO and severe radial spasm (0% vs. 2.0%) [31].

These results suggest that the traumatic process leading to RAO is multifactorial, not just related to the diameter of the entry hole, and while the ease of a Slender introducer is obvious, sheathless catheters may have an advantage in reducing overall vascular trauma. In addition, because Slender introducers have a much thinner wall layer, it's important to handle them carefully to avoid damage (kinking, wrinkling, dislodging) during insertion and manipulation.

Kinking usually occurs at the junction of the shaft and hub (Fig. 18.7a) when a maximum angle of 30–40% is exceeded and can be prevented by taping the hub to the skin during the procedure. Due to the blunt angle at which kinking is expected, these introducers are absolutely not suitable for femoral use. However, DRA also poses a serious risk of kinking for Slender introducers because the angle between the distal and forearm radial arteries is close to the limit of what this introducer can withstand. Kinking can sometimes occur due to the reduced ability of the introducer shaft to overcome longitudinal resistance (Fig. 18.7b). It can be prevented by making a small skin incision and lubricating the shaft with saline prior to sheath insertion.

Unfortunately, in order to maximize the inner lumen diameter, most newer guidewire catheters are slightly larger than their predecessors. The outer coating has also become thicker and more evenly distributed. Both of these developments have increased the friction between the guiding catheter and the introducer. Combined with the lubricity of the Glidesheath Slender, this can cause the introducer to dislodge during manipulation of the guiding catheter. This problem can be avoided by taping the introducer (or its side port) during the procedure.

While the Glidesheath Slender was the first of its kind and was a significant breakthrough for Slender operators, other manufacturers have since developed similar products, focusing on addressing the limitations of the original device. For example, the RAIN sheath (Cordis) appears to have solved the kinking problems by using a proprietary material without sacrificing the thinner wall properties and promises to be a viable competitor to the Glidesheath Slender.

18.5 Slender Devices

As the inner lumen of the guiding catheter narrows, device compatibility may become an issue. With 5 Fr guiding catheters, most PCI procedures can be successfully performed. This is very useful for DRA. Some techniques, such as kissing balloon and crushing stent techniques, require additional lumen for the multiple devices used. To overcome these limitations, the devices themselves should be further miniaturized. The list of devices with 5 Fr compatibility, a feature once considered necessary to claim a Slender "quality" label, is growing by the day. All drug-eluting stents, all compliant and semi-compliant balloons (even in the larger sizes), and all microcatheters are now 5 Fr compatible. Among the specialty balloons, non-compliant balloons (except OPN NC balloons), and intravascular lithotripsy balloons [32], scoring balloons are also 5 Fr compatible. Rotational atherectomy burrs up to 1.5 mm diameter are 5 Fr compatible, while orbital atherectomy catheters are not. Intravascular ultrasound probes are 5 Fr compatible only when electronically (not mechanically) rotated. Strictly speaking, optical coherence tomography catheters are also 5 Fr compatible, but this is not recommended because contrast flushing is suboptimal when using 5 Fr guiding catheters.

In fact, many 5 Fr-compatible interventional products have been incorporated into daily practice in such a way that they are no longer referred to as Slender. Of course, downsized devices can also be used with 6 Fr or larger catheters, as contrast injection and device manipulation are even easier.

As the bar continues to get smaller, a few outstanding devices deserve special recognition. One is an ultrathin angioplasty balloon (Kaneka) that can be advanced on a 0.010″ guidewire instead of the standard 0.014″. Thus, the overall thickness of the system is thinner, the crossing profile of the balloon is smaller, and two such balloons can be accommodated in a 5 Fr guiding catheter, allowing, for example, the kissing balloon technique [33].

Sometimes operators do not feel comfortable using 5 Fr guiding catheters for fear of not being able to manage potential complications. For example, coronary perforation is a life-threatening complication that can occur in any procedure, but more commonly in complex procedures (heavily calcified lesions and/or chronic total occlusions), and requires immediate treatment with a covered stent. Until recently, covered stents were either 6 Fr or 7 Fr compatible due to their "sandwich" structure consisting of two metal scaffolds and a layer of polyurethane. More recently, 5 Fr-compatible covered stents have become available, such as the BeGraft (Bentley) or the PK Papyrus (Biotronik). In particular, the PK Papyrus-covered stent consists of a single ultrathin (60 μm) cobalt chromium strut covered on the abluminal side with an electrospun polyurethane matrix. Its crossing profile is 1.25 mm, and it is 5 Fr compatible up to size 4.0. Its safety and efficacy have been shown to be excellent [34].

Finally, a very innovative device specifically designed for Slender PCI is the Slender Integrated Delivery System (IDS) (Svelte Medical): this stent delivery system incorporates the coronary wire directly onto the shaft of the balloon. By eliminating the need for an internal lumen for the guidewire, the overall system crossing profile is reduced to the lowest currently available (0.031″) (Fig. 18.8). The Slender IDS mounts a sirolimus-eluting stent with thin cobalt chromium struts that can be delivered not only with 5 Fr guiding catheters but even with 4 Fr catheters. Furthermore, this device allows the crushing stenting technique with both 5 Fr and 6 Fr guid-

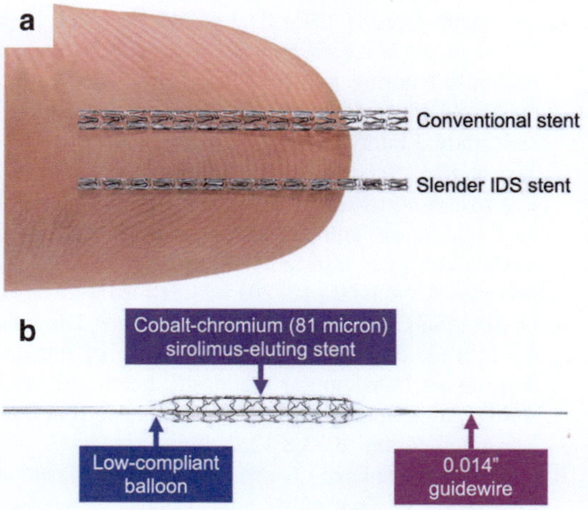

Fig. 18.8 (**a**) When crimped onto the balloon, the Slender IDS (Svelte Medical) sirolimus-eluting stent has the lowest crossing profile (0.031″) available. (**b**) The delivery system consists of a semi-compliant balloon, a cobalt-chromium (81 micron) sirolimus-eluting stent, and a 0.014″ wire, soldered directly to the tip of the balloon

ing catheters [35]. Safety and clinical efficacy were demonstrated in the OPTIMIZE trial, in which the vast majority of patients were treated by TRA with direct stent implantation and excellent results were achieved [36].

References

1. Kiemeneij F, Laarman GJ. Percutaneous transradial artery approach for coronary stent implantation. Catheter Cardiovasc Diagn. 1993;30:173–8.
2. Neumann FJ, Sousa-Uva M, Ahlsson A, Alfonso F, Banning AP, Benedetto U, et al. ESC/EACTS Guidelines on myocardial revascularization. Eur Heart. 2018;40(2):87–165.
3. Lawton JS, Tamis-Holland JE, Bangalore S, Bates ER, Beckie TM, Bischoff JM, et al. 2021 ACC/AHA/SCAI guideline for coronary artery revascularization: a report of the American College of Cardiology/American Heart Association Joint Committee on clinical practice guidelines. J Am Coll Cardiol. 2022;79:e21–e129.
4. Kotowycz MA, Johnston KW, Ivanov J, Asif N, Almoghairi AM, Choudhury A, et al. Predictors of radial artery size in patients undergoing cardiac catheterization: insights from the Good Radial Artery Size Prediction (GRASP) study. Can J Cardiol. 2014;30:211–6.
5. Saito S, Ikei H, Hosokawa G, Tanaka S. Influence of the ratio between radial artery inner diameter and sheath outer diameter on radial artery flow after transradial coronary intervention. Catheter Cardiovasc Interv. 1999;46:173–8.
6. Gwon HC, Doh JH, Choi JH, Lee SH, Hong KP, Park JE, et al. A 5Fr catheter approach reduces patient discomfort during transradial coronary intervention compared with a 6Fr approach: a prospective randomized study. J Interv Cardiol. 2006;19:141–7.
7. Zwaan EM, Koopman AG, Holtzer CA, Zijlstra F, Ritt MJ, Amoroso G, et al. Revealing the impact of local access-site complications and upper extremity dysfunction post transradial percutaneous coronary procedures. Neth Heart J. 2015;23:514–24.
8. Di Serafino L, Pyxaras SA, Mangiacapra F, Dierickx K, Toth G, Bartunek J, et al. Influence of transradial versus transfemoral diagnostic heart catheterisation on peripheral vascular endothelial function. EuroIntervention. 2013;8:1252–8.
9. Ikari Y, Matsukage T, Yoshimachi F, Masutani M, Saito S. Transradial and slender percutaneous coronary intervention: less invasive strategy in PCI. Cardiovasc Interv Ther. 2010;25:60–4.
10. Kiemeneij F, Yoshimachi F, Matsukage T, Amoroso G, Fraser D, Claessen BE, et al. Focus on maximal miniaturisation of transradial coronary access materials and techniques by the Slender Club Japan and Europe: an overview and classification. EuroIntervention. 2015;10:1178–86.
11. Kiemeneij F. Left distal transradial access in the anatomical snuffbox for coronary angiography (ldTRA) and interventions (ldTRI). EuroIntervention. 2017;13:851–7.
12. Lee JW, Park SW, Son JW, Ahn SG, Lee SH. Real-world experience of the left distal transradial approach for coronary angiography and percutaneous coronary intervention: a prospective observational study (LeDRA). EuroIntervention. 2018;14:e995–1003.
13. Grossman PM, Gurm HS, McNamara R, Lalonde T, Changezi H, Share D, et al. Percutaneous coronary intervention complications and guide catheter size: bigger is not better. JACC Cardiovasc Interv. 2009;2:636–44.
14. Dahm JB, Vogelesang D, Hummel A, Staudt A, Volzke H, Felix SB. A randomized trial of 5 vs. 6 French transradial percutaneous coronary interventions. Catheter Cardiovasc Interv. 2002;57:172–6.
15. Lefevre T, Morice MC, Bonan R, Dumas P, Louvard Y, Karrillon G, et al. Coronary angiography using 4 or 6 French diagnostic catheters: a prospective, randomized study. J Invasive Cardiol. 2001;13:674–7.
16. Kaluski E, Moussa ID, Heuser RR, Kern MJ, Weisz G, Klapholz M, et al. Automated contrast injectors for angiography: devices, methodology, and safety. Catheter Cardiovasc Interv. 2009;74:459–64.
17. Chahoud G, Khoukaz S, El-Shafei A, Azrak E, Bitar S, Kern MJ. Randomized comparison of coronary angiography using 4F catheters: 4F manual versus "Acisted" power injection technique. Catheter Cardiovasc Interv. 2001;53:221–4.
18. Takeshita S, Tanaka S, Saito S. Coronary intervention with 4-French catheters. Catheter Cardiovasc Interv. 2010;75:735–9.
19. Mamas M, D'Souza S, Hendry C, Ali R, Iles-Smith H, Palmer K, et al. Use of the sheathless guide catheter during routine transradial percutaneous coronary intervention: a feasibility study. Catheter Cardiovasc Interv. 2010;75:596–602.
20. Yoshimachi F, Torii S, Naito T. A novel percutaneous coronary intervention technique for chronic total occlusion: Contralateral angiography with a single guiding catheter. Catheter Cardiovasc Interv. 2016;87:E229–32.
21. Takeshita S, Saito S. Transradial coronary intervention using a novel 5-Fr sheathless guiding catheter. Catheter Cardiovasc Interv. 2009;74:862–5.
22. Amoroso G, van Dullemen A, Westgeest P, van Duinen M. "Virtual" 3 Fr transradial coronary stenting with the 5 Fr Meito Masamune sheathless guiding catheter: feasibility and safety in an outpatient setting. J Invasive Cardiol. 2016;28:109–14.
23. Yoshimachi F, Takagawa Y, Terai H, Takahashi A, Shimada Y, Katsuki T, et al. The V3 registry investigators. A prospective multicenter study using a Virtual 3 Fr percutaneous coronary intervention system: the V3 registry. J Invasive Cardiol. 2017;29:16–23.

24. Isawa T, Horie K, Tada N, Toyoda S. Initial experience with a novel sheathless guiding catheter (hyperion SheathLess) for transradial coronary intervention. J Invasive Cardiol. 2022;34:E490–5.
25. Colletti G, Auslender J, De Meester A, Aminian A, Kayaert P, Ungureanu C. Feasibility and safety of performing complex coronary interventions by distal radial artery using the railway sheathless vascular system. J Invasive Cardiol. 2020;32:459–62.
26. Ashraf T, Panhwar Z, Habib S, Memon MA, Shamsi F, Arif J. Size of radial and ulnar artery in local population. J Pak Med Assoc. 2010;60:817–9.
27. Aminian A, Dolatabadi D, Lefebvre P, Zimmerman R, Brunner P, Michalakis G, et al. Initial experience with the Glidesheath Slender for transradial coronary angiography and intervention: a feasibility study with prospective radial ultrasound follow-up. Catheter Cardiovasc Interv. 2014;84:436–42.
28. Yoshimachi F, Kiemeneij F, Masutani M, Matsukage T, Takahashi A, Ikari Y. Safety and feasibility of the new 5 Fr Glidesheath Slender. Cardiovasc Interv Ther. 2016;31:38–41.
29. Aminian A, Saito S, Takahashi A, Bernat I, Jobe RL, Kajiya T, et al. Comparison of a new slender 6 Fr sheath with a standard 5 Fr sheath for transradial coronary angiography and intervention: RAP and BEAT (Radial artery patency and bleeding, efficacy, adverse evenT), a randomised multicentre trial. EuroIntervention. 2017;13:e549–56.
30. Aminian A, Sgueglia GA, Wiemer M, Kefer J, Gasparini GL, Ruzsa Z, et al. Distal versus conventional radial access for coronary angiography and intervention: the DISCO RADIAL trial. JACC Cardiovasc Interv. 2022;15:1191–201.
31. Horie K, Tada N, Isawa T, Matsumoto T, Taguri M, Kato S, et al. A randomized comparison of incidence of radial artery occlusion and symptomatic radial artery spasm associated with elective transradial coronary intervention using 6.5-Fr Sheathless Eaucath guiding catheter vs. 6.0-Fr glidesheath slender. EuroIntervention. 2018;13:2018–25.
32. Sgueglia GA, Gioffrè G, Piccioni F, Gaspardone A. Slender distal radial five French coronary shockwave lithotripsy. Catheter Cardiovasc Interv. 2019;94:395–8.
33. Matsukage T, Masutani M, Yoshimachi F, Takahashi A, Katsuki T, Saito S, et al. A prospective multicenter registry of 0.010- inch guidewire and compatible system for chronic total occlusion: the PIKACHU registry. Catheter Cardiovasc Interv. 2010;75:1006–12.
34. Kandzari DE, Sarao RC, Waksman R. Clinical experience of the PK Papyrus covered stent in patients with coronary artery perforations: results from a multi-center humanitarian device exemption survey. Cardiovasc Revasc Med. 2022;43:97–101.
35. Verheye S, Khattab AA, Carrie D, Stella P, Slagboom T, Bartunek J, et al. Direct implantation of rapamycin-eluting stents with bioresorbable drug carrier technology utilising the Svelte coronary stent-on-a-wire: the DIRECT II study. EuroIntervention. 2016;12:e615–22.
36. Kereiakes DJ, Feldman RL, Ijsselmuiden AJJ, Saito S, Amoroso G, Zidar JP, et al. Safety and effectiveness of the SVELTE fixed-wire and rapid exchange bioresorbable- polymer sirolimus-eluting coronary stent systems for the treatment of atherosclerotic lesions: results of the OPTIMIZE randomized study. Circ Cardiovasc Interv. 2021;14:e010609.

19 Sheathless Methods

Stefan Harb and Giuseppe Colletti

19.1 Introduction

The vessels of the human cardiovascular system are organized according to a fractal geometry. Their sizes correlate with the volume of blood transported, and at bifurcations they decrease in size according to a predetermined set of statistical properties as described by Finet et al. [1, 2].

When gaining invasive access to the cardiovascular system, it' is important to choose an access site where the vessel can accommodate the devices that are planned to be used. The access site should be situated above a bony structure such as the femoral head [3] or the radius to allow for carefully dosed compression that remains the gold standard for achieving patent hemostasis, as vascular closure devices, despite their wide availability, cannot prevent rare but serious and potentially fatal bleeding complications [4]. In fact, the smaller the vessel, the easier it is to achieve hemostasis with compression alone.

As interventional devices have evolved and become smaller over time, a shift from traditional femoral access to the safer and more convenient transradial access (TRA) has become possible. And today, with the advent of distal radial access (DRA), we are on the verge of yet another reduction in vessel size for cardiovascular catheterization (Fig. 19.1).

However, despite the amazing miniaturization of our devices, we still need enough space in our guiding catheters to maneuver them safely, especially in complex scenarios. Avoiding the introducer sheath, the so-called sheathless approach, is an effective strategy to take advantage of a larger inner lumen while preserving the vessel integrity by reducing the overall outer diameter to arterial lumen ratio (Fig. 19.2).

S. Harb (✉)
University Heart Center, Medical University of Graz, Graz, Austria

G. Colletti
Cardiovascular Department, Clinique Saint Joseph, Arlon, Belgium

G. A. Sgueglia (ed.), *Distal Radial Access*, https://doi.org/10.1007/978-3-031-89925-6_19

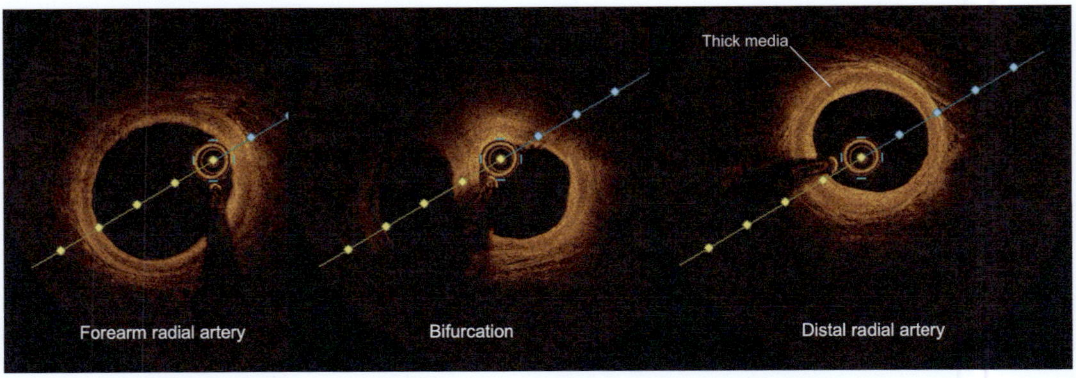

Fig. 19.1 Optical coherence tomography images of the radial artery at the wrist level (left), of its bifurcation with superficial palmar branch and distal radial artery (middle), and of the distal radial artery (right); the prominent media is noticeable suggesting a high potential for spasm; Finet's law would roughly apply in this example: forearm radial diameter is about 3.5 mm, and the diameters of the two vessels seen in the bifurcation are about 2 mm and 2.5 mm and actually (2 + 2.5) × 0.678 is about 3.05, but as can be guessed from the thick media, functional state makes diameters vary widely

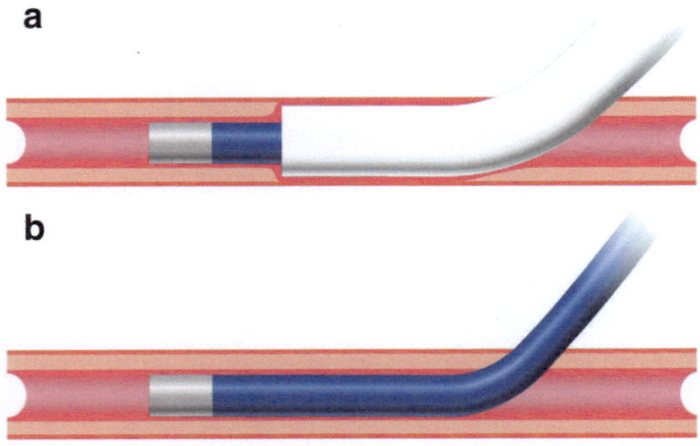

Fig. 19.2 (**a**) In a small radial artery, the use of an introducer sheath may damage the vessel wall. (**b**) Sheathless approach is an effective strategy to take advantage of a larger inner lumen while preserving the vessel integrity by reducing the overall outer diameter to arterial lumen ratio

19.2 Anatomical Features Favoring a Sheathless Approach in Distal Radial Access

There are fundamental geometric differences in the anatomical course of the radial artery at its conventional and distal puncture sites that may be relevant to the arterial access. In conventional TRA, the needle entry angle to the skin is approximately the same as the entry angle to the artery. However, in the anatomical snuffbox, the artery runs from dorsal to palmar and follows the round dorsal shape of the scaphoid bone, approaching the skin layer first before diving deeper again, so the entry angle to the artery can vary greatly depending on which of its "uphill," "hilltop," or "downhill" tracts is being punctured (Fig. 19.3). The entry angle also depends on the flexion, abduction, and grip position of the hand, which is actually used to stretch the artery and bring it closer to the skin level. In the anatomical snuffbox, with the needle oriented medially and with an entry angle to the skin of 30–45°, access to the artery is more coaxial (Fig. 19.4). Although DRA may be more complex to perform compared to conventional TRA, we speculate that the more coaxial access to the artery may significantly contribute to reduce complications related to mechanical factors such as bleeding due to tearing at the arteriotomy or intimal dissection when the needle tip touches the posterior wall.

Another important morphologic difference between the forearm and distal radial arteries is its size according to the fractal geometry of our vascular system [5–11]. Sex is independently associated with vessel diameter, with men having larger vessels compared to women (Table 19.1) [5, 7].

This is important because in conventional TRA, the sheath-to-artery ratio is an independent predictor of radial artery occlusion (RAO), radial

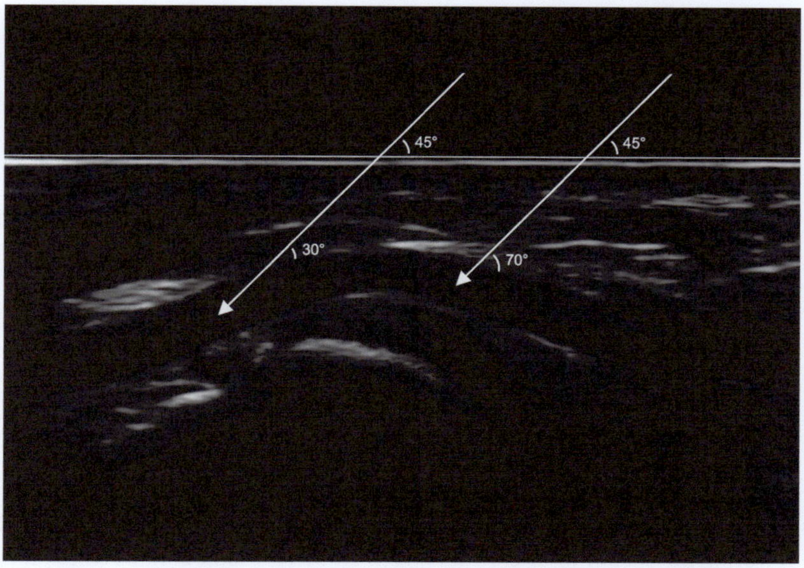

Fig. 19.3 Given the curvilinear course of the distal radial artery, the same angle of entry to the skin corresponds to a different angle of entry to the artery

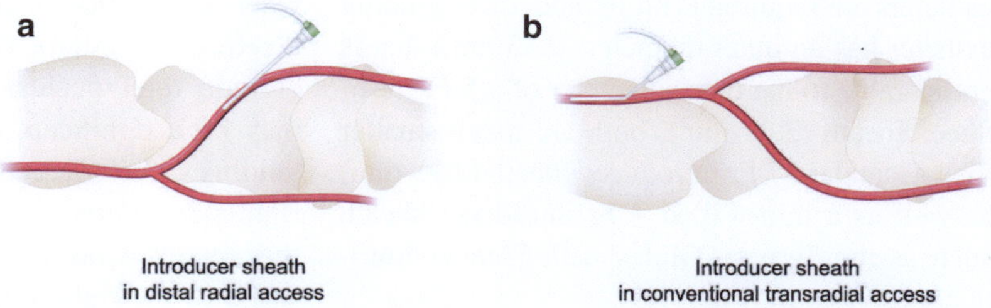

Fig. 19.4 (**a**) Distal radial artery puncture in the anatomical snuffbox allows for more coaxial insertion of the introducer sheath compared to (**b**) radial artery puncture at the wrist level

Table 19.1 Radial artery diameter at conventional and distal puncture sites

Study	Year	Country	Wrist RA diameter (mm)	Distal RA diameter (mm)
Kim et al. [5]	2018	South Korea		2.57 ± 0.50 65 ± 0.46 (male) 2.40 ± 0.53 (female)
Lee et al. [6]	2018	South Korea	3.06 ± 0.54 (left) 3.07 ± 0.48 (right)	2.41 ± 0.50 (left) 2.36 ± 049 (right)
Naito et al. [7]	2019	Japan	2.62 ± 0.60	2.04 ± 0.43 2.04 ± 0.60 (male) 1.96 ± 0.44 (female)
Norimatsu et al. [8]	2019	Japan	3.1 ± 0.4	2.6 ± 0.5
Hadjivassiliou et al. [9]	2020	Canada	2.55 ± 0.39	2.34 ± 0.36
Mizuguchi et al. [10]	2020	Japan	2.7 ± 0.5	2.4 ± 0.5
Yu et al. [11]	2020	China	2.13 ± 0.6	1.71 ± 0.5

RA radial artery

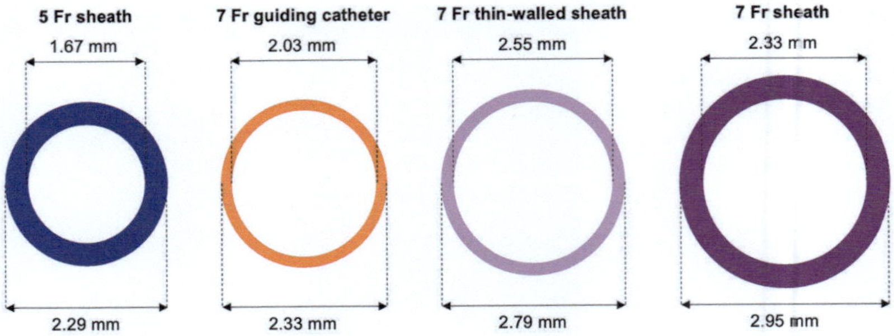

Fig. 19.5 Outer and inner diameters of various introducer sheaths and a 7 Fr guiding catheter, showing that a 5 Fr sheath and a 7 Fr sheath are comparable. (Reproduced from Colletti et al. [18])

artery spasm, and forearm access site complications [12–15].

Attaining a lower device-to-artery ratio may be less achievable with DRA. If thin-walled sheath technology has had a positive impact on lowering the sheath-to-artery ratio [16, 17], there is a great additional potential for a sheathless approach, especially when larger-bore guiding catheters are required [18]. In fact, a 7 Fr guiding catheter has an outer diameter (2.33 mm) that is comparable to the outer diameter of a 5 Fr introducer sheath (2.29 mm); both are much smaller than a standard 7 Fr introducer sheath (2.95 mm) as well as a thin-walled 7 Fr introducer sheath such as the Terumo Glidesheath Slender introducer (2.79 mm) (Fig. 19.5).

In addition, the absence of a sheath may provide greater stability to the overall system once the target coronary ostium has been cannulated. Because the sheathless guiding catheter tends to anchor to the entry site in the skin, especially as the area dries, it reduces the overall risk of losing position throughout the procedure, primarily by minimizing the sliding motion that can occur in an introducer sheath.

In patients undergoing transradial percutaneous coronary intervention (PCI), sheathless approach with a dedicated 6.5 Fr guiding catheter system was associated with a lower incidence of radial artery occlusion and radial artery spasm in a randomized comparison with a 6 Fr thin-walled introducer sheath/guiding catheter combination [19]. No differences in vascular injury were observed in a prospective study comparing the use of a 7 Fr sheathless approach (a 90 cm 7 Fr guiding catheter advanced over a 100 cm 6 Fr multipurpose catheter used as a dilatator) with the use of a 6 Fr introducer sheath/guiding catheter combination [20].

Sheathless approach may potentially allow for a more successful coronary cannulation because the guide can be inserted deeper into the skin compared to an approach through a sheath. This may well compensate for the greater distance of the DRA, especially in taller patients or when using a 90-cm guiding catheter to advance a retrograde microcatheter in the treatment of chronic total occlusion (CTO) lesions. There may be a significant difference in the required guiding catheter length between the left- and the right-side approaches. In the left-sided approach, the vessels tend to be straighter and shorter, while in the right-sided approach, the pathway tends to be more tortuous and consequently longer.

19.3 Development of the Sheathless Approach

Vascular access without a sheath was the first method used for arterial catheterization, as sheaths had not yet been invented.

Initially, access was obtained using Sone's cut-down approach, which involved arteriotomy and selective preparation of the vessel, usually the distal brachial artery, surrounding it with rubber tubes for clamping, puncture, wiring, careful incision, and catheter insertion. Sutures were used for hemostasis, and scar tissue hindered easy re-access.

Later, the Seldinger technique was introduced [21, 22]. This involved percutaneous puncture of the artery with a needle to insert a guidewire, and after a proper nick and some preparation with a hemostat, a bare catheter was twisted in over the guidewire. Trauma to the entry site was unavoidable. Pigtail catheters, with their tapered tips, were used to fill the space between larger guides and the guidewire to reduce this trauma. Compression was required to achieve hemostasis, a time-consuming maneuver responsible for additional local trauma with potential complications, too.

After the invention of the hemostatic valve, working through a sheath was widely adopted, and the femoral artery became the access site of choice. The increase in diameter with the addition of the sheath did not seem to be a problem compared to the convenience of easy access, rapid catheter exchange, and avoidance of troublesome back bleeding. At the time, 6 Fr was considered a small caliber. Because the sheath and its dilator usually had a smooth transition, vascular trauma was reduced, and bleeding complications were fewer but still common [23].

As radial access became popular to reduce such bleeding complications, the smaller vessel size led to further miniaturization of the devices. While 5 Fr and even 4 Fr catheters were sufficient for angiography, conventional balloons and stents for PCI still required at least a 6 Fr guiding catheter. The revival of the sheathless approach effectively reduced the outer diameter while maintaining the same inner lumen of the catheter.

More recently, thin-walled sheaths have become an option to reduce the outer diameter and still benefit from the advantages of sheath and hemostatic valve. Nevertheless, the sheathless approach offers a significantly lower ratio of outer diameter to arterial lumen [24].

As proponents of radial access have traditionally sought to reduce vascular injury, a wealth of knowledge has been gained from conventional TRA that can be applied to DRA [25]. Special techniques have been developed to facilitate guide passage through the small and angulated vessels of the upper extremity: pigtail-assisted tracking [26] and balloon-assisted tracking (BAT) [27] have helped avoid the "razor effect" that poses a risk to the endothelium, especially when larger-bore guiding catheters are required. Indeed, symptomatic occlusion of a coronary artery by a strip of arterial intima scratched by the exposed tip of a guiding catheter advancing through a radial artery spasm has been reported [28].

Today, computed tomography angiography can detect excessive angulations, anomalies, and occlusions of upper extremity arteries, and vascular ultrasound can help assess the course and size of the vessel at the access site and avoid puncturing calcified segments, thereby increasing successful access rates. Remarkably, this information is available non-invasively and prior to the procedure, allowing a more targeted and efficient approach through careful planning of the procedures, selection of the appropriate access site and guiding catheters, which, especially in complex procedures, can optimize performance at the coronary level and minimize complications.

19.4 The Evolving Need for Large-Bore Catheters

According to the fractal principle of vessel geometry, it is safer to access a smaller distal vessel for any PCI. However, this must be balanced with the need for space in the guiding catheter to accommodate the tools needed for PCI, which are usually a combination of the following: guidewires, balloons, stents, an imaging probe, and some specialty devices such as laser catheters, lithotripsy balloons, and tools for orbital and rotational atherectomy.

And it is always necessary to keep in mind a strategy for unexpected emergencies that may require rapid delivery of rescue tools to the coronary intervention site, i.e., perfusion balloons and covered stents, so that a safety margin of available space in the guiding catheter must be considered.

Finally, in advanced interventional procedures such as complex, high-risk, and indicated (CHIP) or CTO cases, we need further additional space in the guiding to accommodate tools such as anchor balloons, trapping balloons, guide extensions, dual-lumen microcatheters, or combinations of tools, for instance, an intravascular ultrasound (IVUS) probe and a dual-lumen microcatheter as in the slipstream IVUS technique [29], which allows imaging-guided access to lumina of chronically occluded arteries with blunt stumps or flush ostial occlusions where angiography does not provide sufficient information.

To simplify the procedure and ensure timely success, but also to provide a safety margin for possible emergencies, sufficient "interventional space" is required, i.e., sufficient space in the guiding catheter lumen to accommodate the required devices. A good knowledge of the exact size of different devices can help plan a complex PCI and choose an appropriate combination of devices to avoid lack of "interventional space" in the middle of the procedure.

There are several ways to achieve sufficient "interventional space": (1) add catheters (ping-pong technique) [30], (2) adjust strategy [31], and (3) upsize guiding catheters. These strategies must take into account the patient's vascular anatomy and the bleeding risk associated with larger-bore or additional guiding catheters [32].

19.5 Dedicated Sheathless Systems

19.5.1 Eaucath

The sheathless Eaucath (Asahi) is a dedicated sheathless guiding catheter system consisting of a vessel dilator tapered onto a 0.035-inch guidewire and a dedicated guiding catheter with a reinforced wall that provides excellent support and torqueability and is responsible for a 0.5 Fr larger outer diameter as compared to the corresponding conventional guiding catheter size (Fig. 19.6). The dedicated guiding catheter is available with a variety of shapes and three sizes from 6.5 to 8.5 Fr, although with an outer diameter that compares favorably to the next smaller introducer sheaths (Fig. 19.6).

The inner dilator is screwed into the proprietary guide with a Luer lock providing a reliable and constant distance between the dilator tip and the guiding catheter tip, optimizing the transition between the two, facilitating entry through the skin, and also facilitating advancement through artery angulations on the pathway to the ascending aorta. The catheter has a hydrophilic coating that further enhances its trackability and reduces the incidence of radial artery spasm during catheter manipulation.

It is a common practice to insert a small introducer sheath (Fig. 19.7a), advance a 0.035″ guidewire, and then remove the sheath while applying gentle pressure over the entry site to avoid unnecessary bleeding (Fig. 19.7b). With one clockwise rotation, the vessel dilator is docked with the Eaucath guiding catheter, and both are advanced over the 0.035″ guidewire into the artery while activating the hydrophilic coating with a wet gauze (Fig. 19.7c). When the vessel dilator and the guiding catheter have reached the ascending aorta, the vessel dilator is removed (Fig. 19.7d). After coronary artery cannulation, the proximal end of the guiding catheter may be secured with an adhesive dressing.

The tip of the dilator is not visible on fluoroscopy, so care must be taken to avoid damaging the artery when the guidewire is not sufficiently protruding. With advanced skill, the shape of the guide can be modified by varying the position of the dilator, which may be helpful in approaching an anomalous coronary ostium, always taking care to advance the guidewire distally to prevent damage to the vessel (Fig. 19.8).

19.5.2 Railway

The Railway Sheathless Access System (Cordis) consists of two different long vessel dilators compatible with a 0.021″ and a 0.035″ guidewire, respectively. They are available in 5 to 7 Fr versions to be compatible with any existing guiding catheters, allowing the use of preferred catheters. The kit includes two arterial puncture systems, one bare needle with short bevel and one cannula-over-needle, and a 45 cm long 0.021″ guidewire. The dilators have a lubricious hydrophilic coating in their distal 20 cm and provide a guidewire port at the appropriate distance from the tip for use with the short access guidewire.

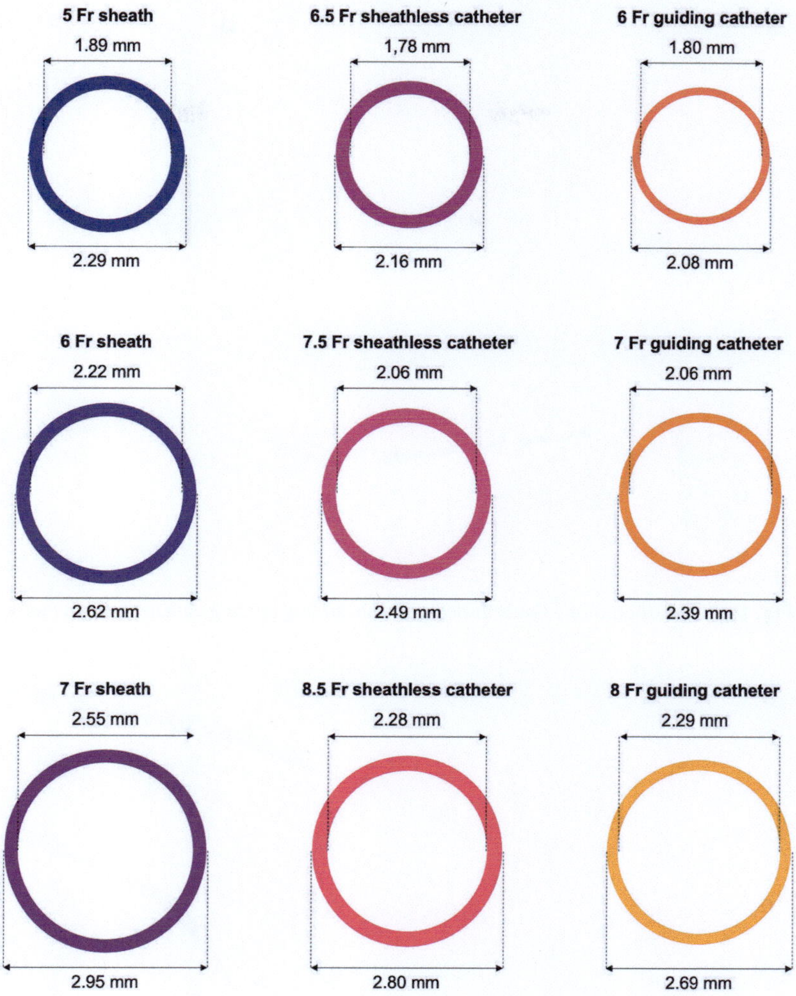

Fig. 19.6 Outer and inner diameters of the Eaucath-dedicated sheathless guiding catheters showing that each has a 0.5 Fr larger outer diameter as compared to the corresponding conventional guiding catheter size yet comparing favorably to the next smaller introducer sheath

The system is designed to facilitate sheathless percutaneous delivery of a guiding catheter from the skin through the subcutaneous tissue into the vessel by eliminating the so-called razor effect through a smooth, atraumatic transition between the tip of the guiding catheter and the tapered dilator. In addition to allowing sheathless access of a guiding catheter, it also improves arterial trackability [33], thus facilitating crossing of complex anatomy [34].

Each of the two vessel dilators in the kit has a different use. The 0.021″ dilator is used to obtain a sheathless access upfront for elective PCI and does not require any device other than those included in the kit. The 0.035″-compatible dilator allows for quick exchange of guiding catheters as well as conversion to a larger-bore sheathless technique after the initial use of a small introducer sheath.

In the upfront sheathless technique for elective PCI cases, the distal radial artery is punctured with one of the two needles supplied with the system. It is recommended that a scalpel be used to make a superficial skin nick at the selected puncture site. The cannula-over-needle is actually more convenient as it allows injection of the spasmolytic cocktail and, if necessary, contrast media, prior to guiding catheter advancement (Fig. 19.9a). On the other hand, the bare needle can ensure selective puncture of the anterior wall of the small artery and safely avoid painful contact with the periosteum of the underlying bone, especially when ultrasound guidance is used. Therefore, the 0.021″ guidewire is advanced, and

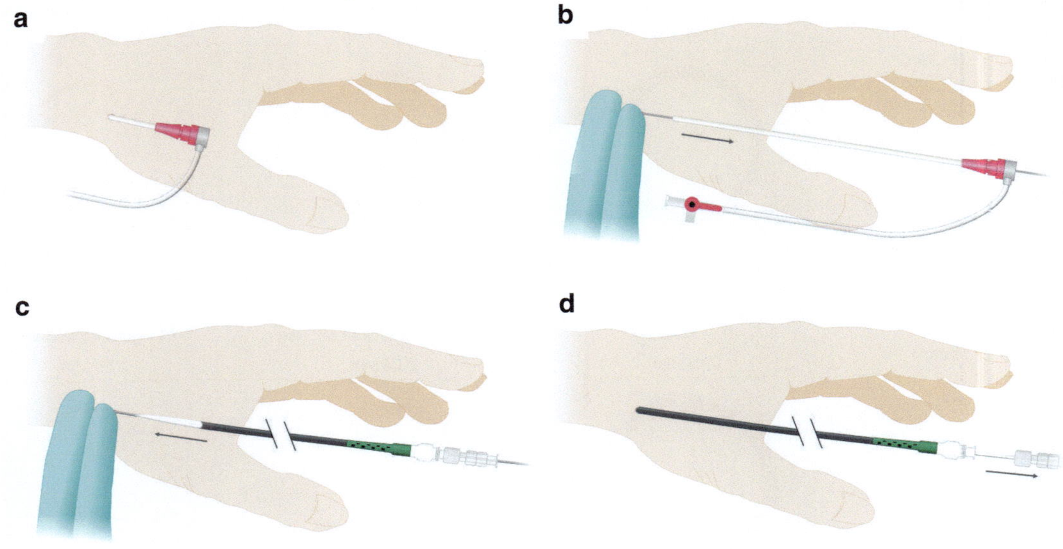

Fig. 19.7 Insertion of the Eaucath-dedicated sheathless guiding catheter system (see text for details)

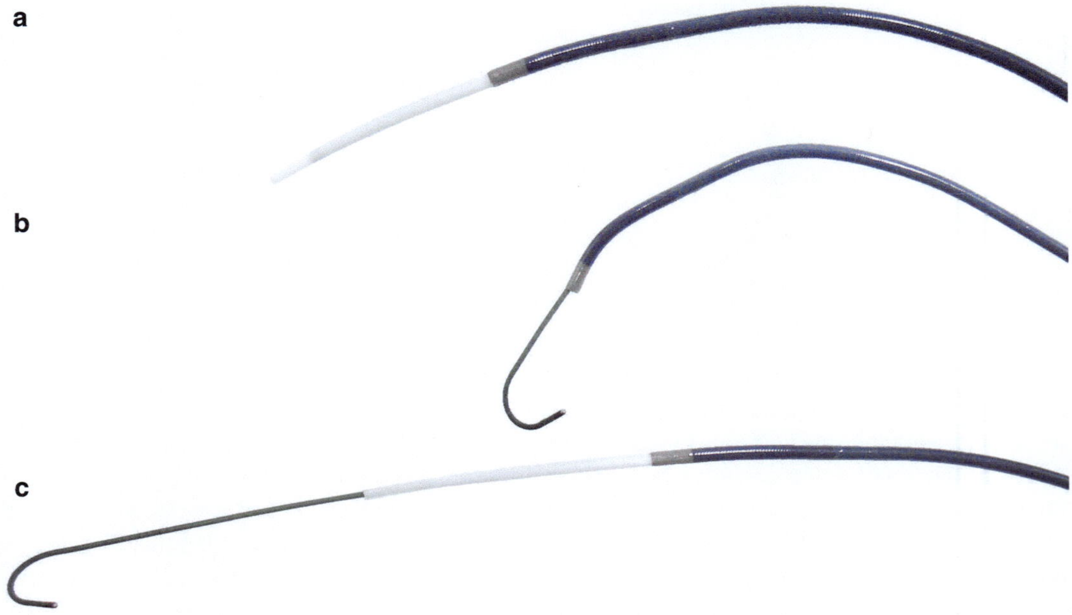

Fig. 19.8 Options for changing the shape of a guide tip by different longitudinal positioning of dilator to help in engaging the coronary ostia in unusual anatomy, keeping in mind that the dilator tip is not radiopaque and must always be protected by a protruding wire to prevent vessel damage

the cannula or the bare needle is removed while applying gentle pressure over the entry site to avoid unnecessary bleeding (Fig. 19.9b). The properly flushed 0.021″ compatible Railway vessel dilator can then be advanced through the skin over the 0.021″ guidewire until the guidewire side port is within approximately 3 cm from the puncture site (Fig. 19.9c). The 0.021″ guidewire can then be removed (Fig. 19.9d), and the guiding catheter can be advanced through the skin

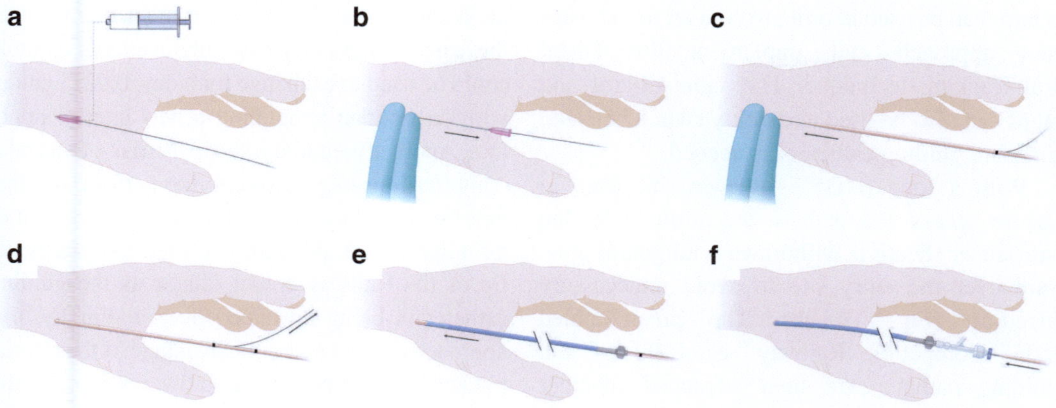

Fig. 19.9 Upfront sheathless approach with the Railway system (see text for details)

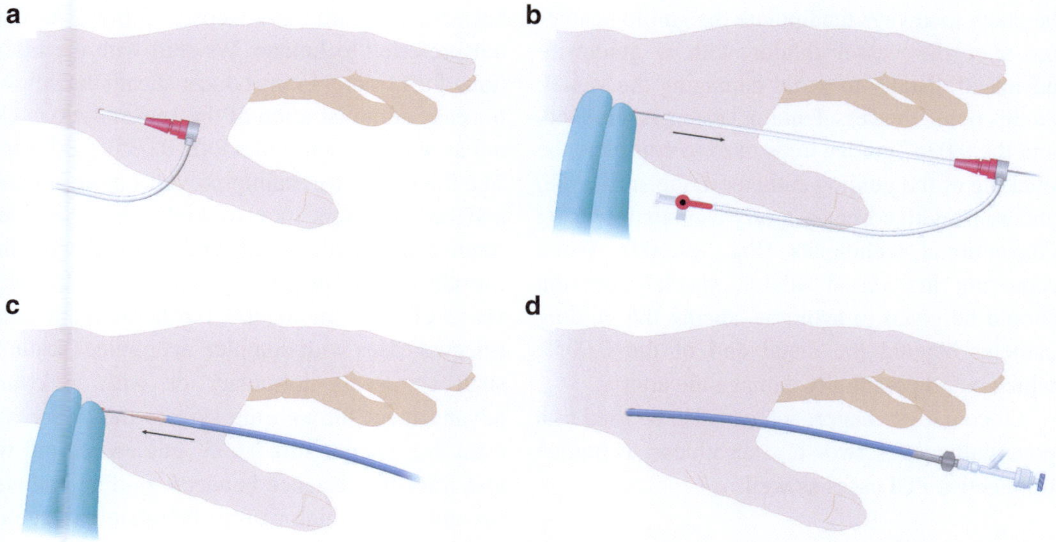

Fig. 19.10 Conversion to ad hoc sheathless percutaneous coronary intervention implementing the Distal RailTracking technique (see text for details)

over the Railway vessel dilator (Fig. 19.9e) with its distal tip securely fixed to avoid trauma to the vessel wall that may otherwise occur if the tip of the dilator moves proximally without the guidewire inside. Once the guiding catheter has been advanced over the vessel dilator sufficiently deep into the artery (the proximal black markers on the dilator indicate the ideal alignment for 90 and 100 cm guiding catheters), the vessel dilator can be retrieved while maintaining the position of the guiding catheter, and a 0.035″ guidewire is used to complete tracking of the guiding catheter to the aortic bulb and facilitate coronary artery cannulation using conventional techniques. The 0.035″ Railway vessel dilator could possibly be inserted into the guiding catheter to facilitate its advance and to fill the space between guide and wire to prevent scraping tissue from the vessel wall and to prevent embolisation (Fig. 19.9f).

In ad hoc PCI cases, where a small introducer sheath was used to perform the diagnostic angiogram (Fig. 19.10a), the 0.035″ Railway vessel dilator can be used in order to convert to a sheathless approach and implement the Distal RailTracking technique. The same dilator and steps can also be used to quickly switch between different guiding catheters as needed.

With a long 0.035″ guidewire in place to secure access and path to the aortic bulb, the introducer sheath is withdrawn with gentle pressure over the entry site to avoid unnecessary bleeding (Fig. 19.10b). The preassembled 0.035″-compatible Railway vessel dilator and guiding catheter are then advanced together through the skin (Fig. 19.10c) up to the subclavian artery over the 0.035″ guidewire while securing its proximal end. Because the tip of the Railway is not visible on fluoroscopy, care must be taken to always manipulate the guiding catheter over the vessel dilator with a guidewire advanced distally to avoid damaging the vessel. At this point, the vessel dilator system is removed, and the 0.035″ guidewire is used to complete the tracking of the guiding catheter to the aortic bulb and assist with coronary artery cannulation using conventional techniques (Fig. 19.10d). When removing the vessel dilator, special attention should be given to avoid advancing the guiding catheter beyond the distal end of the 0.035″, which could potentially damage the artery.

Of course, this approach can also be used as a potentially safer two-step sheathless technique for elective PCI cases as well.

19.6 Distal RailTracking Technique

With the Railway system, the upfront sheathless approach for elective PCI cases saves the cost of one introducer sheath and may appear simpler because it requires fewer steps. However, based on our extensive experience with the device, this approach has many problems besides these minimal advantages. The pathway through the skin and subcutaneous tissue may not be easy at times, and the 0.021″ guidewire may not provide sufficient support in such cases, with the risk of damage and potential complication (e.g., guidewire or vessel rupture) or simply the impossibility of advancing the dilator further because of some acute bends of the wire. In the latter case, the available cannula could be used to exchange for a new 0.021″ guidewire rather than attempting a new arterial puncture. Another potential issue is the risk of vascular complications (e.g., dissection or perforation) that may be caused by the involuntary advancement of the unprotected, pointed, and therefore traumatic tip of the Railway vessel dilator as the guiding catheter is being advanced over it. Finally, this approach doesn't take full advantage of the arterial tracking capabilities of the Railway vessel dilator, hence potentially exposing the patient to an unwarranted increased risk of vascular complications.

The Distal RailTracking technique on the other side might seem more time-consuming because there are more steps to follow, but it is our preferred technique. We start with the insertion of a 4 Fr or 5 Fr introducer sheath that allows for easy administration of the spasmolytic cocktail as well as the use of a long 0.035″ guidewire. The thicker wire certainly provides more support and has less tendency to kink when we then remove the small sheath and proceed with the introduction of the guiding catheter and Railway vessel dilator combination. Furthermore, in some selected cases with complex anatomical features such as severe tortuosity or with awkward advancement through the skin to the artery, we even use a super stiff 0.035″ guidewire, and we also vary the distance between guiding catheter tip and vessel dilator tip to facilitate passage of severe angulations.

Distal RailTracking has already been shown to be feasible and safe for complex PCIs in a small prospective registry [18] and continues to perform extremely well in our daily practice. Another prospective study performing the exact same steps described for the Distal RailTracking, but with conventional TRA, demonstrated its efficacy and safety, showing an extremely low rate of both vascular and procedural complications [35].

To minimize trauma to the vessels of the upper extremity, we advocate the use of long exchange wires to allow the tip of the wire to remain in the aortic sinus during guidewire exchange. And we also avoid unnecessary razor effects in these delicate vessels by extending the dilator to the aortic arch, paying attention to the black markers on the proximal end that confirm the correct position for either 90 cm or 100 cm guidewire catheters. Thus, in our practice, RailTracking has routinely replaced historical alternative sheathless techniques, which we still describe.

19.7 Alternative Sheathless Techniques

Over the years, the lack of a dedicated system has encouraged the development of alternative solutions to achieve sheathless insertion of conventional guiding catheters. All techniques used to improve the arterial trackability of guiding catheters can potentially be used to achieve a sheathless access, as they are designed to reduce the "razor effect" by providing a more gradual transition from the tip of the guiding to the guidewire. Instead of a dedicated vessel dilator, an inner smaller bore catheter or an inflated balloon has been successfully used. The use of hydrophilic-coated guidewires and catheters is certainly helpful in these situations [36].

19.7.1 Balloon-Assisted Tracking

For the BAT technique, a 15–20-mm-long balloon, appropriately sized for the guiding catheter used (e.g., 2 mm balloon for a 6 Fr guiding catheter), is held inflated at low pressure (3–6 atm), partially protruding from the guiding catheter distal tip [27, 37]. The entire system is gently advanced over a 0.014″ coronary guidewire.

In this technique, a radial puncture is performed in a standard manner. After the mini-guidewire is advanced through the needle or the cannula into the radial artery, the needle or the cannula is removed, and the dilator of a small-size introducer sheath is advanced over the mini-guidewire to dilate the tract between the skin and the artery (Fig. 19.11). The mini-guidewire is removed, and a 0.014″ coronary guidewire is inserted through the dilator and advanced into the vessel under fluoroscopic guidance. While applying gentle pressure over the entry site to avoid

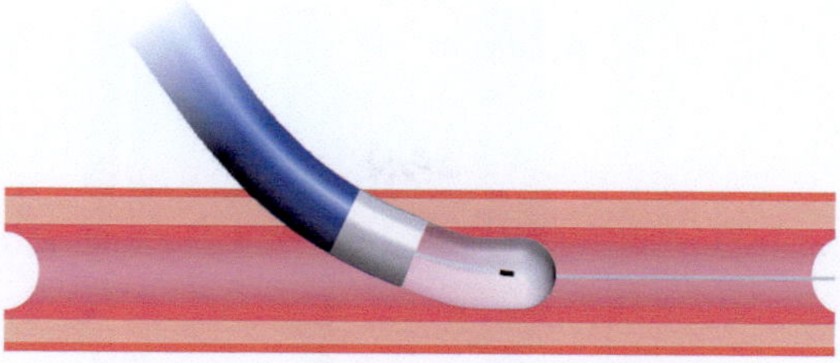

Fig. 19.11 Balloon-assisted tracking technique for sheathless catheter insertion

unnecessary bleeding, the dilator is removed, and the guiding catheter with the balloon inside is loaded and advanced over the 0.014″ coronary guidewire. The low support of the coronary guidewire is certainly a limitation of this technique due to the increased risk of kinking or fracture and potential access site complications.

Initial placement of a small introducer sheath (≤5 Fr), as described in the literature [24], is highly recommended as it allows for the balloon and catheter combination to slide more efficiently through the subcutaneous planes, thus reducing the risk of guidewire kinking or fracture. If it is difficult to advance the inflated balloon and guiding catheter through the skin and underlying tissues, the same balloon can be advanced deflated and the channel dilated. A small skin nick may also assist in advancing the balloon and guiding catheter.

The BAT technique has also been used to increase the success rate of radial access in difficult vascular anatomy, including very small radial arteries, significant tortuosity, complex loops, and severe radial artery spasm. If needed this setup allows for easy dilatation to overcome obstructive stenosis of the arm-artery.

19.7.2 Mother and Child

Techniques using smaller but longer diagnostic catheters loaded inside any guiding catheter have also been described to improve guiding catheter advancement [26] by providing a stepped transition from the tip of the guiding to the guidewire inside the artery (Fig. 19.12).

While this approach has the advantage of being performed over a more supportive 0.035″

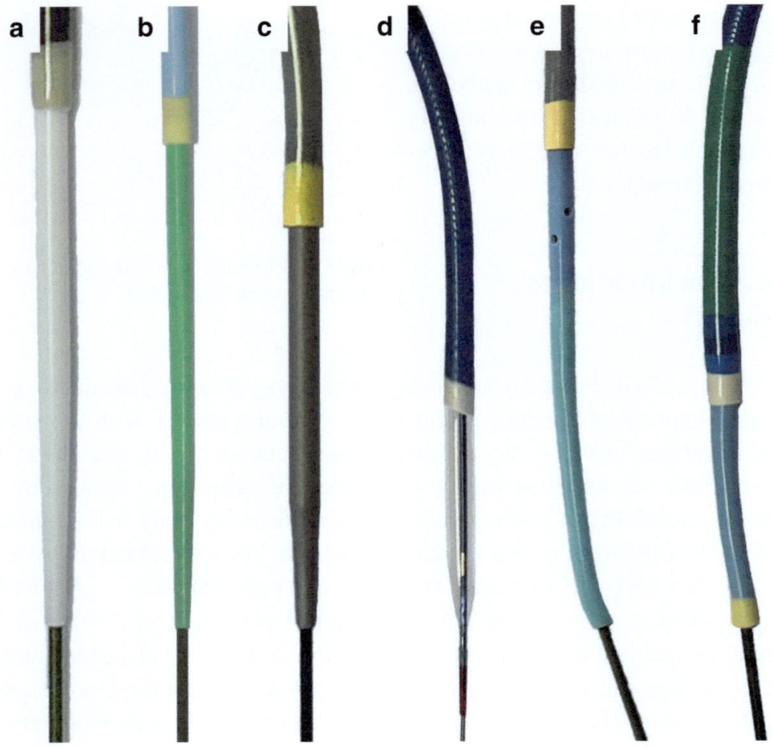

Fig. 19.12 Guidewire to catheter transition according to available sheathless techniques: (**a**) Asahi Eaucath sheathless guiding catheter 7.5 Fr. (**b**) Cordis Vista Brite Tip guiding catheter 6 Fr and Cordis Railway 6 Fr. (**c**) Boston Scientific Mach 1 guiding catheter 7 Fr and Cook Medical Flexor long dilator 7 Fr. (**d**) B. Braun Serpia guiding catheter 6 Fr and Boston Scientific Emerge 2 × 15 mm (balloon-assisted tracking). (**e**) Boston Scientific Mach 1 guiding catheter 6 Fr and longer (110 cm) Terumo Radifocus Optitorque Pigtail 5 Fr (pigtail-assisted tracking). (**f**) Medtronic Launcher guiding catheter and longer (125 cm) Cordis Vista Brite Tip guiding catheter 6 Fr (child and mother)

guidewire, the transitions between guidewire, inner catheter, and guiding catheter are not as smooth as in the BAT technique or when dedicated tapered tip devices are used. To partially compensate for this problem, the use of a straight diagnostic catheter such as a multipurpose or Judkins right has been recommended [38, 39].

19.7.3 Pigtail-Assisted Tracking

The use of a 125-cm pigtail catheter straightened by the 0.035″ guidewire inside the intended guiding catheter has been favored because of its slightly tapered tip compared to other straight diagnostic catheters (Fig. 19.12) [26].

It is a common practice to obtain vascular access and first insert a small introducer sheath, advance a 0.035″ guidewire, and then remove the sheath while applying gentle pressure over the entry site to avoid unnecessary bleeding. The two catheters are then advanced simultaneously into the artery while being held together to avoid excessive vessel trauma in case the guiding catheter needs to advance ahead of the pigtail catheter tip if it is hindered by the subcutaneous tissue.

19.7.4 Extra Vessel Dilator

An even better, but still expensive, solution is to use a tapered vessel dilator from a longer sheath, such as the Flexor series (Cook Medical) [39]. As with other customized solutions, the use of an additional vascular dilator offers great compatibility with most available guiding catheters in an extended size range (Fig. 19.12). In fact, this approach has been used to safely deliver an 8 Fr guiding catheter for transradial CTO PCI [40]. In another report from Japan, an 8 Fr sheathless guiding catheter was advanced over a dedicated 6.5 Fr sheathless guiding catheter and its vessel dilator to perform transradial coronary directional atherectomy [41].

19.8 General Remarks

As mentioned previously, one of the major limitations of sheathless techniques is the risk of kinking of the guiding catheter, particularly at the puncture site. This can occur in cases where there is significant friction or resistance when advancing or rotating the guiding catheter and is a consequence of anatomical factors such as long subcutaneous route to the artery, presence of fibrotic scar tissue such as after trauma or surgery, significant calcification, and/or tortuous course of the artery. To overcome these problems, our first suggestion is the Distal RailTracking technique over a stiff guidewire.

However, if the skin is very resistant to advancement of the sheathless catheter, a small incision should be made with the scalpel touching the dilator and the blade turned upward to avoid contact with the artery (Fig. 19.13). This will not damage the tip of the guiding catheter and will allow it to pass smoothly into the artery. Alternatively, a needle tip can be used instead of a scalpel to carefully loosen up the skin around the guide at the entry site. However, nicking the skin may lead to instability of the guiding catheter position. Wetting the guiding catheter with saline will reduce friction and prevent temperature rise at the entry site when the guide is moved. Alternatively, commercial lubricants intended for use with atherectomy systems may sometimes be helpful in difficult situations to facilitate the passage of large-bore guiding catheters that don't have a hydrophilic coating [42, 43]. A wet guide

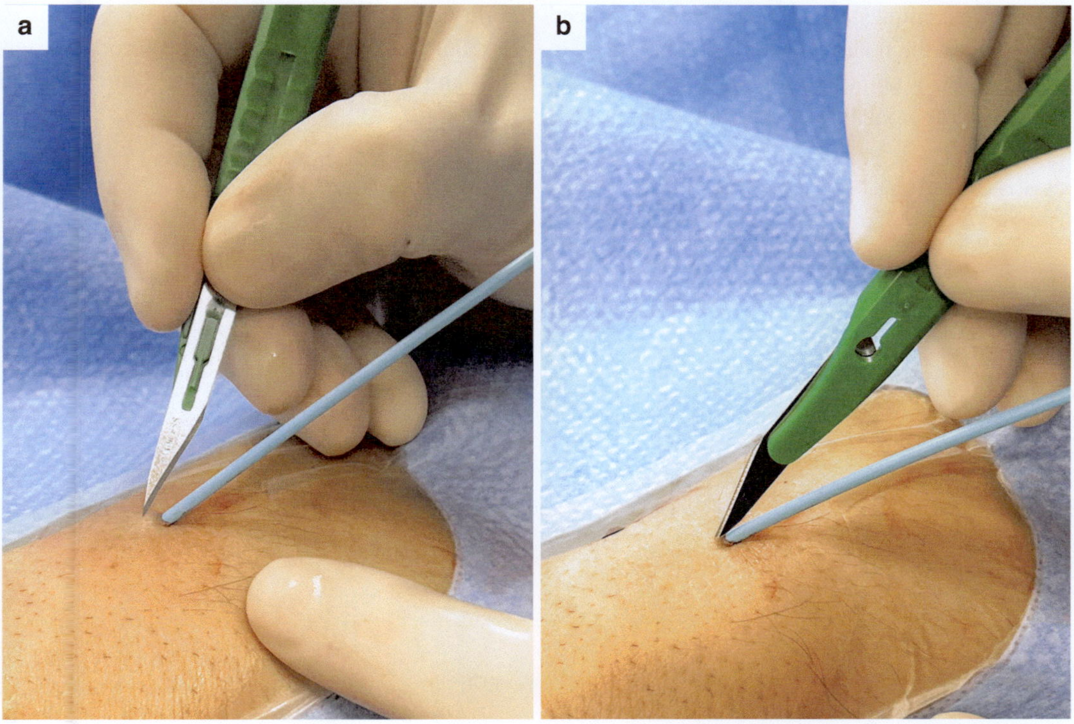

Fig. 19.13 (**a**) Incorrect and (**b**) correct position of the scalpel blade to make a small skin incision to favor the advancement of the sheathless catheter

allows for a "safety clutch" effect, i.e., the guide will slide out during heavy breathing or coughing of the patient, which may prevent damage to the coronary ostium. Once the entry site is dry, the sheathless guidewire may provide a more stable position due to a slight anchoring effect.

19.9 Outlook for the Future of Sheathless Distal Radial Access

Radial access has shown a greater benefit in high-risk patients who are increasingly undergoing complex revascularization procedures. These procedures often require multiple interventional devices and larger-bore guiding catheters. In addition, the associated risk of access site complications is expected to be higher than in simpler situations and therefore most likely to benefit from DRA, although unfortunately this may not occur due to the smaller artery diameter potentially limiting the use of larger introducer sheaths.

Sheathless access now encompasses a full range of techniques and devices that may indeed fully unlock the potential of DRA. And DRA, in turn, can fully empower sheathless. In fact, the sheathless approach may warrant a large-bore catheter option in most cases but also conventional procedures for those whose artery would not tolerate a sheath. It's also a strategy to enhance a slender interventional practice (Figs. 19.14 and 19.15).

Device improvements would be very well received and may implement some relevant iterations to effectively enable the systematic use of these techniques.

In particular, longer devices to compensate for the slightly more distant puncture site when performing DRA may well become the new standard, allowing unrestricted access to distal coronary segments even in taller patients and in those with complex or variant anatomy that defines a longer pathway to the coronary arteries.

Also, given the poorly studied but potentially harmful consequence of systematic advancement of an open-ended catheter in small and tortuous vessels, the use of a vascular dilator may become an elegant routine for safe catheter advancement to the aorta. In addition, an iteration of the currently available devices that allows for accurate visualization and evolute deliverability could significantly extend the benefits of the RailTracking technique to the coronary arteries and significantly change current PCI technique.

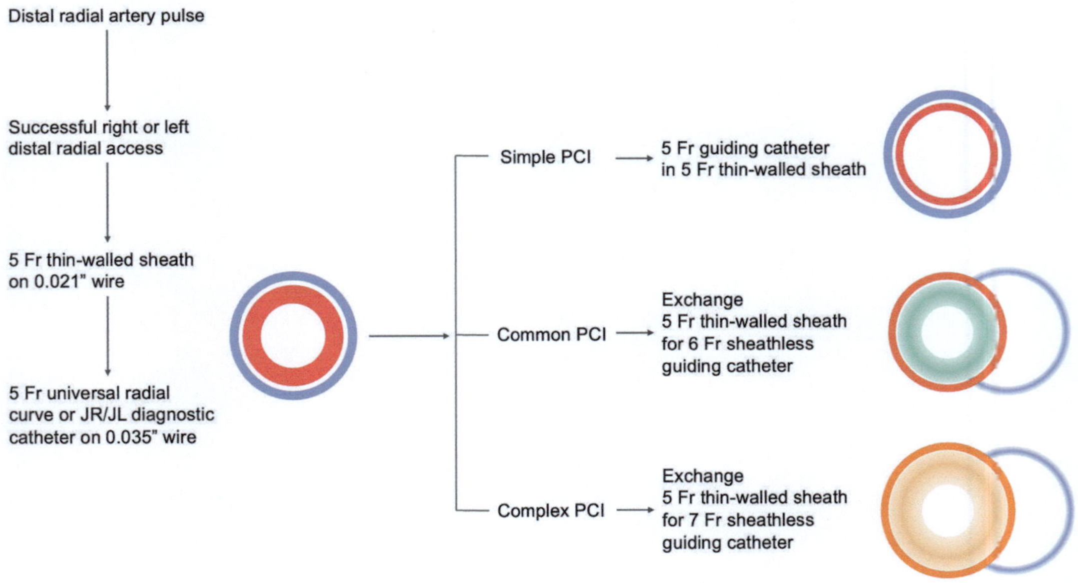

Fig. 19.14 Everyday algorithm for coronary angiography/percutaneous coronary intervention with the Railway system, proposed by S. Harb. The long dilator components are represented by their color

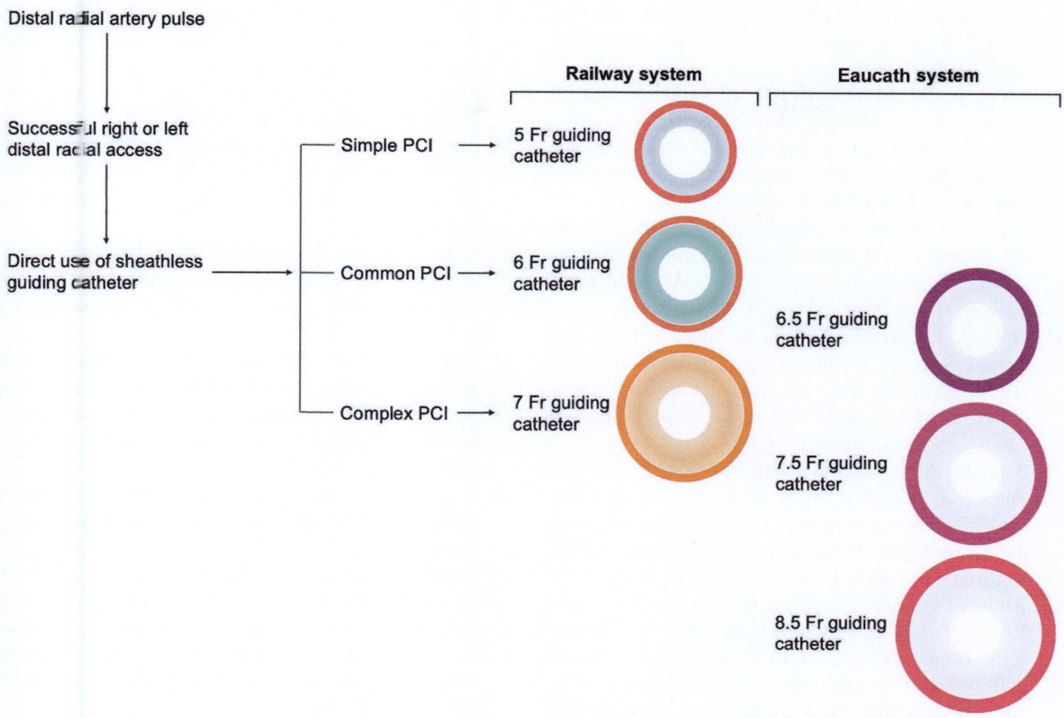

Fig. 19.15 Algorithm for planned percutaneous coronary intervention with the Railway or the Eucath sheahtless system, proposed by S. Harb. The long dilator components are represented by their color

References

1. Zielinski J, Nowosielski JM. Finet's law as a special case of the generalised Murray's law. SN Comput Sci. 2020;1:42.
2. Finet G, Gilard M, Perrenot B, Rioufol G, Motreff P, Gavit L, et al. Fractal geometry of arterial coronary bifurcations: a quantitative coronary angiography and intravascular ultrasound analysis. EuroIntervention. 2008;3:490–8.
3. Mengal MN, Ashraf T, Hassan Rizvi SN, Badini A, Karim M. Assessment of femoral artery bifurcation level with conventional angiography. Cureus. 2018;10:e3479.
4. Noori VJ, Eldrup-Jørgensen J. A systematic review of vascular closure devices for femoral artery puncture sites. J Vasc Surg. 2018;68:887–99.
5. Kim Y, Ahn Y, Kim MC, Sim DS, Hong YJ, Kim JH, et al. Gender differences in the distal radial artery diameter for the snuffbox approach. Cardiol J. 2018;25:639–41.
6. Lee JW, Park SW, Son JW, Ahn SG, Lee SH. Real-world experience of the left distal transradial approach for coronary angiography and percutaneous coronary intervention: a prospective observational study (LeDRA). EuroIntervention. 2018;14:e995–1003.
7. Naito T, Sawaoka T, Sasaki K, Iida K, Sakuraba S, Yokohama K, et al. Evaluation of the diameter of the distal radial artery at the anatomical snuff box using ultrasound in Japanese patients. Cardiovasc Interv Ther. 2019;34:312–6.
8. Norimatsu K, Kusumoto T, Yoshimoto K, Tsukamoto M, Kuwano T, Nishikawa H, et al. Importance of measurement of the diameter of the distal radial artery in a distal radial approach from the anatomical snuffbox before coronary catheterization. Heart Vessel. 2019;34:1615–20.
9. Hadjivassiliou A, Cardarelli-Leite L, Jalal S, Chung J, Liu D, Ho S, et al. Left distal transradial access (ldTRA): a comparative assessment of conventional and distal radial artery size. Cardiovasc Intervent Radiol. 2020;43:850–7.
10. Mizuguchi Y, Izumikawa T, Hashimoto S, Yamada T, Taniguchi N, Nakajima S, et al. Efficacy and safety of the distal transradial approach in coronary angiography and percutaneous coronary intervention: a Japanese multicenter experience. Cardiovasc Interv Ther. 2020;35:162–7.
11. Yu W, Hu P, Wang S, Yao L, Wang H, Dou L, et al. Distal radial artery access in the anatomical snuffbox for coronary angiography and intervention: a single center experience. Medicine. 2020;99:e18330.
12. Saito S, Ikei H, Hosokawa G, Tanaka S. Influence of the ratio between radial artery inner diameter and

sheath outer diameter on radial artery flow after transradial coronary intervention. Catheter Cardiovasc Interv. 1999;46:173–8.
13. Uhlemann M, Möbius-Winkler S, Mende M, Eitel I, Fuernau G, Sandri M, et al. The Leipzig prospective vascular ultrasound registry in radial artery catheterization: impact of sheath size on vascular complications. JACC Cardiovasc Interv. 2012;5:36–43.
14. Rashid M, Kwok CS, Pancholy S, Chugh S, Kedev SA, Bernat I, et al. Radial artery occlusion after transradial interventions: a systematic review and meta-analysis. J Am Heart Assoc. 2016;5:e002686.
15. Garg N, Madan BK, Khanna R, Sinha A, Kapoor A, Tewari S, et al. Incidence and predictors of radial artery occlusion after transradial coronary angioplasty: Doppler-guided follow-up study. J Invasive Cardiol. 2015;27:106–12.
16. Aminian A, Iglesias JF, Van Mieghem C, Zuffi A, Ferrara A, Manih R, et al. First prospective multicenter experience with the 7 French Glidesheath slender for complex transradial coronary interventions. Catheter Cardiovasc Interv. 2017;89:1014–20.
17. Aminian A, Saito S, Takahashi A, Bernat I, Jobe RL, Kajiya T, et al. Comparison of a new slender 6 Fr sheath with a standard 5 Fr sheath for transradial coronary angiography and intervention: RAP and BEAT (radial artery patency and bleeding, efficacy, adverse evenT), a randomised multicentre trial. EuroIntervention. 2017;13:e549–56.
18. Colletti G, Auslender J, De Meester A, Aminian A, Kayaert P, Ungureanu C. Feasibility and safety of performing complex coronary interventions by distal radial artery using the railway sheathless vascular system. J Invasive Cardiol. 2020;32:459–62.
19. Horie K, Tada N, Isawa T, Matsumoto T, Taguri M, Kato S, et al. A randomised comparison of incidence of radial artery occlusion and symptomatic radial artery spasm associated with elective transradial coronary intervention using 6.5 Fr SheathLess Eaucath guiding Catheter vs. 6.0 Fr Glidesheath Slender. EuroIntervention. 2018;13:2018–25.
20. Batchelor W, Dahya V, McGee D, Katopodis J, Dixon W, Campbell J, et al. Ultrahigh-resolution ultrasound characterization of access site trauma and intimal hyperplasia following use of a 7F sheathless guide versus 6F sheath/guide combination for transradial artery PCI: results of the PRAGMATIC trial. Am Heart J. 2018;198:75–83.
21. Seldinger SI. Catheter replacement of the needle in percutaneous arteriography; a new technique. Acta Radiol. 1953;39:368–76.
22. Conti CR. Coronary arteriography. Circulation. 1977;55:227–37.
23. Mamas MA, Ratib K, Routledge H, Neyses L, Fraser DG, de Belder M, et al. Influence of arterial access site selection on outcomes in primary percutaneous coronary intervention: are the results of randomized trials achievable in clinical practice? JACC Cardiovasc Interv. 2013;6:698–706.
24. Mamas MA, George S, Ratib K, Kwok CS, Elkhazin A, Sandhu K, et al. 5-Fr sheathless transradial cardiac catheterization using conventional catheters and balloon assisted tracking; a new approach to downsizing. Cardiovasc Revasc Med. 2017;18:28–32.
25. Mamas MA, Fraser DG, Ratib K, Fath-Ordoubadi F, El-Omar M, Nolan J, et al. Minimising radial injury: prevention is better than cure. EuroIntervention. 2014;10:824–32.
26. Garg N, Sahoo D, Goel PK. Pigtail assisted tracking of guide catheter for navigating the difficult radial: overcoming the "razor effect". Indian Heart J. 2016;68:355–60.
27. Patel T, Shah S, Pancholy S, Rao S, Bertrand OF, Kwan T. Balloon-assisted tracking: a must-know technique to overcome difficult anatomy during transradial approach. Catheter Cardiovasc Interv. 2014;83:211–20.
28. Rozado J, Pascual I, Avanzas P, Moris C. Coronary embolism after iatrogenic radial endarterectomy. J Invasive Cardiol. 2016;28:E54–5.
29. Komiyama H, Takano M, Miyakuni T, Ikeda T, Matsushita M, Inami T, et al. Combination use of intravascular ultrasound and dual-lumen microcatheter guide for chronic total occlusion guidewire manipulation; a practical method. Clin Pract. 2019;16:1015–20.
30. Brilakis ES, Grantham JA, Thompson CA, DeMartini TJ, Prasad A, Sandhu GS, et al. The retrograde approach to coronary artery chronic total occlusions: a practical approach. Catheter Cardiovasc Interv. 2012;79:3–19.
31. Brilakis ES, Mashayekhi K, Tsuchikane E, Abi Rafeh N, Alaswad K, Araya M, ert al. Guiding principles for chronic total occlusion percutaneous coronary intervention: a global expert consensus document. Circulation. 2019;140:420–33.
32. Zivelonghi C, van Kuijk JP, Poletti E, Suttorp MJ, Eefting FD, Rensing BJ, et al. A "minimalistic hybrid algorithm" in coronary chronic total occlusion revascularization: procedural and clinical outcomes. Catheter Cardiovasc Interv. 2020;95:97–104.
33. Ungureanu C, Gasparini GL, Aminian A, Blaimont M, Dumitrascu S, Lepièce C, et al. RailTracking: a novel technique to overcome difficult anatomy during transradial approach. J Invasive Cardiol. 2022;34:E757–62.
34. Ungureanu C, Carlier S, Ghafari C, Auslender J, de Meester de Ravestein A, Colletti G. Successful crossing of complex radial and brachial artery anatomy using a new approach: railtracking. Am J Case Rep. 2022;23:e934760.
35. Raje V, Krathen C, Sanghvi K. Evaluation of railway sheathless access system for transradial coronary and peripheral interventions. Cardiovasc Revasc Med. 2021;22:91–7.
36. Barbeau GR. Radial loop and extreme vessel tortuosity in the transradial approach: advantage of hydrophilic-coated guidewires and catheters. Catheter Cardiovasc Interv. 2003;59:442–50.

37. Merella P, Lorenzoni G, Saderi L, Sotgiu G, Casu G. Vascular assisted tracking for challenging transradial percutaneous intervention. Cardiovasc Revasc Med. 2021;29:38–42.
38. Patel T, Shah S, Pancholy S. "Combo" technique for the use of 7F guide catheter system during transradial approach. Catheter Cardiovasc Interv. 2015;86:1033–40.
39. Kwan TW, Cherukuri S, Huang Y, Pancholy S, Daggubati R, Liou M, et al. Feasibility and safety of 7F sheathless guiding catheter during transradial coronary intervention. Catheter Cardiovasc Interv. 2012;80:274–80.
40. Dautov R, Ribeiro HB, Abdul-Jawad Altisent O, Nombela-Franco L, Gibrat C, Nguyen CM, et al. Effectiveness and safety of the Transradial 8Fr Sheathless approach for revascularization of chronic total occlusions. Am J Cardiol. 2016;118:785–9.
41. Niizeki T, Iwayama T, Kumagai Y, Tohara S, Tsuchikane E. Usefulness of the Transradial 8Fr Sheathless guiding catheter approach in directional coronary atherectomy. Clin Med Insights Case Rep. 2022;15:11795476221075497.
42. Singh A, Awar M, Ahmed A, Fischman DL, Walinsky P, Savage MP. Facilitated stent delivery using applied topical lubrication. Catheter Cardiovasc Interv. 2007;69:218–22.
43. Repanas T, Christopoulos G, Brilakis ES. Administration of ViperSlide™ for treating severe radial artery spasm: case report and systematic review of the literature. Cardiovasc Revasc Med. 2015;16:243–5.

Complex Coronary Procedures

20

Juan F. Iglesias and Pierfrancesco Agostoni

20.1 Introduction

Transradial access (TRA) is the standard vascular access site for coronary angiography and percutaneous coronary intervention (PCI) in all patient and lesion subsets, unless there are procedural contraindications [1, 2]. Compared to transfemoral access (TFA), TRA for PCI has been shown to significantly reduce the risks of major bleeding, major vascular complications, major adverse cardiac events (MACE) and all-cause mortality [3, 4] while improving patient comfort and healthcare costs [5]. In recent years, the growing adoption of TRA has progressively paved the way for its use in patients undergoing complex coronary interventions, despite the scarcity of clinical evidence due to the absence or under-representation of complex coronary lesion subsets in the majority of studies supporting the current "radial first" strategy for PCI endorsed by recent international guidelines [1, 2]. While most coronary interventions can be performed safely and effectively by TRA using 5 Fr or 6 Fr sheaths and guiding catheters, the small size of the radial artery is still perceived by many operators as an important limitation to the use of large-bore guiding catheters (≥7 Fr), restricting the use of TRA for PCI of highly complex coronary lesions such as chronic total occlusions (CTO), left main coronary artery (LMCA) disease, heavily calcified lesions requiring advanced plaque modification techniques, or complex bifurcation lesions.

Distal radial access (DRA) in the anatomical snuffbox or dorsum of the hand has recently emerged as a valid alternative vascular access site to conventional TRA for coronary angiography and PCI, with the goal of further reducing the incidence of procedure-related vascular complications [6–8]. However, most recent randomized controlled trials (RCTs) evaluating the safety and feasibility of DRA compared to conventional TRA have included a relatively low-risk patient population undergoing mainly diagnostic procedures and non-complex interventions using 5 Fr or 6 Fr sheaths and guiding catheters [6–8], thus preventing extrapolation of these study results to higher-risk patient and lesion subgroups undergoing complex coronary interventions using large-bore (≥7 Fr) sheaths and guiding catheters. Currently available evidence on DRA in complex PCI is therefore limited to case reports, case series, small single-center studies, and multicenter registries. The aim of this chapter is to provide a comprehensive review of the existing evidence and future perspectives regarding the use of DRA for complex coronary interventions.

J. F. Iglesias (✉)
Department of Cardiology, Geneva University Hospitals, Geneva, Switzerland
e-mail: juanfernando.iglesias@hcuge.ch

P. Agostoni
Hartcentrum, Ziekenhuis Netwerk Antwerpen, Middelheim, Antwerp, Belgium

G. A. Sgueglia (ed.), *Distal Radial Access*, https://doi.org/10.1007/978-3-031-89925-6_20

20.2 Transradial Access for Complex Coronary Interventions

There is currently no standardized definition for complex or high-risk coronary interventions [9]. Complex PCI commonly refers to a wide range of coronary interventions for complex anatomic lesion subsets, such as multivessel coronary artery disease (CAD), calcified lesions, LMCA disease, bifurcation lesions, in-stent restenosis, CTO, or saphenous vein graft disease, performed in patients with high-risk baseline comorbidities, such as diabetes mellitus, cardiogenic shock, valvular heart disease, acute coronary syndrome, chronic renal failure, or impaired left ventricular systolic function, all of which have been shown to increase the risk of stent- and patient-related adverse outcomes [9]. Despite its associated increased risk of bleeding events, vascular complications, and adverse clinical outcomes [10, 11], TFA has long been considered the preferred access site for complex PCI [12–14] mainly due to the anticipated better support (due to broader operator experience with TFA procedures and guiding catheter shapes originally designed for TFA) and the potential need for large-bore (≥7 Fr) guiding catheters to facilitate the use of dedicated devices, which have been associated with higher procedural success rates in complex PCI [15]. The use of large-bore TRA for the treatment of highly complex coronary lesions has been limited by historically lower operator confidence in TRA for complex PCI and by the smaller size of the radial artery and resulting sheath-to-artery mismatch, which may lead to an increased risk of radial artery occlusion (RAO) [16, 17].

The introduction of novel technologies, including thin-walled radial introducer sheaths (Glidesheath Slender, Terumo; Prelude Ideal, Merit Medical; RAIN, Cordis; Braidin, APT Medical) and sheathless vascular systems (Eaucath, Asahi; Railway, Cordis) have facilitated the use of large-diameter guiding catheters for PCI through TRA by reducing the outer sheath-inner artery diameter mismatch that predisposes to RAO (see also Chaps. 18 and 19). In the first prospective multicenter study of 60 patients undergoing large-bore PCI for complex coronary lesions (CTO, 25%; LMCA disease, 33%; heavily calcified lesions, 15%; complex bifurcation lesions, 27%) through TRA using the thin-walled 7Fr radial Glidesheath Slender sheath [18], procedural success was high (97%), and the incidence of major complications such as major bleeding (0%), vascular access site complications (4.7%), symptomatic radial spasm (11%), and RAO at discharge as assessed by vascular ultrasound (4.8%) were relatively low. The Complex Large-Bore Radial Percutaneous Coronary Intervention (COLOR) multicenter, international, prospective study was the first RCT to compare TRA with TFA for PCI of complex coronary lesions using 7 Fr guiding catheters [19]. Among 388 patients undergoing complex PCI (CTO, 58%; LMCA disease, 14%; heavily calcified lesions, 19%; complex bifurcation lesions, 9%) with a 7 Fr Glidesheath Slender radial sheath, TRA was associated with a significant reduction in the primary composite endpoint of clinically relevant Bleeding Academic Research Consortium (BARC) 2, 3 or 5 access site bleeding or vascular complications requiring intervention at discharge (3.6% vs. 19.1%, $p < 0.001$), a difference driven by a lower risk of BARC 3 major bleeding and vascular complications without compromising procedural success (86.0% vs. 89.2%, $p = 0.29$). Importantly, there were no significant differences between TRA and TFA in terms of access site crossover rates (3.6% vs. 2.6%, $p = 0.56$), procedure time, contrast volume used, or radiation dose. Overall, these results confirm the feasibility and safety of TRA using large 7 Fr guide catheters for complex PCI.

20.3 Distal Radial Access for Complex Coronary Interventions

In recent years, several single- and multicenter RCTs have established DRA as a valid alternative vascular access site to conventional TRA for coronary angiography and/or PCI [6–8]. In a recent meta-analysis including 6208 patients from 14 RCTs [20], DRA for coronary angiography and/or PCI using almost exclusively <7 Fr access sheath sizes was associated with a significant 68% and 64% reduction in the risk of RAO at hospital discharge or last available follow-up, respectively, and a 49% reduction in the risk of major hematoma compared to conventional TRA, at the expense of an almost threefold increased risk of access site crossover. However, these studies included a high proportion of diagnostic and non-complex PCI procedures, mostly using 5 Fr or 6 Fr catheters in low-risk patient populations. In the Distal vs. Conventional Radial Access (DISCO RADIAL) trial, the largest RCT to date comparing DRA with conventional TRA using the 6 Fr Glidesheath Slender introducer sheath in 1309 patients undergoing coronary angiography and/or PCI [8], DRA did not meet the study's prespecified criterion for superiority with respect to the primary endpoint of forearm RAO at hospital discharge compared to conventional TRA (0.3% vs. 0.9%, $p = 0.29$) due to the extremely low rate of RAO in the control TRA arm. However, DRA was associated with significantly higher rates of access site crossover (7.4% vs. 3.5%, $p = 0.002$) and radial artery spasm (5.4% vs. 2.7%, $p = 0.015$) but shorter hemostasis time compared to conventional TRA. The DISCO RADIAL trial included mostly low-risk patients (6 Fr introducer sheath, >99%; diagnostic coronary angiography, 64%; LMCA PCI, 9%), and extrapolation of these results to higher-risk patients undergoing PCI for complex coronary lesions remains uncertain. In particular, the use of large-bore (≥7 Fr) sheaths or guiding catheters required for some complex coronary interventions may potentially be hampered by the smaller size of the distal compared to the forearm radial artery, which has been associated with an increased risk of radial artery spasm and access site crossover [8]. Therefore, due to the lack of randomized data, current evidence on the potential benefits of DRA for complex coronary interventions is limited to small single-center observational studies and post hoc analyses from multicenter registries, as available RCTs of DRA have mostly included patients undergoing coronary angiography and/or non-complex coronary interventions [6–8]. In addition, the results of these studies should be interpreted with caution due to important differences in patient baseline risk, proportion of large-bore (≥7 Fr) sheaths and guiding catheters used, study endpoint definitions, or timing and assessment technique of RAO.

The feasibility and safety of large-bore DRA for complex PCI using the 7 Fr Railway sheathless vascular access were evaluated in a small, single-center study of 20 patients undergoing PCI for distal LMCA disease (8 patients), complex non-LMCA bifurcation lesions (7 patients), and CTO (4 patients) with severely calcified lesions requiring rotational atherectomy (RA, 9 patients), intravascular lithotripsy (2 patients), and modified or super high-pressure noncompliant balloons (3 patients) [21]. The procedural success rate was 95% with no access site crossover, major bleeding, distal and forearm RAO at 24 h, or vascular access site complications, and severe radial spasm was reported in only one patient (5%). In a single-center retrospective observational study of 102 patients undergoing complex PCI (LMCA, 34%; CTO, 25%; bifurcation lesions, 64%; RA, 11%) through DRA (right, 89%) using a 7 Fr thin-walled sheath (Braidin, APT Medical, China) [22], puncture and procedural success rates were high (92% and 98%, respectively), and the incidence of forearm and distal RAO at 24 h and 30 days was relatively low (2.2% and 3.3%, respectively). Radial artery spasm was reported in two (2.2%) patients, and vascular complications were limited to one (1.1%) patient with arterio-venous fistula at follow-up. Collectively, these findings suggest the safety and efficacy of large-bore DRA using dedicated vascular access systems for complex coronary interventions, but dedicated RCTs are needed to confirm these observational findings. The ongoing multicenter, international, prospective Distal Versus Conventional Radial Access for Complex Large-bore Percutaneous Coronary Intervention (DISCO COMPLEX) trial (NCT05490238) is the first randomized RCT

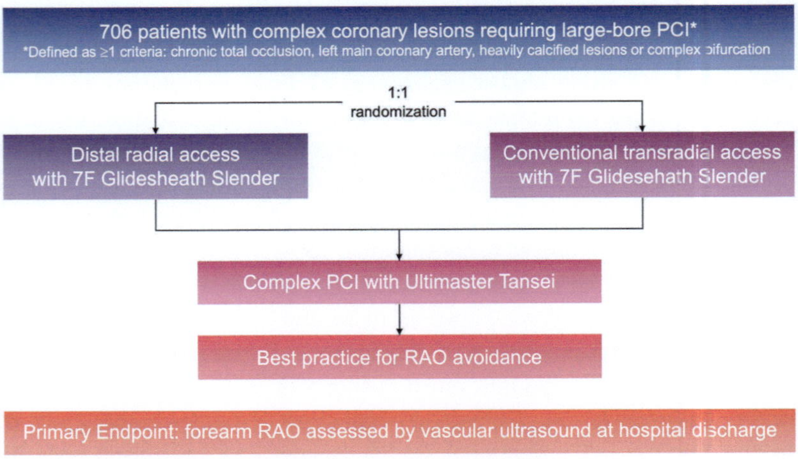

Fig. 20.1 Design of the distal versus conventional radial access for complex large-bore percutaneous coronary intervention (DISCO COMPLEX) randomized controlled trial

designed to evaluate the superiority of large-bore DRA over conventional TRA with respect to forearm RAO rates at hospital discharge in 708 patients undergoing complex PCI using a 7Fr Glidesheath Slender introducer sheath (Fig. 20.1).

In recent years, the use of DRA has also been studied in specific subgroups of patients undergoing PCI for complex CAD, including those with CTOs, LMCA, severely calcified coronary lesions, or complex non-LMCA bifurcation lesions.

20.3.1 Chronic Coronary Occlusions

CTO-PCI has traditionally been performed using TFA to facilitate the use of large-bore guiding catheters and to increase device support. In recent years, TRA has been increasingly used for CTO-PCI despite initial concerns about its safety and efficacy due to a lack of robust clinical evidence [19]. In a meta-analysis of 9 observational studies including 10,590 patients undergoing CTO-PCI [23], TRA was associated with similar technical success rates (78.7% vs. 78.5%, $p = 0.24$), lower risk of access site complications [0. 7% vs. 1.8%; odds ratio (OR), 0.34; 95% confidence interval (CI), 0.22–0.51, $p < 0.001$], and major bleeding (0.2% vs. 0.9%; OR, 0.22; 95% CI, 0.10–0.45, $p < 0.001$) and a similar risk of in-hospital mortality compared to TFA. However, due to the non-randomized design of the included studies, TRA was attempted in patients with lower baseline risk profiles and less complex CTO lesions, as indicated by lower Japan-CTO (J-CTO) scores (2.3 ± 1.2 vs. 2.5 ± 1.3, $p < 0.001$) than those treated with TFA.

Several studies have suggested the feasibility of large-bore TRA for CTO-PCI. In the first prospective, multicenter experience with the 7 Fr Glidesheath Slender sheath for complex coronary interventions, which included 60 patients [18], CTO-PCI was performed in 15 (25%) patients, and a bi-radial 7 Fr slender approach was even used for retrograde CTO techniques in 4 patients. In the randomized COLOR trial comparing 7 Fr TRA to TFA for complex PCI [19], 109 (56%) of 388 patients underwent CTO-PCI (mean J-CTO score, 2.0) via TRA using a 7 Fr Glidesheath Slender introducer sheath. The Femoral or Radial Approach in Treatment of Coronary Chronic Total Occlusion (FORT-CTO) trial was the first dedicated RCT to compare TRA with TFA for CTO-PCI [24]. In 610 CTO patients (mean J-CTO score, 2.1) undergoing PCI with predominantly large-diameter guiding catheters (7 Fr, 76%) by highly experienced operators, TRA was found to be non-inferior to TFA in terms of procedural success (84% vs. 86%, $p = 0.563$) but was associated with significantly fewer access site complications (2.0% vs. 5.6%, $p = 0.019$). In addition, there were no significant differences between TFA and TRA in terms of procedure time, contrast volume, or radiation dose, confirming the safety and feasibility of TRA for CTO-PCI.

The use of a unilateral or bilateral DRA approach for CTO-PCI has been reported in case reports and several small observational studies or post hoc subgroup analyses from large registries [25–29]. However, interpretation of the available evidence is limited by the small total number of patients included, the use of different introducer sheath types and sizes, and heterogeneity in study endpoint definitions, such as technical and procedural success rates. In the first prospective, multicenter, observational study evaluating the feasibility and safety of left DRA for CTO-PCI using a 7 Fr Glidesheath Slender sheath, which included 41 patients (mean age, 68; male, 76%; mean J-CTO score, 2.2), successful left DRA (83%) and technical success rates (90.3%) were high [26]. However, 17% of CTO patients required crossover to another access site, mainly due to weak or absent pulse in the anatomic snuffbox or excessive vessel tortuosity that did not allow wire advancement. The primary endpoint of procedural success was 78%. Importantly, there was no major bleeding, vascular access site complications, radial artery spasm, major sheath kinking, or left distal RAO at 24 h using a "patent hemostasis protocol." At a 1-month follow-up, left distal RAO as assessed by vascular ultrasound was only 4.3%. Overall, these findings demonstrate that large-bore left DRA for CTO-PCI using a 7 Fr Slender approach is feasible and safe, with high procedural success and low access site complication rates when performed by highly experienced DRA and CTO operators.

In a recent analysis from the prospective, multicenter, international Prospective Global Registry for the Study of Chronic Total Occlusion Intervention (PROGRESS-CTO), DRA was used in only 4% of all TRA for CTO-PCI between 2018 and 2019, but its use increased during the study period (13% in 2019) [27]. In a head-to-head comparison of patients undergoing CTO-PCI via DRA ($n = 120$; mean age, 63; left, 81%; 7 Fr guide catheter, 39%; male, 81%; mean J-CTO score, 2.4) or conventional TRA ($n = 2625$), technical success rates were similar between DRA and conventional TRA patients (91% vs. 86%, $p = 0.14$). Procedural success was higher (91% vs. 84%, $p = 0.05$), and radiation dose and incidence of coronary perforation were lower in patients treated with DRA compared to conventional TRA, while in-hospital and 12-month MACE, vascular access site complications and access site bleeding rates did not differ between DRA and conventional TRA patients (Fig. 20.2). Overall, the real-world data from the large PROGRESS-CTO registry confirm that the use of DRA for CTO PCI is increasing, is safe, and is associated with similar procedural success and complication rates as conventional

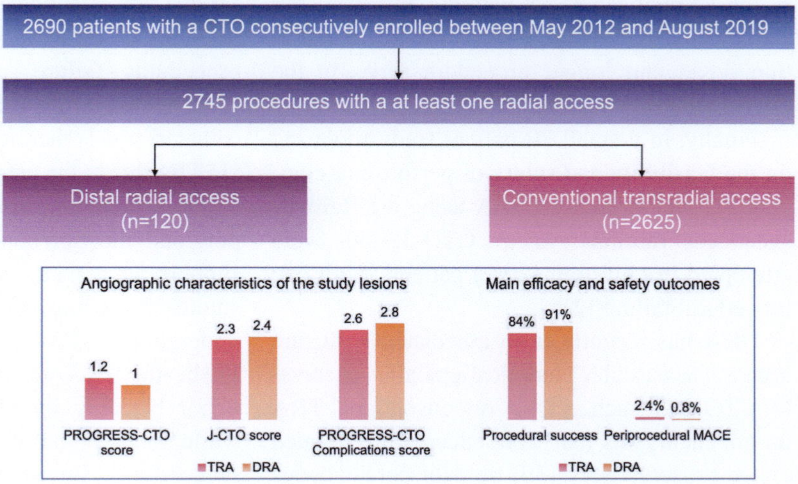

Fig. 20.2 Distal radial access in the Prospective Global Registry for the Study of Chronic Total Occlusion intervention (PROGRESS CTO) international registry

TRA. However, RAO rates during follow-up were not reported. In a single-center Chinese registry of 298 patients who underwent CTO-PCI via DRA (mean age, 61 years; male, 87%; mean J-CTO score, 2.6), mainly using a Glidesheath Slender sheath (7 Fr, 18.5%) by a single experienced operator, technical (94%) and procedural (93.5%; antegrade approach, 96.5%) success rates were high, while major access site vascular complications occurred in only 0.7% of patients. RAO rate was extremely low (0.5%), but detailed information on the modality used to assess RAO was not reported [28]. In a recent retrospective multicenter study of 337 consecutive patients undergoing CTO PCI [29], DRA (n = 80; mean age, 64; male, 65%; J-CTO score ≥ 2, 90%) was associated with significantly lower contrast volumes used and area product radiation doses but longer procedure and fluoroscopy times compared to conventional TRA. Procedural outcomes were similar between DRA and conventional TRA, including procedural (91% vs. 83%, $p = 0.10$) and clinical (88% vs. 80%, $p = 0.16$) success rates, while access site vascular complications were numerically less frequent in patients treated with DRA compared to those treated with conventional TRA, including the incidence of large hematoma and RAO as assessed by vascular ultrasound (1.3% vs. 2.7%, $p = 0.45$). Long-term clinical outcomes after CTO-PCI via DRA or conventional TRA were similar at up to 1 year of follow-up. These differences persisted in a propensity score matching analysis of 88 patients, but were not statistically significant, except for lower radiation doses and longer procedure times in the DRA patients.

Finally, in a small 20-patient study reporting on the feasibility and safety of performing complex PCI via large-bore DRA using the Railway sheathless vascular system, CTO lesions were attempted in only four (20%) patients, with one procedural failure [21].

DRA has recently been associated with rare access site vascular complications after successful CTO-PCI, such as DRA or conventional TRA pseudoaneurysms that were successfully treated either conservatively [30] or with percutaneous thrombin injection [31]. These findings highlight that although DRA is an attractive approach for CTO-PCI, it is not free of conventional vascular complications. Overall, the available non-randomized evidence supports the feasibility and safety of DRA for CTO-PCI using large-bore guiding catheters. However, dedicated larger prospective RCTs are needed to evaluate potential differences in outcomes with large-bore DRA compared to conventional TRA for CTO-PCI, particularly with respect to the occurrence of RAO.

A special consideration when using DRA for CTO-PCI is that the distance between the access site and the coronary ostium is the longest with DRA compared to TRA or TFA. In specific settings, such as retrograde CTO procedures using epicardial collaterals or bypass grafts as retrograde conduits, which often require shorter guide catheters (typically 90 cm), the use of DRA as a standard access site for CTO-PCI could therefore be relatively contraindicated due to the potential lack of sufficient length to achieve successful procedures and should be carefully evaluated before the procedure, taking into account the patient's size and brachiocephalic trunk tortuosity.

20.3.2 Left Main Coronary Artery Disease

LMCA disease remains a challenging lesion subset due to the technical complexity and frequent presence of bifurcation lesions predisposing to procedural failure and complications [32]. LMCA PCI often requires large-bore guiding catheters and is therefore traditionally performed via TFA due to the perceived practical limitations of TRA, including limited guiding catheter support and the potential need for hemodynamic support. In a meta-analysis of 8 observational studies including 3316 patients (TRA, 41%) undergoing LMCA PCI using predominantly <7 Fr sheaths, TRA was shown to reduce the risk of major bleeding by 69% compared with TFA, while maintaining similar rates of procedural success and clinical outcomes, including target lesion revascularization, myocardial infarction, stent thrombosis, and all-cause mortality [33]. In an updated meta-analysis of 12 non-randomized studies including 17,258 patients (TRA, 46%) undergoing LMCA PCI, TRA was associated with a significant reduction in the risk of access site bleeding (OR, 0.11; 95% CI, 0.04–0.26, $p < 0.0001$), major bleeding (OR, 0. 44; 95% CI, 0.27–0.69, $p = 0.0005$), access site or vascular complications (OR, 0.26; 95% CI, 0.17–0.40, $p < 0.00001$), and in-hospital mortality (OR, 0.49; 95% CI, 0.31–0.79, $p = 0.004$), while there were no significant differences in procedural success rates between TRA and TFA [34]. A small, retrospective, single-center Chinese study demonstrated the feasibility and safety of large-bore TRA for LMCA PCI [35]. Among 82 patients undergoing LMCA PCI via TRA using a 7.5 Fr sheathless guiding catheter, the procedural success rate was high (98%), and vascular complications occurred in only three patients (4%). In addition, there is limited data from the existing studies regarding the feasibility of large-bore TRA using thin-walled 7Fr Glidesheath Slender introducer sheaths for LMCA PCI. In a prospective, multicenter, observational registry of 60 patients undergoing 7 Fr TRA for complex PCI, 20 (33%) of patients were treated for unprotected distal LMCA lesions with provisional side-branch stenting in 16 patients, dual stenting in 3 patients, and kissing balloon inflation in 19 patients [18]. In the COLOR randomized trial comparing large-bore 7 Fr TRA with TFA for complex coronary interventions, LMCA PCI (ostial, 29%; distal, 57%) was performed in 31 (16%) of patients with large-bore 7 Fr TRA [19].

Currently, there is limited evidence regarding the feasibility and safety of DRA for LMCA PCI. Due to the lack of randomized data, the available evidence is mostly limited to a few successful cases reporting the use of DRA with 6 Fr [36–38] or standard 7 Fr [39] guiding catheters for complex LMCA PCI with two-stent techniques [39] or in a patient presenting with ST-segment elevation myocardial infarction complicated by cardiogenic shock [38]. Importantly, the number of patients undergoing LMCA PCI via DRA in the existing RCTs and large registries is very limited, precluding extrapolation of these results to this high-risk patient population. In the DISCO RADIAL trial, which compared DRA with conventional TRA for coronary angiography and/or PCI using a 6 Fr introducer sheath, only 8% of the total PCI patient population underwent LMCA PCI via DRA [8]. In a South Korean registry of 106 patients undergoing bifurcation PCI via DRA using predominantly 6 Fr sheaths, LMCA PCI was performed in only 11 (10%) patients [40]. Similarly, in the large Distal Transradial Access as Default Approach for Coronary Angiography and Interventions (DISTRACTION) registry, which included a total of 3683 consecutive patients who underwent coronary procedures via DRA using mostly 6 Fr sheaths (99%) in Brazil, only 70 (2%) patients were treated for LMCA disease [41]. Finally, in a study reporting the first experience with the 7 Fr sheath-free vascular access for complex PCI via DRA [21], 8 (40%) of 20 patients were treated for distal LMCA disease. These studies have confirmed the feasibility of large-bore DRA for LMCA PCI, but due to the overall small number of patients undergoing DRA with large-bore sheaths and guiding catheters in these studies, the safety and efficacy of large-bore (≥7 Fr) DRA compared to conventional TRA for LMCA PCI awaits confirmation in dedicated trials.

20.3.3 Heavily Calcified Coronary Lesions

TFA has long been the preferred approach for PCI in patients with severely calcified coronary lesions due to the anticipated need for large-bore guiding catheters to accommodate large RA burr sizes for plaque modification. However, patients undergoing RA have an increased risk of recurrent ischemic and bleeding complications after PCI [42] and therefore represent a subset of patients who may potentially benefit from TRA. Recently, atherectomy techniques have evolved toward the preferred use of smaller (1.25–1.5 mm) burr sizes, allowing RA to be routinely performed by large-bore TRA using 7 Fr or

7.5 Fr guide catheters, which are compatible with most radial arteries when inserted through a thin-walled sheath [18] or using a sheathless approach [43]. Retrospective studies have confirmed the increased use of TRA for complex PCI of severely calcified coronary lesions. In a retrospective study of 126 patients undergoing RA [44], procedural success rates and clinical outcomes, including in-hospital mortality or myocardial infarction, were similar between TRA and TFA, but TRA was associated with a lower risk of major access site bleeding complications compared with TFA (2% vs. 16%, $p = 0.012$). However, smaller guide catheter diameters and RA burr sizes (1.39 vs. 1.53, $p = 0.001$) were used in the TRA group. In a large retrospective study of 8622 patients from the British Cardiovascular Intervention Society (BCIS)-National Institute of Cardiovascular Outcomes Research (NICOR) database who underwent RA for heavily calcified coronary lesions [14], TRA was associated with similar rates of 30-day mortality, procedural success, major adverse cardiac and cerebrovascular events, and net adverse clinical events but significantly lower rates of in-hospital major bleeding (OR, 0.62; 95% CI, 0.40–0.98, $p = 0.04$) and major access site complications (OR, 0.05; 95% CI, 0.01–0.38, $p = 0.004$) compared to TFA. In a meta-analysis of 9153 patients undergoing RA from five observational studies [45], TRA was associated with a significant reduction of 55% in major access site bleeding and radiation exposure compared with TFA, but there were no significant differences in procedural success rates and procedure time, or in clinical outcomes, including in-hospital all-cause mortality, MACE, stent thrombosis, and myocardial infarction, between the TRA and TFA groups. The total number of patients undergoing PCI for heavily calcified coronary lesions with large-bore (≥7 Fr) TRA in available studies is limited. In a multicenter observational study of 60 patients undergoing large-bore TRA for complex PCI [18], RA was performed in ten patients (17%) using the 7 Fr Glidesheath Slender sheath. The maximum RA burr size was 1.5 mm in five patients, 1.75 mm in four patients, and 2.0 mm in one patient. In the COLOR randomized trial comparing large-bore 7Fr TRA with TFA for complex coronary interventions [19], 40 (21%) of the 388 patients enrolled were treated for heavily calcified coronary lesions via TRA using the 7Fr Glidesheath Slender introducer sheath.

Since most of the devices needed to treat heavily calcified coronary lesions are compatible with 5 Fr (coronary lithotripsy balloons) [46], 6 Fr (1.25–1.5 mm RA burr, 1.25 mm orbital atherectomy crown), or 7 Fr standard and 7.5 Fr sheathless (1.75 mm RA burr) guiding catheters, complex coronary interventions could theoretically be performed using DRA. However, there is limited evidence regarding the feasibility and safety of DRA for PCI of severely calcified coronary lesions. In a registry of 20 patients who underwent large-bore DRA using the 7 Fr Railway sheathless vascular access [21], RA was successfully used in 9 patients, intracoronary lithotripsy in 2 patients, and modified or super-high-pressure noncompliant balloons in 3 patients. Recently, the feasibility of intracoronary lithotripsy via DRA using a 5 Fr sheathless guiding catheter has also been reported [46].

20.3.4 Non-left Main Complex Bifurcation Lesions

Coronary bifurcation lesions are seen in up to 20% of patients undergoing PCI and remain one of the most challenging lesion subsets in interventional cardiology. Bifurcation PCI is associated with an increased risk of procedure failure and long-term MACE compared to PCI of non-bifurcation lesions [47]. Previous studies have shown that conventional TRA is a feasible alternative to TFA for non-LMCA bifurcation PCI [12]. Provisional side-branch stenting is currently the preferred strategy for bifurcation PCI [47], and most coronary bifurcation lesions can therefore be safely and effectively treated using 5 Fr or 6 Fr sheaths and guiding catheters, which can be accommodated by most radial arteries. However, the treatment of complex coronary bifurcation lesions may require a two-stent implantation strategy [47] or the use of multiple large balloons for kissing balloon inflation, which may pose potential challenges for TRA given its practical limitations such as guide catheter support and device size compatibility. In a single-center retrospective study of 805 patients undergoing complex bifurcation PCI with a two-stent technique (crush, 72%, T-Stent, 16%; culotte 10%) for true bifurcation coronary lesions TRA using predominantly 6 Fr guide catheters was associated with similar in-hospital and long-term clinical outcomes (including MACE, cardiac death, myocardial infarction, target vessel revascularization, and stent thrombosis), shorter hospital stay, and fewer bleeding complications (any BARC bleeding, 3.9% vs. 9.1%, $p < 0.01$) compared to TFA [48].

There is a paucity of studies reporting the feasibility and safety of large-bore TRA for complex non-LMCA bifurcation lesions. In the first prospective, multicenter, observational study to demonstrate the feasibility and safety of complex PCI via TRA using the thin-walled 7Fr Glidesheath Slender sheath [18], 16 (27%) of 60 patients underwent non-LMCA bifurcation PCI (two-stent technique, 16%; kissing balloon, 16%). In the COLOR randomized trial, which demonstrated a significant reduction in clinically relevant access site bleeding or vascular complications with large-bore TRA compared to TFA [19], only 13 (7%) of 388 patients underwent complex PCI of bifurcation lesions (Medina 1,1,1, 54%) via TRA using the thin-walled 7Fr Glidesheath Slender sheath.

Evidence regarding the feasibility and safety of DRA for complex non-LMCA bifurcation lesions is limited. In a single-center observational study of 106 patients undergoing PCI of bifurcation lesions (true bifurcation lesions, 40%) using predominantly a 6 Fr (95%) guiding catheter through left DRA [40], successful bifurcation PCI was achieved in 100% of patients without access site crossover, and no major bleeding complications, distal or forearm RAO, forearm hematoma, or mortality were observed at 30 days. Available data on large-bore (≥7 Fr) DRA for complex non-LMCA bifurcation lesions are limited. In the first study of the 7 Fr sheathless vascular access for complex PCI via DRA [21], 7 (35%) of 20 patients had non-LMCA complex bifurcation lesions. These results suggest the feasibility of large-bore DRA for PCI in this high-risk lesion subset, but larger studies are needed to confirm the safety and efficacy of DRA compared to conventional TRA for PCI of complex bifurcation lesions.

20.4 Conclusions

In recent years, several single- and multicenter RCTs have established DRA as a valid alternative vascular access site to conventional TRA for coronary angiography and/or PCI, but these studies have mostly included patients undergoing diagnostic procedures and/or PCI of non-complex coronary lesions using ≤6 Fr sheaths or guiding catheters. The available evidence on the safety and efficacy of DRA for PCI of complex coronary lesions, such as CTO, LMCA disease, severely calcified coronary lesions, or complex bifurcation lesions, is therefore limited to case reports, case series, small single-center studies, and multicenter registries that have included a limited number of patients treated with large-bore (≥7 Fr) sheaths and guiding catheters. Overall, these studies have demonstrated the feasibility and safety of DRA for complex PCI, but dedicated RCTs are needed to confirm these promising results. The ongoing DISCO COMPLEX RCT (NCT05490238) will determine the potential superiority of large-bore DRA over conventional TRA with respect to forearm RAO rates in patients undergoing complex PCI using the 7 Fr Glidesheath Slender introducer sheath.

References

1. Neumann FJ, Sousa-Uva M, Ahlsson A, Alfonso F, Banning AP, Benedetto U, et al. 2018 ESC/EACTS Guidelines on myocardial revascularization. Eur Heart J. 2019;40:87–165.
2. Lawton JS, Tamis-Holland JE, Bangalore S, Bates ER, Beckie TM, Bischoff JM, et al. 2021 ACC/AHA/SCAI guideline for coronary artery revascularization: executive summary: a report of the American College of Cardiology/American Heart Association Joint

Committee on clinical practice guidelines. J Am Coll Cardiol. 2022;79:197–215.
3. Ferrante G, Rao SV, Jüni P, Da Costa BR, Reimers B, Condorelli G, et al. Radial versus femoral access for coronary interventions across the entire spectrum of patients with coronary artery disease: a meta-analysis of randomized trials. JACC Cardiovasc Interv. 2016;9:1419–34.
4. Gargiulo G, Giacoppo D, Jolly SS, Cairns J, Le May M, Bernat I, et al. Effects on mortality and major bleeding of radial versus femoral artery access for coronary angiography or percutaneous coronary intervention: meta-analysis of individual patient data from 7 multicenter randomized clinical trials. Circulation. 2022;146:1329–43.
5. Amin AP, House JA, Safley DM, Chhatriwalla AK, Giersiefen H, Bremer A, et al. Costs of transradial percutaneous coronary intervention. JACC Cardiovasc Interv. 2013;6:827–34.
6. Eid-Lidt G, Rivera Rodríguez A, Jimenez Castellanos J, Farjat Pasos JI, Estrada López KE, Gaspar J. Distal radial artery approach to prevent radial artery occlusion trial. JACC Cardiovasc Interv. 2021;14:378–85.
7. Tsigkas G, Papageorgiou A, Moulias A, Kalogeropoulos AP, Papageorgopoulou C, Apostolos A, et al. Distal or traditional transradial access site for coronary procedures: a single-center, Randomized Study. JACC Cardiovasc Interv. 2022;15:22–32.
8. Aminian A, Sgueglia GA, Wiemer M, Kefer J, Gasparini GL, Ruzsa Z, et al. Distal versus conventional radial access for coronary angiography and intervention: the DISCO RADIAL trial. JACC Cardiovasc Interv. 2022;15:1191–201.
9. Riley RF, Henry TD, Mahmud E, Kirtane AJ, Brilakis ES, Goyal A, et al. SCAI position statement on optimal percutaneous coronary interventional therapy for complex coronary artery disease. Catheter Cardiovasc Interv. 2020;96:346–62.
10. Doyle BJ, Ting HH, Bell MR, Lennon RJ, Mathew V, Singh M, et al. Major femoral bleeding complications after percutaneous coronary intervention: incidence, predictors, and impact on long-term survival among 17,901 patients treated at the Mayo Clinic from 1994 to 2005. JACC Cardiovasc Interv. 2008;1:202–9.
11. Smilowitz NR, Kirtane AJ, Guiry M, Gray WA, Dolcimascolo P, Querijero M, et al. Practices and complications of vascular closure devices and manual compression in patients undergoing elective transfemoral coronary procedures. Am J Cardiol. 2012;110:177–82.
12. Chung S, Her SH, Song PS, Song YB, Hahn JY, Choi JH, et al. Trans-radial versus trans-femoral intervention for the treatment of coronary bifurcations: results from coronary bifurcation stenting registry. J Korean Med Sci. 2013;28:388–95.
13. Maeremans J, Walsh S, Knaapen P, Spratt JC, Avran A, Hanratty CG, et al. The hybrid algorithm for treating chronic total occlusions in Europe: the RECHARGE registry. J Am Coll Cardiol. 2016;68:1958–70.
14. Watt J, Austin D, Mackay D, Nolan J, Oldroyd KG. Radial versus femoral access for rotational atherectomy: A UK observational study of 8622 patients. Circ Cardiovasc Interv. 2017;10:e005311.
15. Tanaka Y, Moriyama N, Ochiai T, Takada T, Tobita K, Shishido K, et al. Transradial coronary interventions for complex chronic total occlusions. JACC Cardiovasc Interv. 2017;10:235–43.
16. Saito S, Ikei H, Hosokawa G, Tanaka S. Influence of the ratio between radial artery inner diameter and sheath outer diameter on radial artery flow after transradial coronary intervention. Catheter Cardiovasc Interv. 1999;46:173–8.
17. Yoo BS, Yoon J, Ko JY, Kim JY, Lee SH, Hwang SO, Choe KH. Anatomical consideration of the radial artery for transradial coronary procedures: arterial diameter, branching anomaly and vessel tortuosity. Int J Cardiol. 2005;101:421–7.
18. Aminian A, Iglesias JF, Van Mieghem C, Zuffi A, Ferrara A, Manih R, et al. First prospective multicenter experience with the 7 French Glidesheath slender for complex transradial coronary interventions. Catheter Cardiovasc Interv. 2017;89:1014–20.
19. Meijers TA, Aminian A, van Wely M, Teeuwen K, Schmitz T, Dirksen MT, et al. Randomized comparison between radial and femoral large-bore access for complex percutaneous coronary intervention. JACC Cardiovasc Interv. 2021;14:1293–303.
20. Ferrante G, Condello F, Rao SV, Maurina M, Jolly S, Stefanini GG, et al. Distal vs conventional radial access for coronary angiography and/or intervention: a meta-analysis of randomized trials. JACC Cardiovasc Interv. 2022;15:2297–311.
21. Colletti G, Auslender J, De Meester A, Aminian A, Kayaert P, Ungureanu C. Feasibility and safety of performing complex coronary interventions by distal radial artery using the railway Sheathless vascular system. J Invasive Cardiol. 2020;32:459–62.
22. Zong B, Liu Y, Han B, Feng CG. Safety and feasibility of a 7F thin-walled sheath via distal transradial artery access for complex coronary intervention. Front Cardiovasc Med. 2022;9:959197.
23. Megaly M, Karatasakis A, Abraham B, Jensen J, Saad M, Omer M, et al. Radial versus femoral access in chronic total occlusion percutaneous coronary intervention. Circ Cardiovasc Interv. 2019;12:e007778.
24. Gorgulu S, Kalay N, Norgaz T, Kocas C, Goktekin O, Brilakis ES. Femoral or radial approach in treatment of coronary chronic total occlusion: a randomized clinical trial. JACC Cardiovasc Interv. 2022;15:823–30.
25. Kim Y, Hyun DY, Cho KH, Kim MC, Sim DS, Hong YJ, et al. Snuffbox approach for coronary chronic total occlusion intervention using a 7-French sheath. Chonnam Med J. 2019;55:175–6.
26. Gasparini GL, Garbo R, Gagnor A, Oreglia J, Mazzarotto P. First prospective multicentre experience with left distal transradial approach for coronary chronic total occlusion interventions using a 7 Fr Glidesheath Slender. EuroIntervention. 2019;15:126–8.

27. Nikolakopoulos I, Patel T, Jefferson BK, Sheikh AM, Jaber W, Samady H, et al. Distal radial access in chronic total occlusion percutaneous coronary intervention: insights from the PROGRESS-CTO registry. J Invasive Cardiol. 2021;33:E717–22.
28. Lin CJ, Lee WC, Lee CH, Chung WJ, Hsueh SK, Chen CJ, et al. Feasibility and safety of chronic total occlusion percutaneous coronary intervention via distal transradial access. Front Cardiovasc Med. 2021;8:673858.
29. Achim A, Szigethy T, Olajos D, Molnár L, Papp R, Bárczi G, et al. Switching from proximal to distal radial artery access for coronary chronic total occlusion recanalization. Front Cardiovasc Med. 2022;9:895457.
30. Gitto M, Brizzi S, Cozzi O, Gohar A, Maurina M, Spaca P, et al. Radial artery pseudoaneurysm complicating distal transradial access for chronic total occlusion recanalization. Cardiovasc Revasc Med. 2022;40S:279–81.
31. Budassi S, Zivelonghi C, De Roover D, Scott B, Agostoni P. Distal radial pseudoaneurysm after chronic total occlusion percutaneous coronary intervention resolved by percutaneous thrombin injection. Cardiovasc Revasc Med. 2020;21(11S):134–7.
32. Naganuma T, Chieffo A, Meliga E, Capodanno D, Park SJ, Onuma Y, et al. Long-term clinical outcomes after percutaneous coronary intervention for ostial/mid-shaft lesions versus distal bifurcation lesions in unprotected left main coronary artery: the DELTA Registry (drug-eluting stent for left main coronary artery disease): a multicenter registry evaluating percutaneous coronary intervention versus coronary artery bypass grafting for left main treatment. JACC Cardiovasc Interv. 2013;6:1242–9.
33. Ando T, Aoi S, Ashraf S, Villablanca PA, Telila T, Briasoulis A, et al. Transradial versus transfemoral percutaneous coronary intervention of left main disease: a systematic review and meta-analysis of observational studies. Catheter Cardiovasc Interv. 2019;94:264–73.
34. Goel S, Pasam RT, Raheja H, Gotesman J, Gidwani U, Ahuja KR, et al. Left main percutaneous coronary intervention-radial versus femoral access: a systematic analysis. Catheter Cardiovasc Interv. 2020;95:E201–13.
35. Zhao H, Banerjee S, Chen H, Li H. Transradial percutaneous coronary intervention for left main bifurcation lesions using 7.5-Fr sheathless guide catheter. Medicine. 2018;97:e0678.
36. Kim Y, Jeong MH, Kim I, Kim MC, Sim DS, Hong YJ, et al. Intravascular ultrasound-guided percutaneous coronary intervention with drug-eluting stent for unprotected left main disease via left snuffbox approach. Korean Circ J. 2018;48:532–3.
37. Yoshimachi F, Kawamura Y, Nagamatsu H, Karasawa Y, Murotani N, Kasai S. Distal radial approach treating a left main lesion during hemostasis of the forearm radial artery on the same side in a case of unstable angina. J Cardiol Cases. 2021;25:52–4.
38. Oliveira MDP, Navarro EC, de Sá GA, Caixeta A. Unprotected left main primary PCI via distal Transradial access in the setting of STEMI-Related Cardiogenic shock. Heart Views. 2021;22:146–9.
39. Kim Y, Jeong MH, Kim MC, Sim DS, Hong YJ, Kim JH, Ahn Y. Successful percutaneous coronary intervention with two-stent technique for unprotected true left main bifurcation lesion via left snuffbox approach. J Invasive Cardiol. 2019;31:E55.
40. Lee OH, Roh JW, Im E, Cho DK, Jeong MH, Choi D, Kim Y. Feasibility and safety of the left distal radial approach in percutaneous coronary intervention for bifurcation lesions. J Clin Med. 2021;10:2204.
41. Oliveira MD, Navarro EC, Caixeta A. Distal transradial access for coronary procedures: a prospective cohort of 3,683 all-comers patients from the DISTRACTION registry. Cardiovasc Diagn Ther. 2022;12:208–19.
42. Cockburn J, Hildick-Smith D, Cotton J, Doshi S, Hanratty C, Ludman P, et al. Contemporary clinical outcomes of patients treated with or without rotational coronary atherectomy – an analysis of the UK central cardiac audit database. Int J Cardiol. 2014;170:381–7.
43. Kassimis G, Patel N, Kharbanda RK, Channon KM, Banning AP. High-speed rotational atherectomy using the radial artery approach and a sheathless guide: a single-centre comparison with the "conventional" femoral approach. EuroIntervention. 2014;10:694–9.
44. Yin WH, Tseng CK, Tsao TP, Jen HL, Huang WP, Huang CL, et al. Transradial versus transfemoral rotablation for heavily calcified coronary lesions in contemporary drug-eluting stent era. J Geriatr Cardiol. 2015;12:489–96.
45. Khan AA, Panchal HB, Zaidi SIM, Papireddy MR, Mukherjee D, Cohen MG, et al. Safety and efficacy of radial versus femoral access for rotational Atherectomy: a systematic review and meta-analysis. Cardiovasc Revasc Med. 2019;20:241–7.
46. Sgueglia GA, Gioffrè G, Piccioni F, Gaspardone A. Slender distal radial five French coronary shockwave lithotripsy. Catheter Cardiovasc Interv. 2019;94:395–8.
47. Lassen JF, Albiero R, Johnson TW, Burzotta F, Lefèvre T, Iles TL, et al. Treatment of coronary bifurcation lesions, part II: implanting two stents. The 16th expert consensus document of the European Bifurcation Club. EuroIntervention. 2022;18:457–70.
48. Gao Z, Xu B, Yang Y, Kandzari DE, Sun Z, Qiao S, et al. Transradial versus transfemoral method of two-stent implantation for true bifurcation lesions: comparison of immediate and long-term outcomes. J Interv Cardiol. 2014;27:99–107.

21 Ancillary Distal Radial Access

Azeem Latib and Stefano Rigattieri

21.1 Introduction

A secondary or ancillary arterial access is often required in various complex coronary or structural heart interventional procedures. Traditionally, both femoral arteries or both femoral and brachial arteries have been used. More recently, with the proliferation of the radial approach for coronary procedures, there has been a growing interest in the use of the radial artery as an ancillary arterial access, given the striking reduction in vascular complications and access site bleeding compared to the femoral approach that has been consistently demonstrated in coronary procedures. Accordingly, several reports have described the use of the radial approach in a variety of structural heart procedures [1]. Of note, the beneficial effect of the ancillary radial approach in reducing major bleeding compared to the femoral or brachial approach was observed in a multicenter observational registry, with similar procedural success rates between the different approaches [2]. In this chapter, we will discuss the use of the ancillary radial approach, focusing on its use in transcatheter aortic valve implantation (TAVI) procedures, while its use in complex percutaneous coronary intervention, chronic total occlusion, and peripheral interventions will be discussed elsewhere in the book. An overview of the major procedural settings in which the radial approach has been used is shown in Fig. 21.1.

A. Latib (✉)
Division of Cardiology, Montefiore Medical Center, Albert Einstein College of Medicine, New York, NY, USA

S. Rigattieri
Division of Cardiology, Sant'Andrea University Hospital, Rome, Italy

G. A. Sgueglia (ed.), *Distal Radial Access*, https://doi.org/10.1007/978-3-031-89925-6_21

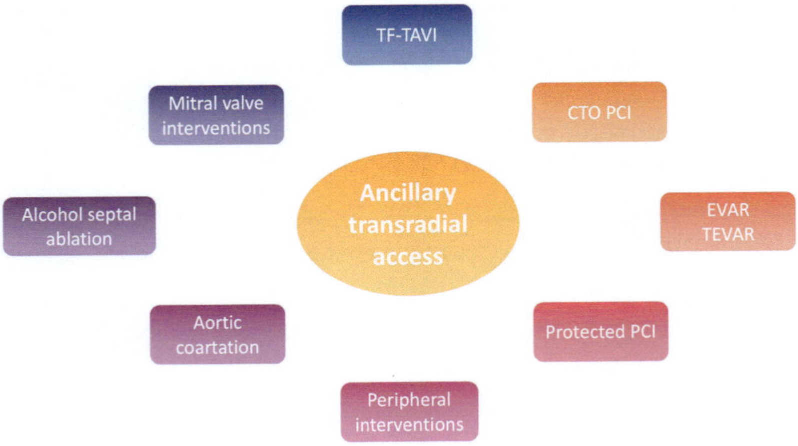

Fig. 21.1 An overview of the contemporary landscape of ancillary transradial approach for percutaneous cardiovascular interventions. *CTO* chronic total occlusion, *EVAR* endovascular aneurysm repair, *PCI* percutaneous coronary intervention, *TAVI* transcatheter aortic valve implantation, *TEVAR* thoracic endovascular aneurysm repair, *TF* transfemoral

21.2 Ancillary Conventional Transradial Access in TAVI: Rationale and Overview of Available Studies

Contemporary TAVI procedures are typically performed through a large-bore percutaneous femoral access or, less commonly, a percutaneous or surgical transaxillary access. Although single-access TAVI has been described [3], in most cases a secondary arterial access is required for the following reasons: (1) performing fluoro- or angio-guided access, (2) performing aortography/invasive hemodynamic monitoring, (3) placing a pigtail catheter (usually in the non-coronary cusp) as a landmark of the aortic annulus, (4) facilitating primary vascular access, (4) facilitating hemostasis of the primary vascular access by inflating a balloon in the common femoral artery, (5) performing angiography of the access site to assess for vascular complications, and finally (6) facilitating management of any complications with balloon/stent implantation. Traditionally, the secondary arterial access has been the contralateral femoral, which, with the crossover technique, allows both angiography of the iliofemoral axis and vascular protection by placing a wire in the superficial femoral artery. However, a major limitation of this approach is the occurrence of vascular complications and bleeding, which may account for up to one quarter of all vascular complications after TAVI [4–6].

Although no randomized comparison of femoral versus radial access in TAVI has ever been performed, several observational studies have demonstrated both the safety and feasibility of radial access, which has been clearly shown to be superior to femoral access in the coronary setting in terms of vascular complications and bleeding in numerous randomized controlled trials and meta-analyses [7]. In a cohort of 462 consecutive patients undergoing TAVI, Allende et al. observed a significantly higher rate of vascular complications and bleeding with femoral than with radial secondary access (5% vs. 0% and 3% vs. 0%, respectively) [4]. Similar results were observed by Wynne et al. in a cohort of 282 patients [8]; however, the secondary transradial access was not suitable for the treatment of primary access bleeding, requiring an urgent contralateral femoral access and highlighting the most important limitation of the secondary radial access, i.e., the lack of adequate length devices and the lack of devices of adequate length. In contrast, such devices (mainly long-shafted balloon catheters) were effectively used by Jackson et al. who successfully managed primary access complications without the need for bail-out contralateral femoral access, although the overall rate of vascular complications related to secondary access was similar in patients with radial versus femoral secondary access (0% vs. 1.6%, p = ns) [9].

A meta-analysis of 6 observational studies including 6373 patients showed that radial access was associated with an approximately 50% reduction in both major bleeding and major vascular complications compared to femoral access [10]. The incidence of access-related vascular complications after radial secondary access or femoral secondary access in TAVR, was assessed in 8851 patients from the multicenter Plug or sUture based vascuLar cloSurE after TAVR (PULSE) registry. Vascular complications occurred in 0.3% of cases in radial secondary access vs 3.2% of cases in femoral secondary access (p<0.001) and were considered major in 0.2% and 1.5% of cases, respectively (p<0.001) [11] . In the TAVI XS, the first randomized clinical trial directly comparing an upper-vs a lower-extremity secondary access in patients undergoing transfemoral TAVI, clinically relevant bleeding occurred in 4.2% of patients in the upper-extremity group vs. 13.4% in the lower-extremity group (p=0.01) [12].

In a multicenter study [5], the 30-day clinical outcomes of 928 patients undergoing TAVI with secondary radial access were compared with a propensity-matched cohort of 2978 patients undergoing TAVI with secondary femoral access; in particular, radial access was associated not only with a significant reduction in bleeding and vascular complications but also with a significant reduction in mortality, stroke, acute kidney injury, and length of hospital stay.

Studies have consistently shown that secondary femoral access for TAVI accounts for 25% of all vascular complications and suggest that radial access is both feasible and safe and is associated with improved 30-day clinical outcomes. The major limitation of secondary radial access is the paucity of devices capable of safely reaching the iliofemoral region from the arm in tall patients or those with severe vessel tortuosity, particularly with covered stents, which now require a contralateral femoral (crossover) approach (Table 21.1). However, in published studies, the need for bailout femoral crossover was rare (less than 1%) and could be safely performed while ensuring balloon hemostasis through the ancillary radial approach; in particular, the ipsilateral retrograde superficial femoral artery approach could be a valid alternative in this setting [13].

Table 21.1 Percutaneous transluminal angioplasty devices suitable for ancillary distal radial access in TAVI

Name	Manufacturer	Category	Max catheter length (cm)	Guidewire diameter	Compatible sheath (Fr)	Diameter (mm)	Length (mm)
Advance 18LP	Cook medical	RX balloon	170	0.018″	5	2–9	20–200
Pacific Xtreme	Medtronic	OTW balloon	180	0.018″	4	4–5	150
Ultraverse 018	BD interventional	OTW balloon	200	0.018″	5–6	4–9	40–300
Lovix	Balton	OTW balloon	170	0.018–0.035″	5–8	1.5–16	20–250
Passeo-35 Xeo	Biotronik	OTW balloon	170	0.0035″	5–6	4–10	20–250
Oceanus 35	iVascular	OTW balloon	200	0.035″	5–6	6–12	20
Sinus Superflex 518	Optimed	Self-expanding nitinol stent	180	0.018″	5	6–10	40–80
Dynetic-35	Biotronik	Balloon-expandable cobalt-chrome	170	0.035″	6	5–10	28–78
VascuFlex	B. Braun	Self-expanding nitinol stent	180	0.018″	5	6–8	40–80

OTW over the wire, *RX* rapid exchange *TAVI* transcatheter aortic valve implantation

21.3 Ancillary Distal Radial Access for TAVI

In recent years, distal radial access (DRA) has emerged as an alternative to conventional transradial access (TRA) for coronary procedures. Like TRA, DRA is associated with a marked reduction in vascular complications and access-related bleeding compared with the femoral approach; moreover, DRA is associated with a lower rate of radial artery occlusion and forearm hematoma compared with TRA, although at the expense of a higher crossover rate and a more technically demanding vascular access [14]. In fact, at the level of the anatomical snuffbox or dorsum of the hand where DRA is performed, the vessel lumen is on average 20% smaller compared to the proximal radial artery; therefore, an echo-guided approach is recommended [15]. Another issue to consider with DRA is that the arteriotomy is 3–5 cm more distal compared to TRA; accordingly, 110 cm coronary catheters are recommended for tall patients [15]. This issue is even more relevant when DRA is chosen for peripheral procedures or as an adjunct to TAVI. In the latter setting, there is only one series in the literature; Achim et al. published the results of a single-center retrospective study of 41 patients with severe aortic stenosis undergoing transfemoral TAVI. No access-related complications were observed at the level of the DRA, whereas seven large-bore access complications were observed, four of which required covered stent placement via ipsilateral superficial femoral artery access [16]. This preliminary study not only demonstrates the feasibility of adjunctive DRA in TAVI but also highlights the major limitation of both TRA and DRA in this setting, which is the inability to treat femoral artery rupture with covered stents. The advantages and disadvantages of different secondary vascular access sites for TAVI are outlined in Table 21.2. With the important exception of vascular complications, the auxiliary femoral access is probably the most comfortable choice for the operator and allows the management of most primary access site complications, including the sealing of femoral artery rupture with covered stents. In contrast, both radial accesses are limited by vessel size and distance from the arteriotomy site; TRA is probably easier to obtain and offers a slightly larger vessel compared to DRA, which in turn may be associated with improved operator comfort (if left-sided access is chosen) and arguably reduced operator radiation exposure, although the latter has not yet been demonstrated in clinical trials.

Finally, DRA can also be used as an alternative to TRA, both for positioning a dual-filter cerebral protection device compatible with a 6 Fr sheath (Sentinel, Boston Scientific) and for coronary protection and chimney technique in procedures considered at high risk of coronary occlusion (Figs. 21.2 and 21.3).

Table 21.2 Advantages and limitations of different ancillary vascular access for TF-TAVI

	Contralateral TFA	Left TRA	Left DRA
Vascular complications	🔴	🟡	🟢
Crossover rate	🟢	🟡	🔴
Radiation exposure	🟢	🔴	🟡
Proximity to arteriotomy site	🟢	🟢	🟡
Compatibility with devices	🟢	🔴	🔴
Vessel size issues	🟢	🟢	🟡
Operator's comfort	🟢	🔴	🟡

DRA distal radial access, *TAVI* transcatheter aortic valve implantation, *TF* transfemoral, *TFA* transfemoral access, *TRA* transradial access, 🟢 optimal, 🟡 fair, 🔴 poor

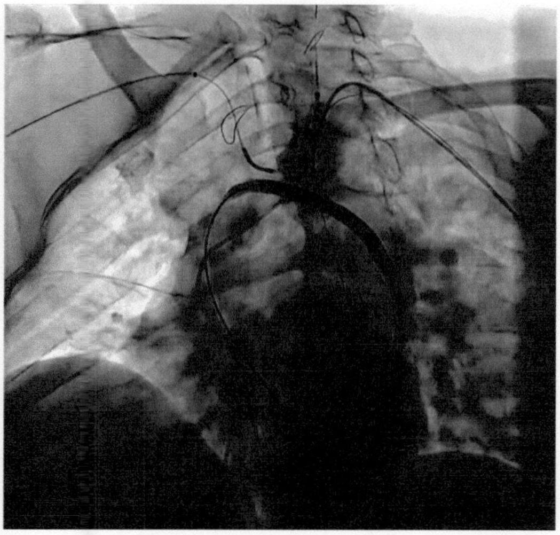

Fig. 21.2 Ancillary right radial access for positioning of a dual-filter cerebral protection device compatible with a 6 Fr sheath (Sentinel, Boston Scientific) and left radial access for pigtail and safety guidewire positioning during the implantation of a Evolut PRO+ (Medtronic) transcatheter aortic valve

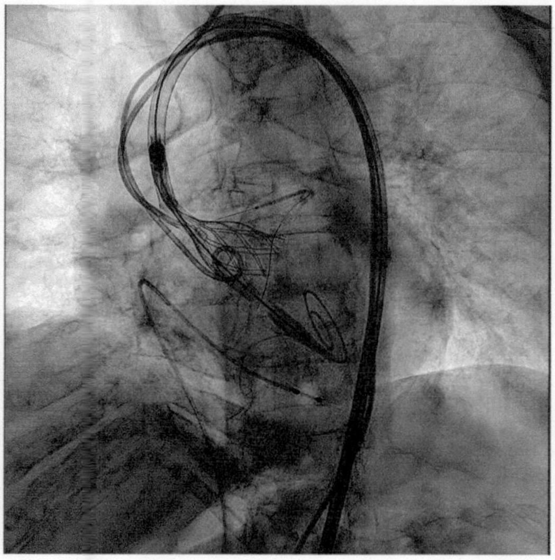

Fig. 21.3 Ancillary radial approach for 0.014″ guidewire and stent positioning in the left main coronary artery during the implantation of a Navitor (Abbott) transcatheter aortic valve deemed at high risk for coronary occlusion due to low left coronary ostium take-off (courtesy of Prof. Andrea Berni, Sant'Andrea University Hospital, Rome, Italy)

21.4 Distal Radial Access in Alternative Access TAVI

Patients with suboptimal femoral access for TAVI may require an alternative approach. Surgical access is being used less frequently, and percutaneous approaches are being used increasingly. Radial access may be particularly useful in two of these approaches:

21.4.1 Transaxillary Access

Transaxillary access is increasingly performed percutaneously with hemostasis performed using suture-based closure devices. Ipsilateral radial access is an integral part of the procedure and is important for:

- Selective baseline subclavian angiography to delineate anatomy and guide arterial puncture.
- Placement of a 0.018″ protection wire.
- Aortography during valve deployment in femoral occlusions.
- Balloon-assisted occlusion during large-bore sheath removal.
- Delivery of a covered stent providing sheath upgrade to a 7 Fr thin-walled sheath.
- Final angiography of the access site to confirm hemostasis.

21.4.2 Transcaval Access

Transcaval access is also an excellent percutaneous option for TAVR in patients with unfavorable femoral access. Typically, transfemoral arterial access is essential to complete the procedure, but transcaval access has been performed in patients with occluded femoral arteries. In these cases, radial access is important for the following:

- Baseline aortography to confirm the transcaval crossing site.
- Placement of a snare to capture the stiff guidewire after crossing and to create a rail to allow exchange of microcatheters and the 0.035″ stiff wire needed to advance the large-bore sheath.
- Aortography during valve implantation.
- Final aortography to confirm closure of the aorto-caval shunt.

21.5 Ancillary Radial Access in Other Structural Interventional Procedures

21.5.1 Mitral Valve Interventions

Transradial access also has a role in transcatheter mitral valve-in-valve and valve-in-ring procedures and may be useful in the following situations:

- Measurement of left ventricular outflow tract gradients during valve implantation.
- Placement of a Sentinel cerebral embolic protection device.
- Snaring of the stiff guidewire during tip-to-base LAMPOON (intentional laceration of the anterior mitral leaflet to prevent left ventricular outflow tract obstruction) procedure.

21.5.2 Alcohol Septal Ablation in Hypertrophic Cardiomyopathy

Alcohol septal ablation is a therapeutic option for patients with symptomatic obstructive hypertrophic cardiomyopathy when medical therapy is either ineffective or intolerable. As an alternative to the conventional double femoral artery approach (one femoral artery for the coronary guide catheter and the other for a pigtail for hemodynamic monitoring in the left ventricle), the use of one (ancillary) or two (main and ancillary) radial arteries has been reported with a similar procedural success rate and a lower incidence of access site complications [17–19]. To the best of our knowledge, no report has been published on the use of DRA, although the latter seems feasible since it usually requires 6 or 7 Fr coronary guiding catheters and 4 or 5 Fr diagnostic pigtail catheters.

21.5.3 Endovascular Repair of Aortic Coarctation

Percutaneous repair of aortic coarctation in adults is usually performed by placing a balloon-expandable bare-metal stent through an 8 Fr femoral approach that accommodates an 8 Fr Gensini catheter used to cross the coarctation retrogradely. Placement of a 6 Fr diagnostic pigtail catheter through an ancillary radial approach may be useful during the procedure as it allows assessment of pressure gradients and aortography in the descending aorta proximal to the coarctation, which is useful during stent placement and clarifies the origin of the left subclavian artery [20]. Although not reported in the literature, DRA may also be a relevant alternative to the conventional TRA in this setting.

21.6 Conclusions

In the evolving field of structural heart interventions, careful selection of vascular access sites is of paramount importance to prevent and eventually treat bleeding and other vascular complications. In addition, with an increasing proportion of younger patients being treated compared to the past, maintaining vascular access sites for future procedures as part of a lifelong strategy is a relevant issue. In this regard, DRA has the advantage of a lower occlusion rate and also preserves the forearm radial artery for future procedures.

References

1. Allende R, Ribeiro HB, Puri R, Urena M, Abdul-Jawad O, del Trigo M, et al. The transradial approach during transcatheter structural heart disease interventions: a review. Eur J Clin Investig. 2015;45:215–25.
2. Cortese B, Rigattieri S, Aranzulla TC, Russo F, Latib A, Burzotta F, et al. Transradial versus transfemoral ancillary approach in complex structural, coronary, and peripheral interventions. Results from the multicenter ancillary registry: a study of the Italian Radial Club. Catheter Cardiovasc Interv. 2018;91:97–102.
3. Aroney NP, Patterson T, Kalogeropoulos A, Allen CJ, Hurrell H, Chehab O, et al. Clinical outcomes following single access transfemoral transcatheter aortic valve implantation. Catheter Cardiovasc Interv. 2022;100:227–32.
4. Allende R, Urena M, Cordoba JG, Ribeiro HB, Amat-Santos I, Delarochellière R, et al. Impact of the use of transradial versus transfemoral approach as secondary access in transcatheter aortic valve implantation procedures. Am J Cardiol. 2014;114:1729–34.
5. Junquera L, Urena M, Latib A, Munõz-Garcia A, Nombela-Franco L, Faurie B, et al. Comparison of transfemoral versus transradial secondary access in transcatheter aortic valve replacement. Circ Cardiovasc Interv. 2020;13:e008609.
6. Fernandez-Lopez L, Chevalier B, Lefèvre T, Spaziano M, Unterseeh T, Champagne S, et al. Implementation of the transradial approach as an alternative vascular access for transcatheter aortic valve replacement guidance: experience from a high-volume center. Catheter Cardiovasc Interv. 2019;93:1367–73.
7. Gargiulo G, Giacoppo D, Jolly SS, Cairns J, Le May M, Bernat I, et al. Effects on mortality and major bleeding of radial versus femoral artery access for coronary angiography or percutaneous coronary intervention: meta-analysis of individual patient data from 7 multicenter randomized clinical trials. Circulation. 2022;146:1329–43.
8. Wynne DG, Rampat R, Trivedi U, De Belder A, Hill A, Hutchinson N, et al. Transradial secondary arterial access for transcatheter aortic valve implantation: experience and limitations. Heart Lung Circ. 2015;24:682–5.
9. Jackson MWP, Muir DF, de Belder MA, Palmer S, Owens WA, Goodwin A, et al. Transradial secondary access to guide valve implantation and manage peripheral vascular complications during transcatheter aortic valve implantation. Heart Lung Circ. 2019;28:637–46.
10. Jhand A, Apala DR, Dhawan R, Katta N, Aronow HD, Daniels MJ, et al. Meta-analysis comparing transradial versus transfemoral secondary access in transcatheter aortic valve implantation. Am J Cardiol. 2020;131:74–81.
11. Grundmann D, Kim W, Kellner C, Adam M, Braun D, Tamm AR, et al. Femoral or radial secondary access in TAVR. JACC Cardiovasc Interv. 2024;17:2923–2932.
12. Versteeg GAA, Rooijakkers MJP, Hemelrijk KI, Vlaar PJ, Overduin DC, van Wely MH, et al. Upper- vs lower-extremity secondary access during transcatheter aortic valve implantation. JAMA Netw Open. 2024;7:e2438578.
13. Sanghvi K, Swarup S, Burns P, Kovach R, Ross R, Soussa T. Prophylactic retrograde distal common femoral access as a bail-out strategy in patients with increased risk for femoral access complication during transfemoral aortic valve replacement. Cardiovasc Revasc Med. 2020;21:481–5.
14. Ferrante G, Condello F, Rao SV, Maurina M, Jolly S, Stefanini GG, et al. Distal vs conventional radial access for coronary angiography and/or intervention: a meta-analysis of randomized trials. JACC Cardiovasc Interv. 2022;15:2297–311.
15. Sgueglia GA, Lee BK, Cho BR, Babunashvili A, Lee JB, Lee JW, et al. Distal radial access: consensus report of the first Korea-Europe transradial intervention meeting. JACC Cardiovasc Interv. 2021;14:892–906.
16. Achim A, Szűcsborus T, Sasi V, Nagy F, Jambrik Z, Nemes A, et al. Distal radial secondary access for transcatheter aortic valve implantation: the minimalistic approach. Cardiovasc Revasc Med. 2022;40:152–7.
17. Blaker N, Bidwell K, Karimianpour A, Miller T, Nielsen C, Fernandes V. Improved outcomes with transradial approach in alcohol septal ablation. J Invasive Cardiol. 2022;34:E726–9.
18. Sawaya FJ, Louvard Y, Spaziano M, Morice MC, Hage F, El-Khoury C, et al. Short and long-term outcomes of alcohol septal ablation with the trans-radial versus the trans-femoral approach a single center-experience. Int J Cardiol. 2016;220:7–13.
19. Isawa T, Tada N, Ootomo T, Sakurai M, Takizawa K, Inoue N. Transradial approach of alcohol septal ablation using a sheathless guiding catheter: a feasibility study. J Invasive Cardiol. 2015;27:E242–7.
20. Dehghani P, Collins N, Benson L, Horlick E. Role of routine radial artery access during aortic coarctation interventions. Catheter Cardiovasc Interv. 2007;70:622–3.

22 Structural Heart Interventions

Carlo Tumscitz and Ignacio M. Seropian

22.1 Introduction

In addition to the diagnosis and treatment of coronary artery disease, transradial access (TRA) is increasingly being used for peripheral vascular procedures, neurointerventions, and selected structural heart disease procedures [1]. Specifically, TRA has been reported as the primary access site for alcohol septal ablation [2], paravalvular leak closure [3], ventricular septal defect closure [4], and endomyocardial biopsy [5]. However, the largest body of evidence relates to balloon aortic valvuloplasty (BAV), a therapeutic procedure designed to treat aortic stenosis by mechanically opening the narrowed valve with an inflated balloon placed across the aortic valve via a femoral vascular access. Alain Cribier first reported this procedure in 1985, nearly two decades before the introduction of transcatheter aortic valve replacement (TAVR) [6]. The common femoral artery was the most commonly used approach with a vascular access of >10 Fr. However, the antegrade femoral vein approach through transseptal approach have also been described but have been performed infrequently due to their higher complexity.

C. Tumscitz (✉)
Azienda Ospedaliero Universitaria di Ferrara, Arcispedale Sant'Anna, Cona, Italy

I. M. Seropian
Hospital Italiano de Buenos Aires, Buenos Aires, Argentina

Currently, clinical guidelines limit the use of BAV to hemodynamically unstable patients or those requiring urgent non-cardiac surgery [7, 8]. However, BAV can significantly improve symptoms in short-term follow-up with less procedural complexity compared to TAVR or surgical aortic valve replacement (SAVR). Therefore, it could be beneficial in improving the overall health status of patients candidates to TAVR (or SAVR), especially when there is a significant risk of futility. For this reason, despite the significant increase in TAVR procedures, there has been an increase in BAV procedures [9]. Finally, patients who are ineligible for TAVR due to futility may experience a significant improvement in the quality of life after BAV.

Therefore, if the BAV technique is simplified to reduce vascular complications compared to the traditional approach, it may be used more frequently and adopted more widely. Traditionally, BAV has been performed through a large-bore femoral access, with brachial or antegrade transseptal access as an alternative for patients with occluded distal aorta or unsuitable femoral access. In 2017, Tumscitz et al. first described radial BAV, a technique that has since gained traction due to its short learning curve and high feasibility [10]. Although initial studies used 9 Fr-compatible balloons, newer-generation balloons with reduced profile and optimal radial force and performance have made this technique accessible to a broader patient population. More recently, distal radial BAV (drBAV) has been

G. A. Sgueglia (ed.), *Distal Radial Access*, https://doi.org/10.1007/978-3-031-89925-6_22

introduced with comparable success rates and efficacy [11]. As detailed elsewhere in this book, distal radial access (DRA) may also be associated with a reduced incidence of radial artery occlusion (RAO) associated with radial BAV, an important consideration for patients with potential future transcatheter interventions.

22.2 How to Perform Distal Radial Balloon Aortic Valvuloplasty

A practical and safe step-by-step guide is presented for performing drBAV. The equipment required are mostly similar to those used for traditional femoral BAV, as detailed in Table 22.1. However, some equipment may vary based on operator preference.

22.2.1 Distal Radial Access

To perform drBAV, DRA is obtained in both arms using a 5 or 6 Fr sheath as described in Chaps. 7 and 8. The procedure can be performed using either the right or left approach. Unfractionated heparin is then administered either intravenously or through the sheath [12] at a dose of 5000 units for most patients, adjusted to 30–50 UI/Kg for extremely obese patients. If two DRA cannot be obtained, the operator can switch to conventional radial or ulnar access, with the DRA preferred for the BAV procedure and the alternative access for blood pressure monitoring.

While single radial access for BAV is possible, it has limitations. For example, it is not possible to simultaneously measure aortic valve gradients through a single access due to the radial anatomy unless a dedicated dual lumen catheter is used. Pressure monitoring is also lost once the balloon dilatation catheter is advanced through the sheath. Pressure drop with rapid pacing cannot be monitored, and there is no contralateral bailout access if severe vessel tortuosity is encountered. As a bailout strategy in single drBAV, a small (≤4 Fr) catheter can be placed in the femoral or brachial artery to continuously monitor blood pressure if no other secondary access is available.

Table 22.1 List of materials needed for distal radial balloon aortic valvuloplasty

Material	Quantity	Purpose
5–6 Fr radial introducer sheath	2	Obtain bilateral distal radial access
0.035″ regular J wire (260 cm)	1	Deliver catheters to aortic valve
5–6 Fr pigtail catheter	2	Measure aortic and left ventricular pressure for gradient calculations
5–6 Fr JR catheter	1	Crossing of the aortic valve
0.035″ straight wire (260 cm)	1	Crossing of the aortic valve
0.035″ extra stiff wire (260 cm, reshaped)	1	Advance balloon dilation catheter
8–10 Fr introducer sheath	1	Advance balloon dilation catheter (size according to balloon)
25–50 ml Luer lock syringe	2	Purge, inflate, and deflate balloon
Pressure line	2	Concomitant measurements of left ventricular and aortic pressure
Alligator clip-style cables	1 pair	0.035″ wire pacing
Lidocaine 2%	5 ml	Bilateral distal radial local anesthesia
Radial hemostatic device	2	Radial hemostasis
Unfractionated heparin	5000 UI	Anticoagulation
Diluted iodinated contrast medium (1:10)	100 ml	Balloon inflation

22.2.2 Aortic Valve Crossing

Multiple catheters can be used to cross the aortic valve from the radial approach. A standard 0.035″ straight wire is used for aortic valve crossing. However, Judkins Right (JR) catheters are preferred, especially from the right radial approach, as they are better aligned with the aortic valve orifice. In addition, JR catheters facilitate left ventricular (LV) pressure measurement and placement of the stiff wire without the need for a pigtail catheter (Fig. 22.1). Once the catheter is in the LV, aortic valve gradients (peak to peak and mean) are calculated. Aortic pressure can be measured in the ascending aorta with a catheter advanced through the contralateral access. However, in many cases, pressure monitoring through the side port of the contralateral radial sheath provides similar accuracy. The operator can first assess whether there are differences between the radial pressure through the sheath and the aortic pressure from the contralateral catheter before advancing it into the LV. It is important to measure baseline and post-BAV gradients to confirm the effectiveness of the balloon dilations (Fig. 22.2).

22.2.3 Large Sheath Insertion

After gradient measurements, an extra stiff 0.035″ wire is advanced to the LV. To avoid ventricular damage, a 3 cm floppy tip, appropriately pigtailed, is recommended. Sometimes preformed TAVR-specific wires are preferred, although they are often more expensive. Once the stiff wire is in the left ventricle, the 5–6 Fr radial sheath is exchanged for an 8–10 Fr sheath, depending on the sheath compatibility of the selected balloon. It is important to advance the sheath within the artery no more than 1–3 cm to avoid pain and spasm. Ideally, a short 5.5 cm 8 Fr sheath is preferred to provide more usable shaft length (Fig. 22.3).

We recommend the use of "low-profile" 8 (or 9) Fr-compatible balloons in the most commonly used sizes (18–24 mm) with a balloon to annulus ratio <1:1 for BAV to reduce major complications. In the Safety and Feasibility of Transradial Mini-invasive Balloon Aortic Valvuloplasty (SOFTLY) registry, most patients were treated with only a 20 mm balloon with satisfactory results (>30% gradient reduction in >80% of cases) [10]. In addition, it is always possible to increase the balloon diameter if the results are unsatisfactory. The operative sheath size compatibility of the most commonly used balloons is summarized in Table 22.2.

22.2.4 Aortic Valve Dilation

The dilatation balloon catheter is primed with saline and diluted contrast prior to use. It is

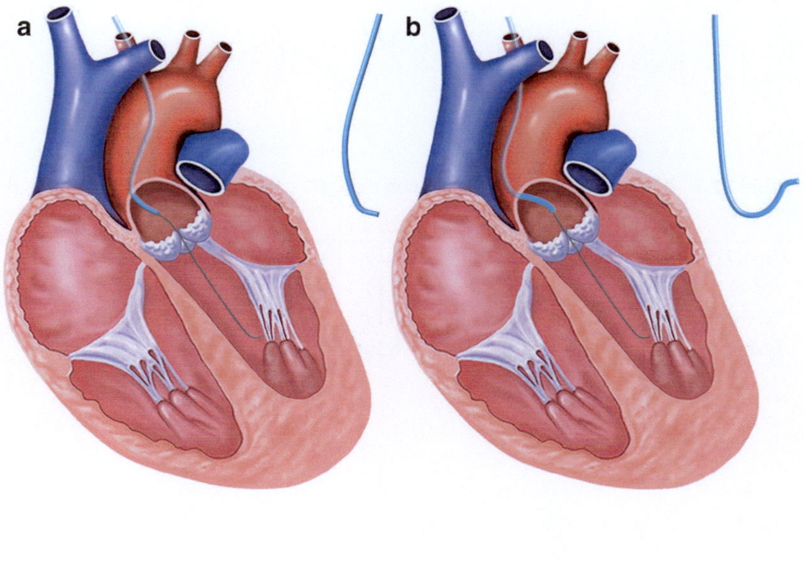

Fig. 22.1 Aortic valve crossing: (**a**) Judkins right (JR) catheters are the first choice because they have better orientation to the aortic valve from the right radial approach. (**b**) Alternatively, an Amplatz left (AL) catheter may be used; in both cases a 0.035″ straight wire is used to cross the aortic valve

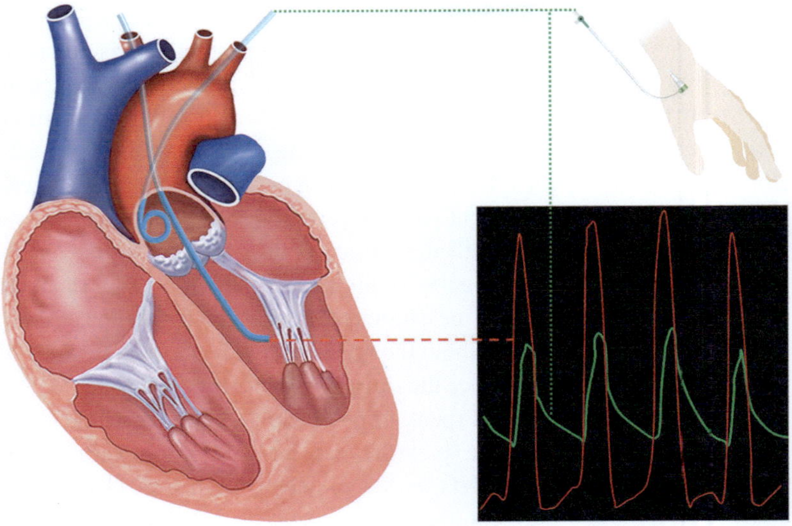

Fig. 22.2 For gradient calculation, aortic pressure can be measured in the ascending aorta with a catheter advanced through the contralateral access, or alternatively pressure can be monitored through the contralateral radial sheath side port with equal accuracy

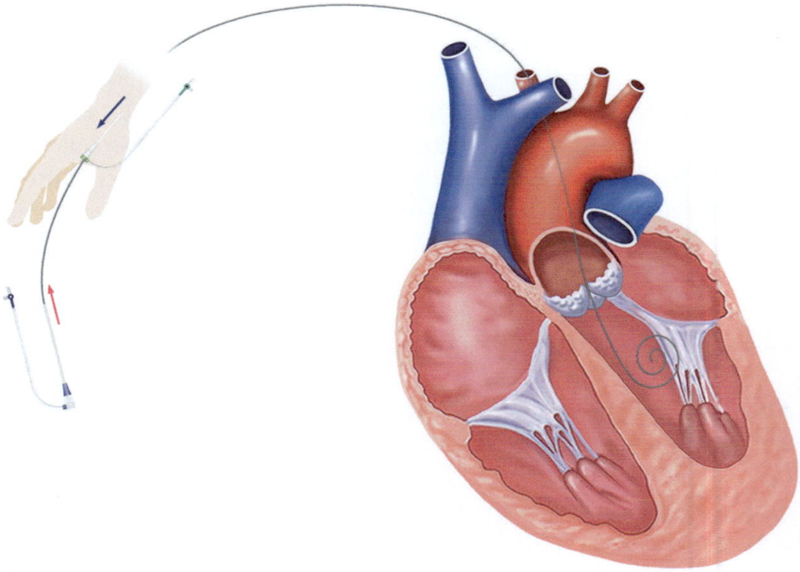

Fig. 22.3 For large sheath insertion, an extra stiff 0.035″ wire is advanced into the left ventricle, and once the stiff wire is in the left ventricle, the 5–6 Fr radial sheath is exchanged for an 8 Fr sheath

Table 22.2 Effective sheath size for balloon dilations catheters commonly used in radial balloon aortic valvuloplasty

	18 mm	20 mm	22 mm	23 mm	24 mm	25 mm
Cristal (Balt)	8 Fr	8 Fr	–	9 Fr	–	10 Fr
VACS II (Osypka)	8 Fr	8 Fr	8 Fr	–	9 Fr	–
Valver (Balton)	8 Fr	8 Fr	–	9 Fr	–	10 Fr
Tyshak II (NuMed)	8 Fr	8 Fr	8 Fr	9 Fr	9 Fr	9 Fr

strongly recommended that a highly diluted solution (approximately 1:10) is used for rapid inflation/deflation. Proper balloon preparation is essential to remove air from the inner tube and balloon to prevent embolization in the event of a rupture. The recommended method for removing air from the balloon is to perform small inflations with a saline contrast solution mixture followed by negative pressure aspiration. However, not all balloon brands allow for preparation prior to balloon insertion into the vasculature, as this can cause loosening of the crossing profile and make balloon insertion into the arterial sheath more difficult. In such cases, we usually prepare the balloon in the ascending aorta [13].

Rapid pacing (180–200 bpm) is often used to stabilize the balloon during inflation, although it is not necessary in all cases. We recommend pacing through the 0.035″ wire to reduce the risk of perforation and to avoid any vascular complications from femoral vein puncture. This technique is similar to that used in TAVR procedures [14] and involves an alligator clip-style cable with one end connected to the subcutaneous tissue via a small intramuscular needle in the groin and the other end connected to the 0.035″ wire a few centimeters proximal to the end of the balloon catheter. To ensure proper stimulation, an external generator capable of delivering at least 15 mA of output current (ideally 25 mA) is used. In addition, both alligator clips must be in contact with the needle/wire, and saline-filled gauze is used to cover the junction to improve conductance. Balloon inflation is typically performed with a 25–50 mL Luer-lock syringe or a percutaneous transluminal angioplasty inflation syringe (Fig. 22.4) [13].

22.2.5 Balloon Retrieval

After deflation, the balloon is withdrawn to the ascending aorta under negative pressure. A 25 mL syringe is filled with 5 mL of contrast and then aspirated to ensure proper refolding and prevent entrapment. The balloon is slowly withdrawn with continuous negative pressure by two operators, one pulling the balloon catheter and the other pushing the wire in a "push and pull" fashion to maintain the position of the wire in the left ventricle. Resistance may be felt at the elbow, and patients may experience pain during the last part of the balloon withdrawal. In such cases, additional analgesia may be administered. The sheath can remain in place unless there is severe resistance at the end of the maneuver, in which case the balloon and sheath can be withdrawn together, leaving the stiff 0.035″ wire in place.

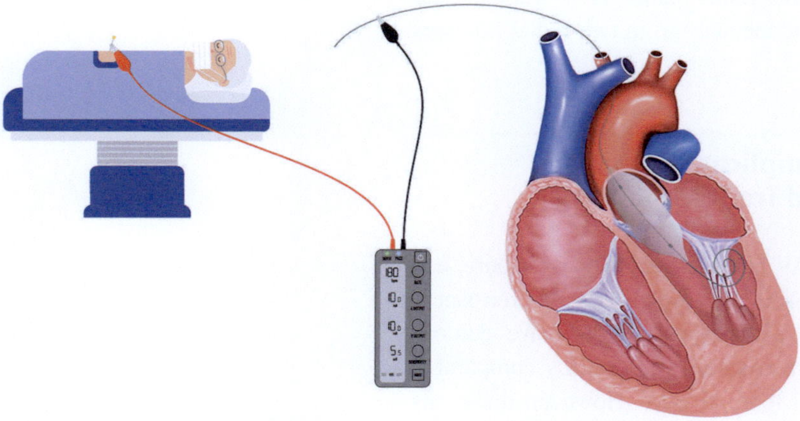

Fig. 22.4 For aortic valve dilation, pacing with the 0.035″ wire reduces the risk of perforation and simplifies the technique. It is performed with alligator clip-style cables with the anode (+, red) connected to the subcutaneous tissue through a small needle and the cathode (–, black) connected to the 0.035″ wire a few centimeters proximal to the end of the balloon catheter

Finally, a pigtail catheter is advanced over the wire into the left ventricle for final gradient measurements. If the results are unsatisfactory, a larger balloon can be used with a sheath upsize based on the operative compatibility chart (Table 22.2).

22.2.6 Hemostasis

Hemostasis is achieved in a regular fashion. Dedicated compression devices may be used but are not mandatory. It is important to warrant a nonocclusive hemostasis due to the higher risk of radial artery occlusion compared to standard 6 Fr coronary procedures.

22.3 Alternatives

This procedure has demonstrated high reproducibility and a low incidence of femoral crossover, even in patients with low body mass index or in the elderly. However, radial BAV may be contraindicated in patients with diffuse calcification of the arm arteries, as often seen in patients with severe chronic kidney disease or on dialysis. In such cases, a classical femoral BAV is the most common alternative, although a "simultaneous double-balloon radial BAV" has been described, in which two smaller balloons (8–12 mm) are inflated simultaneously from two radial accesses [15].

22.4 Complications and Troubleshooting

Although BAV is a relatively new procedure, it is easy to perform. Both prospective and retrospective studies, as reviewed below, have demonstrated excellent safety and efficacy comparable to traditional femoral BAV. However, due to its recent advent, experience with radial BAV is still less than with traditional BAV, which has been in use since 1985. Therefore, further large-scale studies are needed to fully evaluate the efficacy and safety of the procedure.

Advancing an 8–10 Fr balloon across the vertebral and right carotid arteries theoretically carries a higher risk of stroke. However, no increased risk of stroke has been reported. If resistance is encountered at the level of the brachiocephalic trunk, it may be helpful to have the patient look to the left and breathe deeply. Resistance to balloon advancement is generally encountered in the arm during balloon retrieval rather than during advancement. Crossover to the femoral approach is seen in 5% of cases and may be due to inability to achieve radial access, severe bilateral subclavian tortuosity, and spasm or tortuosity impeding balloon advancement.

The most serious complication reported to date with radial BAV is balloon entrapment during inflation requiring surgical removal. This occurred in only one case (0.3%) in the largest multicenter prospective study [16]. Therefore, special attention should be paid to any rupture that occurs during inflation (Fig. 22.5). In the same study, one case (0.3%) of subclavian dissection was observed, which was treated conservatively with no clinical consequences. Other complications included forearm hematoma (0.9%).

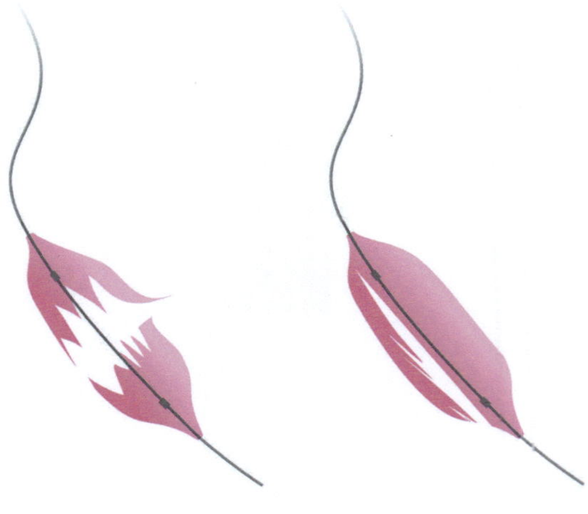

Fig. 22.5 Transverse balloon rupture carries a high risk of balloon entrapment, while longitudinal rupture carries a low risk of balloon entrapment

22.5 Clinical Evidence

Despite being a relatively new technique, multicenter data have demonstrated excellent outcomes and safety, as shown in Table 22.3.

The first prospective pilot study, SOFTLY [10], was a single-center registry at the University of Ferrara in Italy that included 30 patients undergoing conventional transradial BAV. The study population was very elderly, with a median age of 87 years, and BAV was performed prior to cardiac team discussion in half of the patients, while in 20% of the patients, TAVR was already judged futile, and BAV was set as destination therapy. The efficacy endpoint was an invasive mean gradient reduction of at least 30%, which was achieved in 90% of cases, and there were no safety issues such as balloon entrapment or urgent surgery. The rate of radial artery occlusion (RAO) was 20%.

Afterward, SOFTLY II [16] was a multicenter prospective registry in Italy that included 330 patients undergoing radial BAV, making it the largest study to date. Excellent results were also obtained, and the reproducibility of the technique was demonstrated in 16 centers in Italy. The patients were very elderly, with a median age of 88 years and an STS score of 7.5%. Right radial access was used in 60% of cases and DRA in 3%. Crossover to femoral access was only 5%, demonstrating a high success rate in this frail population. A 20 mm balloon was used in almost 90% of cases, and almost all used an 8 or 9 Fr sheath. In terms of safety, only one patient (0.3%) in this large multicenter study experienced balloon entrapment requiring surgical removal. The rate of RAO in this study was lower than in SOFTLY at only 4.6%. Interestingly, in a subset of 192 patients who underwent BAV as a bridge to TAVR, BAV was associated with a significant improvement in frailty as measured by three different scales. The results of SOFTLY II have also been confirmed outside of Italy. A single-center retrospective study from Argentina of 24 slightly younger patients (median age 81 years) showed similar results, with a success rate of 91% (defined as an invasive peak gradient reduction of at least 30%), one (4%) crossover to femoral access, and 8% RAO [17]. In this early experience, patients selected for radial BAV were younger, more robust, and more often male compared to those undergoing femoral BAV during the same study period.

Finally, a single-center substudy from the SOFTLY II registry reported the results of ten patients undergoing radial BAV via DRA. DrBAV showed the same efficacy and safety as conventional radial BAV [11], while RAO was observed in one patient (11%) who completed follow-up. In another single-center registry, 32 patients (80 ± 8 years) underwent drBAV mainly as an emergency indication [18]. Hemodynamic success was achieved in 30 patients (93.75%), and no major complications occurred. At a 30-day follow-up, the radial artery was found to be patent in 94% of the patients.

Table 22.3 Clinical data for radial balloon aortic valvuloplasty

Study	Description	N	Age (years)	Most used sheath size (% use)	Most used balloon size (% use)	Success rate (gradient reduction)	Crossover rate	VARC2 major complications
SOFTLY	Single center, prospective	30	87	9 Fr (100%)	20 mm (100%)	90%	3.3%	0%
SOFTLY II	Multicenter, prospective	330	88	8 Fr (62%)	20 mm (87%)	95%	1.5%	0%
Medina et al.	Single center, retrospective	24	81	8 Fr (46%)	20 mm (50%)	92%	4%	–
Di Cesare et al.	Single center, retrospective	10 (from SOFTLY II)	86	8 Fr (100%)	20 mm (100%)	100%	0%	–

Acknowledgments We thank Dr. Graziella Pompei for her invaluable inspiration and original work that served as the basis for the figures in this chapter.

References

1. Allende R, Ribeiro HB, Puri R, Urena M, Abdul-Jawad O, del Trigo M, et al. The transradial approach during transcatheter structural heart disease interventions: a review. Eur J Clin Investig. 2015;45:215–25.
2. Sawaya FJ, Louvard Y, Spaziano M, Morice MC, Hage F, El-Khoury C, et al. Short and long-term outcomes of alcohol septal ablation with the transradial versus the trans-femoral approach: a single-center experience. Int J Cardiol. 2016;220:7–13.
3. Osken A, Aydin E, Akdemir R, Gunduz H. Percutaneous closure of an aortic prosthetic paravalvular leak with device in a patient presenting with heart failure. Heart Views. 2015;16:56–8.
4. Sanghvi K, Selvaraj N, Luft U. Percutaneous closure of a perimembranous ventricular septal defect through arm approach (radial artery and basilic vein). J Interv Cardiol. 2014;27:199–203.
5. Choudhury T, Lurz P, Schäufele TG, Menezes MN, Lavi S, Tzemos N, et al. Radial versus femoral approach for left ventricular endomyocardial biopsy. EuroIntervention. 2019;15:678–84.
6. Cribier A, Savin T, Saoudi N, Rocha P, Berland J, Letac B. Percutaneous transluminal valvuloplasty of acquired aortic stenosis in elderly patients: an alternative to valve replacement? Lancet. 1986;1:63–7.
7. Vahanian A, Beyersdorf F, Praz F, Milojevic M, Baldus S, Bauersachs J, et al. 2021 ESC/EACTS guidelines for the management of valvular heart disease. Eur Heart J. 2022;43:561–632.
8. Otto CM, Nishimura RA, Bonow RO, Carabello BA, Erwin JP 3rd, Gentile F, et al. 2020 ACC/AHA guideline for the management of patients with valvular heart disease: a report of the American College of Cardiology/American Heart Association Joint Committee on clinical practice guidelines. J Am Coll Cardiol. 2021;77:e25–197.
9. Alkhouli M, Zack CJ, Sarraf M, Bashir R, Nishimura RA, Eleid MF, et al. Morbidity and mortality associated with balloon aortic valvuloplasty: a national perspective. Circ Cardiovasc Interv. 2017;10:e004481.
10. Tumscitz C, Campo G, Tebaldi M, Gallo F, Pirani L, Biscaglia S. Safety and feasibility of transradial mini-invasive balloon aortic valvuloplasty: a pilot study. JACC Cardiovasc Interv. 2017;10:1375–7.
11. Di Cesare A, Tonet E, Campo G, Tumscitz C. Snuffbox approach for balloon aortic valvuloplasty: a case series. Catheter Cardiovasc Interv. 2021;97:E743–7.
12. Pancholy SB. Comparison of the effect of intra-arterial versus intravenous heparin on radial artery occlusion after transradial catheterization. Am J Cardiol. 2009;104:1083–5.
13. Seropian IM, Romeo FJ, Falconi M, Agatiello CR, Berrocal DH. Balloon rupture during aortic valvuloplasty with compliant balloon: predictors and outcomes. Cardiovasc Interv Ther. 2020;35:291–9.
14. Dall'Ara G, Tumscitz C, Grotti S, Santarelli A, Balducelli M, Tarantino F, et al. Contemporary balloon aortic valvuloplasty: changing indications and refined technique. Catheter Cardiovasc Interv. 2021;97:E1033–42.
15. Vassileva A, Valsecchi O, Guagliumi G, Fiocca L, Canova PA, Cereda AF. Bilateral slender transradial aortic balloon valvuloplasty. J Invasive Cardiol. 2018;30:E48–9.
16. Tumscitz C, Di Cesare A, Balducelli M, Piva T, Santarelli A, Saia F, et al. Safety, efficacy and impact on frailty of mini-invasive radial balloon aortic valvuloplasty. Heart. 2021;107:874–80.
17. Medina De Chazal HA, Seropian IM, Romeo F, Chiabrando JG, Valle Raleigh J, Berrocal DH, et al. Balloon aortic valvuloplasty through the novel transradial technique. Minerva Cardiol Angiol. 2021;69:458–63.
18. Achim A, Szűcsborus T, Sasi V, Nagy F, Jambrik Z, Nemes A, et al. Safety and feasibility of distal radial balloon aortic valvuloplasty: the DR-BAV study. JACC Cardiovasc Interv. 2022;15:679–81.

23 Radial Artery Recanalization

Gabriele L. Gasparini and Zoltan Ruzsa

23.1 Introduction

Transradial access (TRA) has become the standard vascular access for coronary interventions because it has been shown to reduce major bleeding, adverse cardiac events, and mortality compared to transfemoral access [1]. However, TRA is not without complications. Among these, radial artery occlusion (RAO) remains its Achilles heel with an incidence ranging from 0.8% to 33% in published reports [2–5]. Actually, RAO has no clinical significance when the palmar arch is complete. Also, RAO is asymptomatic in most cases, but there are case reports and studies of symptomatic RAO and successful radial artery recanalization [6, 7]. Possible mechanisms involved in RAO after transradial catheterization include thrombus formation after vascular injury (dissection, prolonged spasm, and hematoma), occlusive compressive bandage, and distal embolization. When symptomatic RAO is associated with critical hand ischemia, in these cases, conservative treatment is inadequate, and invasive treatment with angioplasty should be considered. Balloon angioplasty and bail-out stenting have good short-term results in symptomatic RAO [6, 7]. In a small number of symptomatic patients with RAO, the cause of hand ischemia was radial artery occlusion along with poor palmar arch (5/15 patients), radial artery occlusion and ulnar artery stenosis (9/15 patients), and radial artery occlusion with distal embolization (1/15 patients [7]. Once occluded, the radial artery is no longer suitable for repeat procedures and requires an alternative vascular access such as the contralateral radial artery (with the subsequent risk of bilateral RAO) or the femoral artery with its drawbacks (prolonged hemostasis, immobilization, etc.) and complications (inguinal hematoma, arteriovenous fistula or pseudoaneurysm, retroperitoneal hemorrhage, etc.). Nevertheless, the possibility of reopening a vascular access thought to be obliterated is an advantage for the operator. The access site for RAO recanalization can be antegrade (common femoral, antegrade brachial, ulnar with crossover access) or retrograde (distal radial or palmar arch technique) (Fig. 23.1) [6–9]. Distal radial access (DRA) was first described as a way to access and recanalize the occluded proximal radial artery segment. Because of the superficial palmar arch that originates proximally to the emergence of the distal radial artery, this segment remains patent by collateralization from the ulnar artery, allowing puncture and retrograde radial artery angioplasty. The first description of successful retrograde radial artery recanalization with balloon dilatation and restoration of vessel patency was reported by Avtandil Babunashvili in 2011 [8].

G. L. Gasparini (✉)
IRCCS Humanitas Research Hospital, Rozzano, Italy

Z. Ruzsa
Department of Internal Medicine, Division of Invasive Cardiology, University of Szeged, Szeged, Hungary

G. A. Sgueglia (ed.), *Distal Radial Access*, https://doi.org/10.1007/978-3-031-89925-6_23

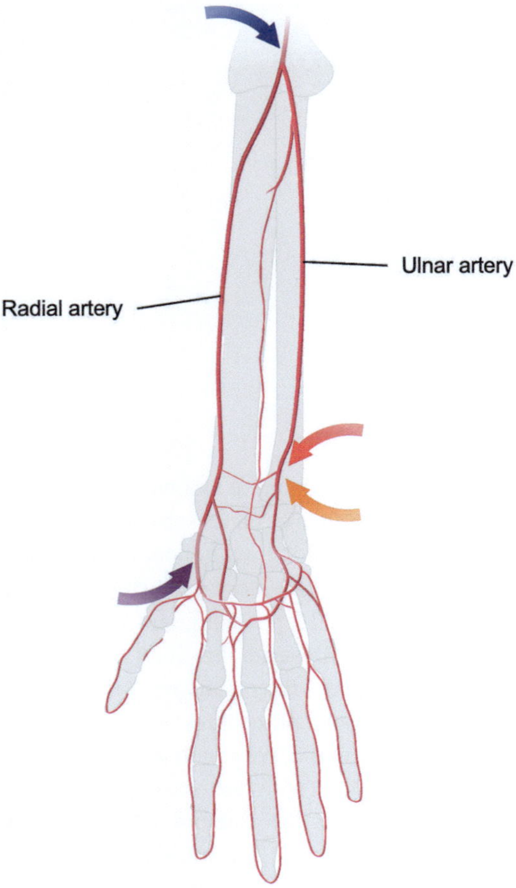

Fig. 23.1 Access sites for radial artery occlusion recanalization: antegrade recanalization through brachial access (blue arrow) or palmar arch technique (purple arrow); retrograde recanalization through distal radial access (fuchsia arrow) or crossover from ulnar access (orange arrow)

Meanwhile, interest in the use of DRA for cardiovascular interventions grew exponentially after the seminal work of Ferdinand Kiemeneij [10]. Several studies have demonstrated its safety and efficacy in percutaneous interventions, and an increasing number of interventionalists are interested in this approach [11–14]. In recent years, a growing number of studies have focused on retrograde recanalization of occluded proximal radial arteries via DRA with promising results [15–23]. This chapter will focus on the technical steps to achieve retrograde RAO recanalization via DRA.

23.2 Patient Preparation, Puncture Sites, and Techniques

After disinfection and local anesthesia, the operators palpate the artery pulsation distal to the occluded radial artery and attempt to puncture distal radial artery. Following DRA palpation, one of the two possible puncture sites can be evaluated accordingly to the site of strongest pulsation in the anatomical snuffbox or in the first intermetacarpal space (dorsum of the hand) (Fig. 23.2). If the pulsation of the DRA is unclear to palpation, ultrasound could be used to guide the puncture. Ultrasonography gives information about the radial artery anatomy and collateral function from the ulnar artery (Fig. 23.3). After optimal arm positioning, the artery can be punctured according to operator preference and/or experience using a 21 G micropuncture needle or alternatively a cannula-over-needle (Fig. 23.4).

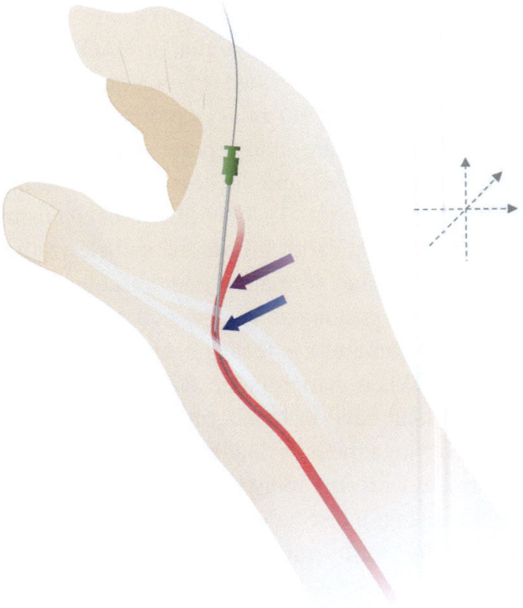

Fig. 23.2 Schematic illustration of the two possible puncture sites for distal radial access: in the anatomical snuffbox (blue arrow) or in the first intermetacarpal space or dorsum of the hand (purple arrow)

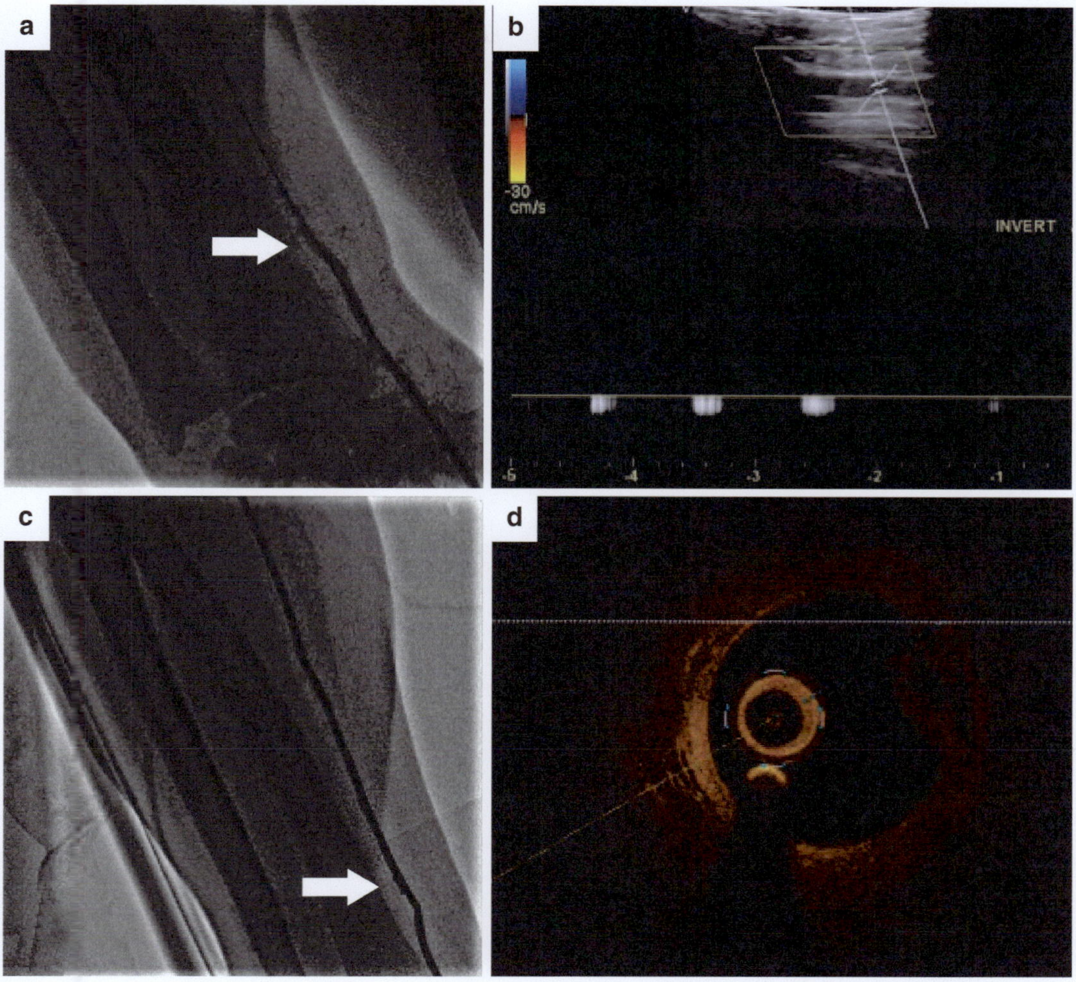

Fig. 23.3 Chronic radial artery occlusion after transradial intervention. (**a**) Selective angiography confirming radial artery occlusion that has been crossed with a Gladius (Asahi) 0.018″ guidewire. (**b**) Vascular ultrasound showing a reverse flow in the distal radial artery. (**c**) Selective angiography after dottering the radial artery with a sheathless guiding catheter. (**d**) Control optical coherence tomography showing non-occlusive intimal injury

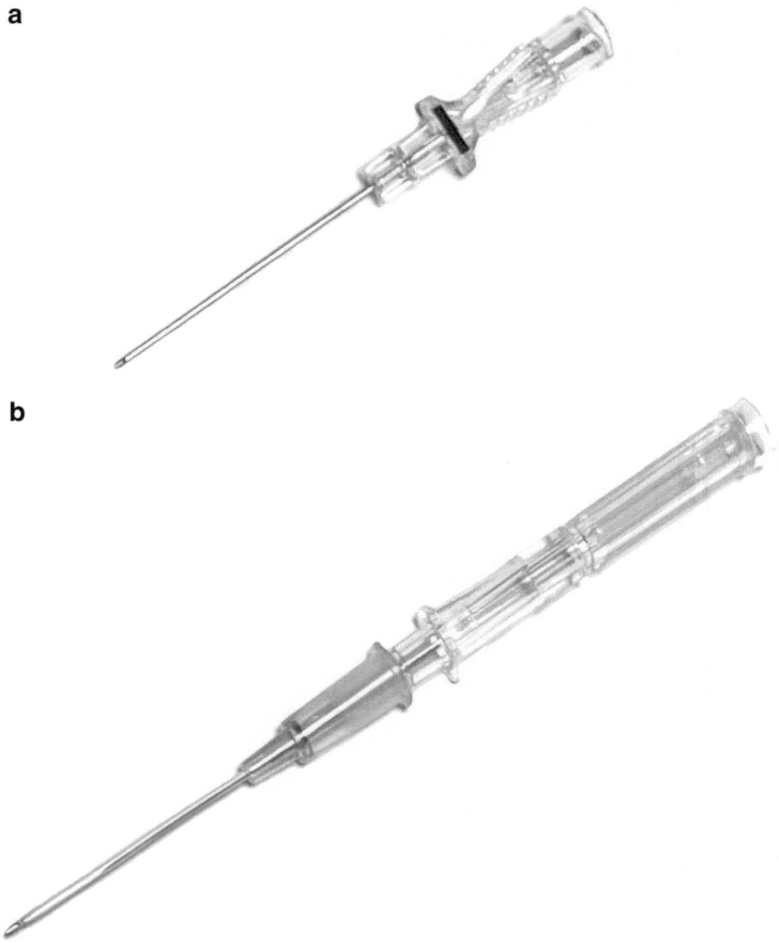

Fig. 23.4 Operator preference or experience helps in using (**a**) 21 G open needle or (**b**) a catheter-covered-needle or cannula-over-needle

23.2.1 Open Needle Micropuncture Technique

After obtaining pulsatile blood flow, a small amount of contrast should be injected through the open needle to better evaluate the occluded segment (Fig. 23.5). After careful evaluation of the anatomic characteristics of the occlusion, wiring of the occluded segment should be the next step. Wiring could be performed using the 21 G open needle (Fig. 23.6), but since the main problem with retrograde RAO recanalization is a guidewire support, advancing a 4 Fr sheath approximately 1–2 cm along the guidewire may be useful if wire crossing of the occluded segment requires more support (Fig. 23.7). Wiring can then be continued through the introducer dilator inserted into the sheath valve. Of the two options above, the most advantageous is chosen on an ad hoc basis, depending on the degree of occlusion and the ability to advance the guidewire. Although the sheath provides more support, in our experience direct wiring through the needle may be safer and no less effective.

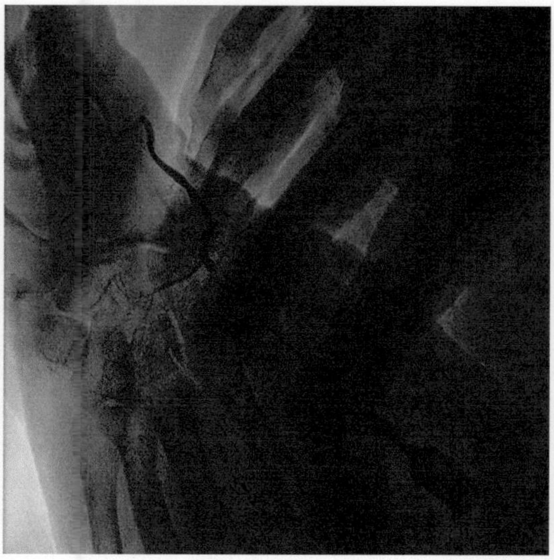

Fig. 23.5 Micropuncture needle technique: a small amount of contrast is injected directly through the open needle to evaluate the occluded segment

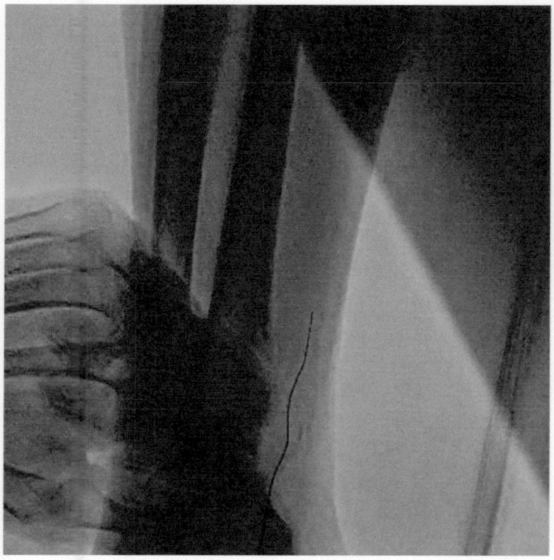

Fig. 23.6 Micropuncture needle technique: wiring of the occluded segment can be achieved directly via the open needle

23.2.2 Cannula-Over-Needle Technique

The over-the-needle technique is not significantly different. After the appearance of blood return, the over-the-needle cannula is advanced a little further, and then the stylet is withdrawn. Under fluoroscopy, the cannula is advanced along the 0.025″ guidewire to stabilize the cannula. After the guidewire is withdrawn, a small amount of contrast is injected to characterize the anatomy of the occluded radial artery (Fig. 23.8). Then, wiring can be continued through the cannula (Fig. 23.9). If crossing the occlusion is not possible through the cannula alone, placement of a 4 Fr sheath approximately 1–2 cm along the guidewire may be useful to increase retrograde support for crossing the occluded segment with a 0.014″ guidewire.

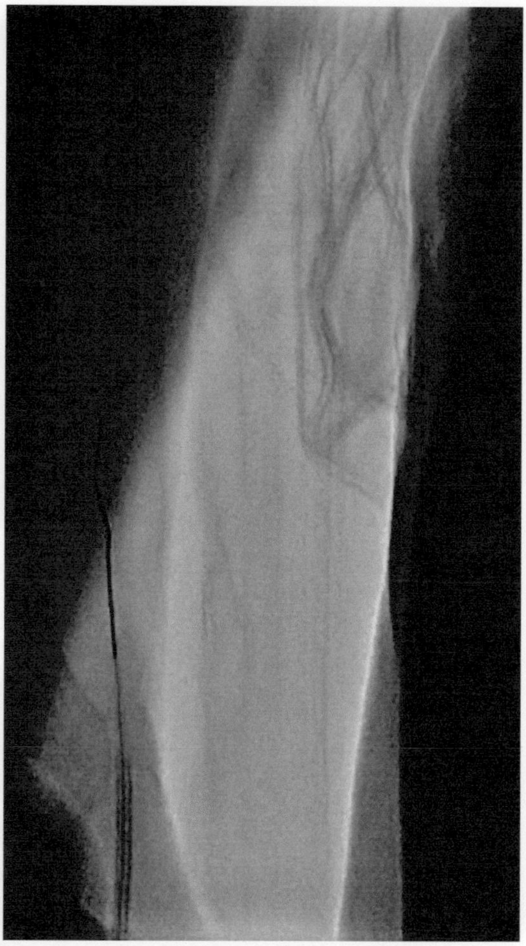

Fig. 23.7 Advancement of 4 Fr sheath (approximately 1–2 cm along the guidewire) can be adopted to achieve more support for guidewire crossing of the occlusion

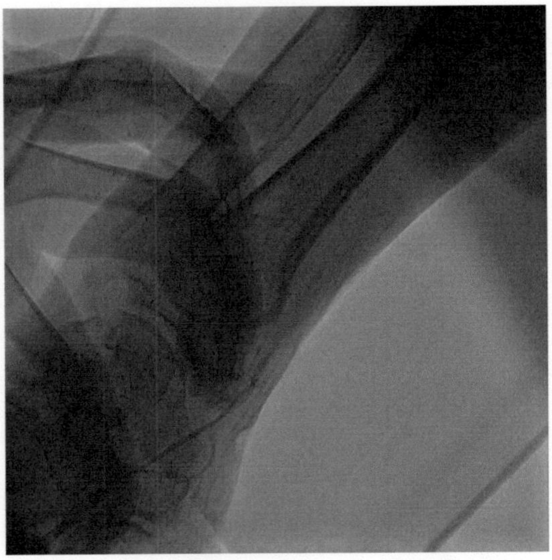

Fig. 23.8 Cannula-over-needle technique: under fluoroscopy the cannula is advanced along the 0.025″ guidewire, then after withdrawing the guidewire, a little amount of contrast is injected for characterizing the anatomy of the occluded radial artery

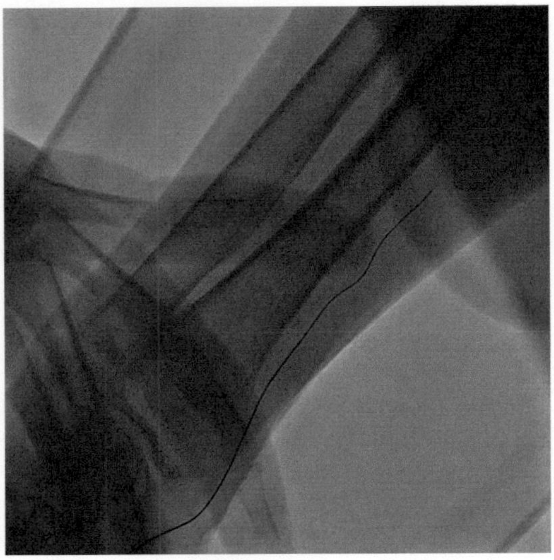

Fig. 23.9 Cannula-over-needle technique: wiring is performed directly via the cannula-over-needle

23.3 Wiring Techniques

Radial artery occlusion recanalization can be luminal or subintimal. The luminal recanalization technique is generally successful in short occlusions but is rarely effective in long occlusions where subintimal angioplasty is required. The rationale for using subintimal angioplasty is to create a subintimal lumen with the guidewire, and after proper balloon angioplasty or passive dilatation with a sheathless guide, the new subintimal space is kept open by blood pressure. Under fluoroscopy, a 0.014″ polymer-coated guidewire with a soft or medium tip load (e.g., Sion Black or Gladius, Asahi Intecc) is advanced through the occlusion, either by intraluminal tracking (microchannel sliding technique) (Fig. 23.10) or by subintimal tracking and re-entry, which can be easily performed with the knuckle technique.

23.3.1 Sliding Technique

The sliding technique is used when microchannels are directly visible or likely to be present and takes advantage of the extreme lubricity of the polymer-jacketed guidewire. The handling must be very gentle with fine movements to achieve intraluminal tracking of the guidewire due to its sliding properties within the microchannel (Fig. 23.11).

23.3.2 Knuckle Technique

A soft/medium tip-load polymer-jacketed guidewire is pushed against the occlusion creating a "tight loop" at its tip, and then the knuckled wire is advanced subintimally through the occlusion until it spontaneously re-enters into the true proximal true lumen (Fig. 23.12).

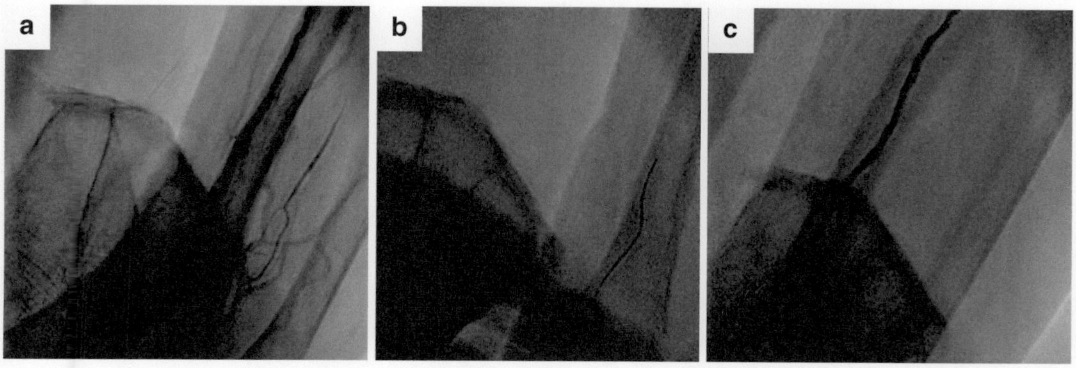

Fig. 23.10 (**a**–**c**) A 0.014″ polymer-jacketed guidewire with soft tip load (Sion Black, Asahi) is advanced through the occlusion by intraluminal microchannel tracking (sliding technique)

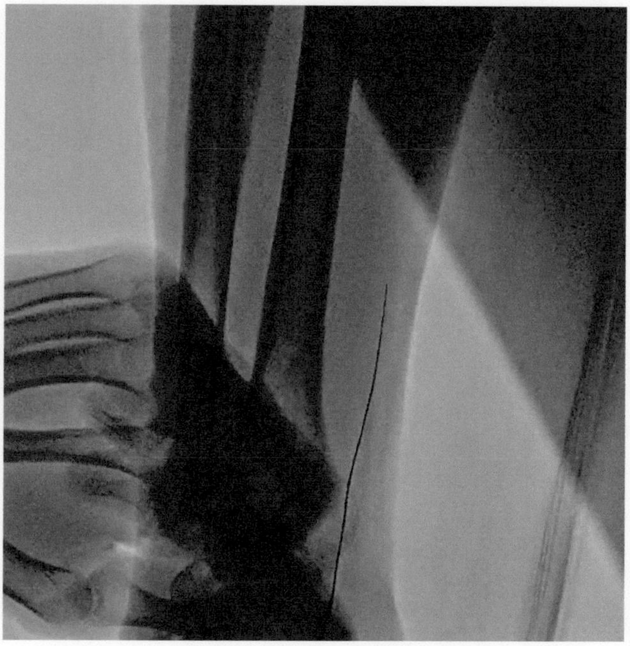

Fig. 23.11 Sliding technique: intraluminal tracking of the guidewire due to its sliding properties within the microchannel

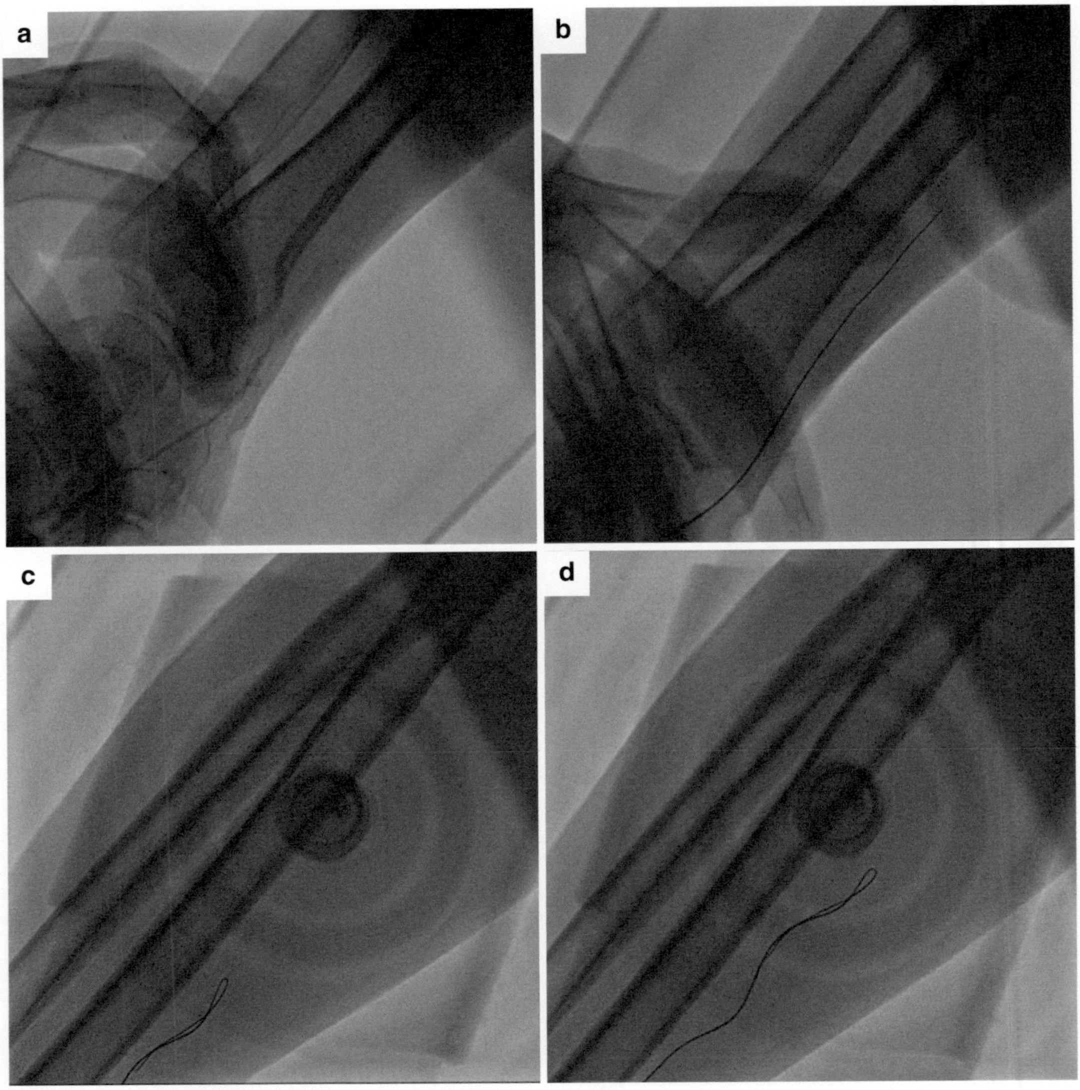

Fig. 23.12 (**a–d**) Knuckling technique: a soft/medium tip-load polymer-jacketed guidewire is pushed against the occlusion creating a "tight loop" at its tip, and then the knuckled wire is advanced subintimally through the occlusion

23.4 Reopening the Occluded Segment

23.4.1 Anterograde Recanalization

The preferred access site for antegrade recanalization is the brachial approach using a 4–5 Fr short sheath. The advantage of this technique is the short distance between the access site and the lesion; the disadvantage is the difficult access. In case of failed guidewire re-entry or passage, the recanalization can be converted to a retrograde technique using the palmar arch technique or DRA.

23.4.2 Retrograde Recanalization

After successful guidewire crossing into the proximal true lumen (i.e., proximal brachial artery), a 6 Fr radial sheath or a sheathless catheter is advanced over the wire through the occlusion (Fig. 23.13) using a push-and-rotate maneuver (similar to dotterization). In the majority of cases, direct advancement of the sheath or sheathless catheter may be sufficient to achieve RAO recanalization, obviating the need for balloon dilatation (Fig. 23.14). The balloon-assisted

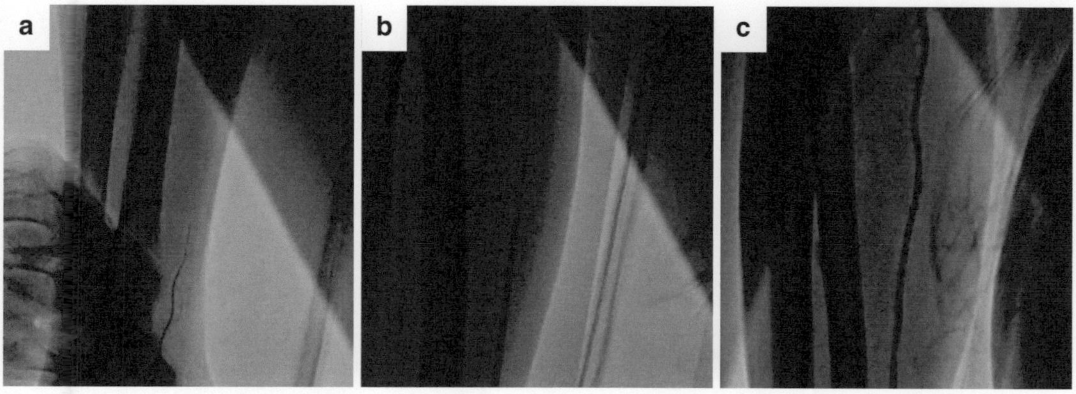

Fig. 23.13 (**a**) Intraluminal tracking with sliding technique. (**b**) A 6 Fr radial sheath is advanced over the wire through the occlusion. (**c**) Radial artery recanalized

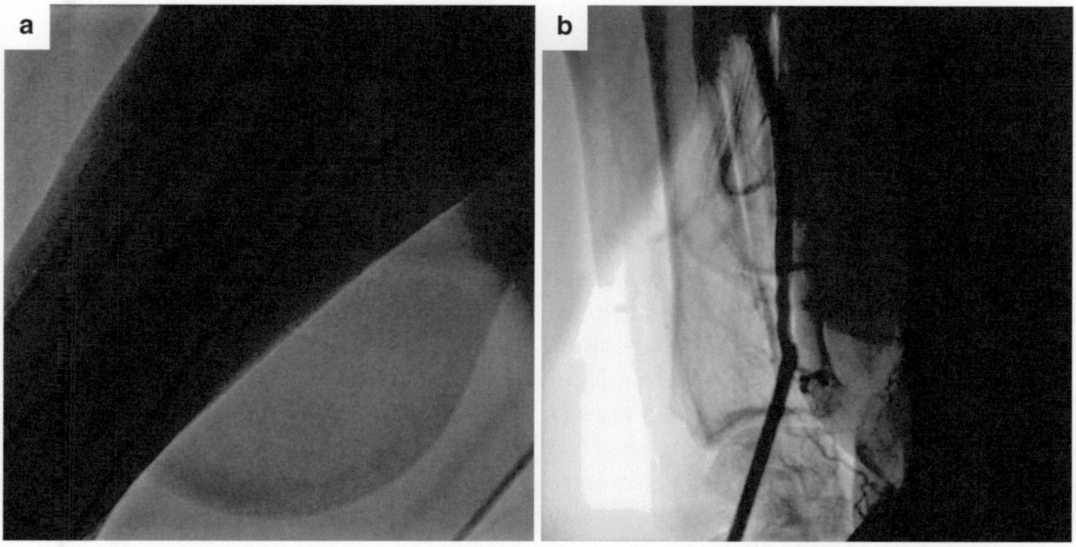

Fig. 23.14 Angiographic results after the direct advancement of the sheathless catheter (**a**) or the radial sheath (**b**) that obviated the need for balloon dilatation

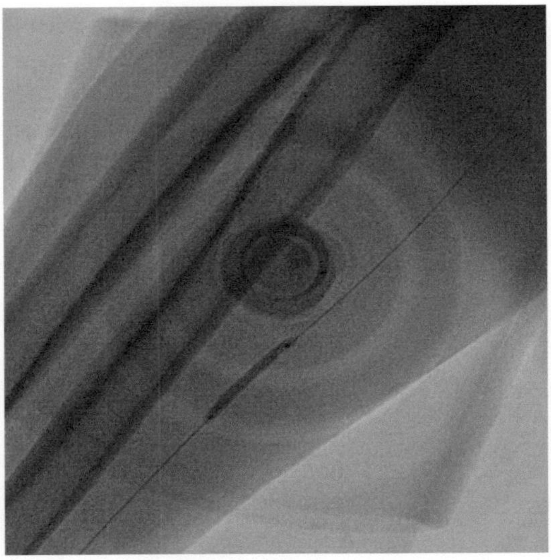

Fig. 23.15 Radial artery angioplasty: after successful crossing of the occluded segment, the guidewire is advanced into the proximal brachial artery, and then a balloon is used to expand the occluded segment

tracking technique may be useful when negotiating the sheathless catheter over the 0.014″ guidewire, which provides less support. Alternatively, after crossing the occluded segment, the guidewire is advanced into the proximal brachial artery, and a balloon is used to repeatedly expand the occluded segment from proximal to distal occlusion (Fig. 23.15) [6]. The diameter of the balloon used can vary from 2.0 to 4.0 mm, while no additional benefits in terms of long-term patency of the radial artery have been reported using drug-coated balloons, probably due to the different mechanism underlying the occlusion (Fig. 23.16). The pathological mechanism of RAO can also be assessed with intravascular imaging. Early occlusions can be treated via DRA, and the thrombus can be aspirated over the sheath or with a guiding catheter (Fig. 23.17). In these cases, balloon angioplasty or stenting is rarely necessary. An important advantage of the DRA technique is the protection against distal embolization provided by the sheath.

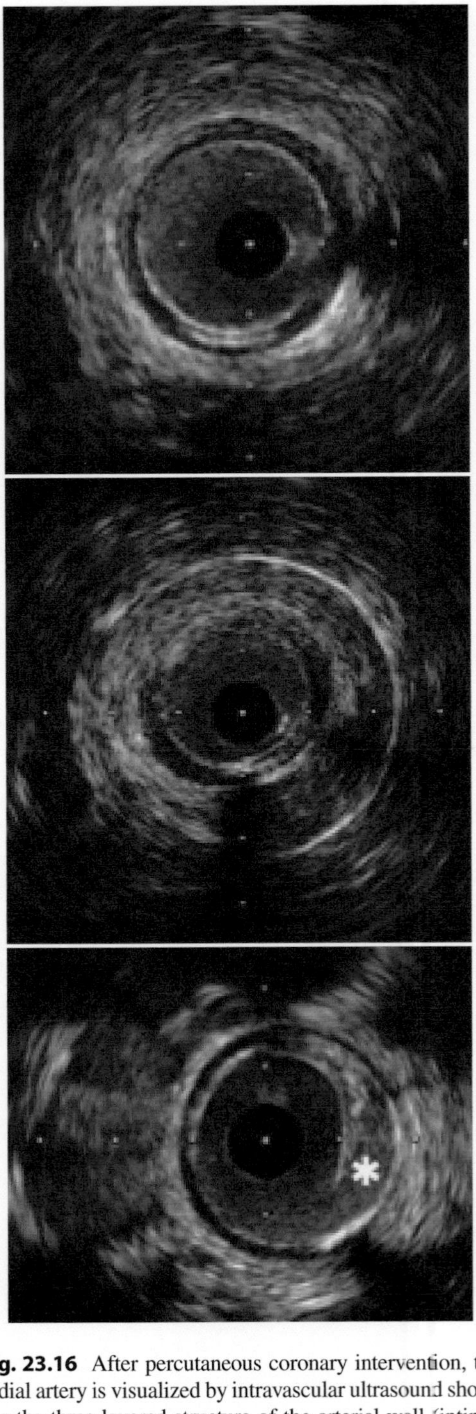

Fig. 23.16 After percutaneous coronary intervention, the radial artery is visualized by intravascular ultrasound showing the three-layered structure of the arterial wall (intima, media, adventitia) suggestive of a normal morphology (asterisk indicates the dissection plane creates adopting a dissection and re-entry technique with a knuckle wire)

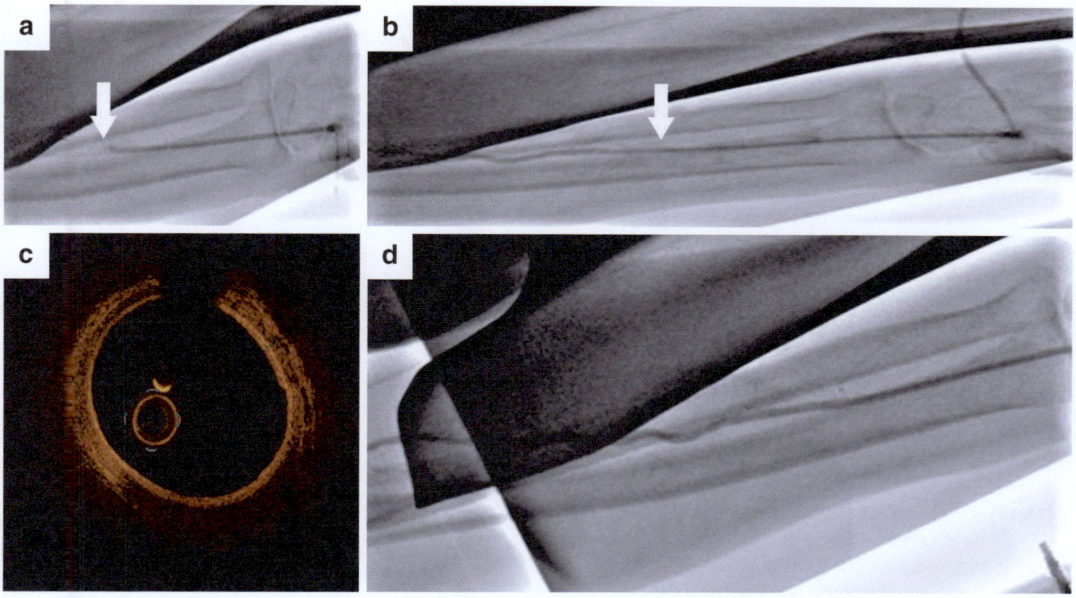

Fig. 23.17 Early radial artery occlusion after transradial catheterization. (**a**) Selective angiography confirming radial artery occlusion that has been crossed with a 0.14″ Progress (Abbott) guidewire. (**b**) Angiography of the radial artery after thrombus aspiration over the sheath. (**c**) Control optical coherence tomography showing the absence of intimal injury. (**d**) Final angiography showing a patent radial artery after the intervention

23.5 Advantages

After retrograde RAO recanalization, all coronary procedures can be performed via DRA. This is especially important in patients with limited vascular access and in patients with previous radial coronary artery bypass grafting [23]. In addition, maintaining radial patency may save an access in a patient who may be a future candidate for a dialysis fistula in the contralateral arm.

23.6 Complications

As RAO recanalization from DRA may be associated with radial artery dissection, radial artery perforation, or digital ischemia, larger registries are needed to evaluate the incidence of these potential complications.

23.7 Patency

One-month arterial patency after retrograde recanalization of RAO has been reported to be >90%, which may allow the radial artery to be used for further ipsilateral transradial catheterization procedures [15, 22]. However, for those patients who do not require immediate cardiac catheterization, retrograde recanalization of the RAO may not be beneficial for maintaining radial artery patency, as evidenced by the low patency rate at a 1-year follow-up (35.9%). Furthermore, the artery should not be used as a bypass conduit for coronary revascularization or for radial artery-cephalic vein arteriovenous fistula in patients on chronic hemodialysis, as both are unproven options [23–25].

References

1. Mason PJ, Shah B, Tamis-Holland JE, Bittl JA, Cohen MG, Safirstein J, et al. An update on radial artery access and best practices for transradial coronary angiography and intervention in acute coronary syndrome: a scientific statement from the American Heart Association. Circ Cardiovasc Interv. 2018;11:e000035.
2. Bernat I, Aminian A, Pancholy S, Mamas M, Gaudino M, Nolan J, et al. Best practices for the prevention of radial artery occlusion after transradial diagnostic angiography and intervention: an international consensus paper. JACC Cardiovasc Interv. 2019;12:2235–46.
3. Rashid M, Kwok CS, Pancholy S, Chugh S, Kedev SA, Bernat I, et al. Radial artery occlusion after transradial interventions: a systematic review and meta-analysis. J Am Heart Assoc. 2016;5:e002686.
4. Hahalis G, Aznaouridis K, Tsigkas G, Davlouros P, Xanthopoulou I, Koutsogiannis N, et al. Radial artery and ulnar artery occlusions following coronary procedures and the impact of anticoagulation: ARTEMIS (Radial and Ulnar ARTEry Occlusion Meta-AnalysIS) systematic review and meta-analysis. J Am Heart Assoc. 2017;6:e005430.
5. Garg N, Madan BK, Khanna R, Sinha A, Kapoor A, Tewari S, et al. Incidence and predictors of radial artery occlusion after transradial coronary angioplasty: doppler-guided follow-up study. J Invasive Cardiol. 2015;27:106–12.
6. Ruzsa Z, Pintér L, Kolvenbach R. Anterograde recanalisation of the radial artery followed by transradial angioplasty. Cardiovasc Revasc Med. 2010;11(266):e1–4.
7. Ruzsa Z, Berta B, Tóth J, Nemes B, Katona A, Hüttl A, et al. Short- and long-term results with a percutaneous treatment in critical hand ischaemia. Catheter Cardiovasc Interv. 2019;93:1301–10.
8. Babunashvili A, Dundua D. Recanalization and reuse of early occluded radial artery within 6 days after previous transradial diagnostic procedure. Catheter Cardiovasc Interv. 2011;77:530–6.
9. Ruzsa Z, Kovács N, Merkely B. Retrograde subintimal recanalization of a radial artery occlusion after coronary angiography using the palmar loop technique. Cardiovasc Revasc Med. 2015;16:259–61.
10. Kiemeneij F. Left distal transradial access in the anatomical snuffbox for coronary angiography (ldTRA) and interventions (ldTRI). EuroIntervention. 2017;13:851–7.
11. Amin MR, Banerjee SK, Biswas E, Paul N, Mahabub EE, Ahmed SF, et al. Feasibility and safety of distal transradial access in the anatomical snuffbox for coronary angiography and intervention. Mymensingh Med J. 2019;28:647–54.
12. Koutouzis M, Kontopodis E, Tassopoulos A, Tsiafoutis I, Katsanou K, Rigatou A, et al. Distal versus traditional radial approach for coronary angiography. Cardiovasc Revasc Med. 2019;20:678–80.
13. Gasparini GL, Garbo R, Gagnor A, Oreglia J, Mazzarotto P. First prospective multicentre experience with left distal transradial approach for coronary chronic total occlusion interventions using a 7 Fr Glidesheath Slender. EuroIntervention. 2019;15:126–8.
14. Achim A, Kákonyi K, Jambrik Z, Nagy F, Tóth J, Sasi V, et al. Distal radial artery access for coronary and peripheral procedures: a multicenter experience. J Clin Med. 2021;10:5974.
15. Sanz-Sánchez J, Regazzoli D, Petriello G, Leone PP, Reimers B, Gasparini GL. The last broken barrier: retrograde radial artery recanalization prior to transradial coronary interventions. Cardiovasc Revasc Med. 2021;28S:125–6.
16. Li F, Shi GW, Zhang BF, Yu XL, Huang HM, Xiao JQ, et al. Recanalization of the occluded radial artery via distal transradial access in the anatomic snuffbox. BMC Cardiovasc Disord. 2021;21:67.
17. Alkhawam H, Windish S, Abo-Salem E. Distal radial artery access among cases with radial artery occlusion for primary percutaneous intervention. Futur Cardiol. 2019;15:169–73.
18. Ali S, Abdullah MS, Abdelrahman K, Ali A, Faisal F, Ali A. Total radial artery occlusion following transradial access: complete recanalization via the anatomical snuffbox. Methodist Debakey Cardiovasc J. 2020;16:314–7.
19. Schulte-Hermes M, Klein-Wiele O, Vorpahl M, Seyfarth M. Feasibility of transradial access for coronary interventions via percutaneous angioplasty of the radial artery in cases of functional radial occlusion. J Invasive Cardiol. 2018;30:355–9.
20. Balaban Y, Elevli MG. It is both possible and safe to perform coronary angiography through the same radial artery, after retrograde recanalization of radial artery occlusion, following a previous coronary angiography. J Interv Cardiol. 2018;31:957–63.
21. Shi G, Li F, Zhang L, Gong C, Xue S, Song Y, et al. Retrograde recanalization of occluded radial artery: a single-centre experience and literature review. J Endovasc Ther. 2022;29:755–62.
22. Achim A, Kákonyi K, Jambrik Z, Olajos D, Nemes A, Bertrand OF, et al. Distal radial artery access for recanalization of radial artery occlusion and repeat intervention: a single center experience. J Clin Med. 2022;11:6916.
23. Sheikh AR, Abdelaal E, Sastry S, Karim S, Zeb M. Novel distal left radial artery access in anatomical snuffbox for recanalization of proximal radial artery total occlusion and percutaneous coronary intervention through left internal mammary artery. Circ Cardiovasc Interv. 2018;11:e006579.
24. Achim A, Leibundgut G. FAME 3 fails to defame coronary artery bypass grafting: what went wrong in the percutaneous coronary intervention arm? Eur J Cardiothorac Surg. 2022;62:ezac036.
25. Nappi F, Bellomo F, Nappi P, Chello C, Iervolino A, Chello M, et al. The use of radial artery for CABG: an update. Biomed Res Int. 2021;2021:5528006.

24 Peripheral Vascular Procedures

Marcelo Guimaraes, Harkanwar S. Gill, and Sasko Kedev

24.1 Introduction

Conventional transradial access (TRA) has emerged as the preferred vascular access for percutaneous coronary procedures over transfemoral approach (TFA) due to its lower risk of death, major adverse cardiovascular events, major bleeding, and vascular complications in a wide range of patients with coronary artery disease. Encouraging results from multicenter trials showing lower local complications compared to femoral access have driven the use of TRA worldwide not only for coronary interventions but also for peripheral endovascular interventions [1–4].

One of the potential advantages of TRA over TFA for peripheral interventions is in patients with bilateral (iliac or femoropopliteal) disease, who are more prone to local vascular access site complications. Indeed, TRA eliminates the need for post-procedural compression or the use of closure devices in the common femoral artery (CFA), which can lead to ischemia or even thrombotic complications if there is atherosclerosis at the CFA puncture site. In addition, TRA allows immediate ambulation after the procedure and facilitates same-day discharge, even with aggressive antithrombotic treatment.

However, repeated percutaneous coronary or endovascular interventions may result in radial artery occlusion (RAO), which has been reported to occur in approximately 1–10% of cases [5]. The rate of RAO usually depends on the relative diameter of the introducer sheath to the inner lumen of the radial artery [6], the duration of hemostatic compression of the radial artery [7], the maintenance of radial artery patency during hemostasis [8], the type of introducer sheath (hydrophilic or hydrophobic) [9], female gender, and the presence of peripheral arterial occlusive disease [10]. Most RAO are asymptomatic and do not affect the patient's quality of life, but it is very important to preserve the radial artery for repeated percutaneous coronary or peripheral interventions.

24.2 Distal Radial Access

Recently, an alternative vascular access has been introduced using the distal portion of the radial artery in the anatomical snuffbox, around the thumb on the dorsal hand [11]. The majority of the ever-growing evidence on distal radial access (DRA) is published in the cardiology literature and focuses on overcoming the current limitations of conventional TRA.

M. Guimaraes · H. S. Gill
Department of Radiology and Radiological Science, Medical University of South Carolina, Charleston, SC, USA

S. Kedev (✉)
Department of Cardiology, Faculty of Medicine, University of Ss. Cyril and Methodius, Skopje, Republic of North Macedonia

G. A. Sgueglia (ed.), *Distal Radial Access*, https://doi.org/10.1007/978-3-031-89925-6_24

Some of the potential advantages of this approach are a larger surface area of bone support below the puncture site and therefore a shorter compression time [12, 13]. Also, with DRA, any potential RAO at the puncture site is distal to the origin of the superficial palmar branch of the radial artery. Therefore, if DRA results in occlusion of the distal radial artery, anterograde blood flow via the superficial palmar arch is preserved (Fig. 24.1). Furthermore, because of its location within the anastomotic network, occlusion of the distal radial artery has essentially no effect on downstream flow [14]. A recent meta-analysis of randomized clinical trials has shown that DRA for percutaneous coronary intervention reduces the risk of RAO and high-grade hematoma compared with conventional TRA [13].

In fact, DRA in the anatomical snuffbox or dorsal hand is gaining interest as a safe alternative to conventional TRA for peripheral interventions as well. Left DRA in the anatomical snuffbox seems to be particularly ergonomic and more patient- and operator-friendly for peripheral procedures.

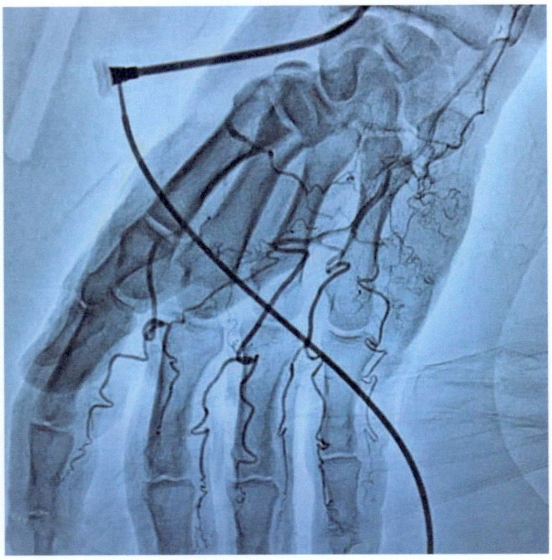

Fig. 24.1 Distal radial access warrants distal flow through the deep palmar arch

Actually, the best practices developed for conventional TRA can be well followed to minimize the risk of radial access complications. The Society of Interventional Radiology Quality Improvement Standards on Radial Artery Access publication of 2021 recommends appropriate patient selection and screening for successful outcomes [15]. To reduce the risk of stroke, caution is recommended in elderly patients with a heavily calcified aortic arch. The risk of hand ischemia and radial artery injury (including avulsion, dissection, and post-procedural occlusion) can be minimized by performing ultrasound examination (measurement of radial access site diameter, inner-to-inner wall) to assess compatibility of the radial access with the outer diameter of the introducer sheath. To minimize the risk of technical failure and access-related complications (including radial artery injury, spasms, and hematomas), all arterial accesses should ideally be obtained under real-time ultrasound guidance. It is highly recommended that a diagnostic forearm angiogram be performed soon after the sheath is secured with a dressing at the DRA site to rule out forearm spasms, kinks, and loops and to prevent radial artery dissection due to branch perforation. The use of fluoroscopy during guidewire and catheter advancement from the wrist to the aortic arch may prevent inadvertent and risky maneuvers [15]. A cocktail of vasodilators and heparin should always be administered to minimize the risk of radial artery spasm and thrombosis [1].

A potential limitation of the DRA approach is the 20% smaller mean diameter of the distal radial artery compared to the radial artery at the wrist [16]. In a Korean study, the distal radial artery was found to be smaller in women than in men (right 2.15 ± 0.38 mm vs. 2.43 ± 0.44 mm, $p < 0.001$; left 2.18 ± 0.39 mm vs. 2.47 ± 0.45 mm, $p < 0.001$), so the puncture may be challenging and a learning curve is required. Certainly, the use of real-time ultrasound guidance may overcome a potentially smaller access site.

The use of the lowest-profile devices compatible with DRA is also important. Table 24.1 shows the correlation between the ideal radial artery puncture site diameter and introducer sheath diameter. Until recently, challenges to the success of peripheral interventions using radial access have included limited wire lengths and long shaft stents/balloons to allow 5 or 6 Fr radial procedures, inadequate torque and support to deliver tools from radial access through tight peripheral artery stenoses or chronic total occlusions, and operator learning curve. The smaller size of the radial artery combined with an increased risk of spasm has potentially limited the use of large sheaths and catheters. A sheathless catheter is an alternative approach to avoid mismatch between the larger sheaths and the radial artery, but the lack of a sheath can complicate catheter exchange, and most of these sheathless catheters are inserted over a 0.035″ guidewire. Fortunately, as shown in Table 24.2, several transradial sheaths, long guide catheters, and wires are now available for the treatment of peripheral artery disease (PAD).

Table 24.1 Radial introducer sheath sizes and corresponding radial artery diameters

Sheath size	Radial artery diameter (mm)
5 Fr slender radial	1.6
5 Fr regular radial	1.8
6 Fr slender radial	2.4
6 Fr regular radial	2.6
7 Fr regular radial	3.1

Table 24.2 Selected radial sheaths, guiding catheters, and wires for transradial peripheral artery disease

Sheaths	5–7 Fr Flexor Shuttle (Cook Medical)	110 cm
	6 Fr R2P Destination Slender (Terumo)	119–149 cm
	6 Fr BRITE TIP RADIANZ (Cordis)	110–135 cm
Guide catheters	6.5–7.5 Fr Sheathless Eaucath (Asahi)	100 cm
	6 Fr MPA VISTA BRITE TIP (Cordis)	125 cm
	8.5 Fr SheathLess PV (Asahi)	120 cm
	7 Fr R2P SlenGuide (Terumo)	120–150 cm
Guide wires	ViperWire Advance 0.014″ (Abbott)	335–475 cm
	V-14 0.014″ and V-18 0.018″ ControlWire (Boston Scientific)	300 cm
	Nitrex 0.035″ (Medtronic)	400 cm
	Glidewire 0.035″ (Terumo)	350–450 cm

24.3 Distal Radial Access Procedure

DRA is a novel approach that can be safely used for percutaneous peripheral interventions in one or both arms by experienced radial operators. The presence of a distal radial artery pulse in the radial fossa is detected by manual palpation, and the diameter of the distal radial artery is assessed by ultrasound. The patient's hand is positioned with its dorsal aspect upward. The artery is punctured under real-time ultrasound guidance at a shallow angle of 30°, preferably in the anatomical snuffbox. Single anterior wall puncture with a 21 G needle is preferred for more distal access, but cannula puncture can also be used.

With either technique, ultrasound guidance and careful manipulation will prevent further advancement of the needle, which could cause pain if it touches the periosteum of the scaphoid or trapezium bone. If good arterial reflux is obtained, 0.021″ nitinol or a 0.025″ hydrophilic guidewire is advanced, and the hydrophilic 4 or 5 Fr sheath is inserted over the guidewire (a small skin incision is usually not necessary) (Fig. 24.2).

An intra-arterial cocktail is administered soon after sheath insertion and side port aspiration to confirm the presence of an intra-arterial position. The cocktail may include a vasodilator (5 mg verapamil) and unfractionated heparin at 50–70 IU/kg, up to a total of 5000 IU, or it may include intra-arterial administration of 200 mcg nitroglycerin and 2.5 mg verapamil and intravenous administration of unfractionated heparin at 50–70 IU/kg, up to 5000 IU. For procedures that may take longer than 1 h, additional administration of 1000 IU of heparin every 30 min should be considered, and the activated clotting time should be monitored and kept between two to three times higher than the baseline.

After insertion of the introducer sheath, diagnostic forearm angiography is performed through the sheath prior to catheter insertion. A solution of 3 mL of contrast mixed with 7 mL of blood is rapidly injected, and fluoroscopy is recorded. The radial artery anatomy is visualized from the lower forearm to the brachial bifurcation, providing a roadmap for safe access and proper material selection. In cases of radial artery spasm, tortuosity and/or radial artery anatomical variations (loops and high take-off radial arteries), a soft 0.014″ or small J 0.035″ hydrophilic guidewire can be used under fluoroscopic guidance to prevent vascular complications and reduce the need for crossover. Once the sheath is properly in place, the procedure through the DRA is similar to the conventional TRA (Tables 24.3 and 24.4).

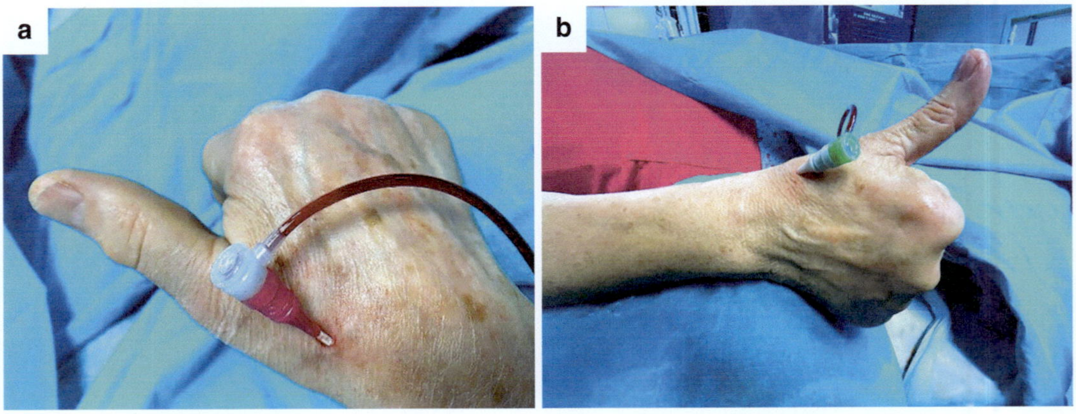

Fig. 24.2 Right distal radial access with thin-walled introducer sheath: (**a**) 5 Fr and (**b**) 6 Fr

Table 24.3 Selected 5/6 Fr balloons for transradial peripheral artery disease

Balloon	Guidewire compatibility	Recommended sheath	Shaft length (cm)	Diameter (mm)	Length (mm)
IN.PACT Admiral DCB (Medtronic)	OTW 0.035″	5–6 Fr	130	4–6	40–250
Stellarex DCB (Philips)	OTW 0.035″	6 Fr	130	4–6	40–200
Lutonix DCB (BD)	OTW 0.018″ and 0.035″	4–5 Fr	130	4–7	40–300
Mustang (Boston Scientific)	OTW 0.035″	5–6 Fr	135	5–10	20–200
EverCross (Medtronic)	OTW 0.035″	5–6 Fr	135	3–10	20–200
Sterling (Boston Scientific)	OTW and Rx 0.018″	4–6 Fr	150	2–10	20–220
NanoCross Elite (Medtronic)	OTW 0.014″	4–6 Fr	150	1.5–6	20–210
Pacific Plus (Medtronic)	OTW 0.018″	4–5 Fr	180	2–7	20–150
SABERX RADIANZ (Cordis)	Rx 0.018″	4–6 Fr	190	4–10	20–300
Ultraverse RX (BD)	Rx 0.014″	4–5 Fr	200	1.25–7	15–300
R2P Metacross (Terumo)	Rx 0.035″	6 Fr	200	3–8	20–200
IN.PACT 018 DCB (Medtronic)	OTW 0.018″	5–6 Fr	200	4–7	40–150

Table 24.4 Selected 6 Fr stent for transradial peripheral artery disease

	Guidewire compatibility	Shaft length (cm)	Diameter (mm)	Length (mm)
Balloon-expandable stents				
iCast Advanta (Getinge)	OTW 0.035″	120	5–6	16–22
Visi-Pro (Medtronic)	OTW 0.035″	135	5–8	17–57
Express LD (Boston Scientific)	OTW 0.035″	135	6–8	17–57
Self-expanding stents				
Viabahn (Gore)	OTW 0.018″	120	5–6	25–250
Epic (Boston Scientific)	OTW 0.035″	120	6–12	20–120
Zilver PTX (Cook Medical)	OTW 0.035″	125	5–8	40–140
Eluvia (Boston Scientific)	OTW 0.035″	130	6–7	40–150
S.M.A.R.T. RADIANZ (Cordis)	Rx 0.018″	190	6–10	20–150
Innova (Boston Scientific)	OTW 0.035″	130	5–8	20–200
EverFlex (Medtronic)	OTW 0.035″	120	5–8	20–200
R2P Misago (Terumo)	Rx 0.035″	200	6–8	40–150

24.4 Distal Radial Access for Carotid Artery Stenting

When performed by experienced operators, carotid artery stenting (CAS) with embolic protection is a proven alternative to carotid endarterectomy in patients with significant carotid disease [17–21]. While the TFA is preferred, TRA has been advocated in specific anatomies potentially associated with high peri-procedural event rate from the femoral catheterization. Indeed, TFA may be difficult in patients with severe PAD or in patients with unfavorable take-off of supra-aortic arteries from dilated aortic arch or in bovine arch. A reported 14% rate of symptomatic strokes contralateral to the vascular territory of the treated carotid stenosis strongly suggests that catheter manipulations in the aorta and aortic arch are a cause of atheroembolic brain lesions, especially when TFA is used [22–24].

In general, TRA or DRA is associated with fewer catheter manipulations in the aortic arch and descending aorta and may be an alternative strategy for CAS. After successful introducer placement and peri-procedural radial artery angiography, diagnostic carotid angiography is performed using a 5 Fr Simmons catheter. There are two methods to reform the naturally reversed curve of the Simmons catheter within the aortic arch.

The first involves passing the catheter over a 0.035″ hydrophilic wire looped in the ascending aorta. This technique is used for a Simmons 1 or Simmons 2 catheter in patients with a very tortuous and dilated aortic arch (Fig. 24.3).

The second method is preferred in most cases for the Simmons 2 catheter. The catheter is advanced into the descending thoracic aorta over a standard guidewire. The curve is reformed by withdrawing the guidewire into the primary curve and prolapsing the catheter into the ascending aorta with counterclockwise rotation. With this maneuver, the catheter forms a loop on itself, often directly engaging the left common carotid artery (CCA) (Fig. 24.4). The catheter can then be rotated and withdrawn into the right CCA.

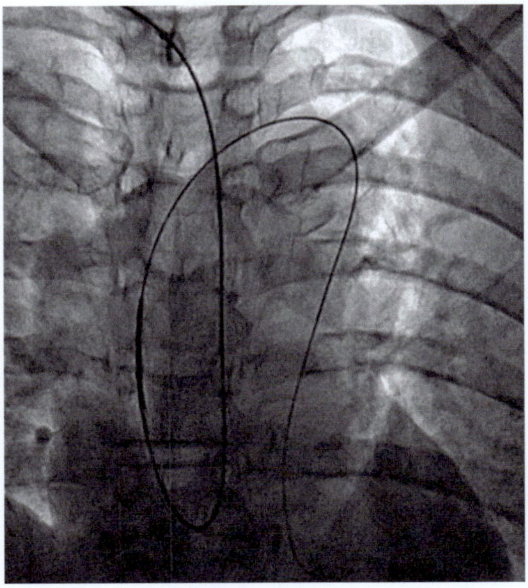

Fig. 24.3 Looping technique of a diagnostic Simmons 2 catheter over a hydrophilic wire in the ascending aorta

If DRA is chosen, CAS is usually performed through a 5 or 6 Fr 90 cm guiding sheath (Shuttle, Cook; Destination, Terumo; or Fubuki, Asahi) (Fig. 24.5). Recently, the thin-wall technology originally developed for lower-profile introducer sheaths has been applied to the production of lower-profile guiding sheaths (Destination Slender, Terumo; and BRITE TIP RADIANZ, Cordis).

There are two different modes of CCA cannulation: anchoring and telescoping. In the anchoring technique, a diagnostic or transfer

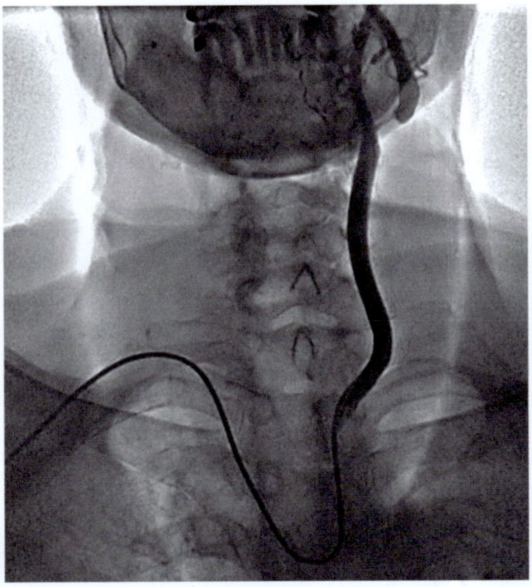

Fig. 24.4 Simmons 2 catheter in the left common carotid artery for diagnostic angiography

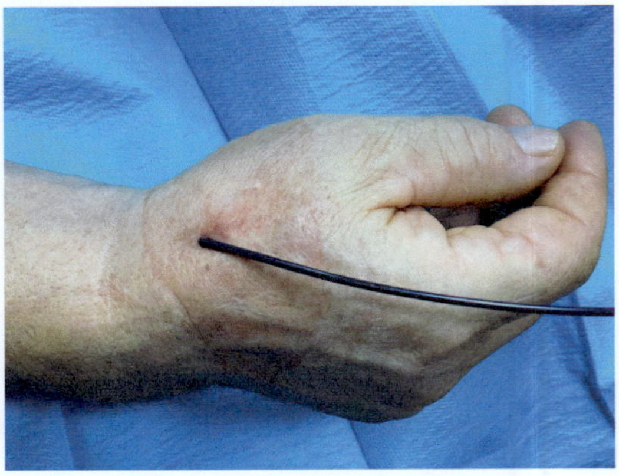

Fig. 24.5 Right distal radial access with a 90 cm 5 Fr guiding sheath

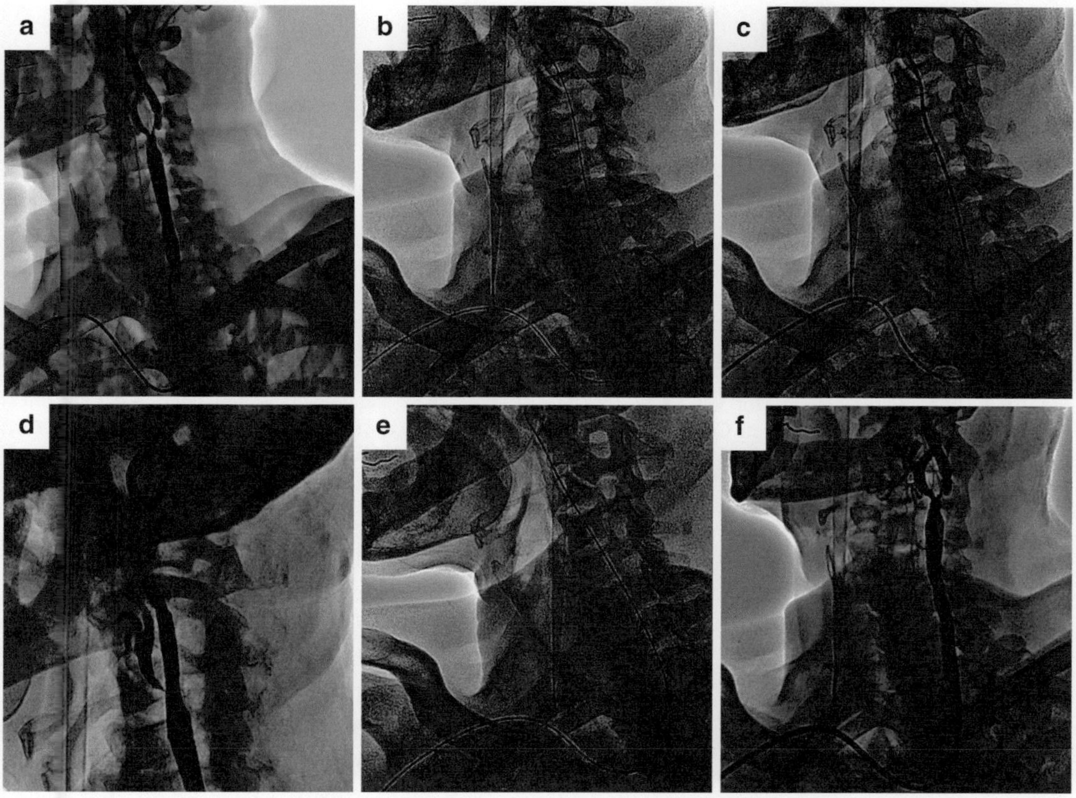

Fig. 24.6 Anchoring technique for left CCA cannulation: (**a**) Simmons 2 catheter in left CCA. (**b**) Glidewire Advantage (Terumo) guidewire in the ECA. (**c**) Transfer catheter (5 Fr JR guiding catheter) in left ECA. (**d**) Amplatz Super Stiff (Boston Scientific) guidewire exchange in left ECA. (**e**) Destination (Terumo) 6 Fr guiding sheath in left CCA. (**f**) Final result after distal radial access stenting of the left internal carotid artery with XACT (Abbott) 6.0–8.0/40 mm stent. *CCA* common carotid artery

catheter is positioned in the external carotid artery (ECA) to insert a replacement guidewire over which a guide sheath is deployed (Fig. 24.6).

In the telescoping technique, a long (125 cm) Simmons 2 wire-braided catheter is positioned inside the introducer sheath as a dilator (Fig. 24.7). This technique is useful for sheath deployment in cases with severe angulations.

Afterward, CAS with distal embolic protection is then performed in the usual manner. Most DRA CAS procedures are performed from the right side. However, in some cases with right ICA lesions, left DRA may be an alternative if the right radial access is not available (Figs. 24.8 and 24.9).

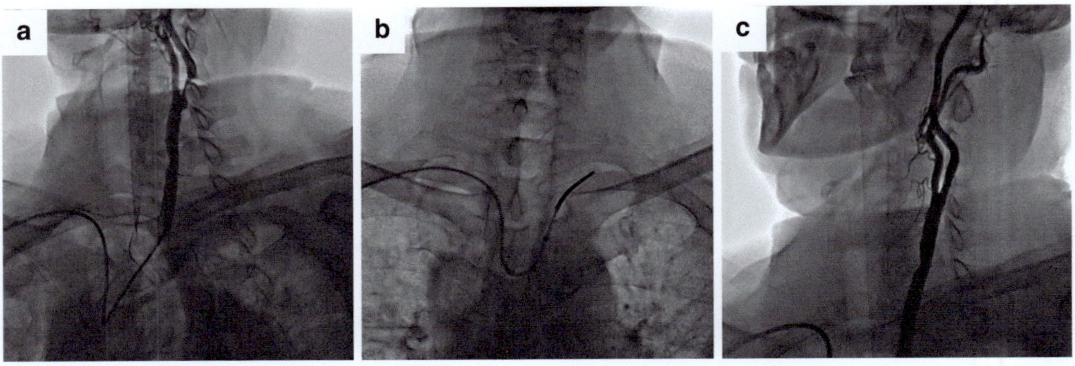

Fig. 24.7 Telescopic technique for left CCA cannulation: (**a**) Simmons 2 catheter in left CCA. (**b**) Simmons 125 cm 6 Fr-braided catheter into Flexor Shuttle (Cook Medical) 6 Fr guiding sheath. (**c**) Final result after distal radial access stenting of the left internal carotid artery with Adapt (Boston Scientific) 4–9/40 mm stent. *CCA* common carotid artery

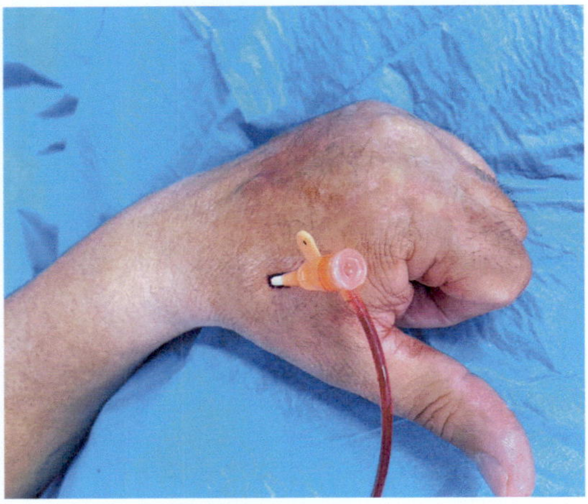

Fig. 24.8 Left distal radial access with a 7 Fr thin-walled introducer sheaths

24.4.1 Advantages of Distal Radial Access Carotid Artery Stenting

1. Alternative access in patients with extensive peripheral vascular disease.
2. Reduction of access site bleeding and vascular complications, particularly in the obese and elderly patients.
3. Patient and operator comfort, especially when using left DRA (more natural arm position and no need for operator to bend over patient).
4. Shorter time of hemostasis achieved.
5. Alternative access in patients with anatomic variations that make cannulation of the CCA difficult from TFA.
6. Easier access in patients with bovine left ICA disease. DRA in patients with right ICA disease and bovine left ICA disease may reduce catheter-induced embolization from the aortic arch [25–28].
7. Early patient mobilization.
8. Reduced nursing cost.

24.4.2 Disadvantages of Distal Radial Access Carotid Artery Stenting

1. Extensive experience with both the DRA and CAS is necessary.
2. Significant learning curve for new radial operators.
3. Sometimes longer procedures for easy TFA CAS with type I aortic arch.
4. Proximal protection and larger devices cannot be used freely in all cases.

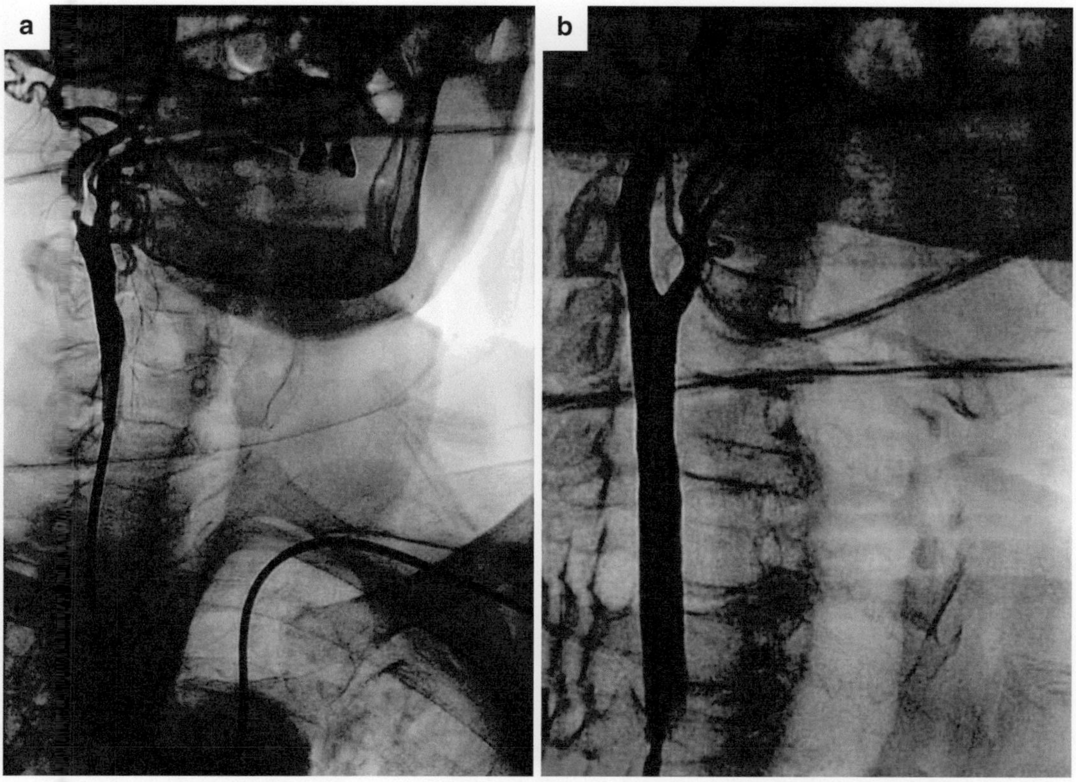

Fig. 24.9 Left distal radial access for (**a**) right internal carotid artery angiography and (**b**) right internal carotid artery stenting

24.5 Distal Radial Access for Subclavian Artery Interventions

Subclavian artery stenosis or chronic total occlusion (CTO) occurs in 2.5% to 7.5% of patients with cardiovascular disease. Although surgery has provided good long-term patency, endovascular techniques have been developed and offer less invasive alternatives [29]. Treatment of complex upper extremity lesions involves the use of single ipsilateral or bilateral conventional TRA or DRA. For single ipsilateral access, the distal radial artery is cannulated as previously described. After sheath insertion, distal forearm angiography is performed, and anti-spasm and antithrombotic medications are administered as described above.

Left DRA could be elegantly used for subclavian CTO angioplasty as part of a bilateral approach. For a bilateral approach, both arms are prepared, and a 5 Fr hydrophilic sheath is placed in the contralateral artery. A JR 4.0 6 Fr guiding catheter is used from the ipsilateral arm, and a 5 Fr Simmons 2 diagnostic catheter is used from the contralateral arm for controlled injections. Occlusion and collaterals are assessed with simultaneous bilateral injections (Figs. 24.10 and 24.11). Contralateral injections are used to confirm proper wire advancement within the lesion. The CTO may be crossed with 0.014″ CTO coronary or dedicated peripheral wires. Predilations are performed with standard semi-compliant coronary balloon catheters. The lesion can then be crossed with the 6 Fr guiding catheter and replaced with a 0.035″ Amplatz 260 mm guidewire (Boston Scientific). Balloon-expandable stents (0.035″ compatible) are then advanced solely by guidewire without the use of a guiding catheter or long guiding sheath. This

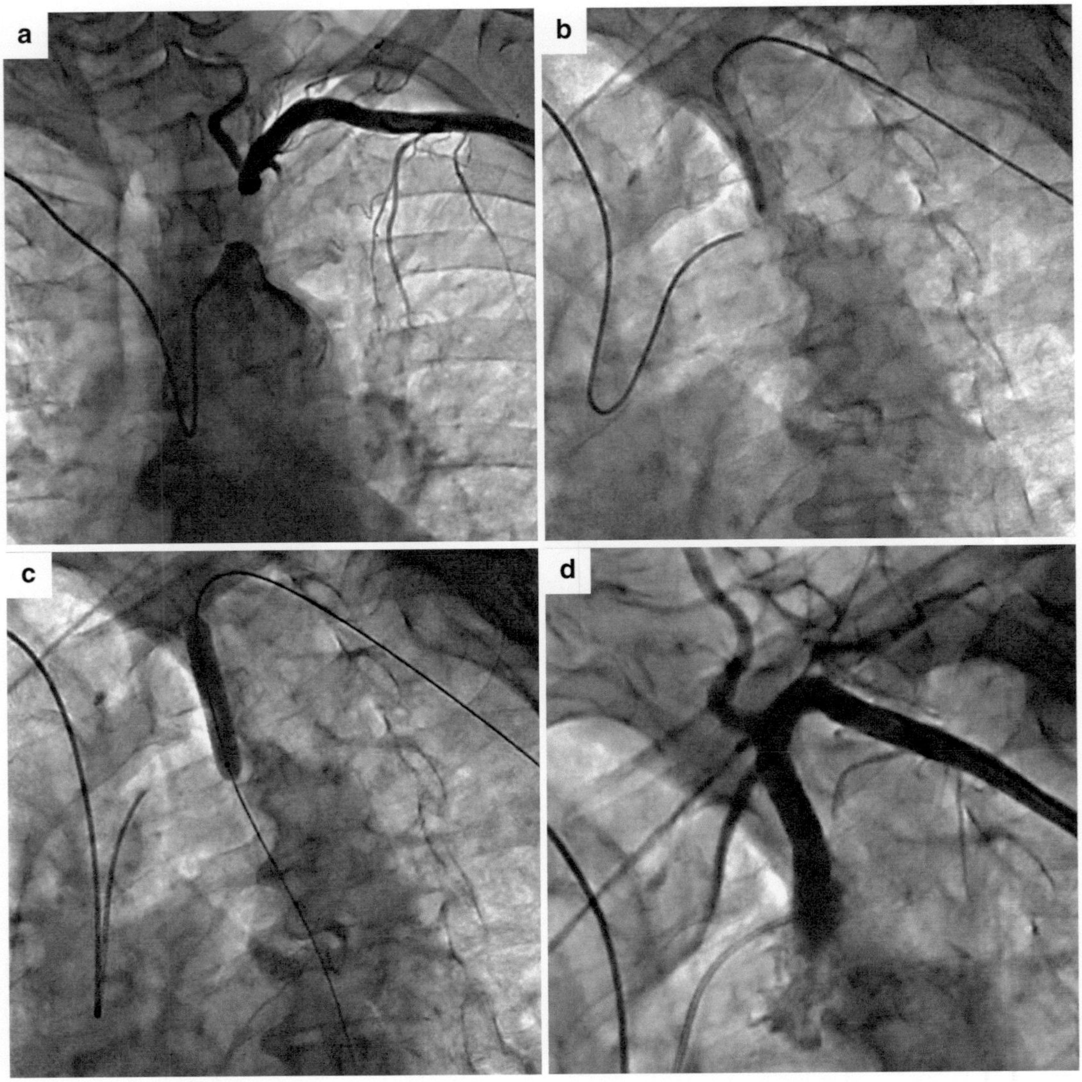

Fig. 24.10 Bilateral distal radial access for subclavian artery stenting: (**a**) Baseline angiography showing chronic total occlusion of the left subclavian artery. (**b**) Balloon angioplasty. (**c**) Guideless Omnilink (Abbott) 8/59 mm stent deployment on 0.035″ guidewire with contralateral guidance. (**d**) Final angiography

technique of guideless retrograde stent delivery eliminates the need for a large-bore guiding catheter or sheath, further reducing the risk of RAO. Correct stent positioning is confirmed with contralateral injections through the Simmons 2 catheter.

24.5.1 Advantages of Guideless Distal Radial Access Subclavian Stenting

1. Smaller catheters are required compared to TFA, and lower-grade radial injury compared to conventional TRA.

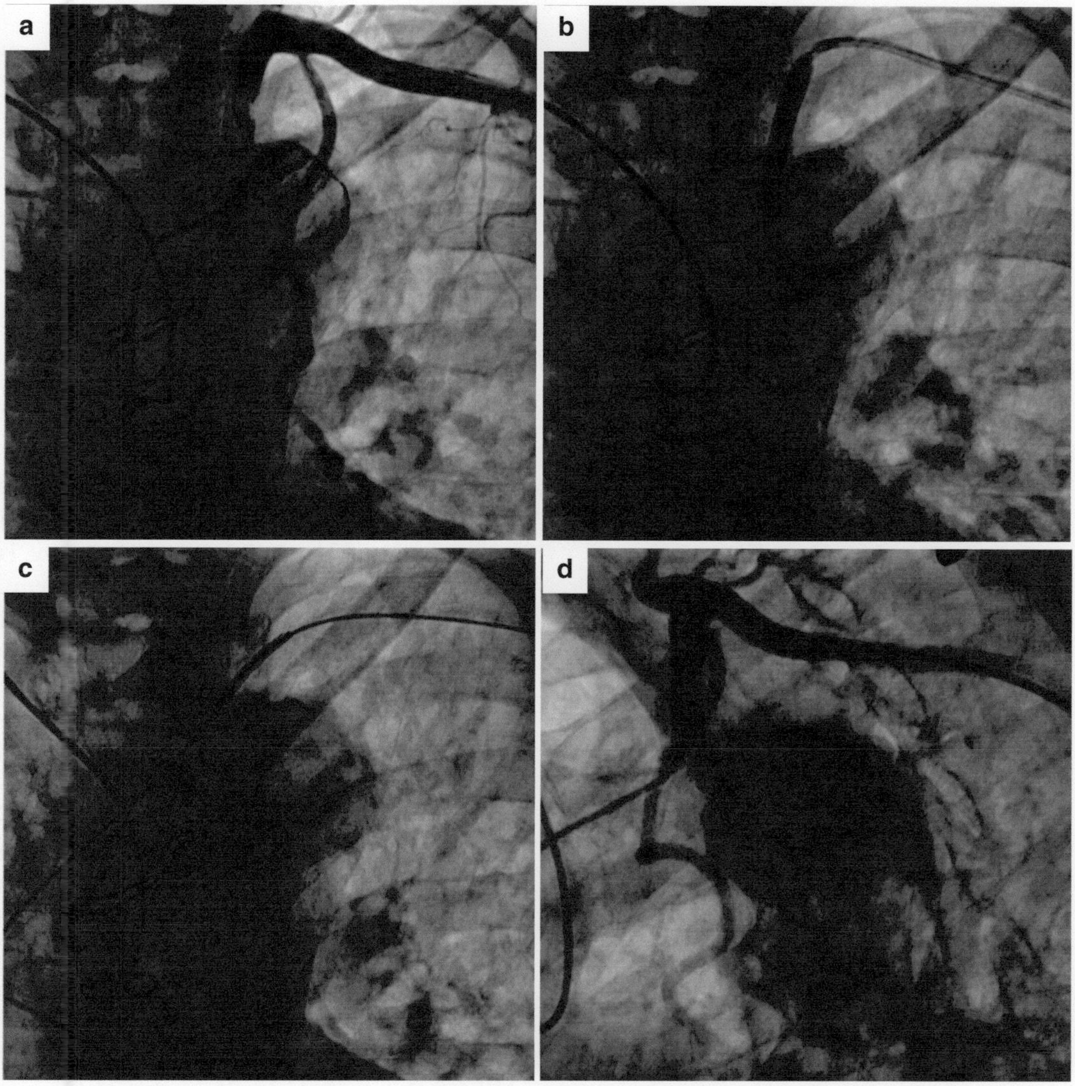

Fig. 24.11 Bilateral distal radial access subclavian artery stenting in patient with coronary steal syndrome after coronary artery by-pass graft surgery: (**a**) Baseline angiography showing ostial lesion of left subclavian artery. (**b**) Predilation with a 5.0/40 mm balloon through 6 Fr guiding catheter from left distal radial access. (**c**) Guideless stent deployment on 0.035″ guidewire with contralateral guidance. (**d**) Final result with preservation of the left internal mammary artery

2. Less aortic arch and descending aorta manipulation than TFA.
3. Ergonomic and more patient- and operator-friendly approach.
4. Bilateral DRA is particularly useful to guide subclavian stenting for CTO as it improves procedural success rate while minimizing access site bleeding and vascular complications associated with TFA.
5. Retrograde DRA facilitates wire crossing through the softer distal cap of the CTO.

24.5.2 Disadvantages of Distal Radial Access Subclavian Percutaneous Interventions

1. Absent or diminished radial pulse on the side of the subclavian occlusion/stenosis. Blind puncture based on anatomy or ultrasound-guided puncture of DRA may be required in some cases.
2. Extensive operator knowledge and expertise in peripheral CTO techniques through TRA.
3. TFA may still be required after failed CTO angioplasty by TRA.

24.6 Distal Radial Access for Iliac Artery Intervention

Of note, PAD results in significant limitations in the quality of life and functional capacity for patients with claudication. It is associated with increased morbidity and mortality in patients with chronic limb-threatening ischemia. Endovascular interventions have become the standard of care for the treatment of lower extremity PAD [30]. The TFA has historically been the preferred access for peripheral diagnostic angiography and intervention, providing easy access and adequate device length for successful revascularization of various lesion types. However, TFA complications occur in 1.4–3.7% of patients, including hematoma, retroperitoneal bleeding, transfusion requirement, pseudoaneurysm, arteriovenous fistula, and arterial thrombosis.

The introduction and widespread use of TRA have extended to the treatment of iliac artery disease. DRA as an alternative to conventional TRA has potential advantages over TFA, particularly in patients with bilateral iliac disease who are more susceptible to local vascular access site complications. It is also more cost-effective due to lower complication rates, earlier ambulation, and shorter hospital stay [31, 32]. Left DRA is particularly comfortable for both the patient and the operator, allowing for a relaxed, natural arm position. It avoids the aortic arch and provides a shorter route to the lower extremity arteries.

The typical distances from the left RA that should be considered while planning the procedure to the iliac arteries (105–125 cm), common femoral artery (120–150 cm), superficial femoral artery (130–170 cm), popliteal artery (150–180 cm), and tibial arteries (200–250 cm) [33, 34].

Recently, we have adopted a novel and very safe technique for iliac artery stenting using single or bilateral DRA. In the bilateral DRA technique, two regular short hydrophilic 6 Fr sheaths are inserted with consequent preprocedural radial artery angiography. Peripheral angiography is performed with a pigtail catheter (110–125 cm). To cross the CTO lesions, a 6 Fr guiding catheter (110–125 cm) and several 0.014″ dedicated CTO wires, usually supported by a microcatheter, are required. After successful wire crossing and predilation, the CTO guidewire is replaced with a 0.035″ Amplatz stiff guidewire. Balloon-expandable stents are preferred in proximal common iliac lesions because of their greater radial strength and more precise deployment compared to self-expanding stents. They are deployed solely on a 0.035″ Amplatz stiff guidewire without the use of a guiding catheter or long sheath. Proper positioning is achieved by contralateral injections from a 110 to 125 cm 5 or 6 Fr JR or MP catheter (Figs. 24.12, 24.13, and 24.14).

For the single DRA technique, a short 6-Fr hydrophilic sheath is inserted into the left or right distal radial artery, and peripheral angiography is performed. Balloon-expandable stents are advanced on 0.035″ Amplatz stiff wire. Angiomarkers are used to ensure proper stent positioning. A variation of this technique can also be used for larger bore 7 Fr-compatible stent graft implantation when indicated (iliac or common femoral artery perforation and bilateral ostial iliac artery disease).

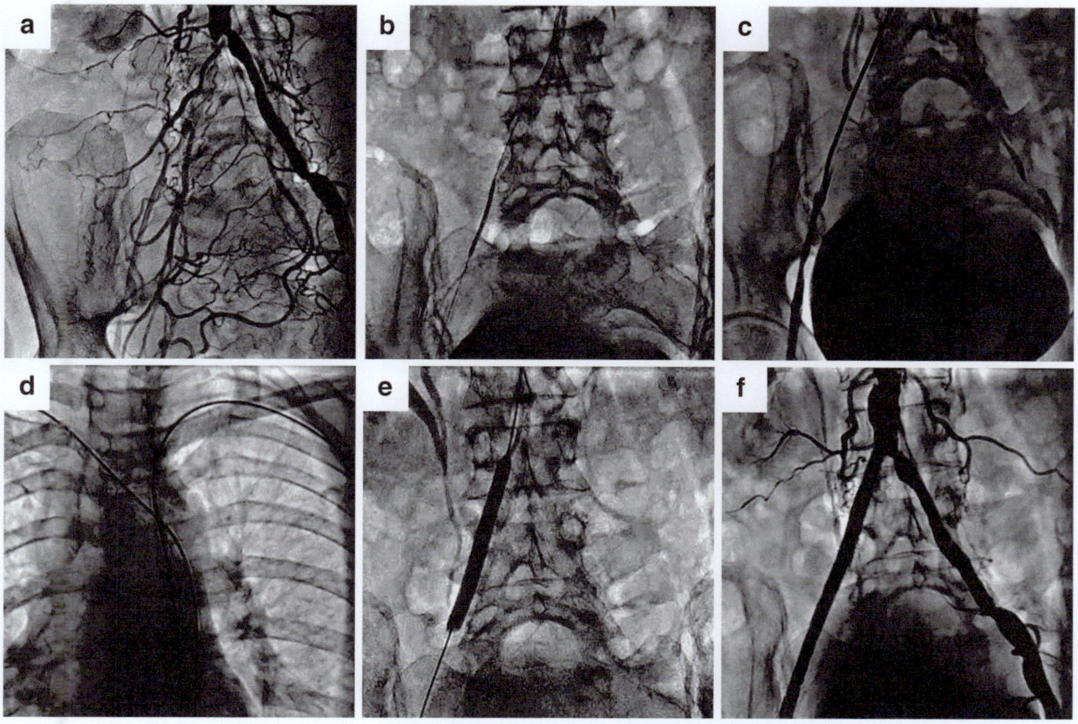

Fig. 24.12 Bilateral distal radial access for iliac artery stenting: (**a**) Baseline angiography showing ostial chronic total occlusion of the right common iliac artery. (**b**) Predilation with small balloon on a 0.014″ guidewire from left distal radial access. (**c**) Predilation result. (**d**) Catheter exchange with a 0.035″ guidewire and advancement of another guidewire from right distal radial access. (**e**) Guideless stent deployment on 0.035″ guidewire with contralateral guidance (JR 4 catheter from right distal radial access). (**f**) Final result

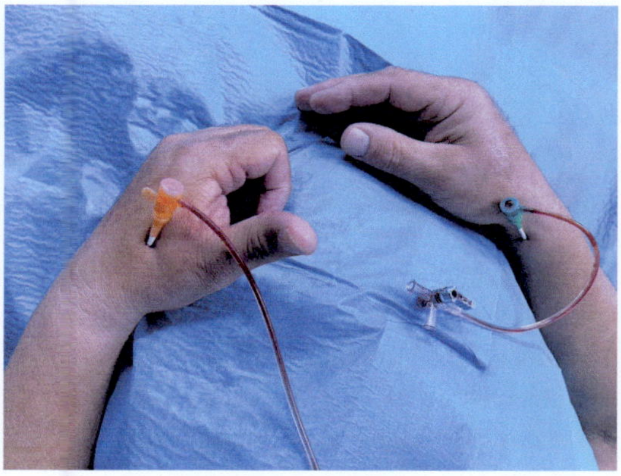

Fig. 24.13 Bilateral access with 7 Fr left distal radial access and 6 Fr right conventional transradial access

24.6.1 Advantages of Distal Radial Access Iliac Stenting

1. Less invasive technique with early patient ambulation and shorter hospital stay.
2. Reduced vascular and bleeding complications.
3. Eliminates the need for large-bore catheters or long sheaths (stent is deployed through 0.035″ guidewire only).
4. Patient and operator comfort, especially when using left DRA (which also provides a shorter distance to the peripheral vessel).

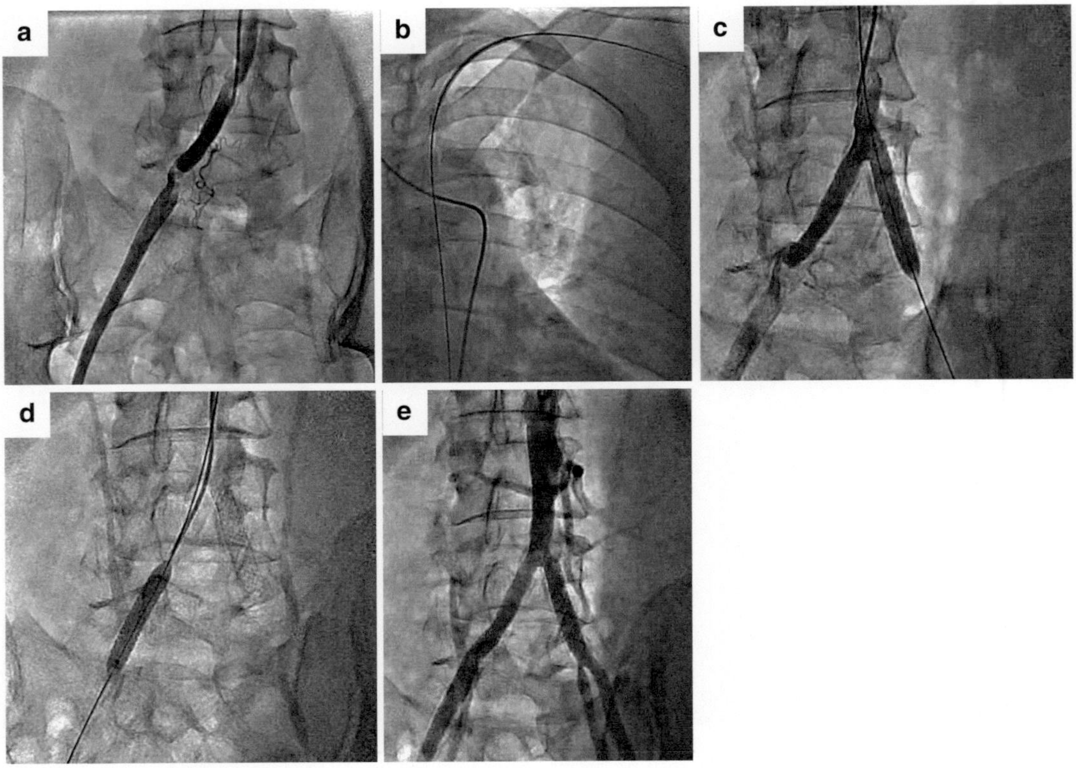

Fig. 24.14 Bilateral access (7 Fr left distal radial access and 6 Fr right conventional transradial access) for iliac artery stenting: (**a**) Baseline angiography showing ostial chronic total occlusion of the left common iliac artery. (**b**) After successful chronic total occlusion crossing and pre-dilation, a guideless Omnilink (Abbott) 9.0/59 mm stent is advanced on 0.035″ wire from left distal radial access. (**c**) Stent deployment in left common iliac artery under guidance from contralateral JR 4 6 Fr guiding catheter. (**d**) Additional deployment of an Omnilink 8.0/39 mm stent in the right iliac artery. (**e**) Final result

24.6.2 Disadvantages of Distal Radial Access Iliac Stenting

1. Lack of dedicated equipment in some cases.
2. Limited compatibility with larger devices.
3. Difficulties with increased tortuosity of the radial/brachial or subclavian arteries and high degree of spasm in elderly or hypertensive patients.

24.7 Arterial Sheath Management

For conventional TRA, patent hemostasis using the Barbeau test is recommended to prevent RAO [15, 35]. However, no method has been reported to achieve reliable patent hemostasis in DRA. The radial sheath is removed immediately after the procedure, and compressive hemostasis is achieved. Compression is applied for approximately 1–2 h (depending on sheath size) with gradual release of compression after the first hour. Patients are usually discharged the following day, but selected cases may be safely discharged the same day after an uneventful procedure.

24.8 Conclusion

We have witnessed a significant increase in radial access procedures worldwide across multiple specialties. Robust data have been published supporting the role of TRA with reduced access site complications, cost-effectiveness, and the ability to treat high-risk bleeding patients. Therefore, it is critical to expand the role of radial access for peripheral artery interventions.

DRA for peripheral interventions is a less invasive technique that allows early patient ambulation and shorter hospital stay. It is more ergonomic and is associated with shorter compression time, less arterial damage at the wrist, and a potential reduction in RAO rate. DRA is associated with improved patient and operator comfort during the procedure, especially for left DRA

The recent availability of long introducer sheaths, 200-cm-long shaft balloons, 200 cm stents, and atherectomy devices has made PAD treatment via DRA possible. There is an ample opportunity for industry innovation in redesigning catheters and devices and shifting the focus from femoral to radial access sites, which is in line with current best practices in coronary interventions.

References

1. Caputo RP, Tremmel JA, Rao S, Gilchrist IC, Pyne C, Pancholy S, et al. Transradial arterial access for coronary and peripheral procedures: executive summary by the transradial committee of the SCAI. Catheter Cardiovasc Interv. 2011;78:823–39.
2. Bertrand OF, Rao SV, Pancholy S, Jolly SS, Rodés-Cabau J, Larose E, et al. Transradial approach for coronary angiography and interventions: results of the first international transradial practice survey. JACC Cardiovasc Interv. 2010;3:1022–31.
3. Pandie S, Mehta SR, Cantor WJ, Cheema AN, Gao P, Madan M, et al. Radial versus femoral access for coronary angiography/intervention in women with acute coronary syndromes: insights from the RIVAL trial. JACC Cardiovasc Interv. 2015;20(8):505–12.
4. Jolly SS, Yusuf S, Cairns J, Niemelä K, Xavier D, Widimsky P, et al. Radial versus femoral access for coronary angiography and intervention in patients with acute coronary syndromes (RIVAL): a randomized, parallel group, multicentre trial. Lancet. 2011;377:1409–20.
5. Stella PR, Kiemeneij F, Laarman GJ, Odekerken D, Slagboom T, van der Wieken R. Incidence and outcome of radial artery occlusion following transradial artery coronary angioplasty. Catheter Cardiovasc Diagn. 1997;40:156–8.
6. Saito S, Ikei H, Hosokawa G, Tanaka S. Influence of the ratio between radial artery inner diameter and sheath outer diameter on radial artery flow after transradial coronary intervention. Catheter Cardiovasc Interv. 1999;46:173–8.
7. Pancholy SB, Patel TM. Effect of duration of hemostatic compression on radial artery occlusion after transradial access. Catheter Cardiovasc Interv. 2012;79:78–81.
8. Pancholy SB, Bertrand OF, Patel T. Comparison of a priori versus provisional heparin therapy on radial artery occlusion after transradial coronary angiography and patent hemostasis (from the PHARAOH study). Am J Cardiol. 2012;110:173–6.
9. Saito S, Tanaka S, Hiroe Y, Miyashita Y, Takahashi S, Satake S, et al. Usefulness of hydrophilic coating on arterial sheath introducer in transradial coronary intervention. Catheter Cardiovasc Interv. 2002;56:328–32.
10. Uhlemann M, Möbius-Winkler S, Mende M, Eitel I, Fuernau G, Sandri M, et al. The Leipzig prospective vascular ultrasound registry in radial artery catheterization: impact of sheath size on vascular complications. JACC Cardiovasc Interv. 2012;5:36–43.
11. Kiemeneij F. Left distal transradial access in the anatomical snuffbox for coronary angiography (ldTRA) and interventions (ldTRI). EuroIntervention. 2017;13:851–7.
12. Aminian A, Sgueglia GA, Wiemer M, Kefer J, Gasparini GL, Ruzsa Z, et al. Distal versus conventional radial access for coronary angiography and intervention the DISCO RADIAL trial. JACC Cardiovasc Interv. 2022;15:1191–201.
13. Ferrante G, Condello F, Rao SV, Maurina M, Jolly S, Stefanini GG, et al. Distal vs conventional radial access for coronary angiography and/or intervention: a metaanalysis of randomized trials. JACC Cardiovasc Interv. 2022;15:2297–311.
14. Sgueglia GA, Santoliquido A, Gaspardone A, Di Giorgio A. First results of the distal radial access Doppler study. JACC Cardiovasc Imaging. 2021;14:1281–3.
15. Gayed A, Yamada R, Bhatia S, Fischman A, Heran MKS, Himes EA, et al. Society of interventional radiology quality improvement standards on radial artery access. J Vasc Interv Radiol. 2021;32(761):e1–21.
16. Lee JW, Son JW, Go TH, Kang DR, Lee SJ, Kim SE, et al. Reference diameter and characteristics of the distal radial artery based on ultrasonographic assessment. Korean J Intern Med. 2022;37:109–18.
17. Brott TG, Hobson RW, Howard G, Roubin GS, Clark WM, Brooks W, et al. Stenting versus endarterectomy for treatment of carotid artery stenosis. N Engl J Med. 2010;363:11–23.
18. Silver FL, Mackey A, Clark WM, Brooks W, Timaran CH, Chiu D, et al. CREST investigators. Safety of stenting and endarterectomy by symptomatic status in the carotid revascularization endarterectomy versus stenting trial (CREST). Stroke. 2011;42:675–80.
19. Gray WA, Yadav JS, Verta P, Scicli A, Fairman R, Wholey M, et al. The CAPTURE registry: predictors of outcomes in carotid artery stenting with embolic protection for high surgical risk patients in the early

post-approval setting. Catheter Cardiovasc Interv. 2007;70:1025–33.
20. Gurm HS, Yadav JS, Fayad P, Katzen BT, Mishkel GJ, Bajwa TK, et al. SAPPHIRE investigators. Long-term results of carotid stenting versus endarterectomy in high-risk patients. N Engl J Med. 2008;358:1572–9.
21. White CJ, Iyer SS, Hopkins LN, Katzen BT, Russell ME, BEACH Trial Investigators. Carotid stenting with distal protection in 4 high surgical risk patients: the BEACH trial: 30 day results. Catheter Cardiovasc Interv. 2006;67:503–12.
22. Hill MD, Brooks W, Mackey A, Clark WM, Meschia JF, Morrish WF, et al. Stroke after carotid stenting and endarterectomy in the carotid revascularization endarterectomy versus stenting trial (CREST). Circulation. 2012;126:3054–61.
23. Macdonald S, Lee R, Williams R, Stansby G. Delphi carotid stenting consensus panel. Towards safer carotid artery stenting: a scoring system for anatomic suitability. Stroke. 2009;40:1698–703.
24. Hammer FD, Lacroix V, Duprez T, Grandin C, Verhelst R, Peeters A, et al. Cerebral microembolization after protected carotid artery stenting in surgical high-risk patients: results of a 2-year prospective study. J Vasc Surg. 2005;42:847–53.
25. Bendszus M, Koltzenburg M, Burger R, Warmuth-Metz M, Hofmann E, Solymosi L. Silent embolism in diagnostic cerebral angiography and neurointerventional procedures: a prospective study. Lancet. 1999;354:1594–7.
26. El-Koussy M, Schroth G, Do DD, Gralla J, Nedeltchev K, von Bredow F, et al. Periprocedural embolic events related to carotid artery stenting detected by diffusion-weighted MRI: comparison between proximal and distal embolus protection devices. J Endovasc Ther. 2007;14:293–303.
27. Barbato JE, Dillavou E, Horowitz MB, Jovin TG, Kanal E, David S, et al. A randomized trial of carotid artery stenting with and without cerebral protection. J Vasc Surg. 2008;47:760–5.
28. Faggioli G, Ferri M, Rapezzi C, Tonon C, Manzoli L, Stella A. Atherosclerotic aortic lesions increase the risk of cerebral embolism during carotid stenting in patients with complex aortic arch anatomy. J Vasc Surg. 2009;49:80–5.
29. AbuRahma AF, Bates MC, Stone PA, Dyer B, Armistead L, Scott Dean L, et al. Angioplasty and stenting versus carotidsubclavian bypass for the treatment of isolated subclavian artery disease. J Endovasc Ther. 2007;14:698–704.
30. Antoniou GA, Chalmers N, Georgiadis GS, et al. A meta-analysis of endovascular versus surgical reconstruction of femoropopliteal arterial disease. J Vasc Surg. 2013;57:242–53.
31. Korabathna R, Yadav SS, Coppola JT, Staniloae CS. Transradial approach to lower extremity interventions. Vasc Health Risk Manag. 2010;6:503–9.
32. Amin AP, Patterson M, House JA, Giersiefen H, Spertus JA, Baklanov DV, et al. Costs associated with access site and same-day discharge among medicare beneficiaries undergoing percutaneous coronary intervention: an evaluation of the current percutaneous coronary intervention care pathways in the United States. JACC Cardiovasc Interv. 2017;10:342–51.
33. Fanaroff AC, Rao SV, Swaminathan RV. Radial access for peripheral interventions. Interv Cardiol Clin. 2020;9:53–61.
34. Chowdhury M, Secemsky EA. Contemporary use of radial to peripheral access for management of peripheral artery disease. Curr Treat Options Cardio Med. 2021;23:17.
35. Barbeau GR, Arsenault F, Dugas L, Simard S, Larivière MM. Evaluation of the ulnopalmar arterial arches with pulse oximetry and plethysmography: comparison with the Allen's test in 1010 patients. Am Heart J. 2004;147:489–93.

25 Neurointervention

Ajit S. Puri, Anna Luisa Kuhn, Kareem El Naamani, Jasmeet Singh, and Pascal Jabbour

25.1 Introduction

In recent years, transradial approach (TRA) has become the preferred access for coronary angiography and percutaneous coronary intervention worldwide, regardless of clinical presentation, based on Class IA indications provided by the 2018 European Society of Cardiology/European Association for Cardiothoracic Surgery Guidelines on Myocardial Revascularization and the 2021 American College of Cardiology/American Heart Association/Society for Cardiovascular Angiography and Interventions Guideline for Coronary Artery Revascularization, demonstrating its superiority over the transfemoral approach [1, 2].

The use of the radial artery has also gained interest in the neurointerventional field following numerous publications in the cardiology literature showing lower rates of access site complications, faster recovery time, and higher patient satisfaction rates compared to the transfemoral approach [3–7]. Notably, TRA also provides direct access to the ipsilateral vertebral artery and easier navigation in type 3 aortic arches [8]. A refinement of conventional TRA is distal radial access (DRA) in the anatomical snuffbox, which has also gained popularity for diagnostic and interventional procedures in the neurointerventional field due to its improved safety, facilitation of left side catheterization, and improved patient-operator ergonomics compared to conventional TRA approach [9, 10]. With a puncture that safeguards palmar collateral flow, DRA limits the risk of hand ischemia and reduces the rate of radial artery occlusion, thus preserving the radial artery for future interventions [11–13]. Understandably, DRA is not without tradeoffs. Compared to the forearm radial artery, the distal radial artery has a smaller diameter, which increases the risk of vasospasm, and a slightly longer distance to the supra-aortic region [8].

In this chapter, we discuss the advantages and disadvantages of DRA, describe the technique and setup used in a DRA procedure, and summarize the different types of neurointerventional procedures performed using DRA.

25.2 Advantages of Distal Radial Access

25.2.1 Radial Artery Occlusion and Hand Ischemia

The use of DRA for endovascular procedures reduces the risk of radial artery occlusion and post-procedural hand ischemia [10, 14, 15]. At

A. S. Puri · A. L. Kuhn · J. Singh
Department of Radiology, Division of Neurointerventional Radiology, University of Massachusetts Medical Center, Worcester, MA, USA

K. El Naamani · P. Jabbour (✉)
Department of Neurosurgery, Thomas Jefferson University Hospital, Philadelphia, PA, USA
e-mail: pascal.jabbour@jefferson.edu

G. A. Sgueglia (ed.), *Distal Radial Access*, https://doi.org/10.1007/978-3-031-89925-6_25

the level of the radial styloid process, and proximal to the anatomical snuffbox, the radial artery bifurcates into the distal radial artery and the superficial palmar artery. The superficial palmar artery anastomoses with the ulnar artery to form the superficial palmar arch, while the distal radial artery crosses the anatomical snuffbox to supply the deep palmar arch of the hand. With DRA, the puncture site is distal to the origin of the superficial palmar branch, so in the event of a distal radial artery occlusion, the superficial palmar branch is not affected, and blood supply to the hand is maintained [14, 16]. Weinberg et al. demonstrated a very low access site complication rate with DRA for neuroendovascular procedures in their series of 120 patients [10]. With this low access site complication rate, DRA not only preserves future procedures but also preserves the radial artery at the level of the wrist for patients requiring arteriovenous fistulas or bypass graft [17]. In cases where cross-over from DRA is eminent, conventional TRA should be the first option before converting to a femoral approach. The main reasons for cross-over from DRA to conventional TRA are spasm and small diameter of the distal radial artery [14].

25.2.2 Patient and Operator Ergonomics

In terms of positioning, DRA offers ergonomic advantages over conventional TRA for both the patient and the operator. From the patient's perspective, DRA can be accessed without the need for hand supination, which is more comfortable, especially for patients with orthopedic limitations (e.g., frozen shoulder) [12]. From the operator's perspective, the natural hand position with DRA allows for easier left-side DRA with the hand adducted to the patient's right groin. This option is essential in the case of a dominant left-sided vertebral artery or a difficult vertebral artery origin [14]. In addition, this option not only avoids bending over the patient, which can be tiring during long procedures in obese patients, but also places the operator at a safer distance from the radiation source [18].

25.2.3 Post-procedural Hemostasis

The location and horizontal plane of the carpal bone relative to DRA site allow for effective hemostasis with light compression in DRA procedures. This is in contrast to the oblique angle of the radial bone relative to the radial artery at the wrist level and the longer duration of compression and higher pressure to achieve hemostasis with conventional TRA procedures. This was remarkably reflected in a significantly shorter post-procedural hemostasis time in Koutouzis et al. comparison of 200 patients undergoing conventional TRA and DRA procedures [19].

25.3 Drawbacks of Distal Radial Access

Although several studies have demonstrated the efficacy and safety of DRA, the rate of access failure and the need to cross-over to another access ranges from 0.3% to 11%. This access failure may be due to several reasons. Compared to conventional TRA, the main limitation of DRA is the small diameter of the distal radial artery, which is a major risk factor for vasospasm. Other reasons for procedure failure and the need for cross-over are the highly tortuous nature of the vessel at the level of the snuffbox, which makes wire advancement difficult, and the instability of the potentially less stable position of patient's hand compared to conventional TRA. Accordingly, DRA is more challenging and requires a steep learning curve even for experienced radial interventionalists [20]. Puncture of the distal radial artery can also be challenging, especially in the early stage, as shown by Kimeneiji et al., who reported a high rate of weak pulse at the anatomic snuffbox that prevented to attempt the puncture [18]. Although this can be overcome with ultrasound-guided cannulation, the perceived longer time may discourage some operators.

25.4 Diagnostic Procedures via Distal Radial Access and Technical Considerations

25.4.1 Patient Preparation

About 15–20 min before the procedure, topical 2.5% lidocaine/prilocaine cream is applied to the snuffbox area and covered with an adhesive dressing. The forearm is placed in an intermediate position between pronation and supination, and the hand is placed tightly against the right hip for a right distal radial approach or over the right groin for a left distal radial approach [11]. Inferiorly and caudally, pads are added to the hand to create a platform on which to place catheters and wires. To bring the artery to the surface of the distal radial fossa, slight ulnar abduction can be achieved either by curling the thumb into the other four fingers or by having the patient grasp a gauze roll [12]. Finally, 2 mL of lidocaine is injected into the periarterial tissue.

25.4.2 Access

Because of the likelihood of having a weak pulse that does not allow cannulation, and considering that the Radial Artery Access with Ultrasound Trial (RAUST) demonstrated that the use of ultrasound reduces access time and complications, ultrasound-guided puncture is highly recommended to achieve rapid and consistent DRA [21]. The distal radial artery puncture is performed with a 20- or 21-gauge needle angled medially toward the radial artery at 30°–50°, and the anterior part of the artery is punctured [19]. Once arterial cannulation is confirmed by arterial blood return, a 0.025″ hydrophilic guidewire is inserted into the radial artery, followed by insertion of a thin-walled 5 Fr 10 cm introducer sheath (Glidesheath Slender, Terumo). Prophylactic antispasmodics (verapamil 2.5 mg and nitroglycerin 200 mcg) are infused through the sheath, and 4000 units of heparin are administered intravenously [18, 19]. Because the arm is positioned closer to the body compared to conventional TRA, table rotation is typically not essential to visualize the right forearm under an anteroposterior view.

25.4.3 Diagnostic Angiography

Once right-side DRA is secured, the first artery encountered when advancing the Sim 2 diagnostic catheter is the right vertebral artery. As the catheter is navigated to the aortic arch, the next step is to select the vessel of interest. Sometimes the guidewire selects the right common carotid artery (CCA) before entering the aortic arch. In this situation, the wire can be pushed close to the carotid bifurcation, and the diagnostic catheter can be tracked into the CCA. This maneuver stabilizes the position of the catheter and allows selection of the internal and/or external carotid artery (ICA and/or ECA) under roadmap guidance. Upon completion of the right-side imaging, the catheter is withdrawn into the CCA and pushed back into the aortic arch to maintain its shape. To prevent dissection, a low threshold should be maintained when the catheter is not pushing back into the aortic arch, but rather traversing the carotid artery. In such cases, it is recommended to retract and twist while pushing. In most cases, the catheter must be reshaped in the ascending or descending aorta before moving to the left side (Fig. 25.1a). If reshaping doesn't work the conventional way, some tricks can be used to get the catheter into position. The first is to push the guidewire and allow it to bounce off the aortic valve. This allows the catheter to be pushed over the wire into the correct shape. The second option is to reshape the catheter in the descending aorta.

When faced with difficulties in manipulating the catheter within the aortic arch following the catheterization of the right vertebral artery, it is

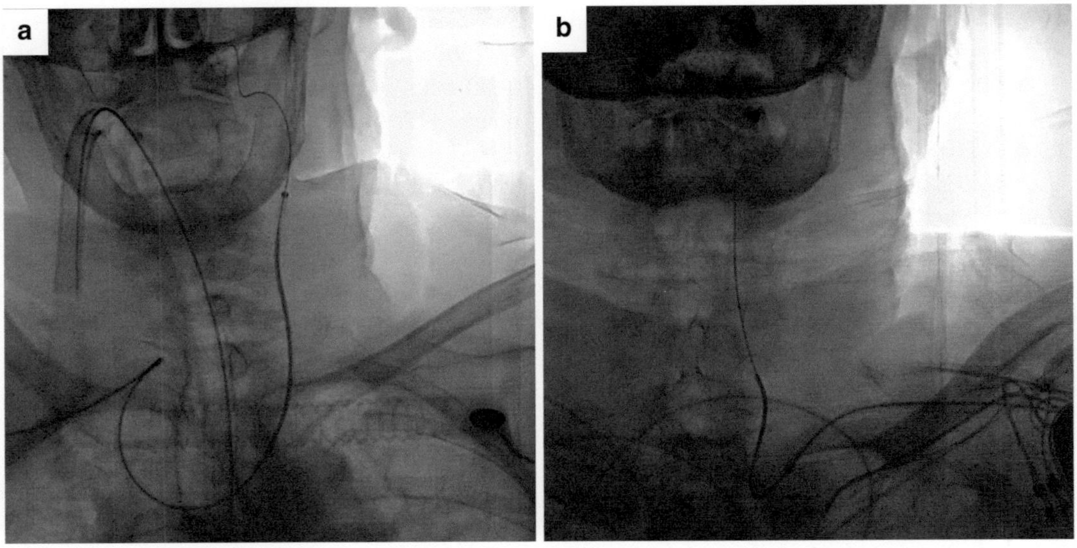

Fig. 25.1 (**a**) Tortuous left intracranial access through right distal radial access. (**b**) Left intracranial access through left distal radial access

advised to proceed from the left side to the right (Fig. 25.1b). It is recommended to keep a Sim 3 catheter or cuff in the left arm at all times to assist with subclavian injections or left vertebral artery catheterization. The left CCA is then catheterized, followed by the right CCA. Sometimes, when a type 3 aortic arch is encountered, the Simmons catheter can be exchanged over a wire for a Berenstein or angled catheter that provides sufficient support for the catheter to select the ICA/ECA.

25.4.4 Radial Artery Spasm

Similar to other radial procedures, vasospasm can be an uncomfortable complication that impedes catheter movement [6, 9, 10]. However, there are several treatment options available. The first option involves vasodilating the arteries by administering an additional injection of calcium channel blockers. If resistance persists, an alternative approach is to replace the catheter with a long radial sheath that extends to the brachial artery. In cases where resistance continues, it is crucial to discontinue the procedure to avoid the risk of a retained catheter. In such instances, the catheter should be flushed while attempting to remove it. This can be facilitated by administering additional calcium channel blockers or by inflating a pressure cuff to the tourniquet level and clamping it for 10 min to induce controlled ischemia, which can trigger flow-mediated vasodilation.

25.4.5 Hemostasis

Puncture site hemostasis is optimally achieved using a PreludeSYNC DISTAL (Merit Medical), which is a specialized wristband equipped with an inflatable bladder [15]. After inflating the bladder, small amounts of air are gradually released until bleeding is observed, at which point 1 cc of air is reinjected. This technique ensures that only the minimum required compression is applied to achieve hemostasis while preserving the distal radial artery for future procedures [14]. To monitor postoperative radial perfusion, the DRA site can be periodically checked, and a pulse oximeter can be placed on the thumb [15, 16].

25.5 Interventions via Distal Radial Access and Technical Considerations

Actually, DRA for neurointerventional procedures is a refinement of conventional TRA. The advantages and disadvantages of vascular access in the anatomical snuffbox for endovascular interventions are similar to those of diagnostic angiography. Prior to the procedure, evaluating the size of the distal radial artery is essential in determining the patient's suitability for this vascular access approach and determining the appropriate catheter setup. Proper ultrasound-guided vascular access will facilitate sheath/catheter insertion and minimize the risk of vasospasm, which could potentially lead to abortion of this treatment approach or possible complications. In addition, depending on the location of the vascular lesion and the choice of treatment device, there are different considerations for precentralization, which are discussed below [22].

25.5.1 Sheath Sizing

The distal radial artery in the anatomical snuffbox is only slightly smaller than the more proximal radial artery on the ventral aspect of the wrist. This small difference allows the use of the same sheath sizes as for conventional TRA [23]. The size of the distal radial artery should be determined by vascular ultrasound prior to the procedure. Ideally, the distal radial artery should be 1 Fr (1 Fr = 0.33 mm) larger than the outer diameter of the sheath to be inserted. This minimizes the risk of vessel stretching and post-procedural radial artery occlusion.

Saito et al. studied the relationship between arterial blood flow and sheath outer diameter and found that the incidence of blood flow reduction is significantly low when the radial artery inner diameter/cannulated sheath outer diameter is ≥1.0 (artery/sheath ratio > 1) [24].

25.5.2 Patient Preparation and Vascular Access

Patient preparation is similar to that described in the DRA diagnostic procedure section. The most common sheath size for DRA procedures is 6 Fr, although 5 Fr and 7 Fr sheaths are used depending on the procedure and choice of catheter setup (Table 25.1) [25]. Some operators use a longer sheath that extends into the brachial or even axillary artery to limit radial artery spasm during catheter manipulation. Alternatively, and if appropriate for the patient's anatomy and the procedure to be performed, a 6 Fr hydrophilic-coated R2P Destination Slender Guiding Sheath (Terumo) can be used, as this device is available in 100 cm lengths with 0.087″ inner diameter and 0.100″ outer diameter.

For procedures where a larger guiding catheter is required, the guiding catheter can be inserted directly into the distal radial artery (sheathless or bareback catheter use). To use a sheathless or bareback guiding catheter, a standard 6 Fr radial sheath is inserted first as previously described, and a 5 Fr diagnostic catheter is navigated into the target vessel. An exchange

Table 25.1 Comparison of the main radial sheaths outer diameters

Sheath	5 Fr	6 Fr	7 Fr
Avanti (Cordis)	2.39 mm	2.68 mm	3.03 mm
RAIN (Cordis)	2.14 mm	2.47 mm	2.80 mm
Glidesheath (Terumo)	2.31 mm	2.63 mm	2.96 mm
Glidesheath slender (Terumo)	2.14 mm	2.44 mm	2.79 mm
Prelude EASE (merit medical)	2.36 mm	2.69 mm	3.07 mm
Prelude IDeal	2.13 mm	2.44 mm	2.77 mm
Arrow (Teleflex)	2.35 mm	2.80 mm	–
PSI radial (Teleflex)	2.44 mm	2.77 mm	3.10 mm

length wire is then securely positioned in a distal segment of the target vessel, and the diagnostic catheter and radial sheath are removed. Another dose of spasmolytics is administered through the radial sheath prior to catheter exchange to prevent vasospasm. The larger caliber guiding catheter is then advanced over the wire into the target vessel. Successful wire exchange when operating from a DRA is critical to reduce vessel manipulation and potential associated vasospasm. Occasionally, catheter delivery into the radial artery can be difficult in patients with taut skin or when there is a step in the transition between the wire, dilator, and catheter. In such cases, a small skin incision at the access site and techniques described in Chap. 19 may ease the process.

Activated clotting time is measured at baseline and throughout the procedure with a target of 250–300 s. Additional intravenous doses of weight-based heparin are administered as needed throughout the procedure.

25.5.3 Procedural Setup for Intracranial Aneurysm Treatment

25.5.3.1 Flow Diverter Placement

In most cases, flow diversion devices are delivered and deployed via a triaxial catheter system. From DRA, deployment of the pipeline embolization device (PED, Medtronic), flow redirection endoluminal device (MicroVention), and Surpass Evolve flow diverter (Stryker) can be delivered using a 6 Fr Benchmark (Penumbra) guiding catheter, 4 Fr Phenom Plus (Medtronic) intermediate catheter, and Phenom 027 (Medtronic) microcatheter. Alternatively, the 6/7 Fr Wahoo (Q'apel) or 6/7 Fr RIST (Medtronic) catheters can be used as guiding catheters.

The Surpass Streamline flow diverter can be placed via DRA using either an AXS Infinity LS (Stryker), Ballast (Balt), or Fubuki (Asahi) guiding sheath for proximal support. For additional support during delivery, an AXS Catalyst 5 (Stryker) distal access catheter or an AXS Offset (Stryker) delivery assist catheter may be used as intermediate catheters [26].

A procedure is illustrated in Fig. 25.2. A radial roadmap was first obtained for safer wire and catheter navigation (Fig. 25.2a). A 5 Fr Sim 2 Glidecath (Terumo) diagnostic catheter was navigated over a 0.035″ Glidewire (Terumo) into the left ICA (Fig. 25.2b). Cerebral angiography revealed a left ophthalmic segment ICA aneurysm measuring 5.2 × 4.7 × 4.9 mm (AP × TR × SI) with a neck width of 2.6 mm (Fig. 25.2b, white arrow). The Glidecath was exchanged over the wire for a 6 Fr Benchmark catheter positioned in the distal cervical left ICA. Alternatively, a 5 Fr Sim Select (Penumbra) catheter could be used with the Benchmark. Using the triaxial technique, a Phenom Plus catheter was placed in the cavernous segment of the left ICA over a Phenom 27 microcatheter and a 0.014" Synchro (Stryker) microwire. The microcatheter was then advanced into the left middle cerebral artery. A 4.25 × 12 mm PED (Medtronic) was successfully placed across the neck of the aneurysm (Fig. 25.2d), with the device extending from the left ICA terminus into the cavernous segment (Fig. 25.2e, white arrows). Follow-up angiograms showed no thromboembolic complications (Fig. 25.2f) and flow stagnation within the aneurysm sac (Fig. 25.2g, white arrow).

25.5.3.2 Woven EndoBridge Placement

A low-profile triaxial catheter system can be used for DRA placement of a Woven EndoBridge (WEB) device, such as the 6 Fr Benchmark guiding catheter and the 5 Fr SOFIA (MicroVention) distal access catheter [27]. The microcatheter is selected according to the size of the WEB device, either a VIA 21, VIA 27, or VIA 33 (MicroVention). If a VIA 33 microcatheter is required due to a larger WEB size, a quadriaxial approach using a Headway DUO (MicroVention) microcatheter within the VIA 33 microcatheter will facilitate its navigation through the intracranial vasculature and into the aneurysm sac [28].

An illustrative case is shown in Fig. 25.3. A radial roadmap was obtained for wire and cathe-

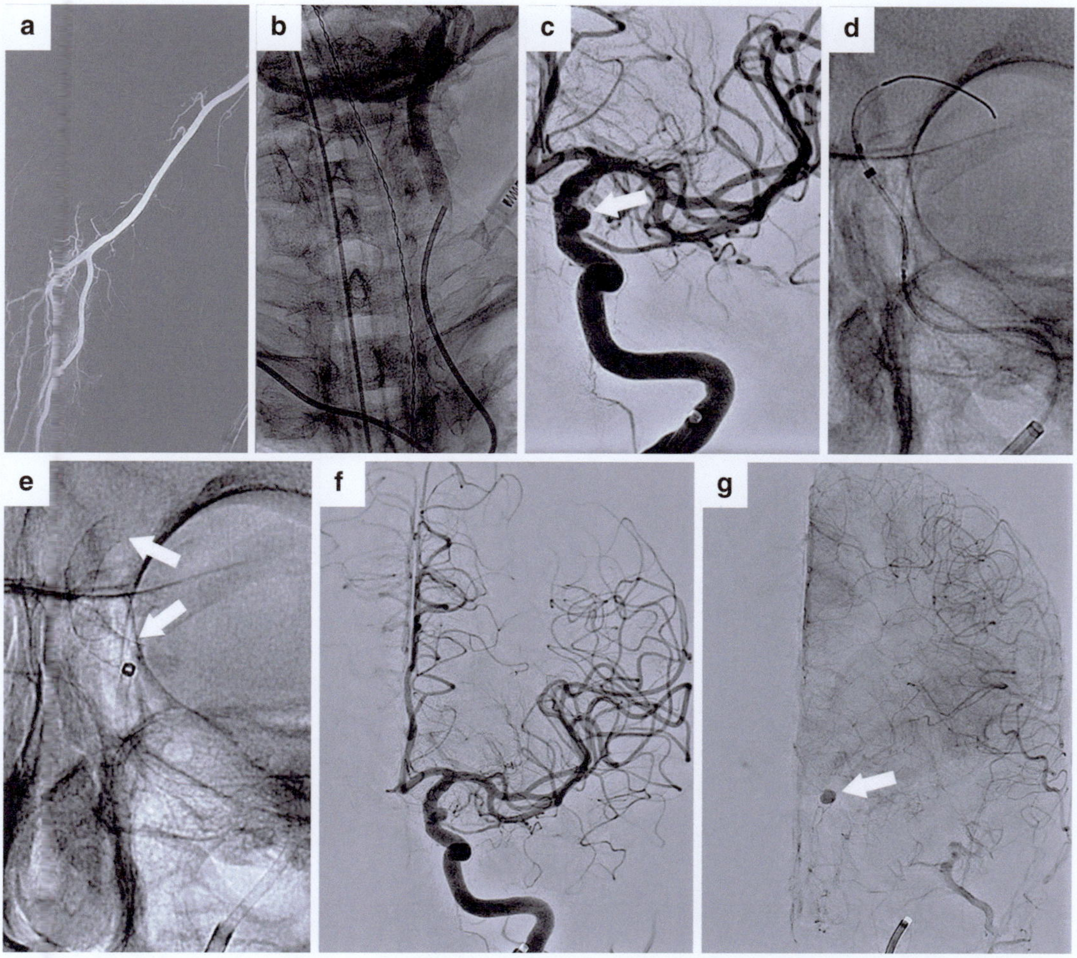

Fig. 25.2 (**a–g**) Flow diverter placement for intracranial aneurysm treatment through distal radial access (see the text for details)

ter navigation (Fig. 25.3a). A 5 Fr Sim 2 Glidecath was navigated over a 0.035″ Glidewire into the right ICA (Fig. 25.3b, white arrows). Using roadmap guidance, the Glidecath was exchanged over the wire for a 6 Fr Benchmark catheter. A cerebral angiogram was obtained demonstrating a wide-necked right middle cerebral artery bifurcation aneurysm measuring 3.3 × 4.8 × 3.8 mm (AP × TR × SI) (Fig. 25.3c, white arrow). Using the triaxial technique, a 5 Fr Sofia distal access catheter was navigated into the right ICA via a VIA 21 microcatheter and 0.014" Synchro microwire. The microwire and microcatheter were advanced into the right-middle cerebral artery. A 5 × 3 mm WEB device was successfully deployed into the aneurysm sac (Fig. 25.3d, white arrow) with the microcatheter in the distal M1 segment (Fig. 25.3d, squiggly arrow), the distal access catheter in the supraclinoid internal carotid artery (Fig. 25.3d, arrowhead), and the guiding catheter in the distal cervical ICA (Fig. 25.3d, thin arrow). The follow-up cerebral angiogram showed proper positioning of the WEB device within the aneurysm sac and incipient contrast enhancement (Fig. 25.3d, white arrow).

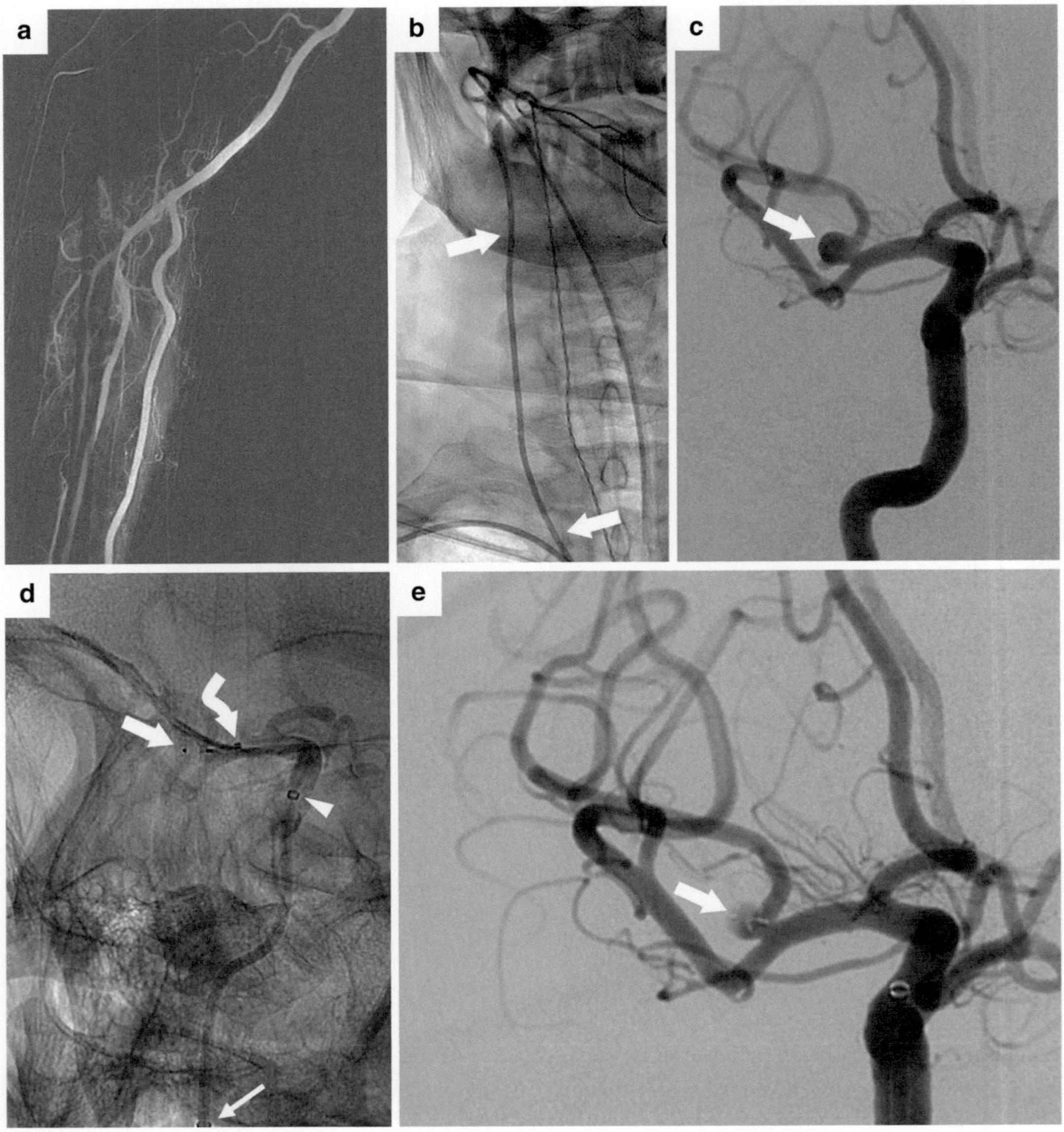

Fig. 25.3 (a–e) Woven EndoBridge (WEB) placement for intracranial aneurysm treatment through distal radial access (see the text for details)

25.5.4 Procedural Setup for Stroke Intervention

25.5.4.1 Anterior Circulation

One case report documented the use of a 6 Fr balloon-tipped catheter for stroke intervention via DRA [29]. At present, balloon-tipped catheters are not designed for DRA, and navigation of the cervical vasculature can be difficult.

A case is illustrated in Fig. 25.4. Under ultrasound guidance, the right distal radial artery was identified in the anatomical snuffbox and deemed suitable for vascular access (Fig. 25.4a). A 6 Fr Glidesheath Slender (Terumo) radial sheath was placed in the right distal radial artery. A radial roadmap was obtained for wire and catheter navigation (Fig. 25.4b). A 5 Fr Sim 2 Glidecath was navigated over a 0.035″ Glidewire into the right CCA. Using roadmap guidance, the Glidecath

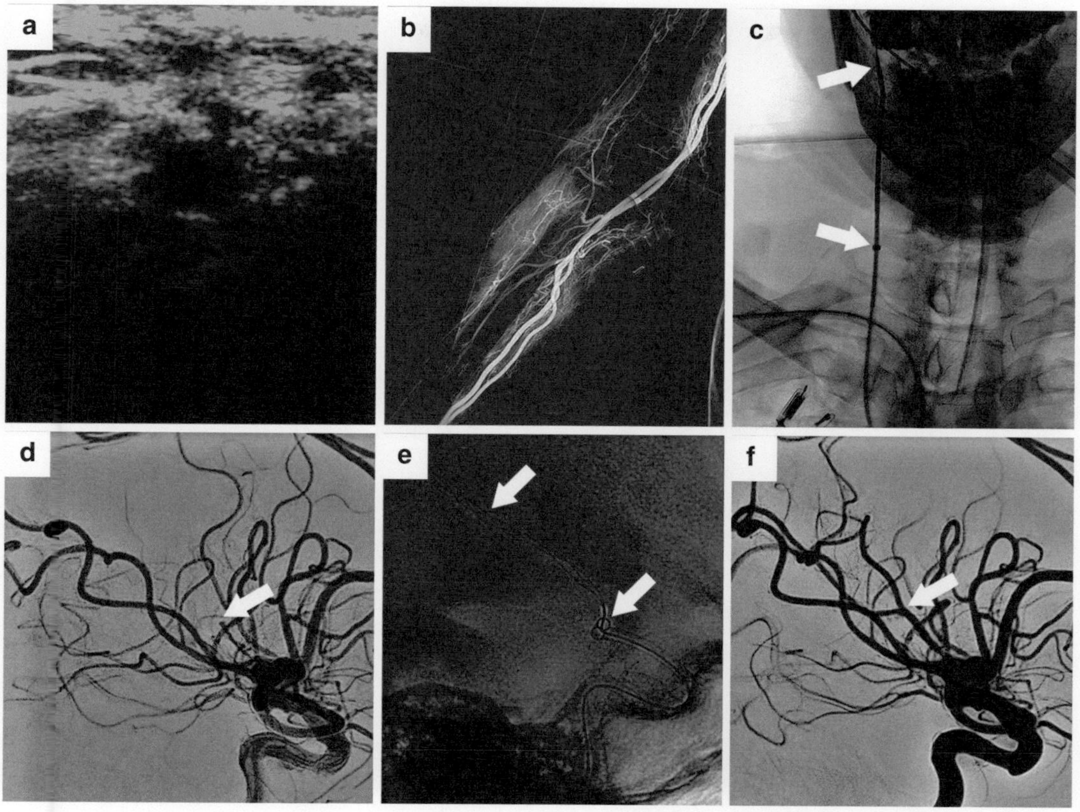

Fig. 25.4 (**a–f**) Distal radial access for anterior circulation stroke intervention (see the text for details)

and 5 Fr sheath were exchanged over the wire for a 6 Fr Infinity (Stryker) guiding catheter (bare-back fashion) and a 5 Fr Berenstein Select catheter, which were placed in the distal right CCA/ICA (Fig 25.4c, white arrows). A cerebral angiogram was obtained showing occlusion of the middle division of the right M2 segment (Fig 25.4d, white arrow). Using the triaxial technique, a large-bore aspiration catheter (Cerenovus) was navigated into the right internal carotid artery via a Trevo Pro 14 (Stryker) microcatheter and a 0.014" Synchro (Stryker) microwire. The microwire and microcatheter were advanced into the middle division of the right-middle cerebral artery. A 3 × 20 mm Trevo XP ProVue (Stryker) thrombectomy device was deployed from the M3 to the proximal M2 segment, and the aspiration catheter was advanced into the middle cerebral artery (Fig. 25.4e, white arrows). The microcatheter was removed. The thrombectomy device was allowed to seat in the clot for 4 min. The device was then withdrawn under continuous aspiration. The follow-up cerebral angiogram showed complete recanalization of the previously occluded vessel (Fig. 25.4e, white arrow).

25.5.4.2 Posterior Circulation

Mechanical thrombectomy of the posterior circulation can be performed using either a right or left vertebral artery approach, depending on the patient's anatomy. A left vertebral approach can sometimes be more easily obtained through ipsilateral DRA. It is important to keep the patient's arm straight at the elbow during the initial catheterization, as the brachial/radial artery may kink in a flexed arm position.

An illustrative case is shown in Fig. 25.5. Computed tomography (CT) angiography 3D reconstructions show a dominant left vertebral artery (Fig. 25.5a, white arrow) and a smaller right vertebral artery caliber (Fig. 25.5a, white

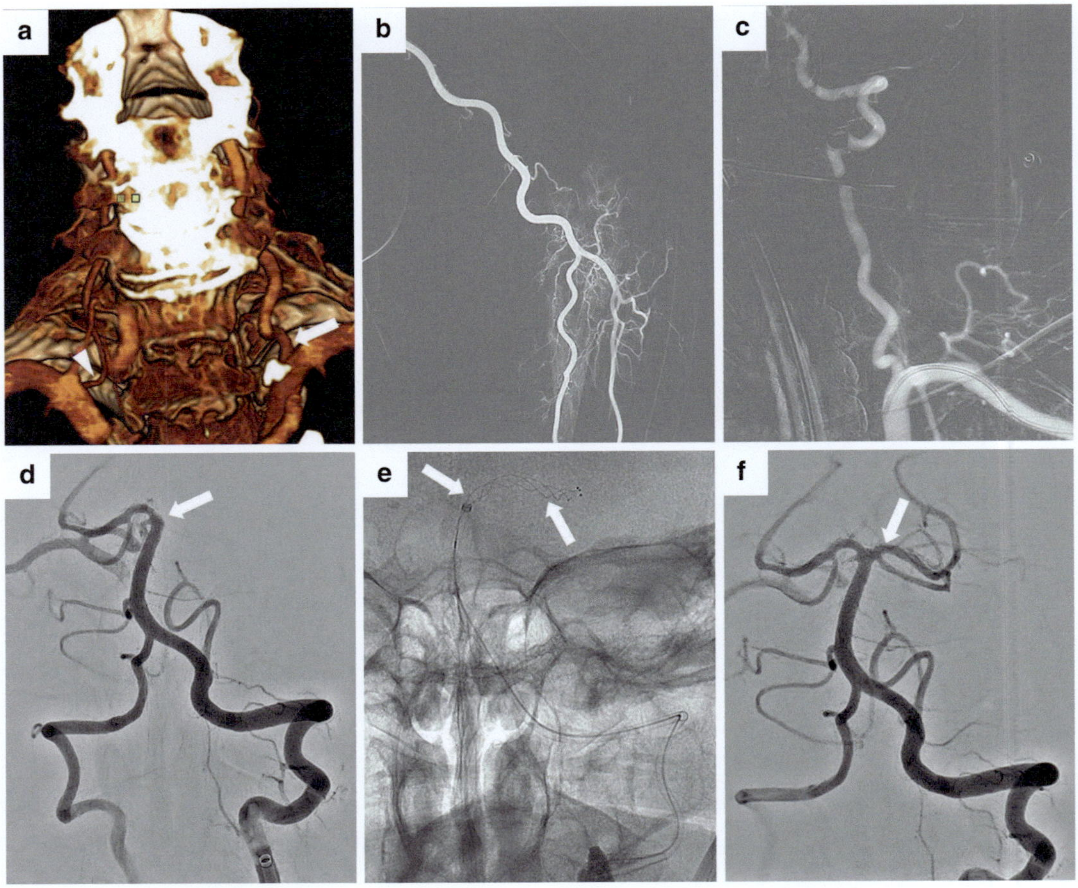

Fig. 25.5 (**a–f**) Distal radial access for posterior circulation stroke intervention (see the text for details)

arrowhead). A radial roadmap was obtained for wire and catheter navigation (Fig. 25.5b). A 5 Fr Sim 2 Glidecath was navigated over a 0.035″ Glidewire into the left subclavian artery, just proximal to the origin of the left vertebral artery. A roadmap view was obtained for wire and catheter navigation (Fig. 25.5c). The Glidecath and 6 Fr radial sheath were exchanged over the wire for a 6 Fr Infinity (Stryker) guiding catheter placed directly into the left distal radial artery (bareback fashion). The Infinity guiding catheter was navigated over a Catalyst 6 (Stryker) aspiration catheter and a Trevo Pro 18 (Stryker) microcatheter and 0.014" Synchro microwire into the left cervical vertebral artery. The cerebral angiogram showed occlusion of the basilar tip and left posterior cerebral artery (Fig. 25.5d, white arrow). The microcatheter was navigated over the microwire into the left posterior cerebral artery. A 4 × 20 mm Trevo XP ProVue thrombectomy device was placed from the left P2 segment into the distal basilar artery, and the aspiration catheter was advanced to the face of the clot (Fig. 25.5d, white arrows). The microcatheter was removed, and the thrombectomy device was allowed to seat in the clot for 4 min. The thrombectomy device assembly and aspiration catheter were then removed with continuous aspiration. The follow-up cerebral angiogram showed complete recanalization of the basilar tip and left posterior cerebral artery (Fig. 25.5d, white arrow).

25.5.5 Procedural Setup for Carotid Artery Stenting

Carotid artery stenting via DRA can be performed using a 6 Fr radial sheath and a 6 Fr Benchmark guiding catheter that can accommodate a Carotid WALLSTENT (Boston Scientific). Other stent systems, such as the Xact or AccuLink stents (Abbott), require a larger guiding catheter, such as the 6 Fr Fubuki with a 0.090″ inner diameter, which can be advanced in a sheathless or bareback fashion via DRA [30]. Alternatively, a 6 Fr Flexor Shuttle (Cook Medical) guiding sheath, a 6 Fr R2P Destination Slender guiding sheath, or 8 Fr Walrus (Q'apel) balloon guiding catheter can be used. The target carotid artery can be selected directly with an appropriate guiding catheter. Alternatively, the target carotid artery can be catheterized with a Sim 2 diagnostic catheter as Glidecath or Impress (Merit Medical), followed by an over-the-wire exchange for the guiding catheter through which the procedure will be performed. A stiff exchange length Glidewire or Glidewire Advantage (Terumo) guidewire can provide good support across the aortic arch. Ideally, the exchange length guidewire is advanced distally into the external carotid artery to provide maximum support.

In some cases, the guidewire may not be positioned sufficiently distal to the target vessel or may prolapse into the aortic arch during the procedure. To mitigate this problem, the use of the "buddy wire technique" with a stiff 0.035″ Glidewire is helpful in navigating the guidewire higher into the desired position. A 0.070″ guiding catheter allows simultaneous navigation of a 0.014″ guidewire and a 0.035″ Glidewire.

In some cases, if the guidewire is retracted proximally during carotid stent deployment, the guiding catheter can be repositioned into the proximal stent by climbing on the inflated angioplasty balloon. This technique can also be used for initial delivery of the guiding catheter after unsuccessful navigation with an inner slip catheter/Glidewire combination or buddy wire technique.

A case of carotid artery stenting in a patient with a bovine aortic arch is presented in Fig. 25.6. The CT angiography maximum intensity projection reconstruction shows a bovine-type aortic arch configuration (Fig. 25.6a, white arrow). A radial roadmap was obtained for wire and catheter navigation (Fig. 25.6b). A 5 Fr Sim 2 Glidecath was navigated over a 0.035″ Glidewire into the right innominate artery and given the bovine aortic arch configuration directly into the left CCA (Fig. 25.6c, white arrows). Cervical angiograms showed >70% stenosis of the left CCA origin with the presence of intraluminal thrombus (Fig. 25.6d, white arrow). Using roadmap guidance, the Glidecath was exchanged over the wire for a 6 Fr Benchmark guiding catheter placed in the distal left CCA just proximal to the carotid bifurcation. A 7.2 mm Emboshield NAV6 (Abbott) protection device was placed in the distal cervical ICA. An 8 × 21 mm Carotid WALLSTENT was then successfully deployed across the stenotic vessel segment. Stent optimization was performed with a 3.5 × 20 mm Sterling (Boston Scientific) balloon (Fig. 25.6e). The follow-up carotid angiogram showed a brisk flow in the left internal carotid artery with excellent luminal gain at the previous site of stenosis (Fig. 25.6f).

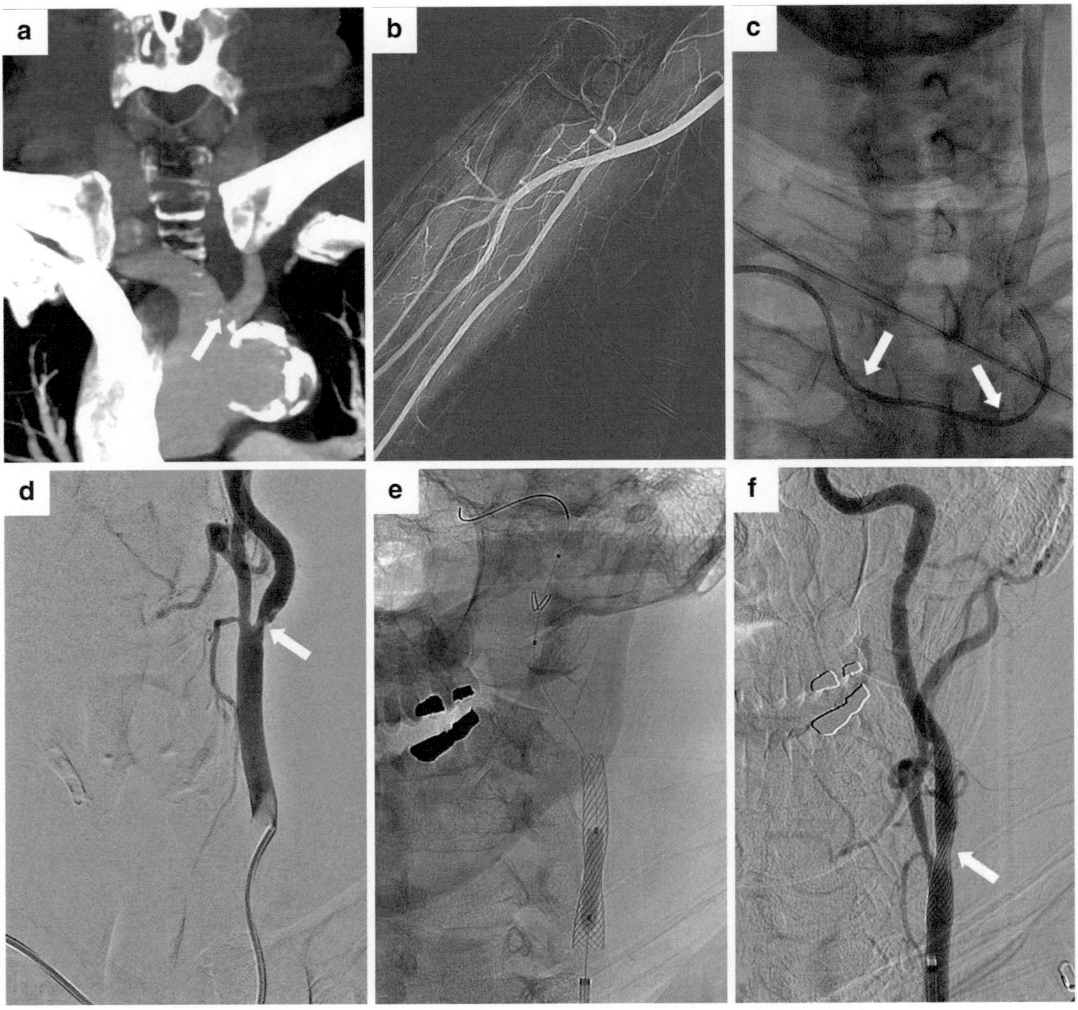

Fig. 25.6 (a–f) Carotid artery stenting in a patient with a bovine aortic arch through right distal radial access (see the text for details)

25.6 Conclusions

In the last years, DRA has gained popularity in the neurointerventional field. With its lower risk of hand ischemia, shorter hemostasis time, improved patient-operator ergonomics, and higher patient satisfaction rates, DRA has emerged as a refinement of conventional TRA. However, DRA has several unique characteristics compared to conventional TRA, including a smaller diameter, a tortuous course in the anatomical snuffbox, a predisposition to vasospasm, and a longer distance to the supra-aortic vessels. Taking these features into account and overcoming the learning curve, DRA has proven to be both effective and safe in diagnostic neurovascular procedures. Recently, DRA has been used in neurovascular procedures for the treatment of cerebrovascular disease. Although still limited, the growing neurointerventional literature increasingly demonstrates its efficacy and safety as an access site for neurovascular interventions.

References

1. Neumann FJ, Sousa-Uva M, Ahlsson A, Alfonso F, Banning AP, Benedetto U, et al. 2018 ESC/EACTS guidelines on myocardial revascularization. Eur Heart J. 2019;40:87–165.
2. Lawton JS, Tamis-Holland JE, Bangalore S, Bates ER, Beckie TM, Bischoff JM, et al. 2021 ACC/AHA/SCAI guideline for coronary artery revascularization: a report of the American College of Cardiology/American Heart Association Joint Committee on clinical practice guidelines. J Am Coll Cardiol. 2022;79(2):e21–129.
3. Valgimigli M, Gagnor A, Calabró P, Frigoli E, Leonardi S, Zaro T, et al. Radial versus femoral access in patients with acute coronary syndromes undergoing invasive management: a randomised multicentre trial. Lancet. 2015;385:2465–76.
4. Brueck M, Bandorski D, Kramer W, Wieczorek M, Höltgen R, Tillmanns H. A randomized comparison of transradial versus transfemoral approach for coronary angiography and angioplasty. JACC Cardiovasc Interv. 2009;2:1047–54.
5. Jolly SS, Yusuf S, Cairns J, Niemelä K, Xavier D, Widimsky P, et al. Radial versus femoral access for coronary angiography and intervention in patients with acute coronary syndromes (RIVAL): a randomised, parallel group, multicentre trial. Lancet. 2011;377:1409–20.
6. Cesaro A, Moscarella E, Gragnano F, Perrotta R, Diana V, Pariggiano I, et al. Transradial access versus transfemoral access: a comparison of outcomes and efficacy in reducing hemorrhagic events. Expert Rev Cardiovasc Ther. 2019;17:435–47.
7. Hamon M, Rasmussen LH, Manoukian SV, Cequier A, Lincoff MA, Rupprecht HJ, et al. Choice of arterial access site and outcomes in patients with acute coronary syndromes managed with an early invasive strategy: the ACUITY trial. EuroIntervention. 2009;5:115–20.
8. Hoffman H, Jalal MS, Masoud HE, Pons RB, Rodriguez Caamaño I, Khandelwal P, et al. Distal transradial access for diagnostic cerebral angiography and neurointervention: systematic review and meta-analysis. AJNR Am J Neuroradiol. 2021;42:888–95.
9. Hamandi M, Saad M, Hasan R, Megaly M, Abbott JD, Dib C, et al. Distal versus conventional transradial artery access for coronary angiography and intervention: a meta-analysis. Cardiovasc Revasc Med. 2020;21:1209–13.
10. Weinberg JH, Sweid A, Khanna O, Mouchtouris N, Asada A, Das S, et al. Access through the anatomical snuffbox for Neuroendovascular procedures: a single institution series. Oper Neurosurg. 2020;19:495–501.
11. Al-Azizi KM, Lotfi AS. The distal left radial artery access for coronary angiography and intervention: a new era. Cardiovasc Revasc Med. 2018;19:35–40.
12. Valsecchi O, Vassileva A, Cereda AF, Canova P, Satogami K, Fiocca L, et al. Early clinical experience with right and left distal transradial access in the anatomical snuffbox in 52 consecutive patients. J Invasive Cardiol. 2018;30:218–23.
13. Soydan E, Akın M. Coronary angiography using the left distal radial approach – an alternative site to conventional radial coronary angiography. Anatol J Cardiol. 2018;19:243–8.
14. Brunet MC, Chen SH, Sur S, McCarthy DJ, Snelling B, Yavagal DR, et al. Distal transradial access in the anatomical snuffbox for diagnostic cerebral angiography. J Neurointerv Surg. 2019;11:710–3.
15. McCarthy DJ, Chen SH, Brunet MC, Shah S, Peterson E, Starke RM. Distal radial artery access in the anatomical snuffbox for neurointerventions: case report. World Neurosurg. 2019;122:355–9.
16. Patel P, Majmundar N, Bach I, Dodson V, Al-Mufti F, Tomycz L, et al. Distal transradial access in the anatomic snuffbox for diagnostic cerebral angiography. AJNR Am J Neuroradiol. 2019;40:1526–8.
17. Lee JW, Park SW, Son JW, Ahn SG, Lee SH. Real-world experience of the left distal transradial approach for coronary angiography and percutaneous coronary intervention: a prospective observational study (LeDRA). EuroIntervention. 2018;14:e995–1003.
18. Kiemeneij F. Left distal transradial access in the anatomical snuffbox for coronary angiography (ldTRA) and interventions (ldTRI). EuroIntervention. 2017;13:851–7.
19. Koutouzis M, Kontopodis E, Tassopoulos A, Tsiafoutis I, Katsanou K, Rigatou A, et al. Distal versus traditional radial approach for coronary angiography. Cardiovasc Revasc Med. 2019;20:678–80.
20. Coughlan JJ, Zebrauskaite A, Arnous S, Kiernan TJ. Left distal trans-radial access facilitates earlier discharge post-coronary angiography. J Interv Cardiol. 2018;31:964–8.
21. Seto AH, Roberts JS, Abu-Fadel MS, Czak SJ, Latif F, Jain SP, et al. Real-time ultrasound guidance facilitates transradial access: RAUST (radial artery access with ultrasound trial). JACC Cardiovasc Interv. 2015;8:283–91.
22. Kühn AL, de Macedo RK, Singh J, Massari F, Puri AS. Distal radial access in the anatomical snuffbox for neurointerventions: a feasibility, safety, and proof-of-concept study. J Neurointerv Surg. 2020;12:798–801.
23. Hadjivassiliou A, Cardarelli-Leite L, Jalal S, Chung J, Liu D, Ho S, et al. Left Distal Transradial Access (ldTRA): a comparative assessment of conventional and distal radial artery size. Cardiovasc Intervent Radiol. 2020;43:850–7.
24. Saito S, Ikei H, Hosokawa G, Tanaka S. Influence of the ratio between radial artery inner diameter and sheath outer diameter on radial artery flow after transradial coronary intervention. Catheter Cardiovasc Interv. 1999;46:173–8.

25. Rao SV, Tremmel JA, Gilchrist IC, Shah PB, Gulati R, Shroff AR, et al. Best practices for transradial angiography and intervention: a consensus statement from the society for cardiovascular angiography and intervention's transradial working group. Catheter Cardiovasc Interv. 2014;83:228–36.
26. Kühn AL, Satti SR, Eden T, de Macedo RK, Singh J, Massari F, et al. Anatomic snuffbox (distal radial artery) and radial artery access for treatment of intracranial aneurysms with FDA-approved flow diverters. AJNR Am J Neuroradiol. 2021;42:487–92.
27. Kühn AL, Singh J, de Macedo RK, Massari F, Moholkar VM, Marwah SK, et al. Distal radial artery (snuffbox) access for intracranial aneurysm treatment using the Woven EndoBridge (WEB) device. J Clin Neurosci. 2020;81:310–5.
28. Dibas M, Adeeb N, Diestro JDB, Cuellar HH, Sweid A, Lay SV, et al. Transradial versus transfemoral access for embolization of intracranial aneurysms with the Woven EndoBridge device: a propensity score-matched study. J Neurosurg. 2022;137:1064–71.
29. Rajah GB, Lieber B, Kappel AD, Luqman AW. Distal transradial access in the anatomical snuffbox for balloon guide-assisted stentriever mechanical thrombectomy: technical note and case report. Brain Circ. 2020;6:60–4.
30. Kühn AL, Singh J, Moholkar VM, Satti SR, Rodrigues KM, Massari F, et al. Distal radial artery (snuffbox) access for carotid artery stenting – technical pearls and procedural set-up. Interv Neuroradiol. 2021;27:241–8.

Part V

Initiating and Progressing Distal Radial Access

26 Learning Curve

Haydn Hoffman and Yongcheol Kim

26.1 Introduction

Radial access has become the preferred choice for many physicians performing cerebral and coronary angiography and intervention. Although radial access in the wrist is familiar to most operators, distal radial access (DRA) in the anatomical snuffbox has many advantages and is well worth adopting [1–3]. Actually, DRA has been described for all kinds of percutaneous coronary procedures and for cerebral angiography and interventions including mechanical thrombectomy, carotid artery stenting, aneurysm embolization, and arteriovenous malformation embolization [4–6]. This chapter illustrates the advantages of DRA, addresses its learning curve, and describes useful tips for improving the achievement of DRA proficiency.

H. Hoffman (✉)
Department of Neurosurgery, State University of New York Upstate Medical University, Syracuse, NY, USA
e-mail: HoffmanH@upstate.edu

Y. Kim
Division of Cardiology, Yonsei University College of Medicine and Cardiovascular Center, Yongin Severance Hospital, Yongin, Republic of Korea

26.2 Advantages of Distal Radial Access

There are several reasons to perform cerebral and coronary procedures via DRA compared to conventional transradial access (TRA). These include increased safety by accessing the radial artery distal to the superficial palmar arch, which reduces the risk of hand ischemia in the event of a radial artery occlusion (RAO). In addition, DRA is more comfortable for patients who are unable to supinate their arm and is ergonomically advantageous when access is obtained on the left side [7, 8]. Also, DRA preserves the proximal radial artery for use in future procedures or surgeries [9]. Finally, the time to achieve hemostasis is shorter with DRA compared to TRA.

26.3 Unique Characteristics of Distal Radial Access

The distal radial artery in the anatomical snuffbox is smaller in caliber than at the wrist level, although studies have shown that this difference is only about 0.3 mm on average [1, 10, 11]. The course of the distal radial artery has a dynamic three-dimensional curvature compared to the relatively linear path of forearm radial artery. It has a slightly medial to lateral trajectory as opposed to the straight course of the artery in the wrist

G. A. Sgueglia (ed.), *Distal Radial Access*, https://doi.org/10.1007/978-3-031-89925-6_26

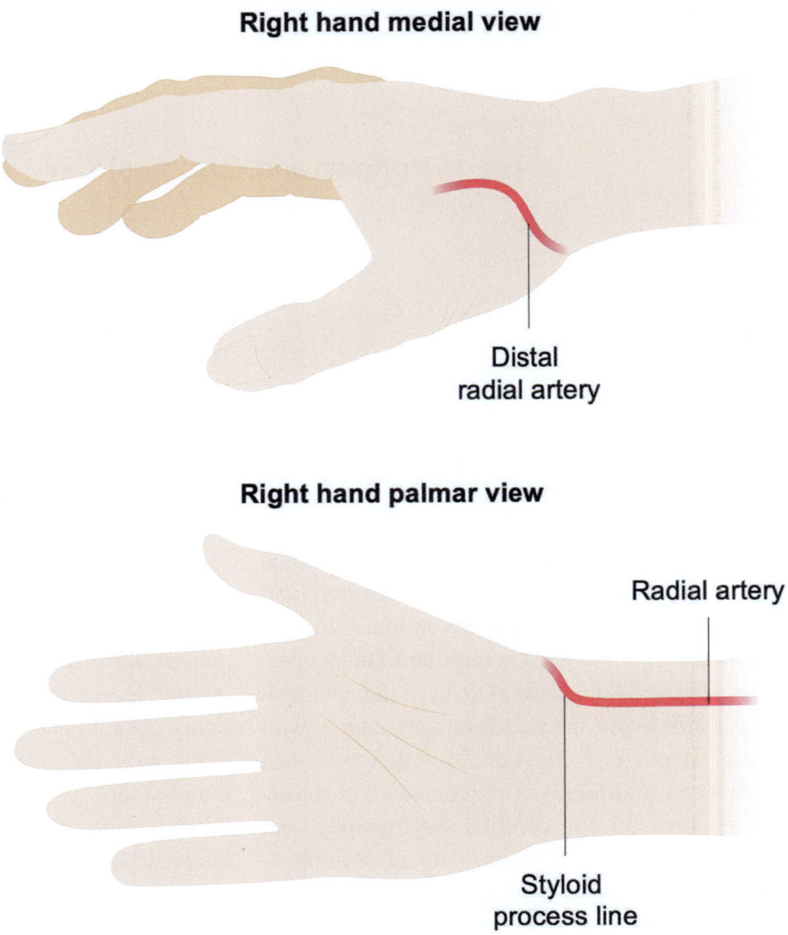

Fig. 26.1 Orthogonal views of the upper extremity show the straight course of the radial artery in the forearm, in contrast to the curved course of the artery in its distal segment in the hand

(Fig. 26.1). The distal radial artery is also more likely to develop spasm with repeated cannulation attempts.

26.4 Evaluating the Distal Radial Learning Curve

An accurate foundation for the development of DRA proficiency is paramount to the expansion of this new vascular access strategy. Indeed, despite the remarkable reduction in RAO demonstrated in randomized clinical trials [12–14] and confirmed by meta-analytic research [15], the adoption of DRA by the interventional community appears to be limited. Reasons for the modest uptake of DRA are largely the same as those that have slowed the adoption of conventional TRA and include inertia in changing routine practice, fear of difficulties in complex situations, and, most importantly, reluctance to learn a new catheterization skill that is both similar to and different from conventional TRA. More importantly, if conventional TRA operators feel uncomfortable changing their practice, this will affect fellows who are not exposed to DRA and are unlikely to incorporate DRA into their interventional practice.

Describing the learning curve for DRA is a task made more challenging by the heterogeneity of often conflicting influences, such as prior conventional TRA experience, use of adjunctive technology, interaction with a skilled DRA operator, and cultural references whose quality ranges from authoritative sources to little more than anecdotes.

26.5 Mastering Distal Radial Access

Despite the learning curve of DRA, high success rates can be achieved when switching to this approach (Tables 26.1 and 26.2). Two studies have specifically evaluated the learning curve of DRA for coronary procedures and cerebral angiography, reporting overall success rates of 95.2% and 98.7%, respectively [16, 20]. Notably, both studies are particularly valuable because they describe the activity of two single operators from their first DRA procedures in an unselected patient population.

The cerebral angiography study focused on the first 75 DRA procedures performed by an operator who had performed approximately 130 diagnostic angiograms using conventional TRA [20]. All DRA were ultrasound-guided using the Seldinger technique, and a 5 Fr thin-walled sheath was used in all cases. In this study, the time from subcutaneous anesthesia to spasmolytic drug administration through the sheath did not change with the increasing number of procedures performed, possibly due to the large scatter of the data, which prevented a linear trend. Nonetheless, locally weighted regression analysis identified the shortest sheath insertion time at procedure number 42, suggesting an improvement in this metric. In another study that retrospectively reviewed data from 85 patients who underwent cerebral angiography via ultrasound-guided DRA by two operators with at least 50 cases of conventional TRA experience, DRA failure was 14.3% in the first and second quarters but decreased to 4.7% and 0% in the third and fourth quarters, respectively [10]. Moreover, after adjusting for covariates in the dedicated learning curve study, sheaths to the first vessel time and procedure time were associated with an increasing case volume [20]. Procedural metrics beyond sheath insertion may be influenced by arm navigation, angiographic catheter manipulation, and vessel of interest selection and are expected to decrease as more angiograms are performed. Similarly, a reduction in fluoroscopy time was observed over 34 cerebral angiograms performed via ultrasound-guided DRA by two neurointerventional specialists and a fellow in selected cases with favorable anatomy and a sufficiently large distal radial artery [21]. Notably, all three operators received formal DRA training prior to the start of the study.

In the interventional cardiology study, data from 1000 consecutive patients undergoing coronary angiography and/or PCI with different sheath sizes were retrospectively analyzed per 100-case stratum [16]. A palpable radial artery was required, and puncture was performed by an experienced transradial operator, mostly on the left side, using either a 20-gauge cannula over needle with the through-and-through puncture technique or a 21-gauge open needle with the anterior wall puncture technique. The DRA success rate, defined as successful sheath placement, increased from 89.5% in the first 200 patients to 96.6% in the later patients, and after the first 200 cases, there was no difference in the DRA success rate per 100-case stratum (p = 0.216). However, the DRA success rate continued to increase to 97–98% in the final 100-case strata (Fig. 26.2a). Notably, in all cases of DRA failure, the switch to conventional TRA was successful. Furthermore, access time and puncture attempts, both defined according to the consensus report of the First Korea-Europe Transradial Intervention

Table 26.1 Overview of available studies with any assessment of distal radial access learning curve

Study	Year	Design	Setting	Number of operators	Experience	Selection	Right DRA	Puncture	Sheath
Roh et al. [16]	2021	Retrospective	Coronary angiography and interventions	1	Experience with TRA	Palpable pulse	5.5%	20 G cannula over needle 21 G open needle	4–7 Fr
Bompotis et al. [17]	2022	Prospective	Coronary angiography and interventions	NA	NA	Absence of precluding conditions	0%	NA	4–7 Fr
Bhambhani et al. [18]	2020	Prospective	Coronary angiography	1	>5000 TRA (DRA training n = 25)	Palpable pulse	100%	20 G cannula over needle	5–6 Fr
Achim et al. [19]	2021	Retrospective	Interventional cardiology procedures	4	>100 TRA	Palpable pulse	89.4%	US-guided	5–8.5 Fr
Tsigkas et al. [13]	2022	Prospective	Coronary angiography and interventions	3	Experience with TRA	Unfavorable conditions excluded	100%	21 G open needle	5–7 Fr
Hoffman et al. [20]	2021	Retrospective	Cerebral angiography	1	~130 TRA	NA	100%	21 G open needle US-guided	5 Fr thin-walled
Brunet et al. [10]	2019	Retrospective	Cerebral angiography	2	>50 TRA	Unfavorable conditions excluded	100%	20 G open needle US-guided	5 Fr thin-walled
Patel et al. [21]	2019	Retrospective	Cerebral angiography	3	Formal DRA training	Distal radial artery >2 mm, normal vascular anatomy	100%	21 G open needle US-guided	5 Fr thin-walled

DRA distal radial access, *NA* not available, *TRA* conventional transradial access, *US* ultrasound

Table 26.2 Main findings of available studies with any assessment of distal radial access learning curve

Study	Year	Procedures	Overall access success	Key secondary finding
Roh et al. [16]	2021	1000	95.2%	Progressive reduction of puncture attempts from 1.52 in the first 100 cases to 1.14 in the last 100 cases ($p < 0.001$) Progressive reduction of access time from 183 s in the first 100 cases to 80 s in the last 100 cases ($p < 0.001$)
Bompotis et al. [17]	2022	1977	90.1%	Significant decrease of failure rate from 20.8% in the first decile to 8.7% in the remaining cases ($p < 0.001$)
Bhambhani et al. [18]	2020	100	77%	Access time reduction from 5.89 min in the first 25 cases to 2.47 min in the last 25 cases ($p < 0.001$)
Achim et al. [19]	2021	1240	97.4%	Progressive reduction of punctures attempts and puncture time over the first 240 cases
Tsigkas et al. [13]	2022	518	78.2%	Progressive reduction of access failure over the quartiles of study duration (from 26.2% to 16.4%)
Hoffman et al. [20]	2021	75	98.7%,	No significant change in access time over the course of the study Progressive reduction of procedure duration over the course of the study ($p < 0.001$)
Brunet et al. [10]	2019	85	91.8%	Access failure reduction from 14.3% in the first two quarters to 4.7% and 0% in the third and fourth quarters
Patel et al. [21]	2019	38	89.5%	Fluoroscopy time decreases over the first 34 cases

Meeting [22], progressively decreased over time ($p < 0.001$ for both, Fig. 26.2b,c). Similarly, in an observational study evaluating left DRA as the default vascular access site in nearly 2000 patients, the failure rate decreased significantly from 20.8% in the first decile to 8.7% in the remaining cases ($p < 0.001$) [17]. A significant progressive reduction in access time was also observed for DRA in a single-operator study comparing two consecutive cohorts of 100 patients each undergoing DRA and conventional TRA for coronary angiography after a training period of 25 patients [18]. In addition, both access time and puncture attempts decreased for each consecutive year of a single operator's contribution to a multicenter registry of 1240 patients undergoing various percutaneous cardiovascular procedures between 2019 and 2021 [19]. In this study, ultrasound-guided puncture was performed in all cases, resulting in an overall DRA success rate of 97.4% (comparable to that reported by the dedicated learning curve study), but inferior performance in the other metrics assessed. Despite the extremely high numbers, the crossover rates in the DRA group of a single-center randomized clinical trial (RCT) comparing DRA with conventional TRA decreased progressively over the quartiles of study duration ($p = 0.073$), suggesting an apparent improvement in DRA proficiency also in a multi-operator context [13].

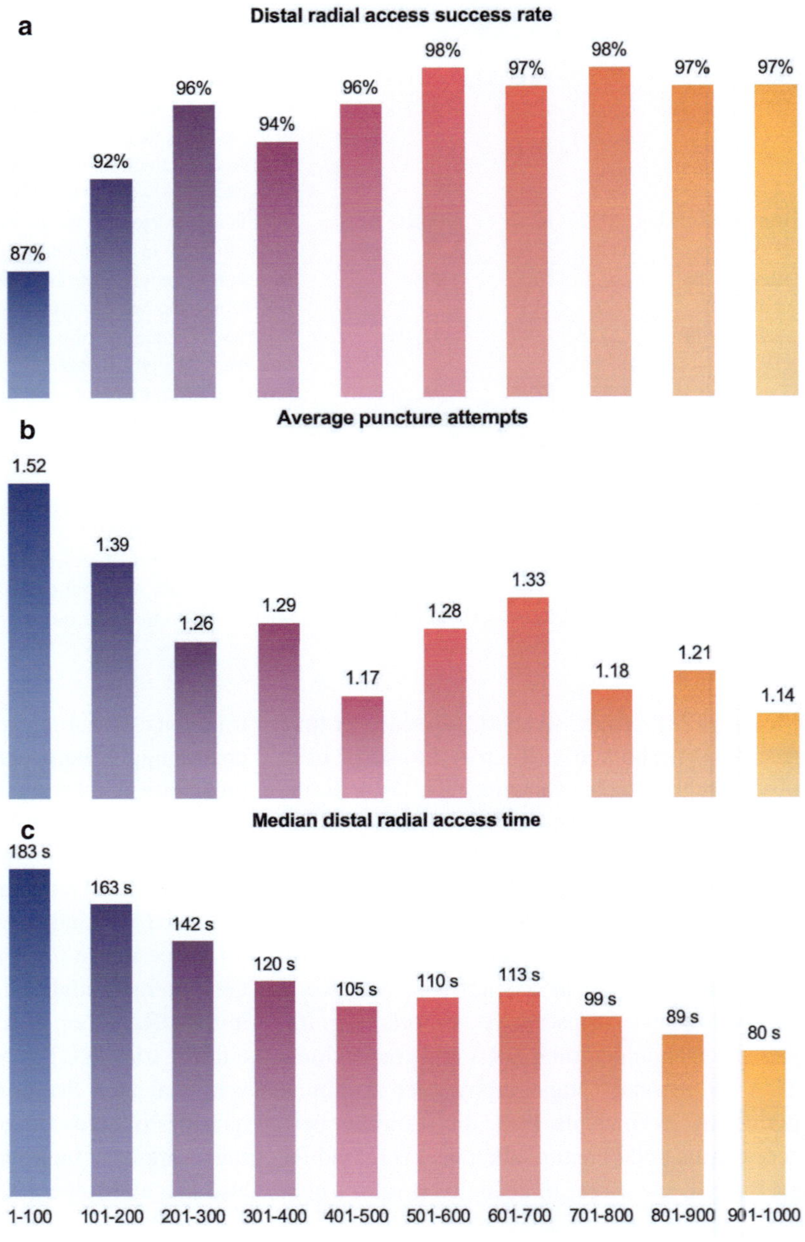

Fig. 26.2 (**a**) Distal radial access success rate per 100-case stratum. (**b**) Average puncture attempts per 100-case stratum. (**c**) Median distal radial access time per 100-case stratum. Data from a study designed to assess the learning curve of distal radial access in patients undergoing coronary angiography or intervention [16]

26.6 Predictors of Distal Radial Access Failure

In the observational registry specifically evaluating the learning curve of DRA in a contemporary interventional cardiology practice, two independent predictors of access failure were identified by multivariable regression analysis, including female sex [odds ratio (OR) 1.84, 95% confidence interval (CI) 1.01–3.39, $p = 0.049$] and systolic blood pressure <120 mmHg (OR 1.87, 95% CI 1.04–3.36, $p = 0.036$) [16]. Outside of learning curve description initiatives, only two RCTs provided an insight on the predictors of DRA failure. In an RCT comparing access success between DRA and conventional TRA in two groups of 450 patients each, (low) body mass index was found to be the only independent predictor of access failure (OR 0.79, 95% CI

0.64–0.97, $p = 0.024$) [23]. In the DISCO RADIAL trial, the largest multicenter trial comparing DRA and conventional TRA in 1307 patients with an indication for coronary angiography or intervention, radial artery spasm (OR 4.4, 95% CI 1.9–10.5, $p < 0.001$) and female sex (OR 2.7, 95% CI 1.5–5.0, $p < 0.01$) were the only independent predictors of crossover identified by stepwise logistic regression analysis [24].

26.7 Side of Distal Radial Access

The interest in left DRA in interventional cardiology has largely been driven by improved ergonomics. The left-sided approach provides an easier way to perform coronary catheterization, but when conventional TRA is chosen, it can be cumbersome for the operator, who must lean over the patient while standing on the right side. Relevantly, DRA eliminates the need for forearm supination and allows the left hand to be in a natural down-facing position, close to the patient's groin. The puncture site is therefore in the same position as with femoral access, making it easier for the operator to stand on the right side of the patient. In contrast, the utility of left DRA is limited in neurointerventions, where a right-sided trajectory is typically more advantageous for catheterization of cerebral vessels, including the left vertebral artery, which is easily accessible from the right radial artery.

In a multicenter registry evaluating the transition to DRA for percutaneous cardiovascular procedures, ultrasound-guided access was similarly successful in the left side (166/172 procedures, 96.5%) and right side (1082/1108 procedures, 97.7%) [19]. Similarly, in a propensity score matching analysis of 182 of 385 coronary procedures performed via DRA with a high proportion of 6 Fr sheaths, the access success rate did not differ between right and left DRA (96.7% for both) [25].

26.8 Comparison with Conventional Transradial Access

In a single-operator record of consecutive conventional TRA coronary procedures performed between 1994 and 1999, the rate of failure was close to 5% after 100 procedures, and it was 3% after 800 procedures [26]. Notably, persisting improvement was observed up to 2400 procedures with the failure rate reaching 1.5%. However, when the first 100 transradial procedures of this large series were performed, they accounted for 51% of all procedures performed by the operator, a figure that increased to 81% for the last 800 procedures, demonstrating that patient selection was occurring and suggesting that the systematic use of the transradial approach in all patients certainly requires more than 50 to 100 procedures to achieve an effective 95% success rate. In an early dual-center study involving four operators, 415 selected patients out of 1008 screened underwent left conventional TRA [27]. In this study, access failure and access time decreased from 14% and 10.2 ± 7.6 min in the first 80 patients to 2% and 2.85 ± 2.53 min in the last 100. In addition, an analysis of the first 1000 transradial coronary angiographies by the same operator showed that the procedural duration continuously decreased from 23.3 min for the first 100 procedures to 13.1 min for the last 100 [28]. Similarly, in a retrospective study describing the transition to a radial-first approach for neurovascular procedures over 5 months that have been divided into four quartiles, access time among 107 cerebral angiography procedures reduced from 10 ± 7 min in the first quartile to 4 ± 3 min in the fourth quartile [29]. Notably, multivariate analysis controlling for ultrasound-guided puncture showed a significant progressive decrease in access time over the fourth quartiles ($p < 0.001$) and no significant change in length with ultrasound-guided puncture ($p = 0.937$).

26.9 Tips for Overcoming the Learning Curve

Although obtaining DRA is somewhat more challenging to achieve, the learning curve can be effectively overcome by implementing simple measures summarized in Table 26.3. Notably, a retrospective study tracking operators transitions from DRA to TRA for cerebral angiograms found similar procedure durations and access time between the two approaches [30].

Radial artery spasm can be reduced by infiltrating the periarterial tissues with a mixture of 2% lidocaine and 200 μg nitroglycerin prior to obtaining access [20]. The use of a nitroglycerin patch has also been suggested [31].

Ultrasound measurement of the distal radial artery prior to puncture is recommended. Most distal radial arteries can accommodate a 6 Fr sheath, which is commonly used for cerebral and coronary interventions.

Also, ultrasound guidance may facilitate DRA, especially during the learning curve. Of note, in a study comparing DRA with or without ultrasound guidance in 137 patients undergoing a coronary procedure, ultrasound-guided DRA was associated with a higher procedural success rate than the standard DRA (97% vs. 87%, $p = 0.038$) [32].

Once access is obtained, a spasmolytic cocktail consisting of 2.5 mg verapamil and 200 μg nitroglycerin is administered through the sheath. At this point, cerebral or coronary angiography can be performed similarly to TRA. Although the DRA is located approximately 5 cm distal to the TRA puncture site at the wrist (Fig. 26.3) and makes angiographic catheter manipulation marginally more difficult, the effect is mostly negligible [30].

Table 26.3 Useful tips to overcome the distal radial access learning curve

Patient selection
Ultrasound guidance
Subcutaneous or transdermic nitroglycerin administration
Use of the smallest sheath for the intended procedure
Spasmolytic cocktail administration right after sheath placement

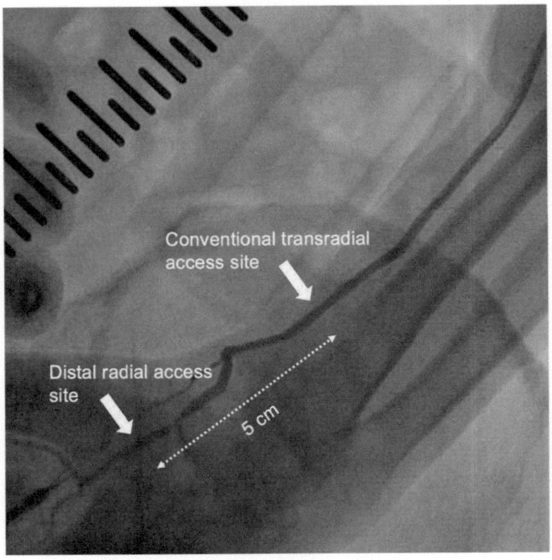

Fig. 26.3 Angiographic measurement of the distance between the typical sites of distal radial access in the anatomical snuffbox and conventional transradial access at wrist

During the procedure, the patency of hand perfusion can be confirmed with continuous pulse oximetry on the right thumb or index finger.

At the end of the procedure, sheath removal and patent hemostasis are similar to conventional TRA, although generally shorter. In fact, the scaphoid and trapezium carpal bones form the floor of the anatomical snuffbox, which may further aid in hemostasis.

26.10 Complications Along the Learning Curve

Overall, low complication rates have been reported during learning of DRA. There were no cases of major adverse events, including symptomatic RAO, in the two dedicated learning curve studies [16, 20]. Notably, in the interventional cardiology study of 1000 patients undergoing coronary angiography or percutaneous coronary intervention, low rates of minor complications were reported, including local numbness (0.2%) and local hematoma not requiring transfusion (3%) [16]. Similarly, in the cerebral angiography study reporting the first 75 cases of one operator's experience with DRA, only 3 (4%) minor complications occurred, including access site hematoma ($n = 1$), radial artery injury with contrast extravasation requiring abortion of the procedure without sequelae ($n = 1$), and, based on a very conservative definition of complication, radial artery spasm requiring administration of additional verapamil to complete the study ($n = 1$) [20]. In a multicenter registry of 1240 patients undergoing various percutaneous cardiovascular procedures by multiple operators, only 15 minor complications were reported: local hematoma ($n = 4$, 0.32%), radial artery occlusion ($n = 5$, 0.4%), and radial artery spasm ($n = 6$, 0.48%) [18].

26.11 Conclusions

There are several advantages to DRA over traditional TRA. From a learning perspective, safety is certainly the most important. In fact, despite the learning curve, the transition to DRA is completely safe, with no major complications reported.

In addition, a high success rate can be achieved after starting DRA practice, especially with commitment, as suggested by the results of dedicated learning curve studies of a single operator. In particular, better metrics have been consistently reported at the beginning of the DRA learning curve compared to what has been previously reported at the beginning of the conventional TRA learning curve.

Selecting the most favorable patient and anatomy and using small devices are useful strategies to shorten the learning curve to the typical 50 training cases. Vascular ultrasound is also a relevant technique to properly assess vascular access options and improve puncture success. Vascular ultrasound also deserves to be properly mastered, which is well worth the effort as it enhances one's interventional practice.

Finally, as with other skills, improvement in DRA persists over time, allowing the benefits associated with this vascular access to be extended to most aspects of interventional cardiovascular medicine.

References

1. Kim Y, Ahn Y, Kim I, Lee DH, Kim MC, Sim DS, et al. Feasibility of coronary angiography and percutaneous coronary intervention via left snuffbox approach. Korean Circ J. 2018;48:1120–30.
2. Kim Y, Lee JW, Lee SY, Bae JW, Lee SJ, Jeong MH, et al. Feasibility of primary percutaneous coronary intervention via the distal radial approach in patients with ST-elevation myocardial infarction. Korean J Intern Med. 2021;36:S53–61.
3. Roh JW, Kim Y, Takahata M, Shiono Y, Kim HY, Jeong MH, et al. Optimal hemostasis duration for percutaneous coronary intervention via the snuffbox approach: a prospective, multi-center, observational study (HEMOBOX). Int J Cardiol. 2021;338:79–82.
4. Rajah GB, Lieber B, Kappel AD, Luqman AW. Distal transradial access in the anatomical snuffbox for balloon guide-assisted stentriever mechanical thrombectomy: Technical note and case report. Brain Circ. 2020;6:60–4.
5. Chivot C, Bouzerar R, Yzet T. Distal radial access for cerebral aneurysm embolization. J Neuroradiol. 2022;49:380–4.
6. Kuhn AL, de Macedo RK, Singh J, Massari F, Puri AS. Distal radial access in the anatomical snuffbox for neurointerventions: a feasibility, safety, and proof-of-concept study. J Neurointerv Surg. 2020;12:798–801.
7. Hoffman H, Jalal MS, Masoud HE, Pons RB, Rodriguez Caamano I, Khandelwal P, et al. Distal transradial access for diagnostic cerebral angiography and neurointervention: systematic review and meta-analysis. AJNR Am J Neuroradiol. 2021;42:888–95.
8. Lee OH, Roh JW, Im E, Cho DK, Jeong MH, Choi D, et al. Feasibility and safety of the left distal radial approach in percutaneous coronary intervention for bifurcation lesions. J Clin Med. 2021;10:2204.
9. Kim Y, Lee SY, Lee DI, Lee JH, Kim SM, Bae JW, et al. Assessment of the conventional radial artery with optical coherent tomography after the snuffbox approach. Cardiol J. 2021;28:849–54.
10. Brunet MC, Chen SH, Sur S, McCarthy DJ, Snelling B, Yavagal DR, et al. Distal transradial access in the anatomical snuffbox for diagnostic cerebral angiography. J Neurointerv Surg. 2019;11:710–3.
11. Saito S, Hasegawa H, Ota T, Takino T, Yoshida Y, Ando K, et al. Safety and feasibility of the distal transradial approach: a novel technique for diagnostic cerebral angiography. Interv Neuroradiol. 2020;26:713–8.
12. Eid-Lidt G, Rivera Rodriguez A, Jimenez Castellanos J, Farjat Pasos JI, Estrada Lopez KE, Gaspar J. Distal radial artery approach to prevent radial artery occlusion trial. JACC Cardiovasc Interv. 2021;14:378–85.
13. Tsigkas G, Papageorgiou A, Moulias A, Kalogeropoulos AP, Papageorgopoulou C, Apostolos A, et al. Distal or traditional transradial access site for coronary procedures: a single-center, randomized study. JACC Cardiovasc Interv. 2022;15:22–32.

14. Aminian A, Sgueglia GA, Wiemer M, Kefer J, Gasparini GL, Ruzsa Z, et al. Distal versus conventional radial access for coronary angiography and intervention: the disco radial trial. JACC Cardiovasc Interv. 2022;15:1191–201.
15. Ferrante G, Condello F, Rao SV, Maurina M, Jolly S, Stefanini GG, et al. Distal vs conventional radial access for coronary angiography and/or intervention: a meta-analysis of randomized trials. JACC Cardiovasc Interv. 2022;15:2297–311.
16. Roh JW, Kim Y, Lee OH, Im E, Cho DK, Choi D, et al. The learning curve of the distal radial access for coronary intervention. Sci Rep. 2021;11:13217.
17. Bompotis GC, Giannopoulos G, Karakanas AI, Meletidou M, Vrachatis D, Lazaridis I, et al. Left distal radial artery access for coronary angiography and interventions: a 12-month all-comers study. J Invasive Cardiol. 2022;34:E505–9.
18. Bhambhani A, Pandey S, Nadamani AN, Tyagi K. An observational comparison of distal radial and traditional radial approaches for coronary angiography. J Saudi Heart Assoc. 2020;32:17–24.
19. Achim A, Kákonyi K, Jambrik Z, Nagy F, Tóth J, Sasi V, et al. Distal radial artery access for coronary and peripheral procedures: a multicenter experience. J Clin Med. 2021;10:5974.
20. Hoffman H, Bunch KM, Mikhailova T, Cote JR, Ashok Kumar A, Masoud HE, et al. Transition from proximal to distal radial access for diagnostic cerebral angiography: learning curve analysis. World Neurosurg. 2021;152:e484–91.
21. Patel P, Majmundar N, Bach I, Dodson V, Al-Mufti F, Tomycz L, et al. Distal transradial access in the anatomic snuffbox for diagnostic cerebral angiography. AJNR Am J Neuroradiol. 2019;40:1526–8.
22. Sgueglia GA, Lee BK, Cho BR, Babunashvili A, Lee JB, Lee JW, et al. Distal radial access: consensus report of the first Korea-Europe transradial intervention meeting. JACC Cardiovasc Interv. 2021;14:892–906.
23. Lin Y, Sun X, Chen R, Liu H, Pang X, Chen J, et al. Feasibility and safety of the distal transradial artery for coronary diagnostic or interventional catheterization. J Interv Cardiol. 2020;2020:4794838.
24. Aminian A, Sgueglia GA, Wiemer M, Kefer J, Gasparini GL, Ruzsa Z, et al. TCT-591 predictors of cross-over for distal radial access: insights from the disco radial study. J Am Coll Cardiol. 2022;80(12 Supplement):B243.
25. Rivera K, Fernández-Rodríguez D, Casanova-Sandoval J, Barriuso I, Zielonka M, Pueyo-Balsells N, et al. Comparison between the right and left distal radial access for patients undergoing coronary procedures: a propensity score matching analysis. J Interv Cardiol. 2022;2022:7932114.
26. Louvard Y, Kumar S, Lefèvre T. Percentage of transradial approach for interventional cardiology in the world and learning the technique. Ann Cardiol Angeiol. 2009;58:327–32.
27. Spaulding C, Lefèvre T, Funck F, Thébault B, Chauveau M, Ben Hamda K, et al. Left radial approach for coronary angiography: results of a prospective study. Catheter Cardiovasc Diagn. 1996;39:365–70.
28. Louvard Y, Krol M, Pezzano M, Sheers L, Piechaud JF, Marien C, et al. Feasibility of routine transradial coronary angiography: a single operator's experience. J Invasive Cardiol. 1999;11:543–8.
29. Vergara-Garcia D, Gomez-Paz S, Robinson TM, Moore J, Ogilvy CS, Thomas AJ. Transition to radial approach for neurovascular procedures is safe and convenient: characterization of a learning experience. Oper Neurosurg. 2020;19:489–94.
30. Hoffman H, Bunch KM, Mikhailova T, Cote JR, Kumar AA, Masoud HE, et al. Comparison of the safety, efficacy, and procedural characteristics associated with proximal and distal radial access for diagnostic cerebral angiography. J Stroke Cerebrovasc Dis. 2022;31:106204.
31. Murai K, Fujino M, Ito S, Imazu M, Arai M, Iwai T, et al. Feasibility of nitroglycerin patch as a pretreatment for the distal radial approach: study protocol for a randomized controlled trial (Drang study). Cardiovasc Revasc Med. 2022;43:43–8.
32. Mori S, Hirano K, Yamawaki M, Kobayashi N, Sakamoto Y, Tsutsumi M, et al. A comparative analysis between ultrasound-guided and conventional distal transradial access for coronary angiography and intervention. J Interv Cardiol. 2020;2020:7342732.

Starting a Distal Radial Access Program

27

Ivo Bernat and James Nolan

27.1 Introduction

Previous chapters have covered many aspects of performing successful distal radial access (DRA), including patient selection and preparation (Chap. 6), conventional or ultrasound guided puncture (Chaps. 7 and 8), post-procedural hemostasis (Chap. 11), prevention and management of complications (Chap. 12,) and description of the learning curve (Chap. 26). We will not revisit these areas in any detail but will instead focus on issues to consider when an experienced radialist decides to start a DRA program and become an expert distalist.

27.2 Before Getting Started

Prior to starting a DRA program, it is beneficial to organize an educational session with all members of the catheterization team to review the published data supporting the new technique; this will ensure that your team understands and supports the new procedural development (an important factor during the learning curve phase). It will also allow the team to become familiar with the new equipment and setup issues before performing the first cases.

Fundamental considerations and questions before starting a DRA program are:

- Why start it when conventional transradial access (TRA) is so well established worldwide and proven to be better for the patient than the femoral approach?
- What can we do to improve the patient experience with DRA over conventional TRA? And are these potential benefits really significant and important?

Correctly performed routine catheterization and intervention with a conventional TRA are associated with a low complication rate and high patient satisfaction. Therefore, there must be good reasons to perform the same procedures using a different approach.

27.3 The Evolving Landscape of Radial Access

Everything in medicine evolves and changes over time, as the following example illustrates. It has taken more than 20 years since the first transradial percutaneous coronary intervention (PCI) from the wrist for this approach to be endorsed by the European Society of Cardiology as a Class I recommendation with Level A evidence over

I. Bernat (✉)
Department of Cardiology, University Hospital and Faculty of Medicine Pilsen, Charles University, Pilsen, Czech Republic

J. Nolan
Cardiovascular Research Group, Keele University, Keele, Staffordshire, UK

G. A. Sgueglia (ed.), *Distal Radial Access*, https://doi.org/10.1007/978-3-031-89925-6_27

femoral access [1]. In a meta-analysis of relevant clinical trials, the incidence of early radial artery occlusion (RAO) was reported to be 7.7% [2]. With numerous improvements, including better post-procedural care, the next three large trials (RAP and BEAT, PROPHET II, and CRASOC), which enrolled more than 5000 patients, reported a reduction in early RAO to 2.7% [3–6]. In 2022, the DISCO-RADIAL randomized trial reported a further reduction in the incidence of RAO in conventional TRA to less than 1% [7]. This positive change in procedure-related adverse events illustrates how something that has been a long-standing problem (over 20 years) has been largely resolved through evolution and optimization of practice.

Indeed, the practice of medicine never stands still. Although the performance of conventional TRA procedures is excellent, there is still room for improvement. According to a recent meta-analysis of 14 trials involving more than 6000 patients, DRA is associated with a beneficial reduction in the risk of RAO and large hematomas compared with conventional TRA [8]. Maintaining radial artery patency is an increasingly important issue for patients undergoing multiple catheterization procedures or those with late-stage renal disease. We believe that the incorporation of DRA into routine clinical practice will further reduce access complication rates with a relatively short learning curve.

In addition to preventing radial access complications, there are other important reasons to use DRA routinely [9]. There are important additional ergonomic and functional benefits to consider. For example, left DRA is more comfortable for the operator and patient than left conventional TRA, especially for right-handed patients (>90% of all procedures), and allows the patient's dominant hand to be used without restriction immediately after the procedure. This is especially beneficial for elective patients in a same-day discharge program. In addition, left arm access facilitates left internal mammary artery cannulation in post-coronary artery bypass graft patients and is associated with lower rates of subclavian tortuosity and anatomical variation, reducing procedural complexity.

In spite of the well-known advantages, access via the left arm is still only used on a sporadic basis. In a large and detailed analysis of nearly 350,000 PCIs from the British Cardiovascular Intervention Society (BCIS) database, left conventional TRA was used in only 4% of procedures [10]. This analysis also confirmed that left conventional TRA was not associated with an increased risk of adverse outcomes and was associated with a significant reduction in in-hospital stroke compared to right conventional TRA (OR 0.52, 95% CI 0.37–0.82, $p < 0.005$). The ergonomic benefits associated with DRA will help overcome resistance to widespread adoption of a left arm approach with proven patient benefit.

Another practical reason to start performing procedures via DRA as soon as possible is easier post-procedure care of the vascular acccess, as distal radial artery compression does not require checking for patent hemostasis and usually requires a shorter and gentler compression protocol [11]. This simplifies follow-up and has the potential to reduce healthcare costs.

27.4 Practical Considerations

Stressful factors for experienced radialists at the beginning of their initial DRA experience may include:

- Risk of technical failure requiring conversion
- Increased risk of spasm
- Limitations associated with the smaller size of the artery
- Concerns about patient discomfort during the learning curve
- Mental block in developing a new skill set

These understandable fears and doubts are a common accompaniment to any new endeavor. However, to an experienced radialist, all the technical aspects of a DRA procedure are very similar and only a few centimeters away from the conventional TRA. It is new, of course, but not very different. The artery is just in a slightly different location and slightly smaller in size (less than half a millimeter in diameter on average).

Once the sheath is in place, all subsequent aspects of performing the catheterization or interventional procedure are virtually identical to conventional TRA. Once the cardiac component of the procedure is completed, the superiority of DRA becomes more apparent for the patient (lower incidence of local complications) and for the staff caring for the artery after the procedure (shorter compression time without the need for patent hemostasis control).

A positive mental attitude with an emphasis on optimizing the work environment is very important, not only at the beginning, but throughout the DRA program. It is important to create a positive, supportive, and empathic environment for the operator and other staff, and for the patient, as excessive stress increases autonomic activation and circulating catecholamines, which increase the propensity for spasm.

Although most of the equipment used for DRA is identical to that used for conventional TRA, there are some important considerations to optimize the performance of the procedure. Given the smaller diameter of the distal vessels, downsizing is important. This can be achieved by using smaller diameter 4 Fr or 5 Fr systems when possible. Thin-walled sheaths minimize arterial stretch at the puncture site and are preferred for DRA. Optimized radial access wires with improved tracking characteristics reduce reliance on PCI wires in difficult anatomy and are easier to deploy from the DRA access site. The use of a dedicated DRA compression device or modification of an existing conventional TRA compression system and a revised compression protocol will be required for hemostasis, and it is important to ensure that team members are familiar with these requirements.

It is important to approach the radial artery at its different puncture sites (wrist and distal) as contiguous vessels that complement each other and are usually interchangeable as access sites. If the operator feels that the quality of the pulse assessed by manual palpation is very similar or the same at the wrist and in the DRA vessels, it is undoubtedly appropriate to start from a distal site. Prior to sterile draping and disinfection, it is advantageous to mark the best palpable pulse sites and thus the anticipated arterial puncture site, preferably as soon as the patient arrives in the cath lab (Fig. 27.1). If the quality of the pulse is significantly reduced distally, it is better to measure the size of the distal radial artery with vascular ultrasound and make a decision based on the findings.

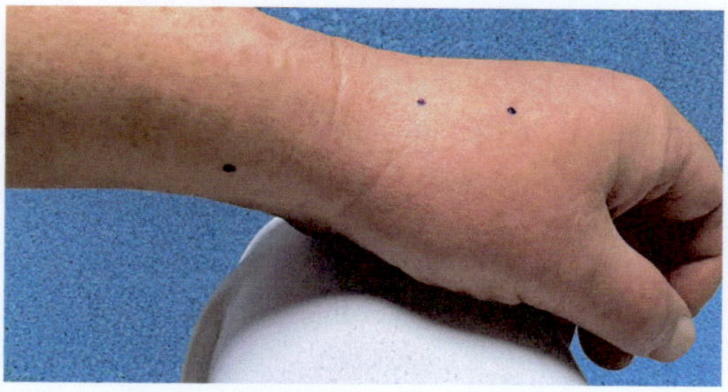

Fig. 27.1 Left radial approach and three possible puncture sites (wrist, anatomical snuffbox, and dorsum of the hand) marked with a skin marker

A potential disadvantage of DRA to consider in tall individuals is the increased distance of the target artery from the puncture site, possibly requiring the use of longer catheters. The distal portion of the radial artery is a small diameter vessel and must be handled carefully and gently, as its diameter is usually smaller than the target coronary artery (the diameter of the coronary artery is usually in the range of 2.5–4.0 mm; the radial artery at the wrist is usually 2.0–3.0 mm). Therefore, the start of the DRA program should be associated with not only technical but also mental preparation.

A wealth of information is now available to help overcome the initial difficulties. It should be emphasized that the subsequent routine DRA program should always be based on this solid foundation.

27.5 Linear Progression for Distal Radial Access

As you begin a DRA program, the following steps will be useful in the early stages of your program. They summarize and supplement the previous text, and most will be helpful in all phases of a DRA program:

Step 1: Ensure a calm and positive atmosphere in the cath lab with stress-reducing staff communication with the patient during preparation for the procedure. Consider light sedation for anxious individuals.

Step 2: Optimize patient selection in the initial phase to avoid those of short stature (who will usually have a small DRA), with a preference for those with an easily palpable pulse. Consider marking the cannulation site after palpation (Fig. 27.1). If the distal radial pulses are not easily palpable, ultrasound guidance is mandatory.

Step 3: After infiltration of a small amount (<1.5 mL) of local anesthesia, proceed to puncture the anterior wall of the artery with a 20–21 G needle at the site of the best pulsation quality. A successful puncture at the first attempt increases the chance of a successful procedure.

Step 4: Careful introduction of the metallic wire into the radial artery followed by introduction of a thin-walled sheath. It is important to ensure that the sheath is not deformed during introduction to reduce the risk of distal sheath fracture at the junction of the thin-walled portion and the fixed end. Once the sheath has been successfully placed, a 0.035″ wire and catheter can be introduced into the ascending aorta (the easiest way to introduce is to approach from the left with the limb straightened as shown in Fig. 27.2). Dedicated 0.035″ wires, such as the Terumo Glidewire Baby-J (Terumo) and the Silverway (Asahi), which are optimized for tracking in the upper limb vessels are available and will reduce the need for PCI guidewire deployment, catheter-assisted tracking, and balloon-assisted tracking in difficult anatomy, and we recommend that operators consider the routine use of these wires. If there is resistance to wire passage, an angiogram is essential to delineate the radial artery anatomy (Fig. 27.3).

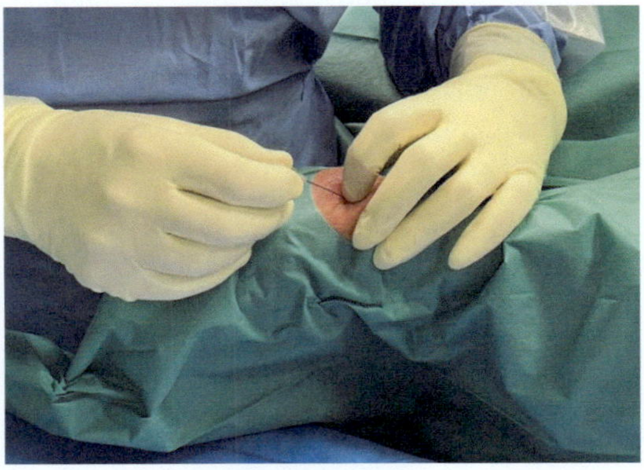

Fig. 27.2 Left distal radial access obtained from the left side of the patient

Step 5: If there is a significant resistance to sheath insertion, make a small (1 mm) skin incision after the tip of the introducer is inserted and before the sheath itself is inserted. This will prevent deformation of the thin-walled sheath tip, which can damage the artery and cause significant pain (Fig. 27.4).

Step 6: After sheath insertion, heparin and spasmolytics are administered using the same protocol as for conventional TRA procedures. The patient's hand can then be positioned to optimize comfort during the procedure. In the case of left DRA, the position of a dorsal distal puncture means that the hand rests with the palm on the abdomen during the procedure, creating a comfortable, stable, and natural position (Fig. 27.5). In contrast, positional stability during left conventional TRA is much more difficult to achieve as the arm must be held in a rotated position to allow access to the sheath. These positional component issues are a major ergonomic advantage associated with the routine use of DRA.

Step 7: If initial insertion of the catheter into the thin-walled sheath is difficult, the most common cause is a kink at the point where the sheath body attaches to the fixed end portion. This can be resolved by pulling back the thin-walled portion for a distance of 1–2 cm.

Step 8: The gentlest initial catheter to introduce into the radial artery due to its low degree of curvature is the 4–5 Fr JR4. The atraumatic nature of this catheter reduces the "razor effect" at the tip, thereby reducing the risk of inducing spasm. With this catheter, it is possible to reliably examine the right coronary artery in most patients and then replace all other catheters along a 210 cm metal wire

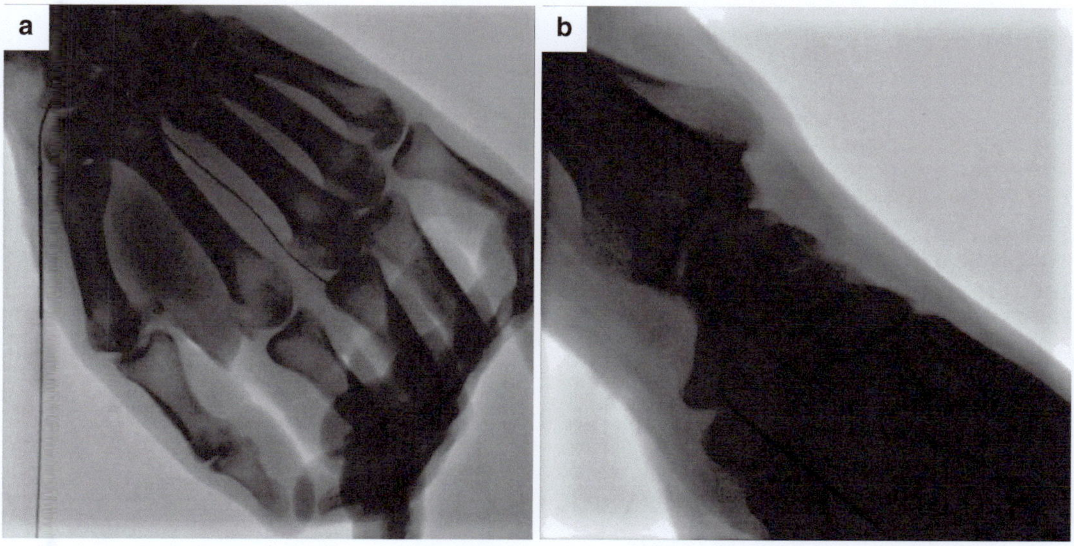

Fig. 27.3 (**a**, **b**) Incorrect tracking of the wire in a common digital artery

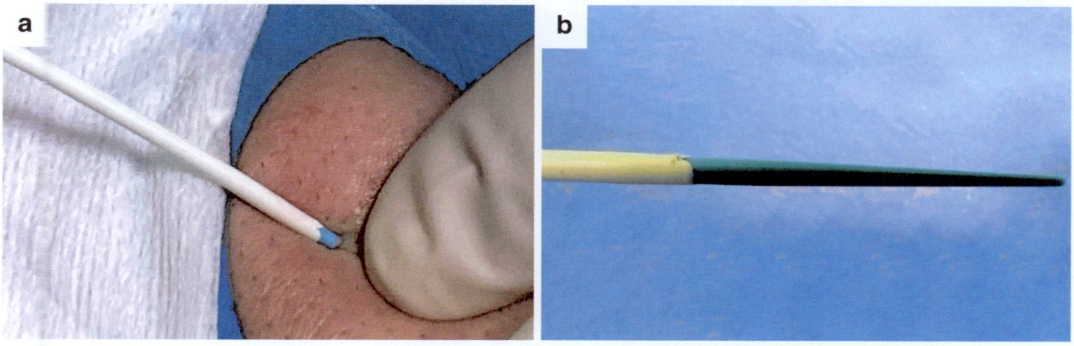

Fig. 27.4 (**a**, **b**) Sheath insertion with potentially dangerous sharp deformation of its tip

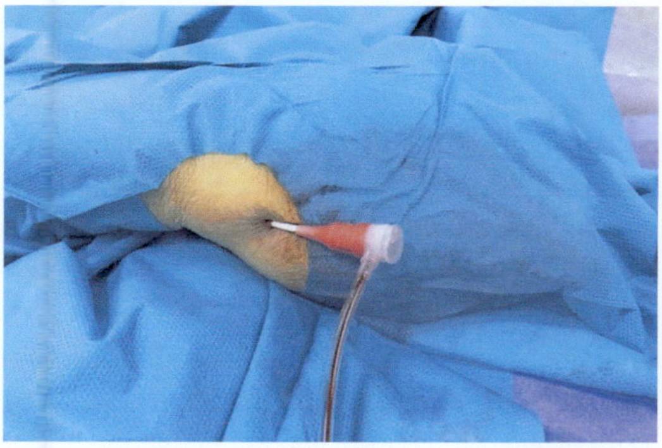

Fig. 27.5 Ergonomic and comfortable position of the left hand in left distal radial access during the procedure

maintained in the ascending aorta. If resistance to the passage of the second catheter is encountered, consider an arm angiogram to guide the next strategy.

Step 9: When changing catheters, it is sometimes helpful (i.e., when the hydrophilic sheath is mobile) to secure the end of this sheath with a sterile patch or manually by a second operator.

Step 10: Excessive initial compression of the distal radial artery at the snuffbox is a risk for dangerous deformation of the thin-walled sheath, which may result in painful dissection

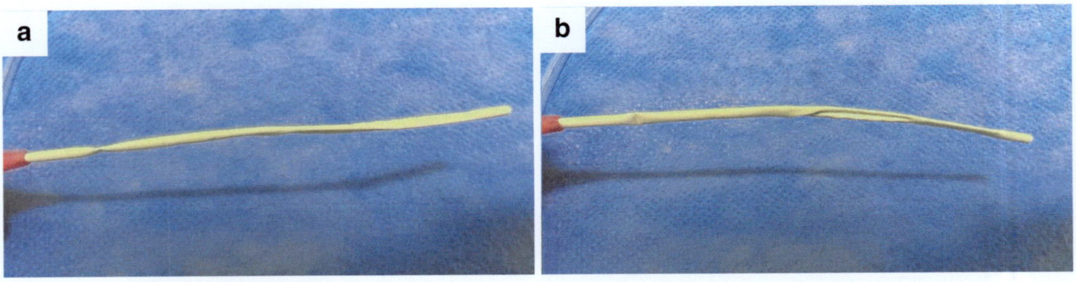

Fig. 27.6 (**a**, **b**) Thin-walled sheath changes in case of high initial compression pressure compression during its removal with potentially dangerous and painful deformation

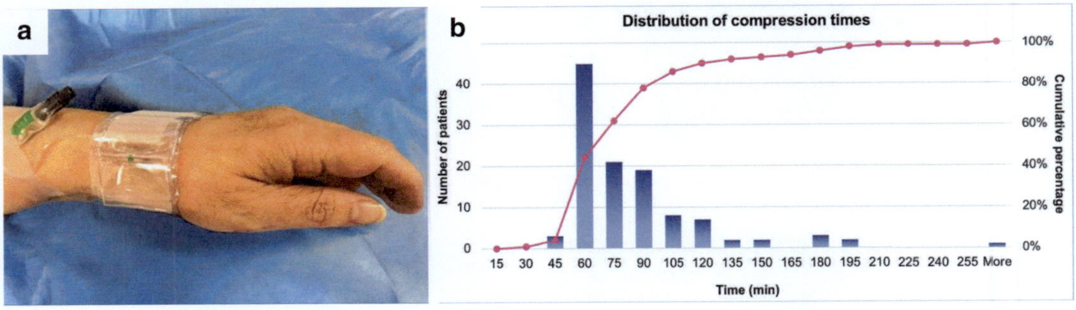

Fig. 27.7 (**a**) Compression with reduced pressure as a prevention of sheath deformation during its removal (here TR Band is initially inflated with only 10 mL of air). (**b**) Frequency and cumulative frequency distribution of compression times showing that approximately 80% of patients had compression times <90 min. (Modified from Horak et al. 2022 [11])

of the artery during sheath removal (Fig. 27.6). Therefore, it is advisable to begin compression of the artery at the end of the procedure with a low initial pressure to avoid this deformation. In addition, this lower initial pressure will help shorten the total compression time (Fig. 27.7).

27.6 Conclusions

In conclusion, DRA has proven advantages over conventional TRA in reducing access site complications and improving ergonomics. These are important benefits for our patients. An additional gain is a reduction in post-procedural care, which minimizes nurse workload. As with all new procedures, there is a learning curve that can be managed by following the steps outlined in this chapter. It is important that all team members are educated about the benefits of a DRA program, as success depends on the entire team, not just the lead operator. For operators who become proficient in DRA, it is possible and not difficult to routinely combine DRA (in the anatomical snuffbox and dorsally distal) with conventional TRA at the wrist. This expands access options for patients requiring repeat procedures. Rotating access sites in the upper limb is advantageous (especially for smaller arteries) and is preferable to repeated sheath insertions from the same puncture site, which can cause more arterial damage and lead to RAO and access problems (Fig. 27.8). With proper preparation and understanding of the technical challenges, a DRA program can be implemented with a real patient benefit.

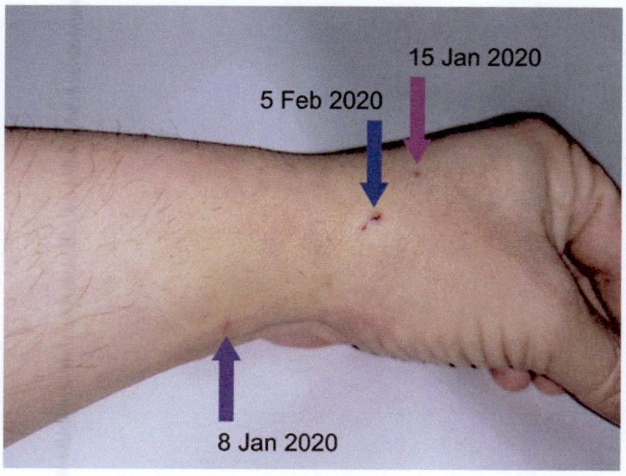

Fig. 27.8 Left hand after three percutaneous coronary interventions performed over 1 month: (day 1) conventional transradial access at the wrist level, (day 8) distal radial access in the dorsum of the hand, and (day 29) distal radial access in the anatomic snuffbox

References

1. Roffi M, Patrono C, Collet JP, Mueller C, Valgimigli M, Andreotti F, et al. 2015 ESC guidelines for the management of acute coronary syndromes in patients presenting without persistent ST-segment elevation: task force for the management of acute coronary syndromes in patients presenting without persistent ST-segment elevation of the European Society of Cardiology (ESC). ESC scientific document group. Eur Heart J. 2016;37:267–315.
2. Rashid M, Kwok CS, Pancholy S, Chugh S, Kedev SA, Bernat I, et al. Radial artery occlusion after transradial interventions: a systematic review and meta-analysis. J Am Heart Assoc. 2016;5:e00268.
3. Aminian A, Saito S, Takahashi A, Bernat I, Jobe RL, Kajiya T, et al. Comparison of a new slender 6 Fr sheath with a standard 5 Fr sheath for transradial coronary angiography and intervention: RAP and BEAT (radial artery patency and bleeding, efficacy, adverse evenT), a randomized multicentre trial. EuroIntervention. 2017;13:e549–56.
4. Pancholy SB, Bernat I, Bertrand OF, Patel TM. Prevention of radial artery occlusion after transradial catheterization: the PROPHET-II randomized trial. JACC Cardiovasc Interv. 2016;9:1992–9.
5. Dangoisse V, Guédès A, Chenu P, Hanet C, Albert C, Robin V, et al. Usefulness of a gentle and short hemostasis using the transradial band device after transradial access for percutaneous coronary angiography and interventions to reduce the radial artery occlusion rate (from the prospective and randomized CRASOC I, II, and III studies). Am J Cardiol. 2017;120:374–9.
6. Bernat I, Aminian A, Pancholy S, Mamas M, Gaudino M, Nolan J, et al. Best practices for the prevention of radial artery occlusion after transradial diagnostic angiography and intervention – an international consensus paper. JACC Cardiovasc Interv. 2019;12:2235–46.
7. Aminian A, Sgueglia GA, Wiemer M, Kefer J, Gasparini GL, Ruzsa Z, et al. Distal versus conventional radial access for coronary angiography and intervention (DISCO RADIAL). JACC Cardiovasc Interv. 2022;15:1191–201.
8. Ferrante G, Condello F, Rao SV, Maurina M, Jolly S, Stefanini GG, et al. Distal vs conventional radial access for coronary angiography and/or intervention: a meta-analysis of randomized trials. JACC Cardiovasc Interv. 2022;15:2297–311.
9. Sgueglia GA, Lee BK, Cho BR, Babunashvili A, Lee JB, Lee JW, et al. Distal radial access: consensus report of the first Korea-Europe transradial intervention meeting. JACC Cardiovasc Interv. 2021;14:892–906.
10. Rashid M, Lawson C, Potts J, Kontopantelis E, Kwok CS, Bertrand OF, et al. Incidence, determinants, and outcomes of left and right radial access use in patients undergoing percutaneous coronary intervention in the United Kingdom: a national perspective using the BCIS dataset. JACC Cardiovasc Interv. 2018;11:1021–33.
11. Horak D, Bernat I, Jirouš Š, Slezák D, Rokyta R. Distal radial access and postprocedural ultrasound evaluation of proximal and distal radial artery. Cardiovasc Interv Ther. 2022;37:710–6.

Current Challenges and Future Opportunities

28

Gregory A. Sgueglia and Juan F. Granada

28.1 Introduction

Over the past three decades, the use of transradial access (TRA) has been increasingly favored over femoral access due to a substantial body of evidence demonstrating its superior benefits for patients, healthcare systems, and physicians (Fig. 28.1) [1–8]. Several meta-analyses have demonstrated that TRA significantly reduces mortality (Fig. 28.2), particularly in the acute phase following coronary interventions (Fig. 28.3). Such a mortality benefit of TRA is also important to consider when performing coronary procedures that are not expected to impact patient survival [9, 10]. In addition, in acute coronary syndromes including ST-elevation myocardial infarction, radial access provides a significant mortality benefit that surpasses many commonly used interventions (Fig. 28.4) [11]. As a results, TRA received the highest level of recommendation in myocardial revascularization guidelines in Europe and the United States [12, 13].

The benefits of TRA demonstrated in coronary interventions have facilitated its acceptance in a wider range of non-coronary diagnostic and interventional procedures as authoritatively described in previous chapters. However, rapid increase in the use of TRA for an expanding range of percutaneous interventions may impact its future use for each individual patient (Fig. 28.5), as success rates decrease by approximately 5% to 10% with each additional access, primarily due to radial artery occlusion (RAO), which is the most common complication of TRA [14]. Initially overlooked due to its mostly asymptomatic presentation, RAO represents a significant limitation to the clinical utility of TRA [15]. To date, preservation of radial artery patency has become one of the most important long-term goals and opportunities for innovation in the field of TRA. Actually, RAO results from a complex interplay of multiple interrelated factors, and a number of strategies have been proposed in an international consensus document

G. A. Sgueglia (✉)
Division of Cardiology, Sant'Eugenio Hospital, Rome, Italy

J. F. Granada
Cardiovascular Research Foundation, New York, NY, USA

G. A. Sgueglia (ed.), *Distal Radial Access*, https://doi.org/10.1007/978-3-031-89925-6_28

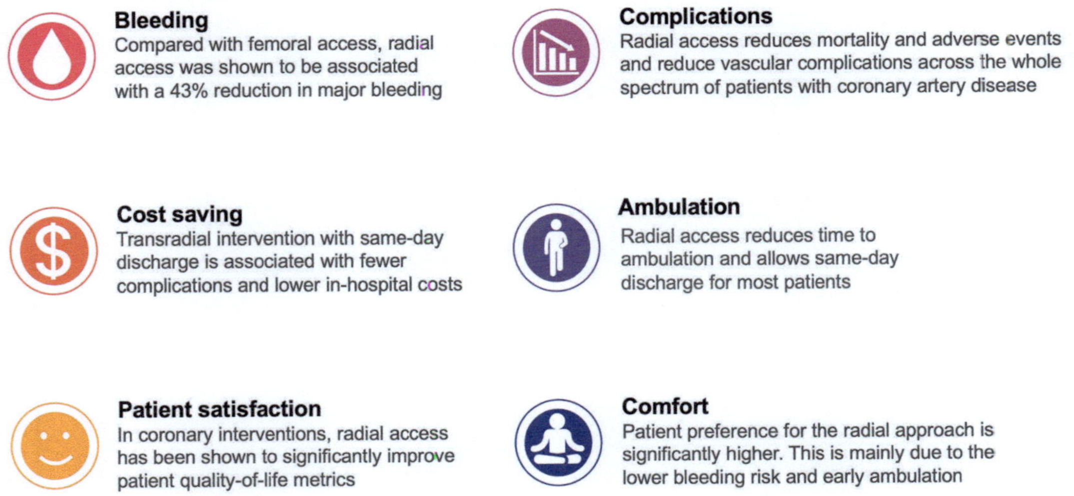

Fig. 28.1 Major advantages of radial access over femoral access include benefits for the patient, the healthcare system, and the operator

Fig. 28.2 In a meta-analysis of 24 studies with 22,843 participants, radial access was shown to significantly reduce mortality and adverse events across the spectrum of patients with coronary artery disease. (Adapted from Ferrante et al. 2016 [9])

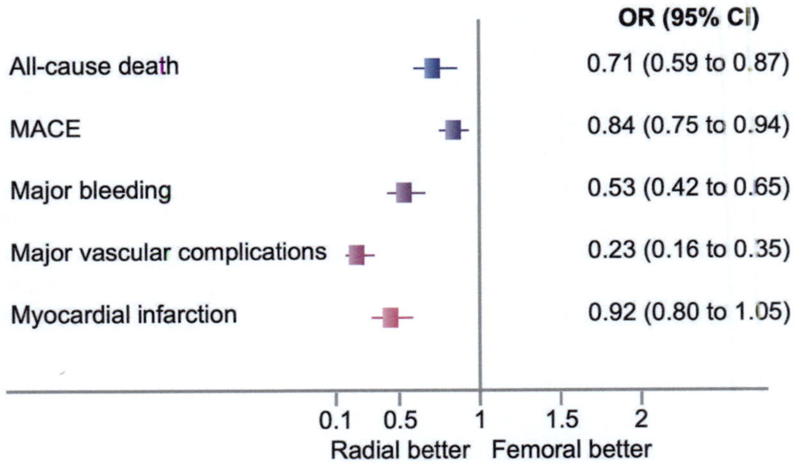

describing a comprehensive set of practices aimed at preventing RAO after TRA [16]. While the effectiveness of these interventions may vary, their combined use is expected to optimally reduce the incidence of RAO.

Distal radial access (DRA) has recently attracted a significant interest in the field of interventional cardiology due to its convenience and safety profile [15, 17]. The DISCO RADIAL trial, the largest randomized controlled trial

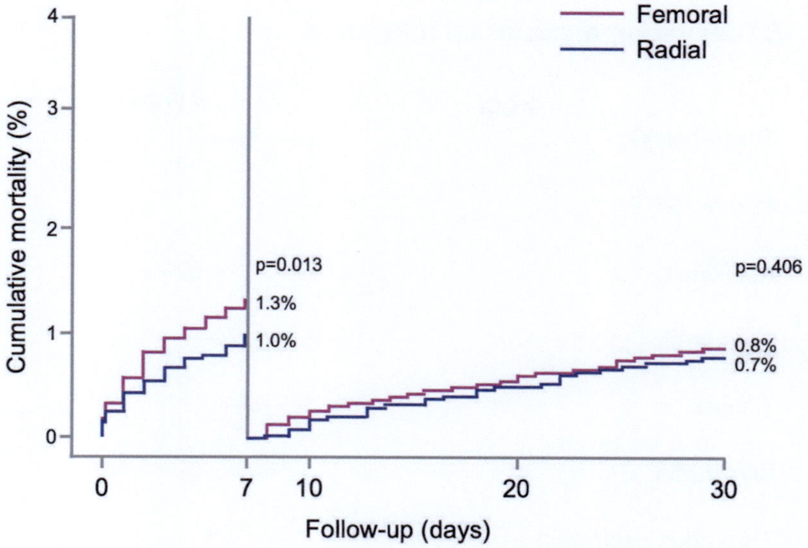

Fig. 28.3 Landmark analysis of all-cause mortality in a meta-analysis of 21,600 individual patient data from 7 multicenter randomized clinical trials shows that the benefit in favor of radial access accrues mainly in the first days after the index procedure. (Adapted from Gargiulo et al. 2022 [10])

(RCT) comparing DRA with conventional TRA, demonstrated that strict adherence to best practices for maintaining radial artery patency significantly reduces the incidence of RAO with traditional TRA [18]. Impressively, RAO rates were found to be three times lower with DRA compared to this intensive strategy.

In addition, a meta-analysis of 14 RCTs comparing DRA with conventional TRA confirmed a substantial and significant reduction in RAO with DRA [19]. Moreover, DRA was associated with fewer access-related adverse events and shorter hemostasis times. However, these benefits appear to be offset by a slightly more difficult access procedure, as evidenced by longer puncture times, more access attempts, and a higher incidence of access site crossover (Fig. 28.6).

On this background, this chapter aims to explore the evolution and future potential of DRA, navigating through clinical adoption, technological advances, and the challenges that lie ahead, with an eye toward the transformative impact DRA may have on the future of interventional practice.

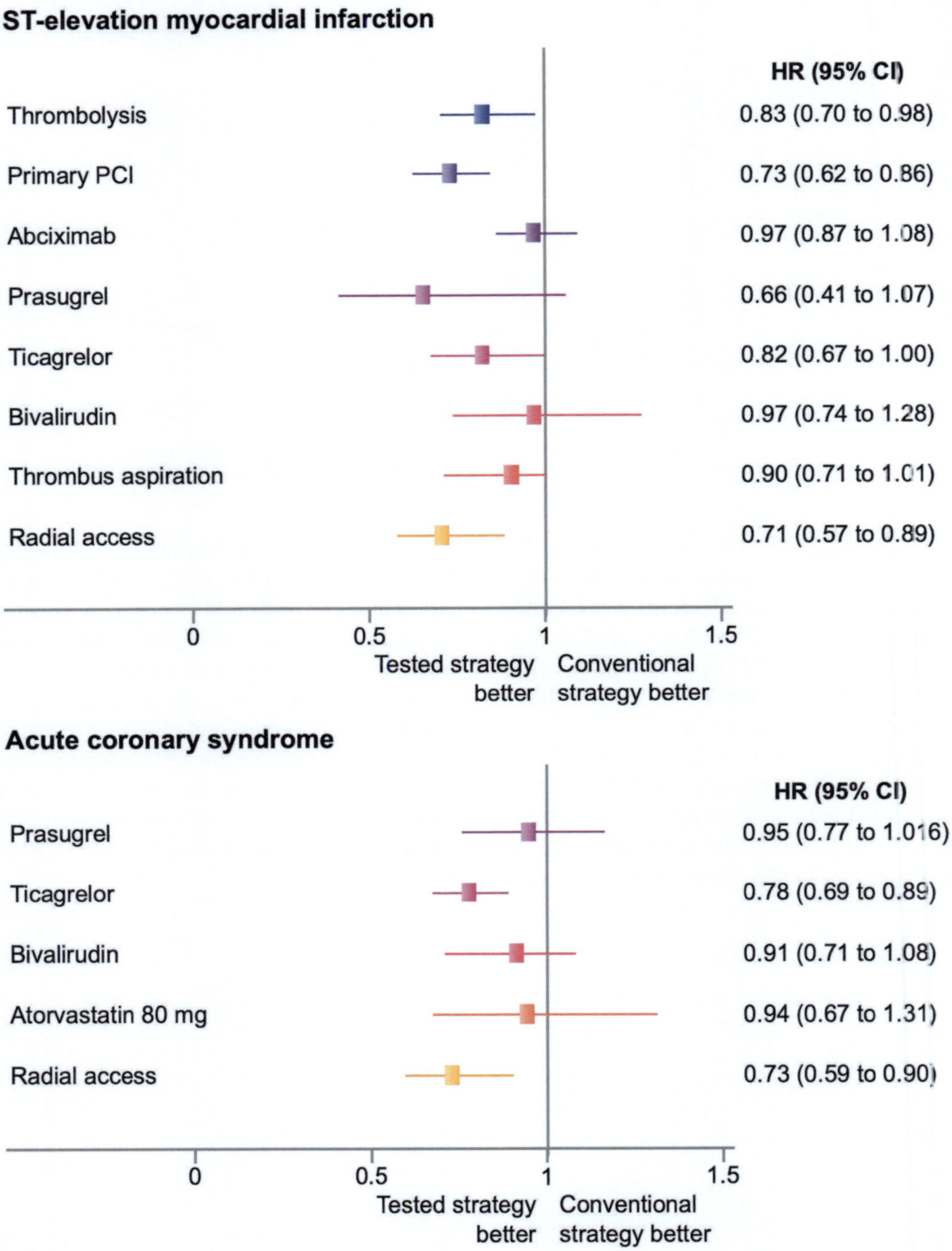

Fig. 28.4 Comparison of the effect of different interventions on mortality in ST-elevation myocardial infarction and acute coronary syndrome [11]

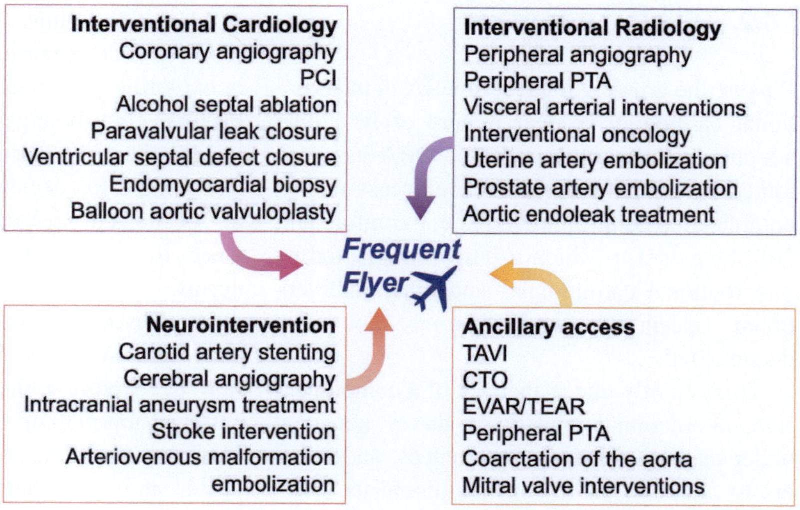

Fig. 28.5 As radial access for percutaneous interventions becomes more widely adopted by interventional cardiology, interventional radiology, and neurointerventional specialists, a growing number of patients are likely to undergo multiple transradial procedures as part of their treatment pathway

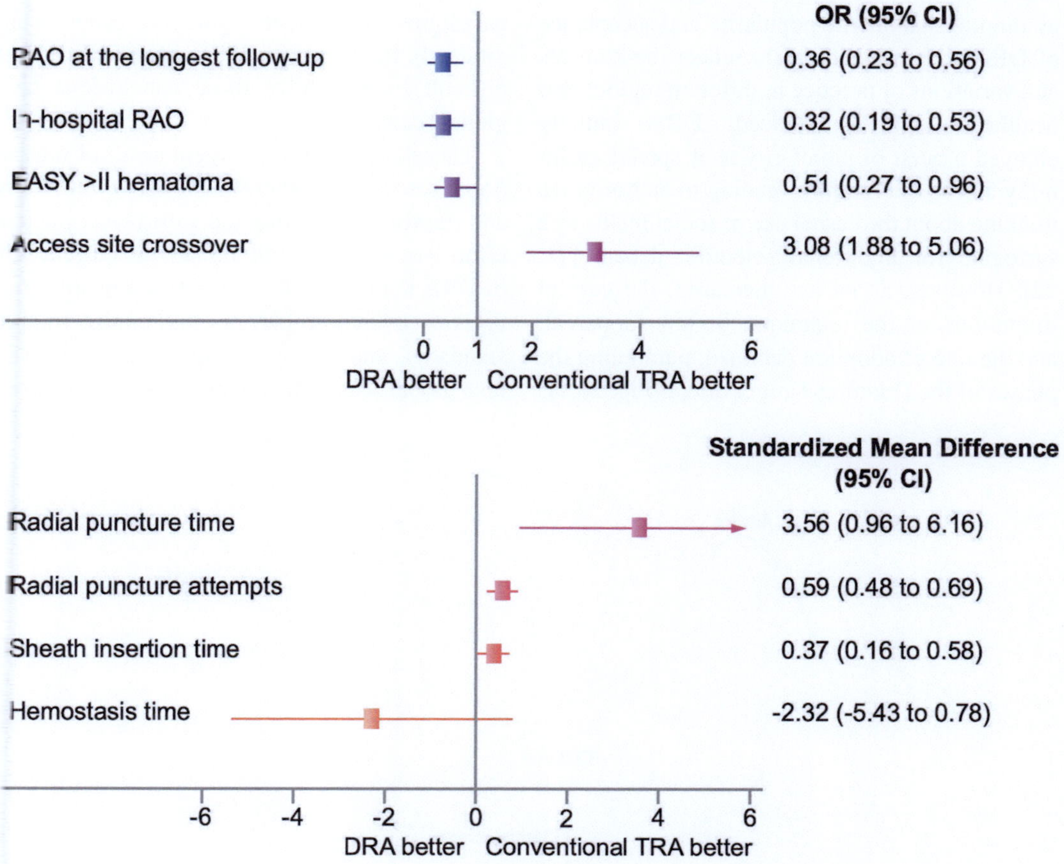

Fig. 28.6 Summary effects of distal radial access versus conventional transradial access in a meta-analysis of 14 studies with 6208 participants. (Adapted from Ferrante et al. 2022 [19])

28.2 Clinical Adoption

Despite the growing interest in DRA in interventional cardiology, a clear picture of its global adoption remains elusive. While DRA has been touted for its potential to reduce access related complications and improve patient comfort [15, 20], the extent to which it has been adopted by interventional cardiologists and other interventional specialists worldwide is not well documented.

This is partly due to the lack of a comprehensive, international registry or survey aimed at understanding practices, preferences, and barriers to adoption among interventionalists. Such data would be critical to identifying both facilitators and barriers to wider adoption of DRA techniques. Also, in the absence of a global outlook, assumptions about the popularity and acceptance of DRA may not accurately reflect the nuances and variations of practice in different regions and healthcare systems. Indeed, DRA initially enjoyed a burst of popularity as it spread amazingly across the Internet, leading to authoritative thinking about the casual use of social media as a surrogate for traditional scientific debate [21, 22]. However, as its use increased, the current limitations of the technique became apparent, and the rate of adoption declined, paralleling the phases of the Dunning-Kruger effect (Fig. 28.7).

Moreover, while the existing literature is robust in data supporting DRA, it often falls short in exploring the reasons for its underutilization. Factors contributing to slow adoption may include the steep learning curve associated with mastering DRA techniques, limited availability of specialized equipment, and a general resistance to change from established procedural norms.

A recent Korean real-world study attempted to shed light on the reasons for DRA underutilization by exploring the perceptions, challenges, and decision-making processes of interventional cardiologists (Table 28.1) [23]. While this multicenter study provided valuable insights into the complexities surrounding DRA adoption, its findings are inherently limited by its regional scope. Indeed, healthcare infrastructure, training paradigms, and patient populations can vary significantly from one country to another, making it difficult to generalize these conclusions on a global scale.

Therefore, there is an urgent need for international research collaboration to truly understand and improve DRA adoption worldwide. Such an effort would not only illuminate the current state of DRA uptake but also identify actionable strategies to overcome barriers, harmonize training standards, and ultimately optimize patient care on a global scale. Most importantly, this perspec-

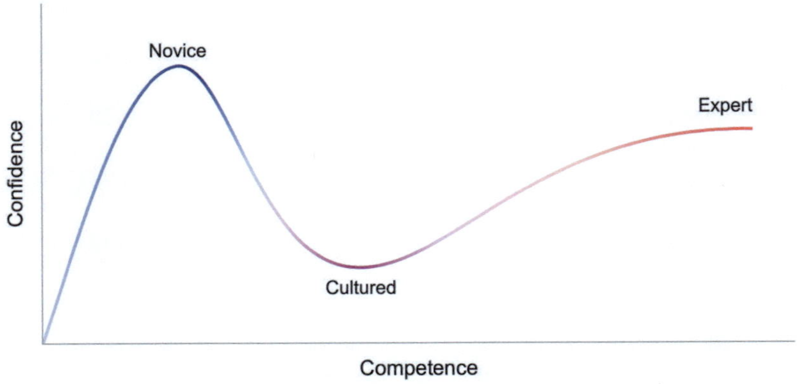

Fig. 28.7 Adoption of distal radial access reflects the Dunning-Kruger effect, a cognitive bias in which novices initially overestimate their competence in overwhelming enthusiasm due to limited awareness of complexity, while increasing knowledge tempers confidence as challenges are recognized. Additional experience boosts confidence in a wider range of applications

Table 28.1 Causes of screening exclusion (*n* = 712) in the KODRA registry [23]

Weak pulse	289 (40.6)
Peripheral arterial disease	95 (13.3)
Acute myocardial infarction	82 (11.5)
Other study enrollment for STEMI	52
STEMI	27
NSTEMI	3
Procedural considerations	63 (8.8)
Staged PCI	32
Chronic total occlusion	16
Left main bifurcation	6
Multivessel disease	3
Need for a larger guiding catheter	6
Hemodynamic instability	56 (7.9)
Cardiogenic shock	47
Cardiac arrest	7
Complete heart block	2
Consent withdrawal	29 (4.1)
Renal failure	28 (3.9)
End-stage renal disease on hemodialysis	24
Chronic kidney disease	2
Acute kidney injury	2
Anatomical problems	27 (3.8)
Tortuosity	14
Restrained both arms	4
Scar on puncture site	3
Wrist fracture	3
Positive Allen's test	2
Failed sheath insertion of small vessel	1
Operator preference	17 (2.4)
Poor cooperation (dementia or delirium)	8 (1.1)
Not reported	7 (1.0)
Follow-up coronary angiography	4 (0.6)
History of coronary artery bypass graft	3 (0.4)
Provocation test	3 (0.4)
Procedural complication	1 (0.1)

NSTEMI non-ST-elevation myocardial infarction, *PCI* percutaneous coronary intervention, *STEMI* ST-elevation myocardial infarction

tive is critical to innovation. Without recognizing these gaps, the development and deployment of novel technological solutions that benefit DRA may be missed or significantly delayed.

28.3 Learning Curve

Robust data analysis in the KODRA registry, through its comprehensive assessment of patient and procedural variables, highlighted two major factors influencing puncture failure: weak distal radial artery pulse and limited operator experience with DRA [23]. These findings address a major gap in the understanding of DRA and provide a significant and practical contribution to its development, increasing operator confidence to effectively navigate the DRA learning curve.

The KODRA registry set operator experience at 100 cases, while another Korean study suggested progressive improvement in technique up to 200 cases [24]. While such numbers may seem intimidating, they reflect the dedication of those who have independently achieved proficiency in distal radial artery conventional puncture. For a more comprehensive description of the DRA learning curve, see the detailed discussion in Chap. 26.

28.4 Ultrasound Guidance

An interesting insight comes from neurointervention, where the diagnostic examination is usually separated from the percutaneous treatment, and the access side is more critical than in other interventional disciplines. In this field, a significantly reduced learning curve has been documented with the adoption of ultrasound-guided techniques for DRA (see Table 26.2) [25–27]. In a study specifically designed for this purpose, the learning curve for ultrasound-guided DRA was found to be largely complete after procedure 33, with some further refinement in performance occurring through procedures 40 and 50 [25]. This finding is very similar to the trend seeing in structural heart procedures. Not only does ultrasound guidance help mitigate the difficulties posed by a weaker distal radial artery pulse, but needs to be integrated into vascular access procedures. Such an approach could be instrumental in realizing the full potential of DRA to benefit a growing patient population.

Interestingly, in the Radial Artery Access with Ultrasound Trial (RAUST) RCT, 698 patients undergoing conventional TRA for a coronary procedure were randomized to puncture with either palpation or real-time ultrasound guidance [28]. In this trial, the number of attempts was reduced with ultrasound guidance (1.65 ± 1.2 vs. 3.05 ± 3.4, $p < 0.0001$), and the first-pass success rate improved (64.8% vs. 43.9%, $p < 0.0001$). The time to access was also reduced (88 ± 78 s vs. 108 ± 112 s, $p = 0.006$). Thus, the RAUST trial demonstrated that ultrasound guidance improves the success and efficiency of radial artery cannulation in patients undergoing TRA.

More recently, in a single-center observational study of patients undergoing percutaneous coronary intervention through DRA, access success was significantly higher with ultrasound guidance compared to conventional puncture (97% vs. 87%, $p = 0.038$) with no significant differences in puncture time [29].

Although modest, the overall data point to ultrasound guidance as a way to significantly improve the efficacy and accuracy of DRA and potentially elevate one's entire interventional practice.

28.5 Promoting Proficiency

As shown in Chap. 3, the three-dimensional geometry of the radial artery in its distal course is more complex than in the forearm and requires a thorough understanding. Optimal knowledge of the normal and variant trajectory of the distal radial artery and its relation to surrounding structures is critical, not only for the initial arterial puncture but also for providing effective and safe hemostasis. Hence, educational effort promoting a better understanding of the distal radial artery anatomy should be directed at the whole cath lab team [17].

However, our knowledge of the anatomy of the distal radial artery in vivo remains incomplete. In fact, current understanding of the anatomy of the distal radial artery in living subjects is somewhat limited. Most of what we know is derived from anatomical atlases that provide detailed plates, each based on a single cadaver dissection. While such resources are undeniably rich in foundational knowledge, they do not capture the diversity or dynamic nature of living anatomy. This gap underscores the need for more extensive in vivo research to improve our understanding of distal radial artery anatomy and its clinical implications. Although computed tomography angiography has provided important insights into the in vivo anatomy, it still doesn't fully overcome the shortcomings due to inherent technical challenges. However, a recently developed method for simultaneous computed tomography angiography of the coronary and radial arteries represents a major breakthrough in this field [30].

Given these complexities, it is evident that the distal radial artery puncture technique remains a challenging aspect of the procedure, and there is currently nothing like an anatomically realistic simulator to accelerate the acquisition of expertise and refinement of skills with the distal radial artery puncture. Yet, it is expected that interaction with an expert DRA operator, possibly with the benefit of some proctoring, can significantly increase an individual's or team's confidence with a different, initially more challenging access route [17].

28.6 Technological Innovation

The distal radial artery presents the challenge of a smaller diameter, typically about 10% smaller than the forearm radial artery at the wrist, according to the current data (Fig. 28.8) [31–39]. This may limit the caliber of catheters that can be used, and currently DRA cannot be universally advocated. Each procedure should be carefully planned using the smallest introducer sheath and catheter combination possible to ensure both safety and efficacy, in accordance with the operator's level of experience and comfort. Yet, all operators would greatly benefit from becoming familiar with slender techniques and exploring sheathless guiding strategies (see Chaps. 18 and 19). Such skills are critical to extending the benefits of DRA to a broader patient population. Over the years, some technological advances

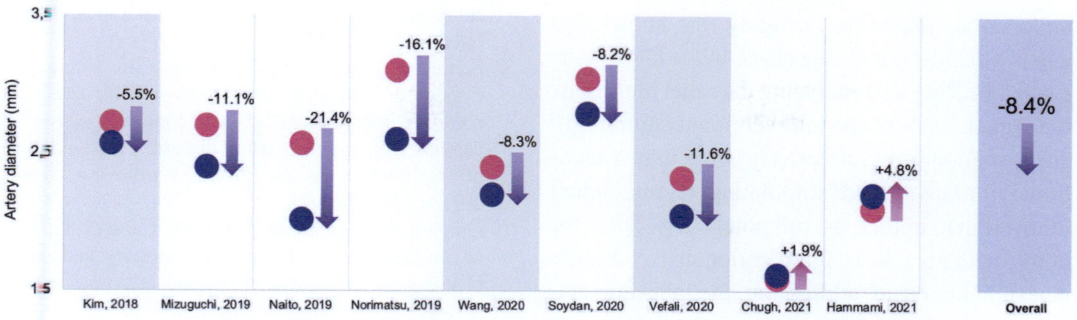

Fig. 28.8 Difference in the diameter of forearm radial artery at the wrist level and distal radial artery in different studies and their pooled summary

have been instrumental in the evolution of DRA, and the introduction of thin-walled introducer sheaths and streamlined systems for sheathless catheter advancement have expanded the scope of DRA to include more complex procedures. However, continued development is important not only to improve the delivery of the existing devices through even smaller arteries but also to inspire the design of novel interventional tools and techniques that require minimal vascular access. Additionally, innovations that simplify distal radial artery puncture would be highly valuable and help make this procedure more accessible and routine for interventionalists. Progress in these areas would represent a significant step forward in expanding the capabilities of DRA.

28.7 Evidence Gap

Available evidence suggests that DRA has a significant potential to replace conventional TRA for most percutaneous coronary procedures. However, our current understanding is far from complete. Challenges such as the suitability of DRA in taller individuals or those with smaller arteries, where conventional catheter lengths may be inadequate and narrower vessels may require sheathless techniques, necessitate further investigation to confirm the efficacy of DRA in these specific patient populations. In addition, assessment of radial artery integrity after DRA and a refined approach to anticoagulation, duration and method of hemostasis, and their interplay are critical factors in maintaining the highest safety protocols. To date, vascular complications associated with DRA have been rare, suggesting a potentially low incidence of access-related adverse events; however, the accuracy of this estimate and its correlation with anticoagulation and hemostasis methods warrant further investigation. In this context, the suitability of DRA in the setting of primary percutaneous coronary intervention requires careful evaluation (see also Chap. 17). The feasibility of using DRA as a routine alternative in the event of failure of conventional TRA or the use of a dual DRA strategy for complex interventions such as chronic total occlusion procedures should be thoroughly evaluated (see also Chap. 20). In addition, the need and methodology for testing patent hemostasis invites further investigation (see also Chap. 11). Finally, the impact of DRA on radiation exposure to both the operator and the patient deserves a detailed study (see also Chap. 14).

28.8 Conclusion

Extensive scientific evidence underscores distal radial access (DRA) as the safest and most effective approach to maintain the benefits of radial access amidst the growing spectrum of interventions utilizing transradial access (TRA). After an initial wave of enthusiasm, the dynamics of DRA adoption and the variables that influence it remain elusive. Intrinsic and extrinsic challenges, such as an inconsistently steep learning curve and operator hesitancy to use DRA, are not fully understood. Therefore, bridging this knowledge gap is a critical upcoming phase in the DRA journey. Collecting and analyzing data that highlights the unmet needs of the interventional community are paramount to effectively directing educational initiatives and stimulating technological innovation to unlock the full potential of DRA for both patients and interventionalists. Future research aimed at addressing the missing evidence will, in parallel, expand the range and scope of DRA in the evolving landscape of percutaneous transcatheter procedures.

References

1. Jolly SS, Yusuf S, Cairns J, Niemelä K, Xavier D, Widimsky P, et al. Radial versus femoral access for coronary angiography and intervention in patients with acute coronary syndromes (RIVAL): a randomised, parallel group, multicentre trial. Lancet. 2011;377:1409–20.
2. Valgimigli M, Frigoli E, Leonardi S, Vranckx P, Rothenbühler M, Tebaldi M, et al. Radial versus femoral access and bivalirudin versus unfractionated heparin in invasively managed patients with acute coronary syndrome (MATRIX): final 1-year results of a multicentre, randomised controlled trial. Lancet. 2018;392:835–48.
3. Rao SV, Cohen MG, Kandzari DE, Bertrand OF, Gilchrist IC. The transradial approach to percutaneous coronary intervention: historical perspective, current concepts, and future directions. J Am Coll Cardiol. 2010;55:2187–95.
4. Hess CN, Krucoff MW, Sheng S, Anstrom KJ, Barham WB, Gilchrist IC, et al. Comparison of quality-of-life measures after radial versus femoral artery access for cardiac catheterization in women: results of the study of access site for enhancement of percutaneous coronary intervention for women quality-of-life substudy. Am Heart J. 2015;170:371–9.
5. Kok MM, Weernink MGM, von Birgelen C, Fens A, van der Heijden LC, van Til JA. Patient preference for radial versus femoral vascular access for elective coronary procedures: the PREVAS study. Catheter Cardiovasc Interv. 2018;91:17–24.
6. Cooper CJ, El-Shiekh RA, Cohen DJ, Blaesing L, Burket MW, Basu A, et al. Effect of transradial access on quality of life and cost of cardiac catheterization: a randomized comparison. Am Heart J. 1999;138:430–6.
7. Mitchell MD, et al. Circ Cardiovasc Qual Outcomes. 2012;5:454–62.
8. Amin AP, House JA, Safley DM, Chhatriwalla AK, Giersiefen H, Bremer A, et al. Costs of transradial percutaneous coronary intervention. JACC Cardiovasc Interv. 2013;68:827–34.
9. Ferrante G, Rao SV, Jüni P, Da Costa BR, Reimers B, Condorelli G, et al. Radial versus femoral access for coronary interventions across the entire spectrum of patients with coronary artery disease: a meta-analysis of randomized trials. JACC Cardiovasc Interv. 2016;9:1419–34.
10. Gargiulo G, Giacoppo D, Jolly SS, Cairns J, Le May M, Bernat I, et al. Effects on mortality and major bleeding of radial versus femoral artery access for coronary angiography or percutaneous coronary intervention: meta-analysis of individual patient data from 7 multicenter randomized clinical trials. Circulation. 2022;146:1329–43.
11. Nagaraja V, Rao SV, George S, Mamas M, Nolan J. Evidence-based arterial access site practice in patients with acute coronary syndromes: has SAFARI-STEMI changed the landscape? Catheter Cardiovasc Interv. 2021;97:1417–21.
12. Neumann FJ, Sousa-Uva M, Ahlsson A, Alfonso F, Banning AP, Benedetto U, et al. 2018 ESC/EACTS guidelines on myocardial revascularization. Eur Heart J. 2019;40:87–165.
13. Lawton JS, Tamis-Holland JE, Bangalore S, Bates ER, Beckie TM, Bischoff JM, et al. 2021 ACC/AHA/SCAI guideline for coronary artery revascularization: a report of the American College of Cardiology/American Heart Association Joint Committee on clinical practice guidelines. J Am Coll Cardiol. 2022;79:e21–129.
14. Sakai H, Ikeda S, Harada T, Yonashiro S, Ozumi K, Ohe H, et al. Limitations of successive transradial approach in the same arm: the Japanese experience. Catheter Cardiovasc Interv. 2001;54:204–8.
15. Sgueglia GA, Di Giorgio A, Gaspardone A, Babunashvili A. Anatomic basis and physiological rationale of distal radial artery access for percutaneous coronary and endovascular procedures. JACC Cardiovasc Interv. 2018;11:2113–9.
16. Bernat I, Aminian A, Pancholy S, Mamas MA, Gaudino M, Nolan J, et al. Best practices for the prevention of radial artery occlusion after transradial diagnostic angiography and intervention: an international consensus paper. JACC Cardiovasc Interv. 2019;12:2235–46.
17. Sgueglia GA, Lee BK, Cho BR, Babunashvili A, Lee JB, Lee JW, et al. Distal radial access: consensus report of the first Korea-Europe transradial intervention meeting. JACC Cardiovasc Interv. 2021;14:892–906.
18. Aminian A, Sgueglia GA, Wiemer M, Kefer J, Gasparini GL, Ruzsa Z, et al. Distal versus conventional radial access for coronary angiography and intervention: the DISCO RADIAL trial. JACC Cardiovasc Interv. 2022;15:1191–201.
19. Ferrante G, Condello F, Rao SV, Maurina M, Jolly S, Stefanini GG, et al. Distal vs conventional radial access for coronary angiography and/or interven-

tion: a meta-analysis of randomized trials. JACC Cardiovasc Interv. 2022;15:2297–311.
20. Sgueglia GA, Santoliquido A, Gaspardone A, Di Giorgio A. First results of the distal radial access Doppler study. JACC Cardiovasc Imaging. 2021;14:1281–3.
21. Capodanno D. Twitterature. EuroIntervention. 2018;14:e959–61.
22. Serruys PW, Onuma Y. Twitterature: will social media have an impact on scientific journals? EuroIntervention. 2018;14:e962–4.
23. Lee JW, Kim Y, Lee BK, Yoo SY, Lee SY, Kim CJ, et al. Distal radial access for coronary procedures in a large prospective multicenter registry: the KODRA trial. JACC Cardiovasc Interv. 2024;17:329–40.
24. Koh JW, Kim Y, Lee OH, Im E, Cho DK, Choi D, et al. The learning curve of the distal radial access for coronary intervention. Sci Rep. 2021;11:13217.
25. Hoffman H, Bunch KM, Mikhailova T, Cote JR, Ashok Kumar A, Masoud HE, et al. Transition from proximal to distal radial access for diagnostic cerebral angiography: learning curve analysis. World Neurosurg. 2021;152:e484–91.
26. Brunet MC, Chen SH, Sur S, McCarthy DJ, Snelling B, Yavagal DR, et al. Distal transradial access in the anatomical snuffbox for diagnostic cerebral angiography. J Neurointerv Surg. 2019;11:710–3.
27. Patel P, Majmundar N, Bach I, Dodson V, Al-Mufti F, Tomycz L, et al. Distal transradial access in the anatomic snuffbox for diagnostic cerebral angiography. AJNR Am J Neuroradiol. 2019;40:1526–8.
28. Seto AH, Roberts JS, Abu-Fadel MS, Czak SJ, Latif F, Jain SP, et al. Real-time ultrasound guidance facilitates transradial access: RAUST (radial artery access with ultrasound trial). JACC Cardiovasc Interv. 2015;8:283–91.
29. Mori S, Hirano K, Yamawaki M, Kobayashi N, Sakamoto Y, Tsutsumi M, et al. A comparative analysis between ultrasound-guided and conventional distal transradial access for coronary angiography and intervention. J Interv Cardiol. 2020;2020:7342732.
30. Tamaoki H, Yoshimachi F, Sakurai T, Shin T, Ikari Y. Simultaneous computed tomographic angiography of the coronary and radial arteries. Cardiovasc Interv Ther. 2020;35:185–93.
31. Kim Y, Ahn Y, Kim I, Lee DH, Kim MC, Sim DS, et al. Feasibility of coronary angiography and percutaneous coronary intervention via left snuffbox approach. Korean Circ J. 2018;48:1120–30.
32. Mizuguchi Y, Izumikawa T, Hashimoto S, Yamada T, Taniguchi N, Nakajima S, et al. Efficacy and safety of the distal transradial approach in coronary angiography and percutaneous coronary intervention: a Japanese multicenter experience. Cardiovasc Interv Ther. 2020;35:162–7.
33. Naito T, Sawaoka T, Sasaki K, Iida K, Sakuraba S, Yokohama K, et al. Evaluation of the diameter of the distal radial artery at the anatomical snuff box using ultrasound in Japanese patients. Cardiovasc Interv Ther. 2019;34:312–6.
34. Norimatsu K, Kusumoto T, Yoshimoto K, Tsukamoto M, Kuwano T, Nishikawa H, et al. Importance of measurement of the diameter of the distal radial artery in a distal radial approach from the anatomical snuffbox before coronary catheterization. Heart Vessel. 2019;34:1615–20.
35. Wang H, Peng WJ, Liu YH, Ma GQ, Wang D, Su B, et al. A comparison of the clinical effects and safety between the distal radial artery and the classic radial artery approaches in percutaneous coronary intervention. Palliat Med. 2020;9:2568–74.
36. Soydan E, Kış M, Akın M. Evaluation of radial artery endothelial functions in transradial coronary angiography according to different radial access sites. Anatol J Cardiol. 2021;25:42–8.
37. Vefalı V, Sarıçam E. The comparison of traditional radial access and novel distal radial access for cardiac catheterization. Cardiovasc Revasc Med. 2020;21:496–500.
38. Chugh Y, Kanaparthy NS, Piplani S, Chugh S, Shroff A, Vidovich M, et al. Comparison of distal radial access versus standard transradial access in patients with smaller diameter radial arteries (the distal radial versus transradial access in small transradial arteries study: D.A.T.A - S.T.A.R study). Indian Heart J. 2021;73:26–34.
39. Hammami R, Zouari F, Ben Abdessalem MA, Sassi A, Ellouze T, Bahloul A, et al. Distal radial approach versus conventional radial approach: a comparative study of feasibility and safety. Libyan J Med. 2021;16:1830600.